TUMOR SUPPRESSOR GENES

Edited by **Yue Cheng**

Tumor Suppressor Genes
Edited by Yue Cheng

Published by InTech
Janeza Trdine 9, 51000 Rijeka, Croatia

Publishing Process Manager Molly Kaliman

Technical Editor Teodora Smiljanic

Cover Designer InTech Design Team

Additional hard copies can be obtained from orders@intechopen.com

Tumor Suppressor Genes, Edited by Yue Cheng
p. cm.
ISBN 978-953-307-879-3

For EU product safety concerns:
IN TECH d.o.o., Prolaz Marije Krucifikse Kozulić 3, 51000 Rijeka, Croatia,
info@intechopen.com or visit our website at intechopen.com.

Meet the editor

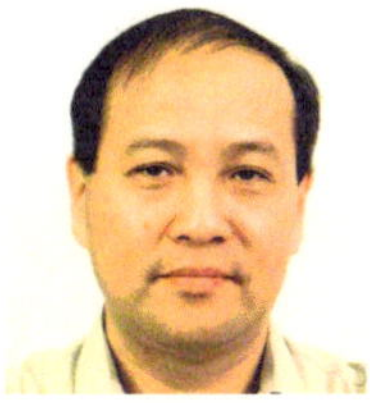

Dr. Yue Cheng is currently a research assistant professor at the Department of Clinical Oncology, University of Hong Kong. He was born in Wenzhou, China, and obtained his PhD degree from the Hong Kong University of Science and Technology. Dr. Cheng began researching tumor suppressor genes in Dr. Eric Stanbridge's laboratory, at the University of California at Irvine. His long-time interest is the study of nasopharyngeal carcinoma, a unique cancer prevalent particularly among the people in southern China, but otherwise rare in most areas around the world. He made landmark achievements by studying tumor suppressive activities in this cancer, and his seminal works provided functional evidence of a tumor suppressive region, mapped on the chromosome 3p21.3 in nasopharyngeal carcinoma. Currently, at least ten candidate tumor suppressor genes have been reported in this region, which is now regarded as one of the most important tumor suppressive areas in the development of many human sporadic tumors. During his career at National Cancer Institute of USA, Dr. Cheng became interested in the study of cancer stem cells. He now works on the exploration of mechanisms of somatic cell reprogramming, and its interactions with cancer development.

Contents

Preface

Tumor suppressor genes (TSGs) play critical roles in many biological processes, including cell cycle control, apoptosis, DNA repair, cell division and differentiation, tumor migration and metastasis, and reprogramming control of somatic cells. TSGs were named so because of their functional roles in original tumor growth control experiments.

Early somatic cell fusion studies of malignant and nonmalignant cell provided the first evidence of a class of negatively acting TSGs, harbored on normal chromosomes that contrast to dominant-acting oncogenes, which play important roles in tumor suppression. The first TSG was isolated from retinoblastoma, although recent evidence has suggested that this gene is also a key regulator of normal developmental events, as addressed in this book. Other important TSGs, such as P53, P16 and PTEN, were subsequently identified based on "two-hit" hypothesis of TSGs as well.

Underlying mechanisms of TSGs have been vigorously investigated over the past 30 years. This book covers the aspects of most fascinating fields, from cell cycle control, signaling pathways, gene dosage effects and epigenetic control of gene expression, to current challenges and future directions in TSG studies. Since tumor suppression is now a huge research field and many novel TSGs have been identified from various human malignancies, it is almost impossible to cover all interesting areas in just one book.

As a classic TSG, P53 is addressed in this book because of its risk on polymorphism and its critical role in apoptosis pathways. P16 and its family that regulate cell cycle and determine cell fate are introduced and reviewed in detail. Some of the chapters focus on the epigenetic control of TSG, notably P16, in lung, pituitary tumors and meningioma. TSG studies in other models, such as transgenic mouse and Drosophila, are also included in this book. Studies on PTEN and other classic TSGs are described in these chapters well. The regulation of an important cellular signaling, TGF-beta, in lung cancer is presented in this book, and readers can find information on other signaling controls of carcinogenesis in different chapters. Furthermore, expression and purification of the human 101F6 protein, encoded by a candidate TSG on the chromosome 3p21.3, is presented as a crystallization trial example. Finally, one chapter discusses a classic approach using cell fusion and chromosome transfer to identify novel TSGs in nasopharyngeal carcinoma.

A wide range of basic, translational, and clinical researches is leading the quest to find promising new ways to use these genes to suppress cancer. An example of such trails in head and neck cancer is presented in this book. Although we are not there yet, ongoing research efforts on TSGs, coupled with advances in gene therapy and other techniques, have the potential to open new avenues in the treatment of human tumors. We hope that this book will be helpful to both researchers and clinicians.

Yue Cheng, PhD
The University of Hong Kong
China

1

Tumor Suppressor Gene p16/INK4A/CDKN2A and Its Role in Cell Cycle Exit, Differentiation, and Determination of Cell Fate

Payal Agarwal, Farruk Mohammad Lutful Kabir, Patricia DeInnocentes and Richard Curtis Bird
College of Veterinary Medicine, Auburn University, Auburn, Al
USA

1. Introduction

Tumor suppressor genes and oncogenes are important regulatory genes which encode proteins regulating transitions in and out of the cell cycle and which also have a role in the gateway to terminal differentiation (Tripathy & Benz, 1992). Defects in tumor suppressor genes and oncogenes result in uncontrolled cell division, which leads to cancer (Tripathy & Benz, 1992). Oncogenes are mutated proto-oncogenes that have a role in malignancy of tumors and most frequently regulate cell cycle re-entry. Gain-of-function mutations result in transformation of proto-oncogenes into dominant oncogenes. Tumor suppressor genes encode proteins that suppress cell growth and most frequently result in exit from the cell cycle. Loss-of-function mutations in tumor suppressor genes result in tumor malignancy and can account for hereditary cancers. Every gene has two alleles present in the genome (with a few exceptions in the hemizygous regions of the sex chromosomes). For tumor suppressor genes to be inactivated either deletion of one allele and somatic mutation of the other allele is required resulting in a loss of heterozygosity (Swellam et al., 2004), or somatic deletion of both of the alleles is required resulting in a complete loss of homozygosity (Quelle et al., 1997). Tumor suppressor genes can also be inactivated by hypermethylation of the gene resulting in promoter suppression so that genes can not be transcribed further (Herman et al., 1997). Telomere shortening and tumor suppressor gene promoter hyper-methylation can be used as potential breast cancer biomarkers (Radpour et al., 2010).

Regulation of cell proliferation and differentiation is important in due course of growth and development of an organism. Cell proliferation is not an infinitely continuous process as cells undergo a finite number of cumulative population doublings (CPDs) in culture before entering replicative senescence (RS) (Hayflick, 1965). Cell replication or growth is controlled by a complex network of signals that control the cell cycle, the orderly sequence of events that all cells pass through as they grow to approximately twice their size, copy their chromosomes, and divide into two new cells. The cell cycle consists of 4 phases; G1, S, G2, and M phase (Enoch & Nurse, 1991). DNA duplication takes place in S phase and cytokinesis in M phase. G1 and G2 are gap phases, which provide the time for cells to ensure suitability of the external and internal environment and preparation for DNA duplication and division. Cell cycle progression from one phase to another is controlled principally by cell cycle proteins; cyclins, the cofactors of cyclin dependent kinases (CDKs), a family of serine/threonine kinases (Afshari & Barrett, 1993). Cyclins are the cell cycle proteins, which bind to CDKs and activate them to function and enhance cell cycle progression (Pines & Hunter, 1991). Cyclin/CDK complexes are specific for each phase transition. In complex eukaryotic cells there are approximately 20 CDK related proteins. Complex combination of all these different CDKs and cyclins in different phases of the cell cycle provide tightly regulated control of cell cycle progression (Satyanarayana & Kaldis, 2009). Levels of CDKs in cells vary little throughout the cell cycle, but cyclins, in contrast are periodically synthesized and destroyed in a timely manner to regulate the CDK's activity during cell cycle (Malumbres & Barbacid, 2009).

Early G1 phase progression is facilitated by CDK4/6 binding with cyclin D family proteins. These complexes phosphorylate members of the retinoblastoma protein (Rb) family (Rb, p130, and p107) (Sherr & Roberts, 1999). Phosphorylation of Rb results in release of E2F protein, which otherwise binds to Rb. E2F is a transcription factor, which activates E2F responsive genes, which are required for further cell-cycle progression in S phase (Weinberg, 1995). CyclinE/CDK2 complexes complete Rb phosphorylation and promote further progression of the cell cycle through late G1 phase. These complexes further activate E2F-mediated transcription and passage through the restriction point to complete G1/S phase transition (Sherr & Roberts, 1999). At the onset of S phase, cyclin A is synthesized, forms a complex with CDK2 and phosphorylates proteins involved in DNA replication (Petersen et al., 1999).

During replication of DNA in S phase of the cell cycle, CDC6 and Cdt1 are recruited to recognition complexes. These factors help in the recruitment of mini-chromosome maintenance (MCM) proteins to replication origins which are known as pre-replicative complexes (preRC). In early S phase, preRC recruits the functional replication complex including DNA polymerase and associated processivity factors such as proliferating cell nuclear antigen (PCNA). Subsequent cell cycle transition takes place through the activity of the CDK1/cyclinA complex initiating prophase of mitosis (Furuno et al., 1999). Finally, activation of CDK1/cyclin B complex activity completes entry into mitosis (Riabowol et al., 1989).

Along with the cyclins and CDKs, other proteins such as the tumor suppressor genes, the retinoblastoma protein (Rb), p53 and transcription factors such as the E2F proteins, play important roles in regulating cell cycle progression. The cell cycle has two important check points that occur at the G1/S and G2/M phase transitions (Hartwell & Weinert, 1989). These check points control cell cycle progression during normal proliferation and during stress, DNA damage, and other types of cellular dysfunction. At these cell cycle check points, cellular CDKs can be inhibited by cyclin-dependent kinase inhibitors (CKIs); thus, inhibiting and regulating cell cycle progression (Morgan, 1997). Rb can remain active suppressing downstream transcription factors if cyclin/CDKs are suppressed and p53 can directly activate CKI gene expression (Udayakumar et al., 2010).

All of the CKIs are proven tumor suppressor genes or suspected of having this potential. Two CKI families which play important roles in regulating cell division are; the INK4 family and the KIP/CIP family (Vidal & Koff, 2000). INK4 family inhibitors inhibit CDK4 and CDK6 in association with cyclin D, while KIPs inhibit CDK1, CDK2 and CDK4 associations with cyclin A, cyclin B, and cyclin E. The INK4 family consists of p16 (INK4A), p15 (INK4B), p18 (INK4C), and p19 (INK4D). The KIP family consists of p21 (CIP1), p27 (KIP1), and p57 (KIP2).

1.1 INK4A/CDKN2A/p16

p16 is an important CKI and a tumor suppressor gene encoded on the 9p21 region of the human genome, chromosome number 4 in mouse, and chromosome 11 in dogs (Serrano et al., 1993; Kamb et al., 1994; Asamoto et al., 1998; Fosmire et al., 2007) at the INK4A/ARF/INK4B locus. This gene locus is a 35kb multigene region which encodes three distinct major tumor suppressor genes, p15, p14ARF, and p16 (Sherr & Weber, 2000). INK4A/ARF/INK4B gene locus is repressed in young and normal cells by polycomb proteins and histone H3 lysine27 (H3K27) trimethylation (Kotake et al., 2007; Kia et al., 2008; Agger et al., 2009) and is induced during aging or by hyperproliferative oncogenic stimuli or stress. The INK4A/ARF locus has been speculated to have a global anti-aging effect by favoring cell quiescence and limiting cell proliferation (Matheu et al., 2009).

The classic role of p16/INK4A/CDKN2A is to check the cell cycle in early G1 phase and inhibit further transition of the cell cycle from G1 to S phase as a component of a multi-protein regulatory complex. During G1 phase, CDK4 and CDK6 form complexes with cyclin D1 which in turn phosphorylate the Rb protein family resulting in additional phosporylation by cyclin E/CDK complexes. These inhibitory phosphorylations of Rb cause release of the E2F transcription factor from Rb/E2F complexes. Rb otherwise inhibits transcription factor E2F (Weinberg, 1995). E2F is a transcription factor which initiates transcription of genes required for S phase such as DNA polymerase, thymidine kinase, dihydrofolate reductase, replication origin binding protein HsOrc1 and MCM (Lukas et al., 1996). Action of p16 inhibits binding of CDK4/6 with cyclin D1 which leaves Rb, and Rb-related proteins like p107 and p103, un-phosphorylated and E2F bound and inactive (Serrano et al., 1993; Walkley & Orkin, 2006). INK4 proteins cause both inhibitory structural changes and block activating structural changes to bound CDKs. p16 binds next to the ATP binding site of the catalytic cleft, opposite to the cyclin binding site, which results in a structural change in the cyclin binding site (Russo et al., 1998). p16/INK4A targets CDK4 and CDK6, rather than the cyclin subunit, and actually competes with cyclin D1 for CDK binding. Binding of p16 results in changes in conformation of CDK proteins so that they can no longer bind cyclin D1 (Russo et al., 1998). p16 distorts the kinase catalytic cleft, interferes with ATP binding, and thus may also deactivate pre-assembled CDK4/6-cyclin D1 complexes blocking their function (Russo et al., 1998). Binding sites for p16 and cyclin D1 on CDK4 are overlapping in some cases and are present near the amino terminus where a majority of the mutations in CDK4 are found. Mutations in the p16 binding site result in diminished capability of p16 binding to CDK4 and also compromise the binding of cyclin D1 to CDK4, which can also lead to melanoma (Coleman et al., 1997; Tsao et al., 1998). Other than inhibiting the pRb/E2F pathway, the very recently reported function of p16 is to downregulate CDK1 expression by upregulating miR-410 and miR-650 (Chien et al., 2011). CDK1 is an indispensable kinase which is most important for cell cycle regulation during G2/M phase (Santamaria et al., 2007). The regulation of CDK1 by p16 is post-transcriptional. Thus, p16 is an important tumor suppressor gene which regulates gene expression at different levels by modifying functional equilibrium of transcription factors, and consequently of miRNAs, and also by binding to post-transcriptional regulators (hnRNP C1/C2 and hnRNP A2/B1) (Souza-Rodrigues et al., 2007). The role of p16 in cell growth can also be attributed by irreversible repression of the hTERT (human telomerase) gene by increasing the amount of histone H3, trimethylated on lysine 27 (H3K27), bound to the hTERT promoter (Bazarov et al., 2010). hTERT encodes the catalytic subunit of telomerase; therefore, p16 induction results in repression of telomerase and thus telomere shortening. Another binding partner important for cell growth inhibition by p16 is GRIM-19 (Gene associated with Retinoid-IFN-induced Mortality-19). GRIM-19 is a tumor suppressor gene mutations of which have been found in primary human tumors. GRIM-19 and p16 synergistically inhibit cell cycle progression via the E2F pathway (Sun et al., 2010).

2. Gene location and mapping of the p16 gene

The region of the human chromosome, 9p21 encompassing the INK4A gene locus, corresponds to regions of dog chromosome 11, mouse chromosome 4, and rat chromosome 5. These regions have been demonstrated to be frequently mutated in various types of cancer (Ruas & Peters, 1998; Sharpless, 2005). The INK4A gene locus also alternatively named the CDKN2B/CDKN2A or INK4A/ARF/INK4B locus, encodes three members of the INK4 family of cyclin dependent kinase inhibitors (CKIs), including p15, p16, and the MDM2 ubiquitin ligase inhibitor p14ARF (Gil & Peters, 2006). p15 has its own reading frame and is physically distinct, but p14ARF and p16 share a common second and third exon but each has a different and unique first exon (Kim & Sharpless, 2006). It has been reported that tandem gene duplication and rearrangement occurred during the evolution of INK4A (p16) and INK4B (p15) that are located 30 kbp apart on the same chromosome (Fig.1) (Sharpless, 2005).

The INK4A gene was initially discovered to have three exons. Subsequent evidence identified an additional exon between the INK4B and INK4A genes, designated as exon1β, that was alternatively spliced from INK4A exon 1α (Mao et al., 1995; Quelle et al., 1995; Stone et al., 1995a). This alternative exon 1β was transcribed from a promoter different from the p16INK4A first exon (exon 1α) and then spliced to the same second and third exons of INK4A to form a transcript, usually shorter than that encoding p16INK4A (Stone et al., 1995b). The 1β transcript encodes a completely different protein from p16 because splicing of exon 1β to exon 2 allows translation from an alternative reading frame resulting in the different protein sequence (Fig. 2) (Quelle et al., 1995; Stone et al., 1995a).

In most mammals this later protein is referred to as p14ARF ('14' indicates molecular weight of the protein and ARF for alternative reading frame). An ortholog of exon1β in mouse and rat is longer than those from other mammals resulting in a larger protein and is designated p19ARF (Quelle et al., 1995). Thus, these two alternative INK4A transcripts (p16 and p14ARF/p19ARF) share a large overlapping nucleotide sequence for the common exons 2 and 3 but result in structurally unrelated proteins due to presence of unique alternative first exons. Both have become important candidates for the study of novel cancer mechanisms.

In dogs, the p16 and p14ARF transcripts derived from INK4A locus have not been fully elucidated. There are no full-length mRNAs or expressed sequence tags (ESTs) available that would completely define these transcripts. In addition this region of the chromosome is extremely GC-rich making it difficult to clone and sequence and causing a gap in the CanFam 2.0 genome assembly (Lindblad-Toh et al., 2005). The biological functions of these two proteins are fairly well understood compared to their genomic structure. Several lines of evidence suggest that both p16 and p14ARF act as potent tumor suppressors apart from their roles as cell cycle regulators during the G1 to S phase transition and p53 mediated cell cycle arrest, respectively.

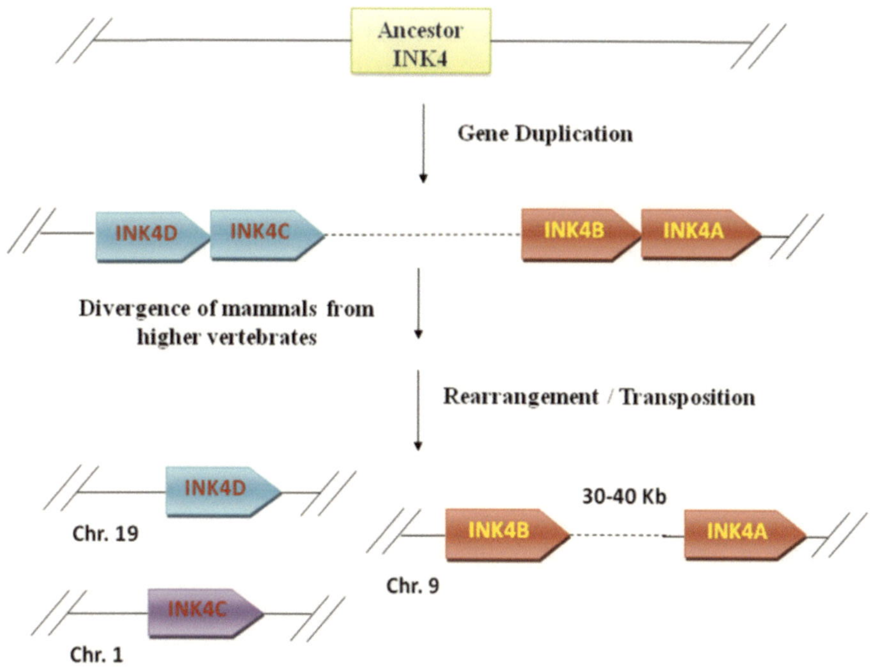

Fig. 1. Evolution of mammalian CKIs. Schematic representation of gene duplication and the evolution of CKIs (p16INK4A, p15INK4B, p18INK4C and p19INK4D) from a single ancestor INK4 gene. The chromosomal localization of INK4 genes are widely conserved across mammals. During the course of evolution, INK4C and INK4D were integrated into different chromosomes while INK4A and INK4B remained located on the same chromosome. Here human chromosomes and corresponding INK4 genes are shown.

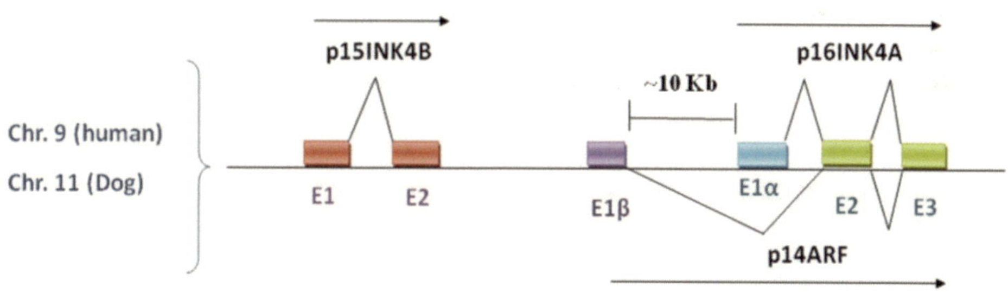

Fig. 2. Alternative splicing of p16INK4A and p14ARF. Exon E1α is spliced to INK4A exons - E2 and E3 forming the p16 mature transcript whereas E1β is alternatively spliced to the same E2 and E3 exons generating the mature p14ARF transcript. The latter produces a different protein from p16 because translation occurs from an alternative reading frame.

Primary melanomas, osteosarcoma and mammary tumor cell lines from dogs have been shown to harbor frequent loss of p16 (Levine & Fleischli, 2000; Koenig et al., 2002; DeInnocentes et al., 2009). Opposing roles of p16 and p14ARF have also been documented, where p16 inactivation attenuates senescence and ageing while p14ARF inactivation induces senescence and aging in skeletal muscle of BubR1 mice (Baker et al., 2008). p16 and p14ARF contribute to reduced growth and survival of B lymphopoiesis and inhibit malignant transformation (Signer et al., 2008). This contrasting behavior could be due to a level of tissue-specific activity of these CKIs.

2.1 Cellular location of p16

The subcellular localization of p16 has been even more cryptic than its genetic behavior and expression. Most studies have supported the localization of this protein both in the nucleus and the cytoplasm. But there are some debates on its specific roles, being in both cellular fractions, and in the context of normal and tumor cell lines. It is generally assumed that p16 is transported to the nucleus and acts as a CKI to regulate the G1 phase cell cycle checkpoint. This phenomenon has been reported in normal cells where the protein was mainly found in the nucleus but not in the cytoplasm (Bartkova et al., 1996). However many tumor cell lines have been shown to harbor p16 in the cytoplasm as well as in the nucleus (Geradts et al., 2000; Nilsson & Landberg, 2006). Two major populations of p16 have been identified in subcellular fractions - one is unphosphorylated or basic in form and the other is phosphorylated or acidic in form and both are generally derived from post-translational modification. The phosphorylated form was found to be associated with CDK4 in normal human fibroblasts (Gump et al., 2003). It has been reported that the localization of the two forms of p16 in both cellular compartments mostly depends on cancer types. In breast cancer cell lines, both forms of p16 were observed in the cytoplasm while the phosphorylated form was predominant in the nucleus (Nilsson & Landberg, 2006). In addition, strong cytoplasmic expression of p16 was observed in many tumor cell lines including primary breast carcinoma associated with a malignant phenotype (Emig et al., 1998; Evangelou et al., 2004) suggesting that the protein might have specific roles for its cytoplasmic localization in certain malignancies. But so far there is no direct evidence for the function of this tumor suppressor in the cytoplasm. One possible mechanism is that p16 can bind to CDK4/6 in the nucleus and the complex is transported to the cytoplasm, inhibiting the association of CDK4/6 with cyclinD in the nucleus and thereby blocking the G1/S phase transition of the cell cycle. In normal cells and epithelial-derived breast carcinoma, a novel substrate for CDK4/6 has been identified which is more prevalent in the cytoplasm than in the nucleus (Kwon et al., 1995). This might cause p16 localization bound to CDK4/6 to the cytoplasm and thus prevent CDK4/6 from acting on the substrate cyclinD1. Another mechanism may be hinted that p16 is mutated in some tumors and resulting in the defective protein being localized in the cytoplasm. However, this speculation is not supported by the fact that p16 is expressed in both the nucleus and the cytoplasm in cell lines with wild-type p16 protein (Craig et al., 1998). Other studies have suggested that the cytoplasmic localization might represent a mechanism for p16 inactivation in various tumors (Evangelou et al., 2004; Nilsson & Landberg, 2006).

2.2 Other INK4 family CKIs – p15, p18, p19

There are two classes of CKIs that interact with cyclin-dependent kinases (CDKs) and reversibly block their enzymatic activities. The first group consists of p21, p27, and p57 and the second group is comprised of p16/INK4A, p15/INK4B, p18/INK4C and p19/INK4D.

The INK4 family CKIs (the second group) generally inhibit the assembly of CDKs by binding to CDK4 or CDK6 (Sherr & Roberts, 1995). Like p15/INK4B and p16/INK4A genes, p18/INK4C and p19/INK4D have been demonstrated to have evolved through tandem gene duplication and rearrangement during the course of evolution. Cross-species observations have suggested that a common vertebrate ancestor containing a single INK4 gene that was duplicated and gave rise to the INK4B-INK4A and INK4C-INK4D gene clusters. After the divergence of mammals and other higher animals from lower vertebrates (~350 million years ago), further gene duplication and rearrangement resulted in the four different INK4 genes (Fig.1) (Gilley & Fried, 2001; Sharpless, 2005). It has been reported that p15 and p16 arose from a common ancestor or single gene locus placed on the same chromosome whereas, p18 and p19 mapped to different chromosomes in humans and other mammals (Guan et al., 1994; Hirai et al., 1995).

Both p18 and p19 proteins share basic structural and biochemical properties with p15 and p16 proteins. All of them consist of repeated ankyrin motifs that play important roles in folding of proteins and in molecular interactions with other proteins such as CDK4/6 (Hirai et al., 1995). The p18 and p19 have not been studied as extensively as p16 and there is also some debate about their roles as independent tumor suppressors (Hirai et al., 1995). Unlike p16 and p15, which are deleted in a number of established tumor cell lines (both human and canine), the expression of p18 and p19 can be readily detected in many cell lines including many different primary tissues (Hirai et al., 1995). For example, both p18 and p19 are uniformly expressed in canine mammary tumor (CMT) cell lines and normal canine fibroblasts (NCF) (Bird et al., unpublished data). Although p15 and p16 differ significantly from each other as one is encoded by two exons and the other by three exons with alternative splicing of the first exon, respectively (Stone et al., 1995a), the two proteins are closely related in their structures and functions. Both have four ankyrin repeats, are involved in similar mechanisms of cell cycle regulation and in some instances may be interchangeable as tumor suppressors (Krimpenfort et al., 2007).

Expression of p18 and p19, have been shown to predominate during early to mid-gestation in mouse development (Zindy et al., 1997) while expression of p15 has been found in later stages of gestation (Zindy et al., 1997). Circumstantially, it appears that different INK4 proteins are not functionally redundant as they appear to be expressed during different periods of development and may also be expressed in distinct tissue-specific profiles. Expression of p15 is down-regulated during human lymphocyte mitogenesis with a marked increase in Rb kinase activity providing a potential role for p15 in cell cycle arrest. p15 mediated growth suppression is induced by TGFβ mediated by SP1 and SP3 transcription factors (Li et al., 1995). p15 and p27 levels were decreased during lymphocyte activation and appear important in maintaining cell quiescence (Lois et al., 1995). Although p15 acts as a tumor suppressor, the frequency of mutations and defects in p15 in tumor cells is lower than p16 (Stone et al., 1995a). Overexpression of p15 can induce cell cycle arrest in cancer cells (Thullberg et al., 2000), TGFβ-mediated cell cycle arrest in human keratenocytes (HaCaT) (Hannon & Beach, 1994), and cell cycle arrest by the pyrido-pyrimidine derivative JTP-70902 in the human colon cancer cell line HT-29 (Yamaguchi et al., 2007). p18 inhibits the CDK-cyclin binding site by distorting the ATP binding site and by misaligning catalytic residues. p18 can also distort the cyclin-binding site of CDKs by reducing the size of the interface of bound cyclin (Jeffrey et al., 2000). A lack of mutations in p18 and p19 has been reported in tumor-derived cell lines and primary tumors, which were mutated for p16 and p15 expression, which shows distinct biological function of evolutionary related INK4 proteins (Zariwala & Xiong, 1996).

The INK4 and CIP cyclin dependent kinase inhibitor families have overlapping roles of cell cycle arrest in mouse embryo fibroblasts. Loss of both INK4 (p15, p16, and p18) and CIP (p21) promotes pRB inactivation, cell immortalization, and H-rasV12/c-myc-induced loss of contact inhibition. However, loss of both families of CKIs is still only weakly able to cause cell immortalization largely due to active apoptosis induction (Carbone et al., 2007). This data strongly supports the concept that both CKI inactivation and apoptosis failure are required to promote a neoplastic phenotype.

2.3 Structure of p16

p16 encodes four or five ankyrin repeats (Russo et al., 1998). Ankyrin repeats are 30 amino acid structural motifs that resemble the letter 'L' with a stem made of a pair of anti-parallel helices with a beta-hairpin region forming the base (Russo et al., 1998). The functional domain of p16 involved in interaction with CDK4/6, is located in the C-terminal half including the III and IV ankyrin repeats and the C-terminal flanking region accompanied by loops 2 and 3 (Fahham et al., 2010). p16 interacts with the N and C lobes of CDK6 and binds to one side of the catalytic cleft opposite to the cyclin binding site. CDK6 bound to p16 is inactive because it can not bind to cyclin and is not phosphorylated; thus, proliferation is suppressed (Russo et al., 1998). p16/INK4A also exerts transcriptional control over cyclin D1. Activating transcription factor-2 (ATF-2) and cAMP-responsive element-binding protein (CREB) induce the cyclinD1 expression by binding to cAMP-response element/activating transcription factor-2 (CRE/ATF-2) binding site at cyclinD1 promoter side, p16 represses the ATF-2 and CREB expression by 40-50%, thus inactivates cyclinD1 independent of its CDK4 inactivating properties (D'Amico et al., 2004).

2.4 p14ARF/p16gamma/p12

As has been noted, the INK4A locus encodes two distinct p16 and p14ARF proteins. However, it has also been reported that besides these two proteins, this gene locus also encodes two additional proteins; p16gamma and p12 (Fig.3).

p14ARF inhibits MDM2, which results in stabilization of the important tumor suppressor p53. p53 is a transcription factor, which activates expression of proteins required for cell-cycle inhibition and apoptosis (Boehme & Blattner, 2009). One of the downstream regulatory protein activations mediated by p53 is p21 up-regulation which checks the cell cycle late in the G1/S phase transition. p53 also acts as a transcription repressor of other genes (Gomez-Lazaro et al., 2004). p53 is more stable in mammary epithelial cells in comparison to fibroblasts in humans, which indicates the importance of p53 in mammary epithelial cell growth (Delmolino et al., 1993). Under normal conditions, p53 is rapidly degraded to keep its protein level low, mediated through the E3 ubiquitin ligase MDM2. Under conditions of stress or other dysfunction, p14ARF binds to MDM2, thus releasing and stabilizing p53 by blocking MDM2. Wild type p53-induced phosphatase 1 (Wip1/Ppm1d) stabilizes MDM2 and downregulates p53, p38MAPK, and p16 expression (Lin et al., 2007; Yu et al., 2007). Disruption of Wip1 activates p53, p16, and p14ARF pathways, through p38MAPK signaling, and suppresses mouse embryo fibroblast transformation by oncogenes *in vivo* (Bulavin et al., 2004). Another mechanism of p14ARF induction and p53 stabilization is stimulation of the DMP1 promoter by HER2/neu growth factor receptor overexpression (Mallakin et al., 2010). HER2/neu activates the DMP1 promoter through the phosphatidylinositol-3'-kinase-Akt-NF-κB pathway, which in turn activates p14ARF transcription (Taneja et al., 2010).

p14ARF expression is not directly involved in the response to DNA damage although p53 negatively regulates p14ARF expression and both of them have an inverse correlation with each other with respect to activity (Stott et al., 1998). Function of p14ARF is not limited to p53 as p14ARF also has other independent roles in cellular systems such as vascular regression in the developing eye (McKeller et al., 2002) and arrest of cell cycle in murine embryo fibroblasts in the absence of p53 (Weber et al., 2000). Loss of p14ARF, results in tumorigenesis by facilitating angiogenesis, which is independent of the p53 pathway (Ulanet & Hanahan, 2010). Other than MDM2, p14ARF also binds to E2F-1, MDMX, HIF1-α, topoisomerase I, c-myc, and nucleophosmine (NPM) (Boehme & Blattner, 2009). p19ARF (the mouse homolog of human p14ARF) is able to induce cell cycle arrest in mammalian fibroblasts analogous to p16 (Quelle et al., 1995).

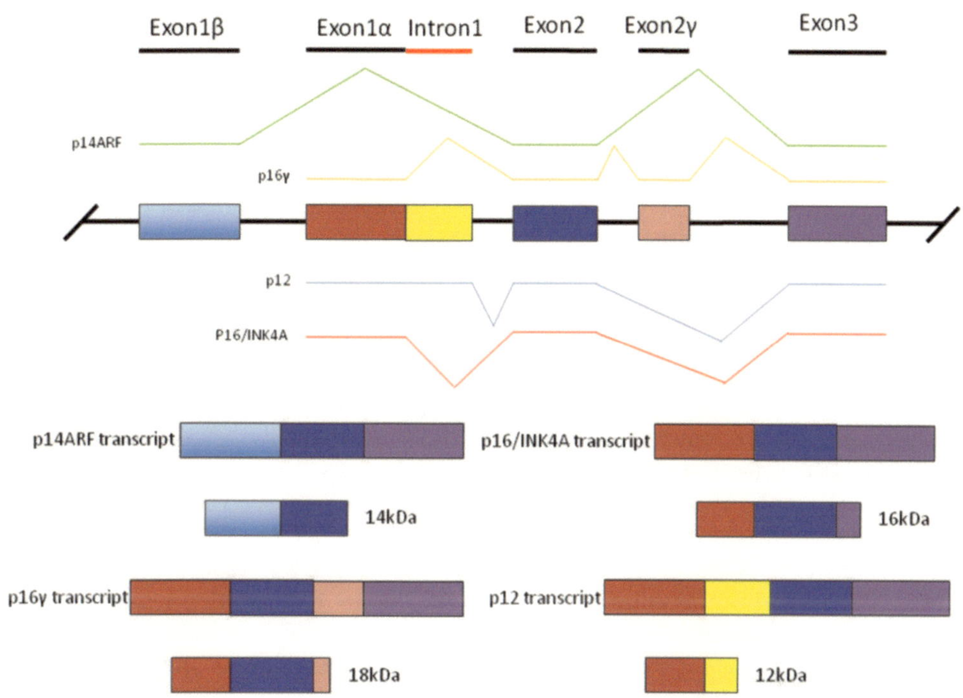

Fig. 3. Transcription from the INK4A/ARF locus. Schematic representation of all the four different transcripts, transcribed from the common INK4A/ARF gene locus. p14ARF and p16/INK4A share exon 2 and exon 3, but differ in their first exons. p14ARF includes exon 1β while p16 includes exon 1α. The stop codon for p14ARF reading frame is located in exon2. The stop codon for the p16/INK4A is located in exon 3. Another transcript transcribed from this locus is p16γ, which has an extra exon (exon2γ) along with all three exons of the p16/INK4A transcript. Exon2γ (197bp) is located in intron 2 between exon 2 and exon 3. p16γ encodes a 18kDa protein. The smallest 12kDa protein encoded from INK4A locus is p12. p12 shares the first exon, exon1α with p16, but first exon of p12 transcribes little longer in intron 1 to give an additional 274bp sequence. Stop codon for p12 is located in the additional intron 1α sequence and introduces an earlier stop codon and encoding a 12kDa protein spite having a longer transcript than p16/INK4A.

E2F induces cell proliferation by activating S phase regulatory proteins but, according to one report, E2F can induce senescence in human diploid fibroblasts by inducing p14ARF expression, which is required for p53 stabilization (Dimri et al., 2000). Id1 encodes a helix-loop-helix transcription factor that is overexpressed in high grade breast tumors and estrogen receptor-negative diseases (Gupta et al., 2007). Overexpression of Id1 or inactivation of the p14ARF-p53-p21 pathway can also revert senescence induced by ras signaling in mouse mammary carcinoma (Swarbrick et al., 2008). Other than facilitating the DNA-damage-induction response of p53, p14ARF also has a role in nucleotide excision repair. p14ARF induces expression of the damaged-DNA recognition protein xeroderma pigmentosum, complementation group C (XPC), by disrupting the interaction of E2F-4 and DRTF polypeptide 1(DP1). p14ARF also reduces the interaction of the E2F-4-p130 repressor complex with the XPC promoter (Dominguez-Brauer et al., 2009). TGF-β activity controls the expression of p14ARF during mouse embryonic development (Freeman-Anderson et al., 2009).

Other than p16 and p14ARF transcription from the INK4A locus, there is one more alternative transcript that has been reported derived from this gene in human lymphoblastic leukemia which is termed as p16 gamma (p16γ)(Fig.3) (Lin et al., 2007). p16γ has been demonstrated to be expressed at both transcriptional and translational levels confirming its functional potential (Lin et al., 2007). p16γ shares the same exon 1α, exon 2, and exon 3 as p16 but with a 197 bp insertion between exon 2 and 3 due to an alternative splicing event that extends exon 2 and concedes a stop codon. p16γ is also an ankyrin-repeat protein and interacts with CDK4. p16γ suppresses E2F activity and induces cell cycle arrest like p16/INK4A. It is not known what functionally distinguishes these 2 transcripts or their encoded proteins.

There is an alternative splice variant of p16 present in human pancreas as well, known as p12 (Fig.3)(Robertson & Jones, 1999). p12 is a 12kd size protein, which is encoded from the same INK4/ARF locus. The p12 gene shares the p16 promoter, 5′UTR, ATG-start codon and exon 1α, and uses the alternative splice donor site to splice to exon 2. The extra sequence encodes a premature stop codon that results in a smaller protein. p12 shares the first ankyrin repeat with p16 but is not predicted to bind to CDK4 or CDK6 based on crystal structure studies. p12 is reported to suppress cell growth but in a pRb-independent mechanism (Sharpless, 2005). When the effect of ectopic expression of all the three transcripts, p16, p14ARF, and p12 was compared, p16 had the most inhibitory effects on cell growth of the human lung cancer cell line A549 (Zhang et al., 2010b).

3. The role of p16

3.1 p16 as a tumor suppressor gene

CKI p16 is an important tumor suppressor gene, defects in which are associated with cancer (Koh et al., 1995). p16 is functional as a growth suppressor gene as introduction of full length p16 cDNA caused marked growth suprression in p16-null human glioma cells (Arap et al., 1995), lung cancer *in vitro* and *in vivo* (Jin et al., 1995), carcinoma cell lines *in vitro* and *in vivo* (Spillare et al., 1996), esophageal cancer cells (Schrump et al., 1996), and human and canine breast cancer cells (Campbell et al., 2000; DeInnocentes et al., 2009). p16 defects are second in frequency only to those in p53 for human malignancies (Baylin et al., 1998). p53 and p16 are thought to work via two independent pathways of growth suppression, but both of them are important in suppressing malignant transformation (Gruis et al., 1995). p16 gene deletions are associated with, and appear permissive for, late-stage, high-grade cancers such as; melanoma, bladder cancer, schistosomal bladder cancer, esophageal cancer, breast cancer, and glioblastoma (Gruis et al., 1995; Izumoto et al., 1995; Zhou et al., 1995; Swellam et al., 2004; DeInnocentes et al., 2009). Deletion of the 9p21 region encoding the p16-INK4A/p14ARF/p15 tumor suppressor loci in humans results in tumor formation in a wide range of tissues (Kamb et al., 1994; Kleihues et al., 1994; Packenham et al., 1995). Loss of heterozygosity (Swellam et al., 2004), loss of homozygosity (Ranade et al., 1995; Quelle et al., 1997), and hypermethylation of the promoter (Herman et al., 1997) in the 9p21 region are all important mechanisms which have been shown to result in loss of p16 expression and promote p16-related neoplasms. Hyper-methylation of the p16 promoter region appears to occur early in neoplastic transformation before development of tumorigenicity in rat respiratory epithelium (Yamada et al., 2010). Loss of p16 is associated with extended life span but is not sufficient for immortality (Loughran et al., 1996; Noble et al., 1996). Frequency of loss of p16 is high in pre-malignant lesions suggesting the importance of loss of p16 activity as an early event in cancer progression (Liggett & Sidransky, 1998) and evaluation of p16 expression could have value as an early prognostic indicator for predicting cancer recurrence (Bartoletti et al., 2007). Hypermethylation of CpG islands in the p16 promoter results in enhanced cell proliferation in human colorectal cancer and can activate DNA demethylation in the invasive region suppressing proliferation but enhancing tumor invasion (Jie et al., 2007). Additionally INK4A/ARF hypermethylation occurs frequently in mammary epithelial cells in high risk women with sporadic breast cancer (Bean et al., 2007; Jing et al., 2007; Sharma et al., 2007).

K-cyclin (ORF72) is a human homolog of cyclinD1 in Kaposi's sarcoma-associated herpesvirus (KSHV/HHV-8) which is oncogenic in immune suppressed individuals. p16 inhibits the unphophorylated CDK6-K-cyclin complex and functional availaibility of K-cyclin for tumorogenesis is largely dependent upon the balance of expression of p16 and CDK6 (Yoshioka et al., 2010). This complex is resistant to CKI p21 and p27 and can phopshorylate both of them explaining the important role of p16 as a tumor suppressor gene in malignancies induced by KSHV and their resistance to multiple CKI activities.

Mutations in the p16 encoding gene have also been reported in other cancer types such as glioblastomas, pancreatic adenocarcinomas, and melanoma-prone pedigrees. Allelic variants of p16 in melanoma-prone pedigrees have been found, which are deficient in interaction with CDK4 and CDK6. p16 allelic variants with decreased CDK interaction capability predisposes these individuals to increased risk of cancer which reinforces the important role of p16 as a tumor suppressor gene (Reymond & Brent, 1995). Mutations in CDK4 prevent p16 binding to CDK4 and have been identified for several noncontiguous amino acid sequences. This suggests there may be multiple binding sites for p16. Such mutated CDK4s have oncogenic potential and occur spontaneously in melanomas and other neoplasms (Ceha et al., 1998).

Matrix metalloproteinases (MMPs) are the zinc-dependent endopeptidases, which are capable of degrading components of the extracellular matrix. The MMP family is composed of at least 20 enzymes. One of the MMP family enzymes is MMP-2, which has been reported to be strongly linked with various types of human cancers such as glioma (Uhm et al., 1996) and astrogliomas (Qin et al., 1998). p16 represses expression of MMP-2 and invasiveness of gliomas (Chintala et al., 1997) by blocking Sp1 to mediate gene transcription of MMP-2 (Wang et al., 2006). Thus, p16 can inhibit the cyclin-CDK complex to suppress the cell cycle can also suppress tumor invasion through other cell regulatory functions.

Rab proteins are members of Ras-related small GTPase family. Rab27A is also linked with human genetic diseases (Seabra et al., 2002). Rab27A is associated with invasive and metastatic breast cancer, which is facilitated by down-regulation of p16 and up-regulation of cyclinD1 (Wang et al., 2008). Concomitant overexpression of p16 and p73 has oncogenic potential and affects the development and growth of breast carcinomas (Garcia et al., 2004).

Alteration of p15 and p16 expression and overexpression of TGF-α are found frequently in schistomal bladder cancers and squamous cell carcinomas (Swellam et al., 2004). Loss of p16 expression has prognostic value in predicting recurrence-free probability in patients affected by low-grade urothelial bladder cancer (Bartoletti et al., 2007). p16 has been reported to be inactive in human colorectal cancer but p16 expression is elevated by the demethylation of the p16 promoter in invasive cancer cells, as these cells cease proliferation at the invasive front (Jie et al., 2007).

β-catenin is the key downstream effector of Wnt signaling and is also a potent oncogene. β-catenin can also inhibit cell proliferation by activating the p14ARF-p53-p21 pathway during trans-differentiation of squamous cell differentiation associated with endometrial carcinoma (Saegusa et al., 2005). p16 is also induced along with loss of pRb expression in trans-differentiation of endometrial carcinoma cells, mediated by β-catenin and p21 (Saegusa et al., 2006). Deletion of p16 has been reported in high-grade B-cell non-Hodgkin's lymphoma (Fosmire et al., 2007) along with increases in Rb phosphorylation at CDK4 phosphorylated sites. Inactivation of p16 has also been reported in high grade non-Hodgkin's lymphoma and is less prevalent in low-grade tumors (Modiano et al., 2007). p16 inactivation is more frequent in blastoid mantle cell lymphoma (Dreyling et al., 1997).

p16 forms a complex with HIF-1α, the transcription factor for the VEGF gene promoter, thus represses the transactivation of VEGF. p16 inhibits VEGF gene expression and inhibits cancer cell induced angiogenesis in breast cancer cells and the loss of p16 is a significant transition in neoplastic development (Zhang et al., 2010a).

3.2 Role of p16 in cell quiescence

p16 checks the cell cycle at the G1/S phase transition and thus has an important role in cell cycle exit and quiescence in a variety of cell systems. Growth suppression by p16 depends upon the presence of functional Rb. Growth in Rb null fibroblasts failed to be suppressed by p16 (Medema et al., 1995). Ectopic p16 expression prevents re-entry into the cell cycle (Lea et al., 2003) and p16 expression can induce a G0-like state in hematopoietic cells (Furukawa et al., 2000). p16 expression is up-regulated by exposure to cellular stressors such as oxidative stress, aging, UV exposure, ionizing radiation, chemotherapeutic agents, telomere dysfunction, and wound healing (Kim & Sharpless, 2006; Natarajan et al., 2006). In response to non-lethal UVC irradiation, only p16 positive cell lines can induce cell cycle delay in comparison to p16 null cell lines (Wang et al., 1996). p16 is induced by MAPK activation, in response to stimulation of the ERK/MAPK pathway through RAS/RAF signaling (Ohtani et al., 2001). RAS activation induces p16 expression through ERK mediated activation of Ets1/2 (Ohtani et al., 2001) and p14ARF through Jun-mediated activation of DMP1 (Sreeramaneni et al., 2005). Histone acetyltransferases (HATs), such as p300/CBP are important transcriptional up-regulators. The GC-rich region in the p16 promoter is the putative binding site for transcription factor Sp1 (Gizard et al., 2005). p300 in-cooperation with Sp1 transcriptionally upregulates p16 expression and induces cell cycle arrest in HeLa cells (Kivinen et al., 1999; Wang et al., 2008). Smooth muscle cells in mature arteries in rat have low rates of proliferation. Suppression of proliferation is dependent on the up-regulated levels of p16 and p27, which makes these cells unable to activate cyclinD1 and cyclinE and their associated kinase activties (Izzard et al., 2002).

p16 has also been associated with a variety of additional cell proliferation control proteins that either bind and suppress its function or compete for p16 targets. SEI-1/p34/TRIP-Br1 protein induces CDK4-mediated Rb phosphorylation through physical binding, independent of p16 (Li et al., 2005). SEI-1 facilitates CDK4 function making it resistant to p16 inhibition. ISOC2 protein binds and co-localizes with p16 inhibiting the function of p16 (Huang et al., 2007). Other than ISOC2, p16 protein has also been found to bind to proliferating cell nuclear antigen (PCNA) and minichromosome maintenance protein 6 (MCM6) (Souza-Rodrigues et al., 2007). The same authors have reported that p16 interacts with DNA polymeraseδ accessory protein PCNA, thus inhibiting the function of DNA polymerase.

p16 is normally localized in the nucleus where it functions as an inhibitor of CDK/cyclin complexes but it has also been reported that p16 can be co-localized in the cytoplasm (Nilsson & Landberg, 2006) . Both cytoplasmic and nuclear p16 bind CDK6 and have a role in cell cycle arrest. Human melanocytes initiate differentiation by activation of the cAMP synthesis pathway. This results in increased association of p16 and p27 with CDK4 and CDK2, respectively, Rb phosphoryalation failure and decreased expression of E2F proteins with decreased DNA-binding activity (Haddad et al., 1999). Senescence induced by the cAMP pathway in these cells can be attributed to the complex formation of CKI/CDK complexes, which cause cell cycle exit (Haddad et al., 1999).

It is known that p16 induces cell cycle arrest via Rb, but there is one more mechanism by which p16 can arrest cell cycle independent of Rb. IκBα is a specific inhibitor of NFκB, which competes with p16 for binding to CDK4 and inhibits its activity (Li et al., 2003). This observation has led to speculation that IκBα could substitute for p16 in CDK4 inhibition in malignant cells. Other than that, in G1 phase, activity of CDKs is required for proper recruitment of mini-chromosome maintenance (MCM) protein to the origin recognition complex. p16 influences CDKs and thus influences prereplicative complex (preRC) at the MCM level resulting in arrest of cell cycle (Braden et al., 2006).

c-myc is a transcription factor that plays an important role in cell proliferation. c-myc can induce cell cycle progression from G1 phase to S phase in quiescent cells (Eilers et al., 1991). Oncogenic activity of altered CDK4 is due to its inability to bind p16 and inhibiting its enzymic activity. The oncogenic activity of c-myc and the CDK4/cyclin D1 complex require each other to effectively transform cells. CDK4 requires Myc protein for proper function and, similary, Myc requires the CDK4 cyclinD complex kinase activity to effect tumor transformation. p16 inhibits the transcription regulatory activity of c-myc by blocking cyclin D1/CDK4 complex formation (Haas et al., 1997).

Introduction of adenovirus expressing p16 in human cancer cell lines result in p16-mediated cytotoxicity and results in apoptosis (Kim et al., 2000). p16 expression and estrogen receptor (ER) gene expression are inversely related (Hui et al., 2000). p16 expressing adenovirus vector resulted in delay in tumor growth in a polyomavirus middle-T antigen model of murine breast carcinoma, in comparison with, p19, p27, p18, and p21 which were ineffective (Schreiber et al., 1999).

In dogs, the p16 and p14ARF transcripts derived from INK4A locus have not been fully elucidated. There are no full-length mRNAs or expressed sequence tags (ESTs) available that would completely define these transcripts. In addition this region of the chromosome is extremely GC-rich making it difficult to clone and sequence and causing a gap in the CanFam 2.0 genome assembly (Lindblad-Toh et al., 2005). The biological functions of these two proteins are fairly well understood compared to their genomic structure. Several lines of evidence suggest that both p16 and p14ARF act as potent tumor suppressors apart from their roles as cell cycle regulators during the G1 to S phase transition and p53 mediated cell cycle arrest, respectively.

3.3 Role of p16 in cell differentiation

Other than senescence and quiescence, p16 also has a role in cell differentiation like other CKIs. Expression of p16 increases by several fold in terminally differentiated human adult brain tissue and p16 is thought to play role in human brain development (Lois et al., 1995). During differentiation of human embryonic teratocarcinoma cells (NT2) into post-mitotic neurons, expression of p16 and p15 protein levels become elevated (Lois et al., 1995). The role of p16 in melanocyte differentiation has also been investigated. Microphthalmia transcription factor (MITF) is able to induce cell cycle arrest prior to cell differentiation by activation of p16 protein (Loercher et al., 2005).

A-type lamins are intermediate filaments which affect gene expression in differentiation and are thought to function through an Rb-dependent mechanism. Rb associates with a number of tissue specific transcription factors in an E2F-independent manner and induces differentiation in those tissues. Rb associates with MyoD and Mef2 in skeletal muscle cells (Sellers et al., 1998; Novitch et al., 1999), CBFA1 and Runx2 in osteocytes (Thomas et al., 2001; Thomas et al., 2004), and C/EBP in adipocytes and during macrophage differentiation (Chen et al., 1996). pRb is essential for muscle and fat cell differentiation (Korenjak & Brehm, 2005) and cellular senescence (Ohtani et al., 2001). Cells lacking A-type lamins do not arrest in the presence of p16 because destabilization of pRb (Nitta et al., 2006). This report suggests a dependence of p16-induced cell cycle arrest on Rb and posits a role for A-type lamins in Rb-dependent cell cycle arrest.

Cyclin, CDKs, and CKIs have been associated with proliferation and differentiation in a variety of cell and tissue systems. CyclinD1, the principle cofactor of p16, targets CDK4/6 and may participate in myoblast differentiation (Rao & Kohtz, 1995). Thus, p16 appears to play a key regulatory role in cell differentiation and senescence through management of cell cycle exit. CDK4/6 also regulates cell division at different stages of erythroid maturation (Malumbres et al., 2004). CDK4 knock-out mice lack postnatal homeostasis of pituitary somato/lactotrophs and pancreatic B cells (Jirawatnotai et al., 2004). CDK6 knock-out mice have mild defects in hematopoeitic cell differentiation. Double deficiency of CDK4/6 in embryos appears to have no effect on organogenesis and associated cell proliferation although they are lethal due to defects in the erythroid lineage (Malumbres et al., 2004). Thus, CDK4/6 are required for many specific tissue differentiation events along with cell cycle progression. For example CDK4 activity is required for pancreatic β-cell proliferation and increased expression of p16, limits the regenerative capacity of β-cells with aging (Krishnamurthy et al., 2006).

Cell proliferation inhibits cell differentiation while, conversely, factors inducing cell cycle exit often lead to differentiation. Cell cycle regulatory proteins are multifunctional and can also affect cell differentiation independent of their role in cell cycle. p21 deficient cells are defective in differentiation although differentiation can resume by transducing cells with p16 to compliment the mutation (Gius et al., 1999). Cyclin-CDK complexes can inhibit differentiation in a kinase-dependent manner. The cyclin D1-CDK4 complex can phosphorylate and inhibit DMP1 or Mef2c transcription factors that are essential for differentiation of skeletal muscle and pre-hypertrophic chondrocytes (Hirai & Sherr, 1996; Lazaro et al., 2002; Arnold et al., 2007). CDK2 and CDK4 can inhibit TGF-β induced growth arrest by phosphorylating Smad3 (Matsuura et al., 2004). p16, as a direct inhibitor of cyclin D1 and CDK4 complexes may thus have an indirect role in cell differentiation.

3.4 Role of p16 in cell senescence

Cell senescence is a permanent cell resting phase and is related to cell aging (Smith & Pereira-Smith, 1996). Senescence can be either induced by DNA replication stress or by oncogene expression but is most often the result of replicative senescence. Accumulation of p16 is associated with replicative senescence. Increased p16 expression has been found in lymphocytes only a few cell doublings before replicative senescence (Chebel et al., 2007). Oncogene induced senescence is linked with elevated p16 and p14ARF expression (Serrano, 1997; Markowski et al., 2010). Deletion of the INK4/ARF gene locus, in K-ras constitutively expressing mice, results in loss of senescence and invasive, metastasizing tumors (Bennecke et al., 2010).

p16 expression has been shown to promote premature cell senescence (Zindy et al., 1997). Level of p16 expression increases as mouse embryonic fibroblasts reaches senescence (Zindy et al., 1997). Immortal fibroblast (NIH3T3) and tumor cell lines frequently lack p16 expression suggesting the removal of p16 as a potential pathway to bypass senescence and also points towards the importance of p16 as a tumor suppressor gene (Kamb et al., 1994; Nobori et al., 1994; Zindy et al., 1997). T box proteins (Tbx2) and polycomb proteins (BMI1, Cbx7, Mel18) have been reported to be repressors of all three genes of the INK4 locus (p16, p14ARF, and p15) (Jacobs et al., 1999; Gil et al., 2004). Repression of the INK4B/INK4A/ARF locus is controlled by methylation of histone 3 at lysine 27, by binding of chromobox 7(CBX7) within the polycomb repressive complex 1 to ANRIL (antisense non-coding RNA of INK4B/INK4A/ARF locus) (Yap et al., 2010). Bmi-1 encodes the polycomb protein, which represses both p16 and p14ARF and is linked with regulation of the replicative life span of human fibroblasts (Itahana et al., 2003). BMI1 protein represses p16 expression by binding directly to the Bmi-1 response element (BRE), within the p16 promoter (Meng et al., 2010), and is dependent on the continued presence of EZH2-containing Polycomb-Repressive Complex 2 (PRC2) complex (Bracken et al., 2007). Enhancer of zeste homolog 2 (EZH2) is a histone methyltransferase and a component of the polycomb group protein complex which represses INK4a/ARF gene expression in pancreatic islet beta cells (Chen et al., 2009).

Under a stress and senescence stimulus EZH2 levels decrease coinciding with up-regulated p16. Coincidently PRC2 and PRC1 complexes, localized at the regulatory domain of p16, are lost when cells enter senescence which in turn results in decreased levels of histone H3K27 trimethylation (H3K27me3) and increased levels of the histone demethylase Jmjd3 with the recruitment of the MLL1 protein (Agherbi et al., 2009). Polycomb proteins are recruited to the INK4/ARF locus through CDC6 and, upon senescence and with an increase in Jmjd3 levels, MLL1 protein is recruited to the locus provoking dissociation of polycomb protein from the INK4/ARF locus. This leads to transcription and replication of the INK4/ARF locus in early S phase prior to reaching senescence (Agherbi et al., 2009). CDC6 is an essential DNA replication regulator. CDC6 overexpression induces increased INK4/ARF tumor suppressor gene expression through epigenetic modification of chromatin at the INK4/ARF locus (Borlado & Mendez, 2008). COOH-terminal-binding protein (CtBP), a physiologically regulated co-repressor, has also been reported to have a significant role in p16 repression. Several of the pathways noted above repress p16 via CtBP-mediated repression as CtBP forms bridges between proteins having PxDLS amino acid motifs including several transcription factors and other proteins involved in transcription (Mroz et al., 2008).

The levels of p27 and p16 proteins are significantly increased in contact-inhibited human fibroblasts while in contrast, levels were low in serum-deprived human fibroblasts but in both cases, even through the mechanisms of growth arrest are different, they both affect the same pathway involving CDK4, cyclin D1, and Rb (Dietrich et al., 1997). Maintenance of p16 and p27 levels have also been shown to contribute to the low levels of proliferation in normal blood vessels (Izzard et al., 2002) and p16 mRNA and protein accumulate in human fibroblasts as they become senescent (Hara et al., 1996).

4. Potential of p16 as a therapeutic or gene therapy target

p16 is an important tumor suppressor gene, deletion of which causes various types of tumors making it an important potential target for cancer gene therapy. It has been reported that p16 positive oropharyngeal squamous cell carcinoma (OPSCC) patients respond more favorably to intensity-modulated radiotherapy treatment in comparison to similar p16 negative tumors (Shoushtari et al., 2010). Infectious delivery of the whole p15/p16/p14ARF locus, in infectious bacterial artificial chromosomes, results in growth suppression in human glioma cells (Inoue et al., 2004). Induction of p16 using the DNA methyltransferase inhibitor zebularine combined with the histone deacetylation (HDAC) inhibitors depsipeptide led to inhibition of cell growth in lung tumor cell lines (Chen et al., 2010). Ectopic p16 introduction in cancer cells alone or with other tumor suppressor genes inhibits cell growth and induces apoptosis and senescence, while p16 gene silencing reduced the p53-mediated response to chemotherapeutic agents in cancers (Derenzini et al., 2009). Histone methyltransferase EZH2 inhibitor 3-deazaneplanocin A and the histone deacetylase inhibitor panobinostat together induce p16, p21, p27, and FBX032 and down-regulates cyclin E and HOXA9 levels, which induces apoptosis in cultured and primary human acute myeloid leukemia (AML) cell line cells (Fiskus et al., 2009). p16 along with the murine granulocyte-macrophage colony-stimulating factor gene (AdGM-CSF) can induce effective anti-tumor immunity (Wang et al., 2002). Exogenous expression of p16 and p53 induce apoptosis in lung carcinoma cells (Bai et al., 2000), leukemia cell line K562 (Rui & Su, 2002), non-small lung cancer (Wu et al., 2000), and pancreatic cancer (Ghaneh et al., 2001). p16 along with p27 inhibits angioplasty-induced neointimal hyperplasia and coronary artery occlusion (Tsui et al., 2001), inhibits proliferation in neointimal hyperplasia (McArthur et al., 2001), and a wide range of other tumor types (Patel et al., 2000). Ectopic expression of p16 by replication-competent adenovirus leads to potent anti-tumor effects in gastric cancer xenografts in nude mice (Ma et al., 2009) while p16 transfection along with cisplatin treatment increased senescence and growth inhibition in non-small cell lung cancer xenografts in mice (Fang et al., 2007). Ectopic p16 expression was able to induce growth arrest in pancreatic carcinoma JF305 cell lines (Ma et al., 2007), human laryngeal squamous cell carcinoma (Liu et al., 2003; Fu et al., 2004), and inhibit experimental lung metastasis in Balb/c nude mice (Kim et al., 2003), inhibit cell growth in nasopharyngeal carcinoma (Lee et al., 2003), and a murine model of head and neck cancer (Rhee et al., 2003), human mesothelioma (Yang et al., 2003), and suppress tumor growth by glioblastoma cells *in vivo* and *in vitro* (Adachi et al., 2002). p16 transfection suppressed growth of Bcap-37 breast cancer cells (Bai et al., 2001), the human melanoma cell line WM-983A (Cheng et al., 1999), human lung adenocarcinomas (Fu et al., 1999), pancreatic cancer (Calbo et al., 2001), and inhibits cardiac hypertrophy *in vitro* and *in vivo* (Nozato et al., 2001). p16 also inhibited cell growth in a human ovarian cancer cell line (Wang et al., 1999), a human gastric cell line (Sun & Lu, 1997), and a small cell lung carcinoma (Sumitomo et al., 1999). All of these diverse examples demonstrate the potent and broadly efficient effects of exogenous p16 expression on cell proliferation in p16 negative cancer cells *in vitro* and *in vivo* and reflects the importance of p16 as regulatory factor and potential target for gene therapy and cancer therapeutics.

5. Conclusions

p16/INK4A/CDKN2A is an important tumor suppressor gene, which is required for the control of unregulated cell growth in many and perhaps most cell types. The INK4A locus is also unique in eukaryotes, where 3 and perhaps 4 transcripts are derived which have similar functions of suppressing cell growth but that work via very different pathways. Most surprising is the utilization of alternative open reading frames from a single gene complex mandating co-evolution of the unrelated protein sequences. Despite these constraints, mutation of p16 is second only to p53 in mutation frequency in a wide range of tumors. This strongly suggests that p16 may have real potential as an important new target for cancer gene therapy. p16 is not just an important cell cycle regulatory protein that helps suppress the cell growth and tumor formation, p16 also has a role in other cell cycle phases. p16 has been reported to play an important role in cell differentiation, cell quiescence, and cell senescence, which makes it not just a tumor suppressor protein but a cell regulatory protein that plays a critical role in regulating terminal differentiation and the aging process. There is a great need to investigate all the subtleties surrounding p16 function and to unravel all the pathways and binding partners of p16. p16 is a promising gene located within a complex gene locus with many roles in cell metabolism.

6. Acknowledgements

The authors would like to acknowledge a wide range of people who have helped directly or indirectly in this research and have helped made this manuscript possible. The authors thank Dr. Bruce F. Smith, Dr. Anthony T. Moss, Dr. Frederik van Ginkel, Allison Church Bird, Dr. Deepa Bedi, Dr. Jeremy Foote, Maninder Sandey, Willie Morris, Jishan Zaman, and Ashley Ladegast for their contributions, support, and encouragement.

7. References

Adachi Y., Chandrasekar, N., Kin, Y., Lakka, S.S., Mohanam, S., Yanamandra, N., Mohan, P.M., Fuller, G.N., Fang, B., Fueyo, J., Dinh, D.H., Olivero, W.C., Tamiya, T., Ohmoto, T., Kyritsis, A.P. & Rao, J.S. (2002). "Suppression of glioma invasion and growth by adenovirus-mediated delivery of a bicistronic construct containing antisense uPAR and sense p16 gene sequences. *Oncogene*, Vol. 21, No.1, pp. (87-95). 0950-9232.

Afshari C.A. & Barrett, J.C. (1993). "Cell cycle controls: potential targets for chemical carcinogens? *Environ Health Perspect*, Vol. 101 Suppl 5, pp. (9-14). 0091-6765.

Agger K., Cloos, P.A., Rudkjaer, L., Williams, K., Andersen, G., Christensen, J. & Helin, K. (2009). "The H3K27me3 demethylase JMJD3 contributes to the activation of the INK4A-ARF locus in response to oncogene- and stress-induced senescence. *Genes Dev*, Vol. 23, No.10, pp. (1171-1176). 1549-5477.

Agherbi H., Gaussmann-Wenger, A., Verthuy, C., Chasson, L., Serrano, M. & Djabali, M. (2009). "Polycomb mediated epigenetic silencing and replication timing at the INK4a/ARF locus during senescence. *PLoS One*, Vol. 4, No.5, pp. (e5622). 1932-6203.

Arap W., Nishikawa, R., Furnari, F.B., Cavenee, W.K. & Huang, H.J. (1995). "Replacement of the p16/CDKN2 gene suppresses human glioma cell growth. *Cancer Res*, Vol. 55, No.6, pp. (1351-1354). 0008-5472.

Arnold M.A., Kim, Y., Czubryt, M.P., Phan, D., McAnally, J., Qi, X., Shelton, J.M., Richardson, J.A., Bassel-Duby, R. & Olson, E.N. (2007). "MEF2C transcription factor controls chondrocyte hypertrophy and bone development. *Dev Cell*, Vol. 12, No.3, pp. (377-389). 1534-5807.

Asamoto M., Hori, T., Baba-Toriyama, H., Sano, M., Takahashi, S., Tsuda, H. & Shirai, T. (1998). "p16 gene overexpression in mouse bladder carcinomas. *Cancer Lett*, Vol. 127, No.1-2, pp. (9-13). 0304-3835

Bai J., Zhu, X., Zheng, X. & Wu, Y. (2001). "Retroviral vector containing human p16 gene and its inhibitory effect on Bcap-37 breast cancer cells. *Chin Med J (Engl)*, Vol. 114, No.5, pp. (497-501). 0366-6999.

Bai X., Che, F., Li, J., Ma, Y., Zhou, Y., Zhai, J. & Meng, L. (2000). "Effects of adenovirus-mediated p16 and p53 genes transfer on apoptosis and cell cycle of lung carcinoma cells. *Zhonghua Bing Li Xue Za Zhi*, Vol. 29, No.5, pp. (354-358). 0529-5807.

Baker D.J., Perez-Terzic, C., Jin, F., Pitel, K., Niederlander, N.J., Jeganathan, K., Yamada, S., Reyes, S., Rowe, L., Hiddinga, H.J., Eberhardt, N.L., Terzic, A. & van Deursen, J.M. (2008). "Opposing roles for p16Ink4a and p19Arf in senescence and ageing caused by BubR1 insufficiency. *Nat Cell Biol*, Vol. 10, No.7, pp. (825-836). 1476-4679.

Bartkova J., Lukas, J., Guldberg, P., Alsner, J., Kirkin, A.F., Zeuthen, J. & Bartek, J. (1996). "The p16-cyclin D/Cdk4-pRb pathway as a functional unit frequently altered in melanoma pathogenesis. *Cancer Res*, Vol. 56, No.23, pp. (5475-5483). 0008-5472.

Bartoletti R., Cai, T., Nesi, G., Roberta Girardi, L., Baroni, G. & Dal Canto, M. (2007). "Loss of P16 expression and chromosome 9p21 LOH in predicting outcome of patients affected by superficial bladder cancer. *J Surg Res*, Vol. 143, No.2, pp. (422-427). 0022-4804.

Baylin S.B., Herman, J.G., Graff, J.R., Vertino, P.M. & Issa, J.P. (1998). "Alterations in DNA methylation: a fundamental aspect of neoplasia. *Adv Cancer Res*, Vol. 72, pp. (141-196). 0065-230X.

Bazarov A.V., Van Sluis, M., Hines, W.C., Bassett, E., Beliveau, A., Campeau, E., Mukhopadhyay, R., Lee, W.J., Melodyev, S., Zaslavsky, Y., Lee, L., Rodier, F., Chicas, A., Lowe, S.W., Benhattar, J., Ren, B., Campisi, J. & Yaswen, P. (2010). "p16(INK4a) -mediated suppression of telomerase in normal and malignant human breast cells. *Aging Cell*, Vol. 9, No.5, pp. (736-746). 1474-9726.

Bean G.R., Bryson, A.D., Pilie, P.G., Goldenberg, V., Baker, J.C., Jr., Ibarra, C., Brander, D.M., Paisie, C., Case, N.R., Gauthier, M., Reynolds, P.A., Dietze, E., Ostrander, J., Scott, V., Wilke, L.G., Yee, L., Kimler, B.F., Fabian, C.J., Zalles, C.M., Broadwater, G., Tlsty, T.D. & Seewaldt, V.L. (2007). "Morphologically normal-appearing mammary epithelial cells obtained from high-risk women exhibit methylation silencing of INK4a/ARF. *Clin Cancer Res*, Vol. 13, No.22 Pt 1, pp. (6834-6841). 1078-0432.

Bennecke M., Kriegl, L., Bajbouj, M., Retzlaff, K., Robine, S., Jung, A., Arkan, M.C., Kirchner, T. & Greten, F.R. (2010). "Ink4a/Arf and oncogene-induced senescence prevent tumor progression during alternative colorectal tumorigenesis. *Cancer Cell*, Vol. 18, No.2, pp. (135-146). 1878-3686.

Boehme K.A. & Blattner, C. (2009). "Regulation of p53--insights into a complex process. *Crit Rev Biochem Mol Biol*, Vol. 44, No.6, pp. (367-392). 1549-7798.

Borlado L.R. & Mendez, J. (2008). "CDC6: from DNA replication to cell cycle checkpoints and oncogenesis. *Carcinogenesis*, Vol. 29, No.2, pp. (237-243). 1460-2180.

Bracken A.P., Kleine-Kohlbrecher, D., Dietrich, N., Pasini, D., Gargiulo, G., Beekman, C., Theilgaard-Monch, K., Minucci, S., Porse, B.T., Marine, J.C., Hansen, K.H. & Helin, K. (2007). "The Polycomb group proteins bind throughout the INK4A-ARF locus and are disassociated in senescent cells. *Genes Dev*, Vol. 21, No.5, pp. (525-530). 0890-9369.

Braden W.A., Lenihan, J.M., Lan, Z., Luce, K.S., Zagorski, W., Bosco, E., Reed, M.F., Cook, J.G. & Knudsen, E.S. (2006). "Distinct action of the retinoblastoma pathway on the DNA replication machinery defines specific roles for cyclin-dependent kinase complexes in prereplication complex assembly and S-phase progression. *Mol Cell Biol*, Vol. 26, No.20, pp. (7667-7681). 0270-7306.

Bulavin D.V., Phillips, C., Nannenga, B., Timofeev, O., Donehower, L.A., Anderson, C.W., Appella, E. & Fornace, A.J., Jr. (2004). "Inactivation of the Wip1 phosphatase inhibits mammary tumorigenesis through p38 MAPK-mediated activation of the p16(Ink4a)-p19(Arf) pathway. *Nat Genet*, Vol. 36, No.4, pp. (343-350). 1061-4036.

Calbo J., Marotta, M., Cascallo, M., Roig, J.M., Gelpi, J.L., Fueyo, J. & Mazo, A. (2001). "Adenovirus-mediated wt-p16 reintroduction induces cell cycle arrest or apoptosis in pancreatic cancer. *Cancer Gene Ther*, Vol. 8, No.10, pp. (740-750). 0929-1903.

Campbell I., Magliocco, A., Moyana, T., Zheng, C. & Xiang, J. (2000). "Adenovirus-mediated p16INK4 gene transfer significantly suppresses human breast cancer growth. *Cancer Gene Ther*, Vol. 7, No.9, pp. (1270-1278). 0929-1903.

Carbone C.J., Grana, X., Reddy, E.P. & Haines, D.S. (2007). "p21 loss cooperates with INK4 inactivation facilitating immortalization and Bcl-2-mediated anchorage-independent growth of oncogene-transduced primary mouse fibroblasts. *Cancer Res*, Vol. 67, No.9, pp. (4130-4137). 0008-5472.

Ceha H.M., Nasser, I., Medema, R.H. & Slebos, R.J. (1998). "Several noncontiguous domains of CDK4 are involved in binding to the P16 tumor suppressor protein. *Biochem Biophys Res Commun*, Vol. 249, No.2, pp. (550-555). 0006-291X.

Chebel A., Chien, W.W., Gerland, L.M., Mekki, Y., Bertrand, Y., Ffrench, P., Galmarini, C.M. & Ffrench, M. (2007). "Does p16ink4a expression increase with the number of cell doublings in normal and malignant lymphocytes? *Leuk Res*, Vol. 31, No.12, pp. (1649-1658). 0145-2126.

Chen H., Gu, X., Su, I.H., Bottino, R., Contreras, J.L., Tarakhovsky, A. & Kim, S.K. (2009). "Polycomb protein Ezh2 regulates pancreatic beta-cell Ink4a/Arf expression and regeneration in diabetes mellitus. *Genes Dev*, Vol. 23, No.8, pp. (975-985). 1549-5477.

Chen M., Voeller, D., Marquez, V.E., Kaye, F.J., Steeg, P.S., Giaccone, G. & Zajac-Kaye, M. (2010). "Enhanced growth inhibition by combined DNA methylation/HDAC inhibitors in lung tumor cells with silenced CDKN2A. *Int J Oncol*, Vol. 37, No.4, pp. (963-971). 1791-2423.

Chen P.L., Riley, D.J., Chen, Y. & Lee, W.H. (1996). "Retinoblastoma protein positively regulates terminal adipocyte differentiation through direct interaction with C/EBPs. *Genes Dev*, Vol. 10, No.21, pp. (2794-2804). 0890-9369.

Cheng J., Lin, C. & Xing, R. (1999). "[Apoptosis of human melanoma cell line WM-983A by p16 gene transduction]. *Zhonghua Zhong Liu Za Zhi*, Vol. 21, No.2, pp. (89-92). 0253-3766.

Chien W.W., Domenech, C., Catallo, R., Kaddar, T., Magaud, J.P., Salles, G. & Ffrench, M. (2011). "Cyclin-dependent kinase 1 expression is inhibited by p16(INK4a) at the post-transcriptional level through the microRNA pathway. *Oncogene*, Vol. 30, No.16, pp. (1880-1891). 1476-5594.

Chintala S.K., Fueyo, J., Gomez-Manzano, C., Venkaiah, B., Bjerkvig, R., Yung, W.K., Sawaya, R., Kyritsis, A.P. & Rao, J.S. (1997). "Adenovirus-mediated p16/CDKN2 gene transfer suppresses glioma invasion in vitro. *Oncogene*, Vol. 15, No.17, pp. (2049-2057). 0950-9232.

Coleman K.G., Wautlet, B.S., Morrissey, D., Mulheron, J., Sedman, S.A., Brinkley, P., Price, S. & Webster, K.R. (1997). "Identification of CDK4 sequences involved in cyclin D1 and p16 binding. *J Biol Chem*, Vol. 272, No.30, pp. (18869-18874). 0021-9258.

Craig C., Kim, M., Ohri, E., Wersto, R., Katayose, D., Li, Z., Choi, Y.H., Mudahar, B., Srivastava, S., Seth, P. & Cowan, K. (1998). "Effects of adenovirus-mediated p16INK4A expression on cell cycle arrest are determined by endogenous p16 and Rb status in human cancer cells. *Oncogene*, Vol. 16, No.2, pp. (265-272). 0950-9232.

D'Amico M., Wu, K., Fu, M., Rao, M., Albanese, C., Russell, R.G., Lian, H., Bregman, D., White, M.A. & Pestell, R.G. (2004). "The inhibitor of cyclin-dependent kinase 4a/alternative reading frame (INK4a/ARF) locus encoded proteins p16INK4a and p19ARF repress cyclin D1 transcription through distinct cis elements. *Cancer Res*, Vol. 64, No.12, pp. (4122-4130). 0008-5472.

DeInnocentes P., Agarwal, P. & Bird, R.C. (2009). "Phenotype-rescue of cyclin-dependent kinase inhibitor p16/INK4A defects in a spontaneous canine cell model of breast cancer. *J Cell Biochem*, Vol. 106, No.3, pp. (491-505). 1097-4644.

Delmolino L., Band, H. & Band, V. (1993). "Expression and stability of p53 protein in normal human mammary epithelial cells. *Carcinogenesis*, Vol. 14, No.5, pp. (827-832). 0143-3334.

Derenzini M., Brighenti, E., Donati, G., Vici, M., Ceccarelli, C., Santini, D., Taffurelli, M., Montanaro, L. & Trere, D. (2009). "The p53-mediated sensitivity of cancer cells to chemotherapeutic agents is conditioned by the status of the retinoblastoma protein. *J Pathol*, Vol. 219, No.3, pp. (373-382). 1096-9896.

Dietrich C., Wallenfang, K., Oesch, F. & Wieser, R. (1997). "Differences in the mechanisms of growth control in contact-inhibited and serum-deprived human fibroblasts. *Oncogene*, Vol. 15, No.22, pp. (2743-2747). 0950-9232.

Dimri G.P., Itahana, K., Acosta, M. & Campisi, J. (2000). "Regulation of a senescence checkpoint response by the E2F1 transcription factor and p14(ARF) tumor suppressor. *Mol Cell Biol*, Vol. 20, No.1, pp. (273-285). 0270-7306.

Dominguez-Brauer C., Chen, Y.J., Brauer, P.M., Pimkina, J. & Raychaudhuri, P. (2009). "ARF stimulates XPC to trigger nucleotide excision repair by regulating the repressor complex of E2F4. *EMBO Rep*, Vol. 10, No.9, pp. (1036-1042). 1469-3178.

Dreyling M.H., Bullinger, L., Ott, G., Stilgenbauer, S., Muller-Hermelink, H.K., Bentz, M., Hiddemann, W. & Dohner, H. (1997). "Alterations of the cyclin D1/p16-pRB pathway in mantle cell lymphoma. *Cancer Res*, Vol. 57, No.20, pp. (4608-4614). 0008-5472.

Eilers M., Schirm, S. & Bishop, J.M. (1991). "The MYC protein activates transcription of the alpha-prothymosin gene. *Embo J*, Vol. 10, No.1, pp. (133-141). 0261-4189.

Emig R., Magener, A., Ehemann, V., Meyer, A., Stilgenbauer, F., Volkmann, M., Wallwiener, D. & Sinn, H.P. (1998). "Aberrant cytoplasmic expression of the p16 protein in breast cancer is associated with accelerated tumour proliferation. *Br J Cancer*, Vol. 78, No.12, pp. (1661-1668). 0007-0920.

Enoch T. & Nurse, P. (1991). "Coupling M phase and S phase: controls maintaining the dependence of mitosis on chromosome replication. *Cell*, Vol. 65, No.6, pp. (921-923). 0092-8674.

Evangelou K., Bramis, J., Peros, I., Zacharatos, P., Dasiou-Plakida, D., Kalogeropoulos, N., Asimacopoulos, P.J., Kittas, C., Marinos, E. & Gorgoulis, V.G. (2004). "Electron microscopy evidence that cytoplasmic localization of the p16(INK4A) "nuclear" cyclin-dependent kinase inhibitor (CKI) in tumor cells is specific and not an artifact. A study in non-small cell lung carcinomas. *Biotech Histochem*, Vol. 79, No.1, pp. (5-10). 1052-0295.

Fahham N., Sardari, S., Ostad, S.N., Vaziri, B. & Ghahremani, M.H. (2010). "C-terminal domain of p16(INK4a) is adequate in inducing cell cycle arrest, growth inhibition and CDK4/6 interaction similar to the full length protein in HT-1080 fibrosarcoma cells. *J Cell Biochem*, Vol. 111, No.6, pp. (1598-1606). 1097-4644.

Fang K., Chiu, C.C., Li, C.H., Chang, Y.T. & Hwang, H.T. (2007). "Cisplatin-induced senescence and growth inhibition in human non-small cell lung cancer cells with ectopic transfer of p16INK4a. *Oncol Res*, Vol. 16, No.10, pp. (479-488). 0965-0407.

Fiskus W., Wang, Y., Sreekumar, A., Buckley, K.M., Shi, H., Jillella, A., Ustun, C., Rao, R., Fernandez, P., Chen, J., Balusu, R., Koul, S., Atadja, P., Marquez, V.E. & Bhalla, K.N. (2009). "Combined epigenetic therapy with the histone methyltransferase EZH2 inhibitor 3-deazaneplanocin A and the histone deacetylase inhibitor panobinostat against human AML cells. *Blood*, Vol. 114, No.13, pp. (2733-2743). 1528-0020.

Fosmire S.P., Thomas, R., Jubala, C.M., Wojcieszyn, J.W., Valli, V.E., Getzy, D.M., Smith, T.L., Gardner, L.A., Ritt, M.G., Bell, J.S., Freeman, K.P., Greenfield, B.E., Lana, S.E., Kisseberth, W.C., Helfand, S.C., Cutter, G.R., Breen, M. & Modiano, J.F. (2007). "Inactivation of the p16 cyclin-dependent kinase inhibitor in high-grade canine non-Hodgkin's T-cell lymphoma. *Vet Pathol*, Vol. 44, No.4, pp. (467-478). 0300-9858.

Freeman-Anderson N.E., Zheng, Y., McCalla-Martin, A.C., Treanor, L.M., Zhao, Y.D., Garfin, P.M., He, T.C., Mary, M.N., Thornton, J.D., Anderson, C., Gibbons, M., Saab, R., Baumer, S.H., Cunningham, J.M. & Skapek, S.X. (2009). "Expression of the Arf tumor suppressor gene is controlled by Tgfbeta2 during development. *Development*, Vol. 136, No.12, pp. (2081-2089). 0950-1991.

Fu X., Zhang, S. & Ran, R. (1999). "[Effect of exogenous p16 gene on the growth of wild-type p53 human lung adenocarcinoma cells]. *Zhonghua Zhong Liu Za Zhi*, Vol. 21, No.2, pp. (102-104). 0253-3766.

Fu Y.J., Liu, S.X. & Xian, J.M. (2004). "[Combination of adenovirus p16(INK4A) gene therapy and ionizing radiation for laryngeal squamous cell carcinoma]. *Sichuan Da Xue Xue Bao Yi Xue Ban*, Vol. 35, No.2, pp. (209-211). 1672-173X.

Furukawa Y., Kikuchi, J., Nakamura, M., Iwase, S., Yamada, H. & Matsuda, M. (2000). "Lineage-specific regulation of cell cycle control gene expression during haematopoietic cell differentiation. *Br J Haematol*, Vol. 110, No.3, pp. (663-673). 0007-1048.

Furuno N., den Elzen, N. & Pines, J. (1999). "Human cyclin A is required for mitosis until mid prophase. *J Cell Biol*, Vol. 147, No.2, pp. (295-306). 0021-9525.

Garcia V., Silva, J., Dominguez, G., Garcia, J.M., Pena, C., Rodriguez, R., Provencio, M., Espana, P. & Bonilla, F. (2004). "Overexpression of p16INK4a correlates with high expression of p73 in breast carcinomas. *Mutat Res*, Vol. 554, No.1-2, pp. (215-221). 0027-5107.

Geradts J., Hruban, R.H., Schutte, M., Kern, S.E. & Maynard, R. (2000). "Immunohistochemical p16INK4a analysis of archival tumors with deletion, hypermethylation, or mutation of the CDKN2/MTS1 gene. A comparison of four commercial antibodies. *Appl Immunohistochem Mol Morphol*, Vol. 8, No.1, pp. (71-79). 1541-2016.

Ghaneh P., Greenhalf, W., Humphreys, M., Wilson, D., Zumstein, L., Lemoine, N.R. & Neoptolemos, J.P. (2001). "Adenovirus-mediated transfer of p53 and p16(INK4a) results in pancreatic cancer regression in vitro and in vivo. *Gene Ther*, Vol. 8, No.3, pp. (199-208). 0969-7128.

Gil J., Bernard, D., Martinez, D. & Beach, D. (2004). "Polycomb CBX7 has a unifying role in cellular lifespan. *Nat Cell Biol*, Vol. 6, No.1, pp. (67-72). 1465-7392.

Gil J. & Peters, G. (2006). "Regulation of the INK4b-ARF-INK4a tumour suppressor locus: all for one or one for all. *Nat Rev Mol Cell Biol*, Vol. 7, No.9, pp. (667-677). 1471-0072.

Gilley J. & Fried, M. (2001). "One INK4 gene and no ARF at the Fugu equivalent of the human INK4A/ARF/INK4B tumour suppressor locus. *Oncogene*, Vol. 20, No.50, pp. (7447-7452). 0950-9232.

Gius D.R., Ezhevsky, S.A., Becker-Hapak, M., Nagahara, H., Wei, M.C. & Dowdy, S.F. (1999). "Transduced p16INK4a peptides inhibit hypophosphorylation of the retinoblastoma protein and cell cycle progression prior to activation of Cdk2 complexes in late G1. *Cancer Res*, Vol. 59, No.11, pp. (2577-2580). 0008-5472.

Gizard F., Amant, C., Barbier, O., Bellosta, S., Robillard, R., Percevault, F., Sevestre, H., Krimpenfort, P., Corsini, A., Rochette, J., Glineur, C., Fruchart, J.C., Torpier, G. & Staels, B. (2005). "PPAR alpha inhibits vascular smooth muscle cell proliferation underlying intimal hyperplasia by inducing the tumor suppressor p16INK4a. *J Clin Invest*, Vol. 115, No.11, pp. (3228-3238). 0021-9738.

Gomez-Lazaro M., Fernandez-Gomez, F.J. & Jordan, J. (2004). "p53: twenty five years understanding the mechanism of genome protection. *J Physiol Biochem*, Vol. 60, No.4, pp. (287-307). 1138-7548.

Gruis N.A., Weaver-Feldhaus, J., Liu, Q., Frye, C., Eeles, R., Orlow, I., Lacombe, L., Ponce-Castaneda, V., Lianes, P., Latres, E. & et al. (1995). "Genetic evidence in melanoma and bladder cancers that p16 and p53 function in separate pathways of tumor suppression. *Am J Pathol*, Vol. 146, No.5, pp. (1199-1206). 0002-9440.

Guan K.L., Jenkins, C.W., Li, Y., Nichols, M.A., Wu, X., O'Keefe, C.L., Matera, A.G. & Xiong, Y. (1994). "Growth suppression by p18, a p16INK4/MTS1- and p14INK4B/MTS2-related CDK6 inhibitor, correlates with wild-type pRb function. *Genes Dev*, Vol. 8, No.24, pp. (2939-2952). 0890-9369.

Gump J., Stokoe, D. & McCormick, F. (2003). "Phosphorylation of p16INK4A correlates with Cdk4 association. *J Biol Chem*, Vol. 278, No.9, pp. (6619-6622). 0021-9258.

Gupta G.P., Perk, J., Acharyya, S., de Candia, P., Mittal, V., Todorova-Manova, K., Gerald, W.L., Brogi, E., Benezra, R. & Massague, J. (2007). "ID genes mediate tumor reinitiation during breast cancer lung metastasis. *Proc Natl Acad Sci U S A*, Vol. 104, No.49, pp. (19506-19511). 1091-6490.

Haas K., Staller, P., Geisen, C., Bartek, J., Eilers, M. & Moroy, T. (1997). "Mutual requirement of CDK4 and Myc in malignant transformation: evidence for cyclin D1/CDK4 and p16INK4A as upstream regulators of Myc. *Oncogene*, Vol. 15, No.2, pp. (179-192). 0950-9232.

Haddad M.M., Xu, W., Schwahn, D.J., Liao, F. & Medrano, E.E. (1999). "Activation of a cAMP pathway and induction of melanogenesis correlate with association of p16(INK4) and p27(KIP1) to CDKs, loss of E2F-binding activity, and premature senescence of human melanocytes. *Exp Cell Res*, Vol. 253, No.2, pp. (561-572). 0014-4827.

Hannon G.J. & Beach, D. (1994). "p15INK4B is a potential effector of TGF-beta-induced cell cycle arrest. *Nature*, Vol. 371, No.6494, pp. (257-261). 0028-0836.

Hara E., Smith, R., Parry, D., Tahara, H., Stone, S. & Peters, G. (1996). "Regulation of p16CDKN2 expression and its implications for cell immortalization and senescence. *Mol Cell Biol*, Vol. 16, No.3, pp. (859-867). 0270-7306.

Hartwell L.H. & Weinert, T.A. (1989). "Checkpoints: controls that ensure the order of cell cycle events. *Science*, Vol. 246, No.4930, pp. (629-634). 0036-8075.

Hayflick L. (1965). "The Limited in Vitro Lifetime of Human Diploid Cell Strains. *Exp Cell Res*, Vol. 37, pp. (614-636). 0014-4827.

Herman J.G., Civin, C.I., Issa, J.P., Collector, M.I., Sharkis, S.J. & Baylin, S.B. (1997). "Distinct patterns of inactivation of p15INK4B and p16INK4A characterize the major types of hematological malignancies. *Cancer Res*, Vol. 57, No.5, pp. (837-841). 0008-5472.

Hirai H., Roussel, M.F., Kato, J.Y., Ashmun, R.A. & Sherr, C.J. (1995). "Novel INK4 proteins, p19 and p18, are specific inhibitors of the cyclin D-dependent kinases CDK4 and CDK6. *Mol Cell Biol*, Vol. 15, No.5, pp. (2672-2681). 0270-7306.

Hirai H. & Sherr, C.J. (1996). "Interaction of D-type cyclins with a novel myb-like transcription factor, DMP1. *Mol Cell Biol*, Vol. 16, No.11, pp. (6457-6467). 0270-7306.

Huang X., Shi, Z., Wang, W., Bai, J., Chen, Z., Xu, J., Zhang, D. & Fu, S. (2007). "Identification and characterization of a novel protein ISOC2 that interacts with p16INK4a. *Biochem Biophys Res Commun*, Vol. 361, No.2, pp. (287-293). 0006-291X.

Hui R., Macmillan, R.D., Kenny, F.S., Musgrove, E.A., Blamey, R.W., Nicholson, R.I., Robertson, J.F. & Sutherland, R.L. (2000). "INK4a gene expression and methylation in primary breast cancer: overexpression of p16INK4a messenger RNA is a marker of poor prognosis. *Clin Cancer Res*, Vol. 6, No.7, pp. (2777-2787). 1078-0432.

Inoue R., Moghaddam, K.A., Ranasinghe, M., Saeki, Y., Chiocca, E.A. & Wade-Martins, R. (2004). "Infectious delivery of the 132 kb CDKN2A/CDKN2B genomic DNA region results in correctly spliced gene expression and growth suppression in glioma cells. *Gene Ther*, Vol. 11, No.15, pp. (1195-1204). 0969-7128.

Itahana K., Zou, Y., Itahana, Y., Martinez, J.L., Beausejour, C., Jacobs, J.J., Van Lohuizen, M., Band, V., Campisi, J. & Dimri, G.P. (2003). "Control of the replicative life span of human fibroblasts by p16 and the polycomb protein Bmi-1. *Mol Cell Biol*, Vol. 23, No.1, pp. (389-401). 0270-7306.

Izumoto S., Arita, N., Ohnishi, T., Hiraga, S., Taki, T. & Hayakawa, T. (1995). "Homozygous deletions of p16INK4A/MTS1 and p15INK4B/MTS2 genes in glioma cells and primary glioma tissues. *Cancer Lett*, Vol. 97, No.2, pp. (241-247). 0304-3835.

Izzard T.D., Taylor, C., Birkett, S.D., Jackson, C.L. & Newby, A.C. (2002). "Mechanisms underlying maintenance of smooth muscle cell quiescence in rat aorta: role of the cyclin dependent kinases and their inhibitors. *Cardiovasc Res*, Vol. 53, No.1, pp. (242-252). 0008-6363.

Jacobs J.J., Kieboom, K., Marino, S., DePinho, R.A. & van Lohuizen, M. (1999). "The oncogene and Polycomb-group gene bmi-1 regulates cell proliferation and senescence through the ink4a locus. *Nature*, Vol. 397, No.6715, pp. (164-168). 0028-0836.

Jeffrey P.D., Tong, L. & Pavletich, N.P. (2000). "Structural basis of inhibition of CDK-cyclin complexes by INK4 inhibitors. *Genes Dev*, Vol. 14, No.24, pp. (3115-3125). 0890-9369.

Jie G., Zhixiang, S., Lei, S., Hesheng, L. & Xiaojun, T. (2007). "Relationship between expression and methylation status of p16INK4a and the proliferative activity of different areas' tumour cells in human colorectal cancer. *Int J Clin Pract*, Vol. 61, No.9, pp. (1523-1529). 1368-5031.

Jin X., Nguyen, D., Zhang, W.W., Kyritsis, A.P. & Roth, J.A. (1995). "Cell cycle arrest and inhibition of tumor cell proliferation by the p16INK4 gene mediated by an adenovirus vector. *Cancer Res*, Vol. 55, No.15, pp. (3250-3253). 0008-5472.

Jing F., Zhang, J., Tao, J., Zhou, Y., Jun, L., Tang, X., Wang, Y. & Hai, H. (2007). "Hypermethylation of tumor suppressor genes BRCA1, p16 and 14-3-3sigma in serum of sporadic breast cancer patients. *Onkologie*, Vol. 30, No.1-2, pp. (14-19). 0378-584X.

Jirawatnotai S., Aziyu, A., Osmundson, E.C., Moons, D.S., Zou, X., Kineman, R.D. & Kiyokawa, H. (2004). "Cdk4 is indispensable for postnatal proliferation of the anterior pituitary. *J Biol Chem*, Vol. 279, No.49, pp. (51100-51106). 0021-9258.

Kamb A., Gruis, N.A., Weaver-Feldhaus, J., Liu, Q., Harshman, K., Tavtigian, S.V., Stockert, E., Day, R.S., 3rd, Johnson, B.E. & Skolnick, M.H. (1994). "A cell cycle regulator potentially involved in genesis of many tumor types. *Science*, Vol. 264, No.5157, pp. (436-440). 0036-8075.

Kia S.K., Gorski, M.M., Giannakopoulos, S. & Verrijzer, C.P. (2008). "SWI/SNF mediates polycomb eviction and epigenetic reprogramming of the INK4b-ARF-INK4a locus. *Mol Cell Biol*, Vol. 28, No.10, pp. (3457-3464). 1098-5549.

Kim M., Katayose, Y., Rojanala, L., Shah, S., Sgagias, M., Jang, L., Jung, Y.J., Lee, S.H., Hwang, S.G. & Cowan, K.H. (2000). "Induction of apoptosis in p16INK4A mutant cell lines by adenovirus-mediated overexpression of p16INK4A protein. *Cell Death Differ*, Vol. 7, No.8, pp. (706-711). 1350-9047.

Kim O., Park, M., Kang, H., Lim, S. & Lee, C.T. (2003). "Differential protein expressions induced by adenovirus-mediated p16 gene transfer into Balb/c nude mouse. *Proteomics*, Vol. 3, No.12, pp. (2412-2419). 1615-9853.

Kim W.Y. & Sharpless, N.E. (2006). "The regulation of INK4/ARF in cancer and aging. *Cell*, Vol. 127, No.2, pp. (265-275). 0092-8674.

Kivinen L., Tsubari, M., Haapajarvi, T., Datto, M.B., Wang, X.F. & Laiho, M. (1999). "Ras induces p21Cip1/Waf1 cyclin kinase inhibitor transcriptionally through Sp1-binding sites. *Oncogene*, Vol. 18, No.46, pp. (6252-6261). 0950-9232.

Kleihues P., Lubbe, J., Watanabe, K., von Ammon, K. & Ohgaki, H. (1994). "Genetic alterations associated with glioma progression. *Verh Dtsch Ges Pathol*, Vol. 78, pp. (43-47). 0070-4113.

Koenig A., Bianco, S.R., Fosmire, S., Wojcieszyn, J. & Modiano, J.F. (2002). "Expression and significance of p53, rb, p21/waf-1, p16/ink-4a, and PTEN tumor suppressors in canine melanoma. *Vet Pathol*, Vol. 39, No.4, pp. (458-472). 0300-9858.

Koh J., Enders, G.H., Dynlacht, B.D. & Harlow, E. (1995). "Tumour-derived p16 alleles encoding proteins defective in cell-cycle inhibition. *Nature*, Vol. 375, No.6531, pp. (506-510). 0028-0836.

Korenjak M. & Brehm, A. (2005). "E2F-Rb complexes regulating transcription of genes important for differentiation and development. *Curr Opin Genet Dev*, Vol. 15, No.5, pp. (520-527). 0959-437X.

Kotake Y., Cao, R., Viatour, P., Sage, J., Zhang, Y. & Xiong, Y. (2007). "pRB family proteins are required for H3K27 trimethylation and Polycomb repression complexes binding to and silencing p16INK4alpha tumor suppressor gene. *Genes Dev*, Vol. 21, No.1, pp. (49-54). 0890-9369.

Krimpenfort P., Ijpenberg, A., Song, J.Y., van der Valk, M., Nawijn, M., Zevenhoven, J. & Berns, A. (2007). "p15Ink4b is a critical tumour suppressor in the absence of p16Ink4a. *Nature*, Vol. 448, No.7156, pp. (943-946). 1476-4687.

Krishnamurthy J., Ramsey, M.R., Ligon, K.L., Torrice, C., Koh, A., Bonner-Weir, S. & Sharpless, N.E. (2006). "p16INK4a induces an age-dependent decline in islet regenerative potential. *Nature*, Vol. 443, No.7110, pp. (453-457). 1476-4687.

Kwon T.K., Buchholz, M.A., Gabrielson, E.W. & Nordin, A.A. (1995). "A novel cytoplasmic substrate for cdk4 and cdk6 in normal and malignant epithelial derived cells. *Oncogene*, Vol. 11, No.10, pp. (2077-2083). 0950-9232.

Lazaro J.B., Bailey, P.J. & Lassar, A.B. (2002). "Cyclin D-cdk4 activity modulates the subnuclear localization and interaction of MEF2 with SRC-family coactivators during skeletal muscle differentiation. *Genes Dev*, Vol. 16, No.14, pp. (1792-1805). 0890-9369.

Lea N.C., Orr, S.J., Stoeber, K., Williams, G.H., Lam, E.W., Ibrahim, M.A., Mufti, G.J. & Thomas, N.S. (2003). "Commitment point during G0-->G1 that controls entry into the cell cycle. *Mol Cell Biol*, Vol. 23, No.7, pp. (2351-2361). 0270-7306.

Lee A.W., Li, J.H., Shi, W., Li, A., Ng, E., Liu, T.J., Klamut, H.J. & Liu, F.F. (2003). "p16 gene therapy: a potentially efficacious modality for nasopharyngeal carcinoma. *Mol Cancer Ther*, Vol. 2, No.10, pp. (961-969). 1535-7163.

Levine R.A. & Fleischli, M.A. (2000). "Inactivation of p53 and retinoblastoma family pathways in canine osteosarcoma cell lines. *Vet Pathol*, Vol. 37, No.1, pp. (54-61). 0300-9858.

Li J., Joo, S.H. & Tsai, M.D. (2003). "An NF-kappaB-specific inhibitor, IkappaBalpha, binds to and inhibits cyclin-dependent kinase 4. *Biochemistry*, Vol. 42, No.46, pp. (13476-13483). 0006-2960.

Li J., Muscarella, P., Joo, S.H., Knobloch, T.J., Melvin, W.S., Weghorst, C.M. & Tsai, M.D. (2005). "Dissection of CDK4-binding and transactivation activities of p34(SEI-1) and comparison between functions of p34(SEI-1) and p16(INK4A). *Biochemistry*, Vol. 44, No.40, pp. (13246-13256). 0006-2960.

Li J.M., Nichols, M.A., Chandrasekharan, S., Xiong, Y. & Wang, X.F. (1995). "Transforming growth factor beta activates the promoter of cyclin-dependent kinase inhibitor p15INK4B through an Sp1 consensus site. *J Biol Chem*, Vol. 270, No.45, pp. (26750-26753). 0021-9258.

Liggett W.H., Jr. & Sidransky, D. (1998). "Role of the p16 tumor suppressor gene in cancer. *J Clin Oncol*, Vol. 16, No.3, pp. (1197-1206). 0732-183X.

Lin Y.C., Diccianni, M.B., Kim, Y., Lin, H.H., Lee, C.H., Lin, R.J., Joo, S.H., Li, J., Chuang, T.J., Yang, A.S., Kuo, H.H., Tsai, M.D. & Yu, A.L. (2007). "Human p16gamma, a novel transcriptional variant of p16(INK4A), coexpresses with p16(INK4A) in cancer cells and inhibits cell-cycle progression. *Oncogene*, Vol. 26, No.49, pp. (7017-7027). 0950-9232.

Lindblad-Toh K., Wade, C.M., Mikkelsen, T.S., Karlsson, E.K., Jaffe, D.B., Kamal, M., Clamp, M., Chang, J.L., Kulbokas, E.J., 3rd, Zody, M.C., Mauceli, E., Xie, X., Breen, M., Wayne, R.K., Ostrander, E.A., Ponting, C.P., Galibert, F., Smith, D.R., DeJong, P.J., Kirkness, E., Alvarez, P., Biagi, T., Brockman, W., Butler, J., Chin, C.W., Cook, A., Cuff, J., Daly, M.J., DeCaprio, D., Gnerre, S., Grabherr, M., Kellis, M., Kleber, M., Bardeleben, C., Goodstadt, L., Heger, A., Hitte, C., Kim, L., Koepfli, K.P., Parker, H.G., Pollinger, J.P., Searle, S.M., Sutter, N.B., Thomas, R., Webber, C., Baldwin, J., Abebe, A., Abouelleil, A., Aftuck, L., Ait-Zahra, M., Aldredge, T., Allen, N., An, P., Anderson, S., Antoine, C., Arachchi, H., Aslam, A., Ayotte, L., Bachantsang, P., Barry, A., Bayul, T., Benamara, M., Berlin, A., Bessette, D., Blitshteyn, B., Bloom, T., Blye, J., Boguslavskiy, L., Bonnet, C., Boukhgalter, B., Brown, A., Cahill, P., Calixte, N., Camarata, J., Cheshatsang, Y., Chu, J., Citroen, M., Collymore, A., Cooke, P., Dawoe, T., Daza, R., Decktor, K., DeGray, S., Dhargay, N., Dooley, K., Dooley, K., Dorje, P., Dorjee, K., Dorris, L., Duffey, N., Dupes, A., Egbiremolen, O., Elong, R., Falk, J., Farina, A., Faro, S., Ferguson, D., Ferreira, P., Fisher, S., FitzGerald, M., Foley, K., Foley, C., Franke, A., Friedrich, D., Gage, D., Garber, M., Gearin, G., Giannoukos, G., Goode, T., Goyette, A., Graham, J., Grandbois, E., Gyaltsen, K., Hafez, N., Hagopian, D., Hagos, B., Hall, J., Healy, C., Hegarty, R., Honan, T., Horn, A., Houde, N., Hughes, L., Hunnicutt, L., Husby, M., Jester, B., Jones, C., Kamat, A., Kanga, B., Kells, C., Khazanovich, D., Kieu, A.C., Kisner, P., Kumar, M., Lance, K., Landers, T., Lara, M., Lee, W., Leger, J.P., Lennon, N., Leuper, L., LeVine, S., Liu, J., Liu, X., Lokyitsang, Y., Lokyitsang, T., Lui, A., Macdonald, J., Major, J., Marabella, R., Maru, K., Matthews, C., McDonough, S., Mehta, T., Meldrim, J., Melnikov, A., Meneus, L., Mihalev, A., Mihova, T., Miller, K., Mittelman, R., Mlenga, V., Mulrain, L., Munson, G., Navidi, A., Naylor, J., Nguyen, T., Nguyen, N., Nguyen, C., Nguyen, T., Nicol, R., Norbu, N., Norbu, C., Novod, N., Nyima, T., Olandt, P., O'Neill, B., O'Neill, K., Osman, S., Oyono, L., Patti, C., Perrin, D., Phunkhang, P., Pierre, F., Priest, M., Rachupka, A., Raghuraman, S., Rameau, R., Ray, V., Raymond, C., Rege, F., Rise, C., Rogers, J., Rogov, P., Sahalie, J., Settipalli, S., Sharpe, T., Shea, T., Sheehan, M., Sherpa, N., Shi, J., Shih, D., Sloan, J., Smith, C., Sparrow, T., Stalker, J., Stange-Thomann, N., Stavropoulos, S., Stone, C., Stone, S., Sykes, S., Tchuinga, P., Tenzing, P., Tesfaye, S., Thoulutsang, D., Thoulutsang, Y., Topham, K., Topping, I., Tsamla, T., Vassiliev, H., Venkataraman, V., Vo, A., Wangchuk, T., Wangdi, T., Weiand, M., Wilkinson, J., Wilson, A., Yadav, S., Yang, S., Yang, X., Young, G., Yu, Q., Zainoun, J., Zembek, L., Zimmer, A. & Lander, E.S. (2005). "Genome sequence, comparative analysis and haplotype structure of the domestic dog. *Nature*, Vol. 438, No.7069, pp. (803-819). 1476-4687.

Liu X.Q., Zeng, R.S., Huang, H.Z. & Liao, G.Q. (2003). "[Expression of p15 and p16 proteins in tongue squamous cell carcinoma and their significances]. *Ai Zheng*, Vol. 22, No.11, pp. (1214-1218). 1000-467X.

Loercher A.E., Tank, E.M., Delston, R.B. & Harbour, J.W. (2005). "MITF links differentiation with cell cycle arrest in melanocytes by transcriptional activation of INK4A. *J Cell Biol*, Vol. 168, No.1, pp. (35-40). 0021-9525.

Lois A.F., Cooper, L.T., Geng, Y., Nobori, T. & Carson, D. (1995). "Expression of the p16 and p15 cyclin-dependent kinase inhibitors in lymphocyte activation and neuronal differentiation. *Cancer Res*, Vol. 55, No.18, pp. (4010-4013). 0008-5472.

Loughran O., Malliri, A., Owens, D., Gallimore, P.H., Stanley, M.A., Ozanne, B., Frame, M.C. & Parkinson, E.K. (1996). "Association of CDKN2A/p16INK4A with human head and neck keratinocyte replicative senescence: relationship of dysfunction to immortality and neoplasia. *Oncogene*, Vol. 13, No.3, pp. (561-568). 0950-9232.

Lukas J., Petersen, B.O., Holm, K., Bartek, J. & Helin, K. (1996). "Deregulated expression of E2F family members induces S-phase entry and overcomes p16INK4A-mediated growth suppression. *Mol Cell Biol*, Vol. 16, No.3, pp. (1047-1057). 0270-7306.

Ma H.B., Wang, X.J., Ma, J., Xia, H., Wang, Z., Li, Z., Han, Z.K. & Wu, C.M. (2007). "[Effect of irradiation-induced pcDNA3.1-Egr.1p-p16 on cell apoptosis and cell cycle of JF305 cells]. *Nan Fang Yi Ke Da Xue Xue Bao*, Vol. 27, No.8, pp. (1183-1186). 1673-4254.

Ma J., He, X., Wang, W., Huang, Y., Chen, L., Cong, W., Gu, J., Hu, H., Shi, J., Li, L. & Su, C. (2009). "E2F promoter-regulated oncolytic adenovirus with p16 gene induces cell apoptosis and exerts antitumor effect on gastric cancer. *Dig Dis Sci*, Vol. 54, No.7, pp. (1425-1431). 1573-2568.

Mallakin A., Sugiyama, T., Kai, F., Taneja, P., Kendig, R.D., Frazier, D.P., Maglic, D., Matise, L.A., Willingham, M.C. & Inoue, K. (2010). "The Arf-inducing transcription factor Dmp1 encodes a transcriptional activator of amphiregulin, thrombospondin-1, JunB and Egr1. *Int J Cancer*, Vol. 126, No.6, pp. (1403-1416). 1097-0215.

Malumbres M., Sotillo, R., Santamaria, D., Galan, J., Cerezo, A., Ortega, S., Dubus, P. & Barbacid, M. (2004). "Mammalian cells cycle without the D-type cyclin-dependent kinases Cdk4 and Cdk6. *Cell*, Vol. 118, No.4, pp. (493-504). 0092-8674.

Malumbres M. & Barbacid, M. (2009). "Cell cycle, CDKs and cancer: a changing paradigm. *Nat Rev Cancer*, Vol. 9, No.3, pp. (153-166). 1474-1768.

Mao L., Merlo, A., Bedi, G., Shapiro, G.I., Edwards, C.D., Rollins, B.J. & Sidransky, D. (1995). "A novel p16INK4A transcript. *Cancer Res*, Vol. 55, No.14, pp. (2995-2997). 0008-5472.

Markowski D.N., von Ahsen, I., Nezhad, M.H., Wosniok, W., Helmke, B.M. & Bullerdiek, J. (2010). "HMGA2 and the p19Arf-TP53-CDKN1A axis: a delicate balance in the growth of uterine leiomyomas. *Genes Chromosomes Cancer*, Vol. 49, No.8, pp. (661-668). 1098-2264.

Matheu A., Maraver, A., Collado, M., Garcia-Cao, I., Canamero, M., Borras, C., Flores, J.M., Klatt, P., Vina, J. & Serrano, M. (2009). "Anti-aging activity of the Ink4/Arf locus. *Aging Cell*, Vol. 8, No.2, pp. (152-161). 1474-9726.

Matsuura I., Denissova, N.G., Wang, G., He, D., Long, J. & Liu, F. (2004). "Cyclin-dependent kinases regulate the antiproliferative function of Smads. *Nature*, Vol. 430, No.6996, pp. (226-231). 1476-4687.

McArthur J.G., Qian, H., Citron, D., Banik, G.G., Lamphere, L., Gyuris, J., Tsui, L. & George, S.E. (2001). "p27-p16 Chimera: a superior antiproliferative for the prevention of neointimal hyperplasia. *Mol Ther*, Vol. 3, No.1, pp. (8-13). 1525-0016.

McKeller R.N., Fowler, J.L., Cunningham, J.J., Warner, N., Smeyne, R.J., Zindy, F. & Skapek, S.X. (2002). "The Arf tumor suppressor gene promotes hyaloid vascular regression during mouse eye development. *Proc Natl Acad Sci U S A*, Vol. 99, No.6, pp. (3848-3853). 0027-8424.

Medema R.H., Herrera, R.E., Lam, F. & Weinberg, R.A. (1995). "Growth suppression by p16ink4 requires functional retinoblastoma protein. *Proc Natl Acad Sci U S A*, Vol. 92, No.14, pp. (6289-6293). 0027-8424.

Meng S., Luo, M., Sun, H., Yu, X., Shen, M., Zhang, Q., Zhou, R., Ju, X., Tao, W., Liu, D., Deng, H. & Lu, Z. (2010). "Identification and characterization of Bmi-1-responding element within the human p16 promoter. *J Biol Chem*, Vol. 285, No.43, pp. (33219-33229). 1083-351X.

Modiano J.F., Breen, M., Valli, V.E., Wojcieszyn, J.W. & Cutter, G.R. (2007). "Predictive value of p16 or Rb inactivation in a model of naturally occurring canine non-Hodgkin's lymphoma. *Leukemia*, Vol. 21, No.1, pp. (184-187). 0887-6924.

Morgan D.O. (1997). "Cyclin-dependent kinases: engines, clocks, and microprocessors. *Annu Rev Cell Dev Biol*, Vol. 13, pp. (261-291). 1081-0706.

Mroz E.A., Baird, A.H., Michaud, W.A. & Rocco, J.W. (2008). "COOH-terminal binding protein regulates expression of the p16INK4A tumor suppressor and senescence in primary human cells. *Cancer Res*, Vol. 68, No.15, pp. (6049-6053). 1538-7445.

Natarajan E., Omobono, J.D., 2nd, Guo, Z., Hopkinson, S., Lazar, A.J., Brenn, T., Jones, J.C. & Rheinwald, J.G. (2006). "A keratinocyte hypermotility/growth-arrest response involving laminin 5 and p16INK4A activated in wound healing and senescence. *Am J Pathol*, Vol. 168, No.6, pp. (1821-1837). 0002-9440.

Nilsson K. & Landberg, G. (2006). "Subcellular localization, modification and protein complex formation of the cdk-inhibitor p16 in Rb-functional and Rb-inactivated tumor cells. *Int J Cancer*, Vol. 118, No.5, pp. (1120-1125). 0020-7136.

Nitta R.T., Jameson, S.A., Kudlow, B.A., Conlan, L.A. & Kennedy, B.K. (2006). "Stabilization of the retinoblastoma protein by A-type nuclear lamins is required for INK4A-mediated cell cycle arrest. *Mol Cell Biol*, Vol. 26, No.14, pp. (5360-5372). 0270-7306.

Noble J.R., Rogan, E.M., Neumann, A.A., Maclean, K., Bryan, T.M. & Reddel, R.R. (1996). "Association of extended in vitro proliferative potential with loss of p16INK4 expression. *Oncogene*, Vol. 13, No.6, pp. (1259-1268). 0950-9232.

Nobori T., Miura, K., Wu, D.J., Lois, A., Takabayashi, K. & Carson, D.A. (1994). "Deletions of the cyclin-dependent kinase-4 inhibitor gene in multiple human cancers. *Nature*, Vol. 368, No.6473, pp. (753-756). 0028-0836.

Novitch B.G., Spicer, D.B., Kim, P.S., Cheung, W.L. & Lassar, A.B. (1999). "pRb is required for MEF2-dependent gene expression as well as cell-cycle arrest during skeletal muscle differentiation. *Curr Biol*, Vol. 9, No.9, pp. (449-459). 0960-9822.

Nozato T., Ito, H., Watanabe, M., Ono, Y., Adachi, S., Tanaka, H., Hiroe, M., Sunamori, M. & Marum, F. (2001). "Overexpression of cdk Inhibitor p16INK4a by adenovirus vector inhibits cardiac hypertrophy in vitro and in vivo: a novel strategy for the gene therapy of cardiac hypertrophy. *J Mol Cell Cardiol*, Vol. 33, No.8, pp. (1493-1504). 0022-2828.

Ohtani N., Zebedee, Z., Huot, T.J., Stinson, J.A., Sugimoto, M., Ohashi, Y., Sharrocks, A.D., Peters, G. & Hara, E. (2001). "Opposing effects of Ets and Id proteins on p16INK4a expression during cellular senescence. *Nature*, Vol. 409, No.6823, pp. (1067-1070). 0028-0836.

Packenham J.P., Taylor, J.A., White, C.M., Anna, C.H., Barrett, J.C. & Devereux, T.R. (1995). "Homozygous deletions at chromosome 9p21 and mutation analysis of p16 and p15 in microdissected primary non-small cell lung cancers. *Clin Cancer Res*, Vol. 1, No.7, pp. (687-690). 1078-0432.

Patel S.D., Tran, A.C., Ge, Y., Moskalenko, M., Tsui, L., Banik, G., Tom, W., Scott, M., Chen, L., Van Roey, M., Rivkin, M., Mendez, M., Gyuris, J. & McArthur, J.G. (2000). "The p53-independent tumoricidal activity of an adenoviral vector encoding a p27-p16 fusion tumor suppressor gene. *Mol Ther*, Vol. 2, No.2, pp. (161-169). 1525-0016.

Petersen B.O., Lukas, J., Sorensen, C.S., Bartek, J. & Helin, K. (1999). "Phosphorylation of mammalian CDC6 by cyclin A/CDK2 regulates its subcellular localization. *Embo J*, Vol. 18, No.2, pp. (396-410). 0261-4189.

Pines J. & Hunter, T. (1991). "Cyclin-dependent kinases: a new cell cycle motif? *Trends Cell Biol*, Vol. 1, No.5, pp. (117-121). 0962-8924.

Qin H., Moellinger, J.D., Wells, A., Windsor, L.J., Sun, Y. & Benveniste, E.N. (1998). "Transcriptional suppression of matrix metalloproteinase-2 gene expression in human astroglioma cells by TNF-alpha and IFN-gamma. *J Immunol*, Vol. 161, No.12, pp. (6664-6673). 0022-1767.

Quelle D.E., Zindy, F., Ashmun, R.A. & Sherr, C.J. (1995). "Alternative reading frames of the INK4a tumor suppressor gene encode two unrelated proteins capable of inducing cell cycle arrest. *Cell*, Vol. 83, No.6, pp. (993-1000). 0092-8674.

Quelle D.E., Cheng, M., Ashmun, R.A. & Sherr, C.J. (1997). "Cancer-associated mutations at the INK4a locus cancel cell cycle arrest by p16INK4a but not by the alternative reading frame protein p19ARF. *Proc Natl Acad Sci U S A*, Vol. 94, No.2, pp. (669-673). 0027-8424.

Radpour R., Barekati, Z., Haghighi, M.M., Kohler, C., Asadollahi, R., Torbati, P.M., Holzgreve, W. & Zhong, X.Y. (2010). "Correlation of telomere length shortening with promoter methylation profile of p16/Rb and p53/p21 pathways in breast cancer. *Mod Pathol*, Vol. 23, No.5, pp. (763-772). 1530-0285.

Ranade K., Hussussian, C.J., Sikorski, R.S., Varmus, H.E., Goldstein, A.M., Tucker, M.A., Serrano, M., Hannon, G.J., Beach, D. & Dracopoli, N.C. (1995). "Mutations associated with familial melanoma impair p16INK4 function. *Nat Genet*, Vol. 10, No.1, pp. (114-116). 1061-4036.

Rao S.S. & Kohtz, D.S. (1995). "Positive and negative regulation of D-type cyclin expression in skeletal myoblasts by basic fibroblast growth factor and transforming growth factor beta. A role for cyclin D1 in control of myoblast differentiation. *J Biol Chem*, Vol. 270, No.8, pp. (4093-4100). 0021-9258.

Reymond A. & Brent, R. (1995). "p16 proteins from melanoma-prone families are deficient in binding to Cdk4. *Oncogene*, Vol. 11, No.6, pp. (1173-1178). 0950-9232.

Rhee J.G., Li, D., O'Malley, B.W., Jr. & Suntharalingam, M. (2003). "Combination radiation and adenovirus-mediated P16(INK4A) gene therapy in a murine model for head and neck cancer. *ORL J Otorhinolaryngol Relat Spec*, Vol. 65, No.3, pp. (144-154). 0301-1569.

Riabowol K., Draetta, G., Brizuela, L., Vandre, D. & Beach, D. (1989). "The cdc2 kinase is a nuclear protein that is essential for mitosis in mammalian cells. *Cell*, Vol. 57, No.3, pp. (393-401). 0092-8674.

Robertson K.D. & Jones, P.A. (1999). "Tissue-specific alternative splicing in the human INK4a/ARF cell cycle regulatory locus. *Oncogene*, Vol. 18, No.26, pp. (3810-3820). 0950-9232.

Ruas M. & Peters, G. (1998). "The p16INK4a/CDKN2A tumor suppressor and its relatives. *Biochim Biophys Acta*, Vol. 1378, No.2, pp. (F115-177). 0006-3002.

Rui H.B. & Su, J.Z. (2002). "Co-transfection of p16(INK4a) and p53 genes into the K562 cell line inhibits cell proliferation. *Haematologica*, Vol. 87, No.2, pp. (136-142). 0390-6078.

Russo A.A., Tong, L., Lee, J.O., Jeffrey, P.D. & Pavletich, N.P. (1998). "Structural basis for inhibition of the cyclin-dependent kinase Cdk6 by the tumour suppressor p16INK4a. *Nature*, Vol. 395, No.6699, pp. (237-243). 0028-0836.

Saegusa M., Hashimura, M., Kuwata, T., Hamano, M. & Okayasu, I. (2005). "Upregulation of TCF4 expression as a transcriptional target of beta-catenin/p300 complexes during trans-differentiation of endometrial carcinoma cells. *Lab Invest*, Vol. 85, No.6, pp. (768-779). 0023-6837.

Saegusa M., Hashimura, M., Kuwata, T., Hamano, M. & Okayasu, I. (2006). "Induction of p16INK4A mediated by beta-catenin in a TCF4-independent manner: implications for alterations in p16INK4A and pRb expression during trans-differentiation of endometrial carcinoma cells. *Int J Cancer*, Vol. 119, No.10, pp. (2294-2303). 0020-7136.

Santamaria D., Barriere, C., Cerqueira, A., Hunt, S., Tardy, C., Newton, K., Caceres, J.F., Dubus, P., Malumbres, M. & Barbacid, M. (2007). "Cdk1 is sufficient to drive the mammalian cell cycle. *Nature*, Vol. 448, No.7155, pp. (811-815). 1476-4687.

Satyanarayana A. & Kaldis, P. (2009). "Mammalian cell-cycle regulation: several Cdks, numerous cyclins and diverse compensatory mechanisms. *Oncogene*, Vol. 28, No.33, pp. (2925-2939). 1476-5594.

Schreiber M., Muller, W.J., Singh, G. & Graham, F.L. (1999). "Comparison of the effectiveness of adenovirus vectors expressing cyclin kinase inhibitors p16INK4A, p18INK4C, p19INK4D, p21(WAF1/CIP1) and p27KIP1 in inducing cell cycle arrest, apoptosis and inhibition of tumorigenicity. *Oncogene*, Vol. 18, No.9, pp. (1663-1676). 0950-9232.

Schrump D.S., Chen, G.A., Consuli, U., Jin, X. & Roth, J.A. (1996). "Inhibition of esophageal cancer proliferation by adenovirally mediated delivery of p16INK4. *Cancer Gene Ther*, Vol. 3, No.6, pp. (357-364). 0929-1903.

Seabra M.C., Mules, E.H. & Hume, A.N. (2002). "Rab GTPases, intracellular traffic and disease. *Trends Mol Med*, Vol. 8, No.1, pp. (23-30). 1471-4914.

Sellers W.R., Novitch, B.G., Miyake, S., Heith, A., Otterson, G.A., Kaye, F.J., Lassar, A.B. & Kaelin, W.G., Jr. (1998). "Stable binding to E2F is not required for the retinoblastoma protein to activate transcription, promote differentiation, and suppress tumor cell growth. *Genes Dev*, Vol. 12, No.1, pp. (95-106). 0890-9369.

Serrano M., Hannon, G.J. & Beach, D. (1993). "A new regulatory motif in cell-cycle control causing specific inhibition of cyclin D/CDK4. *Nature*, Vol. 366, No.6456, pp. (704-707). 0028-0836.

Serrano M. (1997). "The tumor suppressor protein p16INK4a. *Exp Cell Res*, Vol. 237, No.1, pp. (7-13). 0014-4827.

Sharma G., Mirza, S., Prasad, C.P., Srivastava, A., Gupta, S.D. & Ralhan, R. (2007). "Promoter hypermethylation of p16INK4A, p14ARF, CyclinD2 and Slit2 in serum and tumor DNA from breast cancer patients. *Life Sci*, Vol. 80, No.20, pp. (1873-1881). 0024-3205.

Sharpless N.E. (2005). "INK4a/ARF: a multifunctional tumor suppressor locus. *Mutat Res*, Vol. 576, No.1-2, pp. (22-38). 0027-5107.

Sherr C.J. & Roberts, J.M. (1995). "Inhibitors of mammalian G1 cyclin-dependent kinases. *Genes Dev*, Vol. 9, No.10, pp. (1149-1163). 0890-9369.

Sherr C.J. & Roberts, J.M. (1999). "CDK inhibitors: positive and negative regulators of G1-phase progression. *Genes Dev*, Vol. 13, No.12, pp. (1501-1512). 0890-9369.

Sherr C.J. & Weber, J.D. (2000). "The ARF/p53 pathway. *Curr Opin Genet Dev*, Vol. 10, No.1, pp. (94-99). 0959-437X.

Shoushtari A., Meeneghan, M., Sheng, K., Moskaluk, C.A., Thomas, C.Y., Reibel, J.F., Levine, P.A., Jameson, M.J., Keene, K. & Read, P.W. (2010). "Intensity-modulated radiotherapy outcomes for oropharyngeal squamous cell carcinoma patients stratified by p16 status. *Cancer*, Vol. 116, No.11, pp. (2645-2654). 0008-543X.

Signer R.A., Montecino-Rodriguez, E., Witte, O.N. & Dorshkind, K. (2008). "Aging and cancer resistance in lymphoid progenitors are linked processes conferred by p16Ink4a and Arf. *Genes Dev*, Vol. 22, No.22, pp. (3115-3120). 0890-9369.

Smith J.R. & Pereira-Smith, O.M. (1996). "Replicative senescence: implications for in vivo aging and tumor suppression. *Science*, Vol. 273, No.5271, pp. (63-67). 0036-8075.

Souza-Rodrigues E., Estanyol, J.M., Friedrich-Heineken, E., Olmedo, E., Vera, J., Canela, N., Brun, S., Agell, N., Hubscher, U., Bachs, O. & Jaumot, M. (2007). "Proteomic analysis of p16ink4a-binding proteins. *Proteomics*, Vol. 7, No.22, pp. (4102-4111). 1615-9853.

Spillare E.A., Okamoto, A., Hagiwara, K., Demetrick, D.J., Serrano, M., Beach, D. & Harris, C.C. (1996). "Suppression of growth in vitro and tumorigenicity in vivo of human carcinoma cell lines by transfected p16INK4. *Mol Carcinog*, Vol. 16, No.1, pp. (53-60). 0899-1987.

Sreeramaneni R., Chaudhry, A., McMahon, M., Sherr, C.J. & Inoue, K. (2005). "Ras-Raf-Arf signaling critically depends on the Dmp1 transcription factor. *Mol Cell Biol*, Vol. 25, No.1, pp. (220-232). 0270-7306.

Stone S., Dayananth, P., Jiang, P., Weaver-Feldhaus, J.M., Tavtigian, S.V., Cannon-Albright, L. & Kamb, A. (1995a). "Genomic structure, expression and mutational analysis of the P15 (MTS2) gene. *Oncogene*, Vol. 11, No.5, pp. (987-991). 0950-9232.

Stone S., Jiang, P., Dayananth, P., Tavtigian, S.V., Katcher, H., Parry, D., Peters, G. & Kamb, A. (1995b). "Complex structure and regulation of the P16 (MTS1) locus. *Cancer Res*, Vol. 55, No.14, pp. (2988-2994). 0008-5472.

Stott F.J., Bates, S., James, M.C., McConnell, B.B., Starborg, M., Brookes, S., Palmero, I., Ryan, K., Hara, E., Vousden, K.H. & Peters, G. (1998). "The alternative product from the human CDKN2A locus, p14(ARF), participates in a regulatory feedback loop with p53 and MDM2. *Embo J*, Vol. 17, No.17, pp. (5001-5014). 0261-4189.

Sumitomo K., Shimizu, E., Shinohara, A., Yokota, J. & Sone, S. (1999). "Activation of RB tumor suppressor protein and growth suppression of small cell lung carcinoma cells by reintroduction of p16INK4A gene. *Int J Oncol*, Vol. 14, No.6, pp. (1075-1080). 1019-6439.

Sun M. & Lu, Y. (1997). "[Exogenous mtsl/p16 gene suppresses tumorigenicity of human gastric cancer cell line]. *Zhonghua Zhong Liu Za Zhi*, Vol. 19, No.6, pp. (410-413). 0253-3766.

Sun P., Nallar, S.C., Raha, A., Kalakonda, S., Velalar, C.N., Reddy, S.P. & Kalvakolanu, D.V. (2010). "GRIM-19 and p16(INK4a) synergistically regulate cell cycle progression and E2F1-responsive gene expression. *J Biol Chem*, Vol. 285, No.36, pp. (27545-27552). 1083-351X.

Swarbrick A., Roy, E., Allen, T. & Bishop, J.M. (2008). "Id1 cooperates with oncogenic Ras to induce metastatic mammary carcinoma by subversion of the cellular senescence response. *Proc Natl Acad Sci U S A*, Vol. 105, No.14, pp. (5402-5407). 1091-6490.

Swellam M., El-Aal, A.A. & AbuGabel, K.M. (2004). "Deletions of p15 and p16 in schistosomal bladder cancer correlate with transforming growth factor-alpha expression. *Clin Biochem*, Vol. 37, No.12, pp. (1098-1104). 0009-9120.

Taneja P., Maglic, D., Kai, F., Sugiyama, T., Kendig, R.D., Frazier, D.P., Willingham, M.C. & Inoue, K. (2010). "Critical roles of DMP1 in human epidermal growth factor receptor 2/neu-Arf-p53 signaling and breast cancer development. *Cancer Res*, Vol. 70, No.22, pp. (9084-9094). 1538-7445.

Thomas D.M., Carty, S.A., Piscopo, D.M., Lee, J.S., Wang, W.F., Forrester, W.C. & Hinds, P.W. (2001). "The retinoblastoma protein acts as a transcriptional coactivator required for osteogenic differentiation. *Mol Cell*, Vol. 8, No.2, pp. (303-316). 1097-2765.

Thomas D.M., Johnson, S.A., Sims, N.A., Trivett, M.K., Slavin, J.L., Rubin, B.P., Waring, P., McArthur, G.A., Walkley, C.R., Holloway, A.J., Diyagama, D., Grim, J.E., Clurman, B.E., Bowtell, D.D., Lee, J.S., Gutierrez, G.M., Piscopo, D.M., Carty, S.A. & Hinds, P.W. (2004). "Terminal osteoblast differentiation, mediated by runx2 and p27KIP1, is disrupted in osteosarcoma. *J Cell Biol*, Vol. 167, No.5, pp. (925-934). 0021-9525.

Thullberg M., Bartkova, J., Khan, S., Hansen, K., Ronnstrand, L., Lukas, J., Strauss, M. & Bartek, J. (2000). "Distinct versus redundant properties among members of the INK4 family of cyclin-dependent kinase inhibitors. *FEBS Lett*, Vol. 470, No.2, pp. (161-166). 0014-5793.

Tripathy D. & Benz, C.C. (1992). "Activated oncogenes and putative tumor suppressor genes involved in human breast cancers. *Cancer Treat Res*, Vol. 63, pp. (15-60). 0927-3042.

Tsao H., Benoit, E., Sober, A.J., Thiele, C. & Haluska, F.G. (1998). "Novel mutations in the p16/CDKN2A binding region of the cyclin-dependent kinase-4 gene. *Cancer Res*, Vol. 58, No.1, pp. (109-113). 0008-5472.

Tsui L.V., Camrud, A., Mondesire, J., Carlson, P., Zayek, N., Camrud, L., Donahue, B., Bauer, S., Lin, A., Frey, D., Rivkin, M., Subramanian, A., Falotico, R., Gyuris, J., Schwartz, R. & McArthur, J.G. (2001). "p27-p16 fusion gene inhibits angioplasty-induced neointimal hyperplasia and coronary artery occlusion. *Circ Res*, Vol. 89, No.4, pp. (323-328). 1524-4571.

Udayakumar T., Shareef, M.M., Diaz, D.A., Ahmed, M.M. & Pollack, A. (2010). "The E2F1/Rb and p53/MDM2 pathways in DNA repair and apoptosis: understanding the crosstalk to develop novel strategies for prostate cancer radiotherapy. *Semin Radiat Oncol*, Vol. 20, No.4, pp. (258-266). 1532-9461.

Uhm J.H., Dooley, N.P., Villemure, J.G. & Yong, V.W. (1996). "Glioma invasion in vitro: regulation by matrix metalloprotease-2 and protein kinase C. *Clin Exp Metastasis*, Vol. 14, No.5, pp. (421-433). 0262-0898.

Ulanet D.B. & Hanahan, D. (2010). "Loss of p19(Arf) facilitates the angiogenic switch and tumor initiation in a multi-stage cancer model via p53-dependent and independent mechanisms. *PLoS One*, Vol. 5, No.8, pp. (e12454). 1932-6203.

Vidal A. & Koff, A. (2000). "Cell-cycle inhibitors: three families united by a common cause. *Gene*, Vol. 247, No.1-2, pp. (1-15). 0378-1119.

Walkley C.R. & Orkin, S.H. (2006). "Rb is dispensable for self-renewal and multilineage differentiation of adult hematopoietic stem cells. *Proc Natl Acad Sci U S A*, Vol. 103, No.24, pp. (9057-9062). 0027-8424.

Wang C.H., Chang, H.C. & Hung, W.C. (2006). "p16 inhibits matrix metalloproteinase-2 expression via suppression of Sp1-mediated gene transcription. *J Cell Physiol*, Vol. 208, No.1, pp. (246-252). 0021-9541.

Wang J.S., Wang, F.B., Zhang, Q.G., Shen, Z.Z. & Shao, Z.M. (2008). "Enhanced expression of Rab27A gene by breast cancer cells promoting invasiveness and the metastasis potential by secretion of insulin-like growth factor-II. *Mol Cancer Res*, Vol. 6, No.3, pp. (372-382). 1541-7786.

Wang L., Qi, X., Sun, Y., Liang, L. & Ju, D. (2002). "Adenovirus-mediated combined P16 gene and GM-CSF gene therapy for the treatment of established tumor and induction of antitumor immunity. *Cancer Gene Ther*, Vol. 9, No.10, pp. (819-824). 0929-1903.

Wang M., Jiang, S. & Kong, B. (1999). "[Study of the inhibitory effects of retrovirus-mediated p16 gene on human ovarian cancer cell line]. *Zhonghua Fu Chan Ke Za Zhi*, Vol. 34, No.5, pp. (304-307). 0529-567X.

Wang X.Q., Gabrielli, B.G., Milligan, A., Dickinson, J.L., Antalis, T.M. & Ellem, K.A. (1996). "Accumulation of p16CDKN2A in response to ultraviolet irradiation correlates with late S-G(2)-phase cell cycle delay. *Cancer Res*, Vol. 56, No.11, pp. (2510-2514). 0008-5472.

Weber J.D., Jeffers, J.R., Rehg, J.E., Randle, D.H., Lozano, G., Roussel, M.F., Sherr, C.J. & Zambetti, G.P. (2000). "p53-independent functions of the p19(ARF) tumor suppressor. *Genes Dev*, Vol. 14, No.18, pp. (2358-2365). 0890-9369.

Weinberg R.A. (1995). "The retinoblastoma protein and cell cycle control. *Cell*, Vol. 81, No.3, pp. (323-330). 0092-8674.

Wu W., Zhang, X. & Qi, X. (2000). "[Gene therapy with tumor suppressor gene p53 and(or) p16 on the nude mice models of NSCLC in vivo]. *Zhonghua Jie He He Hu Xi Za Zhi*, Vol. 23, No.7, pp. (403-405). 1001-0939.

Yamada Y., Nakata, A., Yoshida, M.A., Shimada, Y., Oghiso, Y. & Poncy, J.L. (2010). "Implication of p16 inactivation in tumorigenic activity of respiratory epithelial cell lines and adenocarcinoma cell line established from plutonium-induced lung tumor in rat. *In Vitro Cell Dev Biol Anim*, Vol. 46, No.5, pp. (477-486). 1543-706X.

Yamaguchi T., Yoshida, T., Kurachi, R., Kakegawa, J., Hori, Y., Nanayama, T., Hayakawa, K., Abe, H., Takagi, K., Matsuzaki, Y., Koyama, M., Yogosawa, S., Sowa, Y., Yamori, T., Tajima, N. & Sakai, T. (2007). "Identification of JTP-70902, a p15(INK4b)-inductive compound, as a novel MEK1/2 inhibitor. *Cancer Sci*, Vol. 98, No.11, pp. (1809-1816). 1349-7006.

Yang C.T., You, L., Lin, Y.C., Lin, C.L., McCormick, F. & Jablons, D.M. (2003). "A comparison analysis of anti-tumor efficacy of adenoviral gene replacement therapy (p14ARF and p16INK4A) in human mesothelioma cells. *Anticancer Res*, Vol. 23, No.1A, pp. (33-38). 0250-7005.

Yap K.L., Li, S., Munoz-Cabello, A.M., Raguz, S., Zeng, L., Mujtaba, S., Gil, J., Walsh, M.J. & Zhou, M.M. (2010). "Molecular interplay of the noncoding RNA ANRIL and methylated histone H3 lysine 27 by polycomb CBX7 in transcriptional silencing of INK4a. *Mol Cell*, Vol. 38, No.5, pp. (662-674). 1097-4164.

Yoshioka H., Noguchi, K., Katayama, K., Mitsuhashi, J., Yamagoe, S., Fujimuro, M. & Sugimoto, Y. (2010). "Functional availability of gamma-herpesvirus K-cyclin is regulated by cellular CDK6 and p16INK4a. *Biochem Biophys Res Commun*, Vol. 394, No.4, pp. (1000-1005). 1090-2104.

Yu E., Ahn, Y.S., Jang, S.J., Kim, M.J., Yoon, H.S., Gong, G. & Choi, J. (2007). "Overexpression of the wip1 gene abrogates the p38 MAPK/p53/Wip1 pathway and silences p16 expression in human breast cancers. *Breast Cancer Res Treat*, Vol. 101, No.3, pp. (269-278). 0167-6806.

Zariwala M. & Xiong, Y. (1996). "Lack of mutation in the cyclin-dependent kinase inhibitor, p19INK4d, in tumor-derived cell lines and primary tumors. *Oncogene*, Vol. 13, No.9, pp. (2033-2038). 0950-9232.

Zhang J., Lu, A., Li, L., Yue, J. & Lu, Y. (2010a). "p16 Modulates VEGF expression via its interaction with HIF-1alpha in breast cancer cells. *Cancer Invest*, Vol. 28, No.6, pp. (588-597). 1532-4192.

Zhang W., Zhu, J., Bai, J., Jiang, H., Liu, F., Liu, A., Liu, P., Ji, G., Guan, R., Sun, D., Ji, W., Yu, Y., Jin, Y., Meng, X. & Fu, S. (2010b). "Comparison of the inhibitory effects of three transcriptional variants of CDKN2A in human lung cancer cell line A549. *J Exp Clin Cancer Res*, Vol. 29, pp. (74). 1756-9966.

Zhou X., Suzuki, H., Shimada, Y., Imamura, M., Yin, J., Jiang, H.Y., Tarmin, L., Abraham, J.M. & Meltzer, S.J. (1995). "Genomic DNA and messenger RNA expression alterations of the CDKN2B and CDKN2 genes in esophageal squamous carcinoma cell lines. *Genes Chromosomes Cancer*, Vol. 13, No.4, pp. (285-290). 1045-2257.

Zindy F., Quelle, D.E., Roussel, M.F. & Sherr, C.J. (1997). "Expression of the p16INK4a tumor suppressor versus other INK4 family members during mouse development and aging. *Oncogene*, Vol. 15, No.2, pp. (203-211). 0950-9232.

2

Susceptibility of Epithelium to PTEN-Deficient Tumorigenesis

Chun-Ming Chen[1,2], Tsai-Ling Lu[1], Fang-Yi Su[1] and Li-Ru You[2,3]
[1]*Department of Life Sciences and Institute of Genome Sciences,*
[2]*VGH-YM Genome Center,*
[3]*Institute of Biochemistry and Molecular Biology,*
National Yang-Ming University, Taipei,
Taiwan

1. Introduction

Phosphatase and tension homolog deleted on chromosome 10, PTEN, is a tumor suppressor gene that is responsible for controlling tumorigenesis in various organs (Li and Sun 1997, Steck et al. 1997, Li et al. 1997, Ali, Schriml and Dean 1999). Functionally, PTEN exhibits phospholipid phosphatase activity and negatively regulates the conversion of phosphatidylinositol 4, 5-diphosphate (PIP2) to PIP3 (Stambolic et al. 1998, Wu et al. 1998). PTEN ablation results in the accumulation of PIP3, which recruits AKT to the cell membrane, where PIP3-dependent protein kinase-1 (PDK1) and mammalian target of rapamycin (mTOR) complex 2 (mTORC2), also known as the Rictor-mTOR complex, activate and phosphorylate AKT at amino acid residues Thr308 and Ser473, respectively (Alessi et al. 1997, Sarbassov et al. 2004, Sarbassov et al. 2005). Consequently, activated AKT acts as a key effector and modulates a variety of downstream signal regulators. One AKT-targeting protein is tuberous sclerosis complex 2 (TSC2) (Inoki et al. 2002, Manning et al. 2002), which is a GTPase-activating protein that forms a complex with TSC1 to block a small GTPase Rheb at GDP-bound status, consequently resulting in mTORC1 (the Raptor-mTOR complex) inhibition. Thus, AKT-mediated TSC1-TSC2 inhibition results in mTORC1 activation, which promotes cell growth and protein translation partly through phosphorylating S6 kinase (S6K) and the eIF-4E-binding protein 1 (4E-BP1) (Brunn et al. 1997, Hara et al. 1997, Brown et al. 1995). Activated mTORC1 and S6K can also regulate PI3K-AKT signaling through a negative feedback mechanism [see Fig 1; reviewed in (Carracedo and Pandolfi 2008, Manning and Cantley 2007)]. In addition, activated AKT can target glycogen synthase kinase 3 (GSK3) (Cross et al. 1995), β-catenin (Fang et al. 2007, He et al. 2007), double minute 2 (Mdm2) (Mayo and Donner 2001, Zhou et al. 2001b), p21 (Zhou et al. 2001a), p27 (Fujita et al. 2002), forkhead-related transcription factors (Brunet et al. 1999), Bcl2-antagonist of cell death (Datta et al. 1997, Peso et al. 1997), and other genes, leading to cellular proliferation, anti-apoptosis, survival, and tumorigenesis [see Fig 1; (Cully et al. 2006, Kishimoto et al. 2003, Manning and Cantley 2007, Dunlop and Tee 2009)].

To model *Pten*-deficient malignancies, conditional *Pten* mutant alleles have been generated in mice. Using tissue-specific Cre-*lox*P-mediated *Pten* gene excision, the roles of *Pten* have been intensively studied across multiple organs in mice. We previously used an inducible

Cre under the control of a ubiquitous promoter, *ROSA26* (*R26*), to examine the susceptibility of all tissues to *Pten*-deficient tumorigenesis in an adult mice strain referred to as *R26-Pten*$^{fx/fx}$. We found that lymphomas accounted for the majority of *Pten*-deficient malignancies (Lu et al. 2007). However, the high incidence and short latency of lymphomas in the *R26-Pten*$^{fx/fx}$ mice limited our analyses of the tumors arising from the epithelial tissues, the most common origin of human cancers. To address the susceptibility of epithelial tissues to *Pten* loss, we performed spatiotemporally controlled *Pten* excision by using a newly generated inducible Cre transgene driven by the keratin 8 (K8) promoter in a mouse strain referred to as *K8-Pten*$^{fx/fx}$. In this epithelial *Pten*-deficient mouse, multiple epithelial tumors arose, and they could be monitored at different time points after *Pten* was ablated.

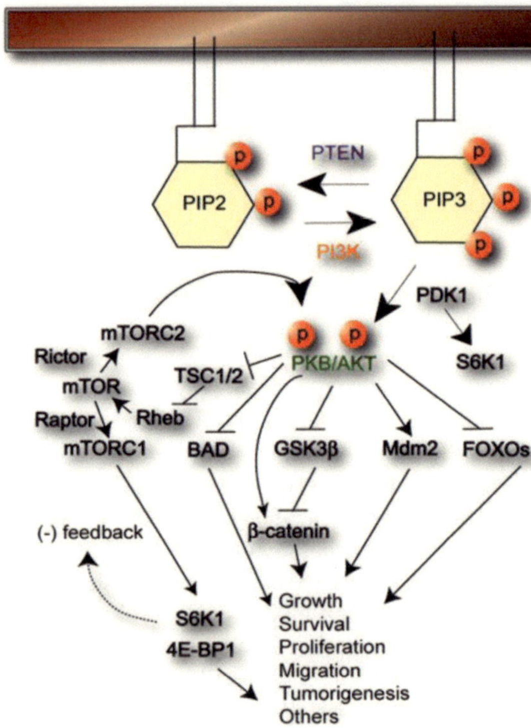

Fig. 1. Schematic illustration of PTEN/PI3K/AKT and their downstream effectors.

2. Genetic tool for conditional genetic manipulation in the epithelial tissues

To develop transgenic mice expressing inducible Cre (CreER^{T}) in epithelial tissues, we generated and characterized the transgenic mouse line *Tg(K18-EGFP, K8-CreER*^{T}*)*, in which the visualized enhanced green fluorescence protein (EGFP) is driven by the K18 upstream regulatory elements and the *CreER*^{T} fusion gene is driven by *K8* (Fig 2). To evaluate the induced *CreER*^{T} recombinase activity after tamoxifen (Tam) administration, *Tg(K18-EGFP,K8-CreER*^{T}*)* mice, hereafter abbreviated as *K18-EG/K8-CE*, were bred with *ROSA26 Cre* reporter (*R26R*$^{LacZ/+}$) mice (Soriano 1999) to generate *K18-EG/K8-CE*$^{tg/+}$*;R26R*$^{LacZ/+}$ bigenic mice.

We monitored K18 promoter-directed EGFP expression in the offspring of C57BL/6 females, which were bred with different lines of *K18-EG/K8-CE* males. We found that lines B, G, and H among eight transgenic lines exhibited strong and consistent EGFP signals in the tail, footpads, and all internal organs lined by simple epithelium (data not shown). Subsequently, these three lines were selected to breed with *R26R*$^{LacZ/+}$ mice to generate double-transgenic mice (referred to *K18-EG/K8CE*$^{tg/+}$;*R26R*$^{LacZ/+}$), which were evaluated by whole mount X-gal staining of inducible *CreER*^{T} recombinase expression driven by the K8 upstream sequence. At 5-6 weeks of age, Tam was intraperitoneally administered to *K18-EG/K8CE*$^{tg/+}$;*R26R*$^{LacZ/+}$ bigenic and control (*R26R*$^{LacZ/+}$) mice, after which we examined inducible Cre activity by assessing X-gal staining, which reflected *LacZ* expression at 10 days after Tam treatment. We found that similar *LacZ* expression patterns were observed among the B, G, and H lines on the *R26R*$^{LacZ/+}$ background.

2.1 Evaluation of inducible Cre activity of *K18-EG/K8-CE*$^{tg/+}$; *R26R*$^{LacZ/+}$ bigenic mice across multiple organs

In the lower respiratory tract of bigenic mice, EGFP- and X-gal-positive staining was clearly observed in the trachea, bronchi, and bronchioles, but not in the alveoli (Fig 2BB′ and CC′). Histological sections of X-gal-stained tissues revealed that inducible Cre activity was mainly restricted in the pseudostratified epithelial cells of the terminal bronchiole (TB) (Fig 2C′) that expressed K8, which colocalized with EGFP fluorescence driven by the K18 upstream sequence (Fig 1B′), but Cre activity was not observed in the pneumocyte lining of the alveolar sac (AS) (Fig 2B and C). In the liver of bigenic mice, intense EGFP- and X-gal-positive staining revealed the organization of bile ducts or gross portal tracts (Fig 2D and E). Intense EGFP- and X-gal-positive staining was also visualized in the gallbladder (GB, Fig 2D and E). Through histological analysis and immunofluorescence staining using an antibody against K8, we found that intense K8 and EGFP expression was detected in the intrahepatic bile duct (BD) compared with that in the surrounding hepatocytes (Fig 2D′). Intensely X-gal-stained cells were mainly observed in the epithelial lining of the intrahepatic BD (Fig 2E′) and gallbladder (data not shown). Furthermore, bright EGFP-positive and intense X-gal-positive signals could be easily visualized in the pancreas, but not in the adjacent spleen (Fig 2F and G), of bigenic mice. Microscopically, pancreatic ducts (PDs) and exocrine acini expressed EGFP and K8 (Fig 2F′), which colocalized with X-gal staining (Fig 2G′).
Along the gastrointestinal tract of bigenic mice, the hind-stomach and intestine also exhibited bright EGFP fluorescence (Fig 2H and J) and the intense blue X-gal staining indicative of LacZ expression (Fig 2I and K). Immunostaining using an antibody against K8, together with EGFP fluorescence, revealed that both K8 and EGFP expression appeared in the epithelial cells of the hind stomach (Fig 2H′) and small intestine (Fig 2J′). Tam-induced LacZ expression was detected in the lower portion of zymogenic and parietal cells in the glandular hind stomach (Fig 2I′) and in crypts of the small intestine (Fig 2K′).
We further examined EGFP and induced LacZ expression in the reproductive tracts of bigenic mice (Fig 3). In the male reproductive tract, the seminal vesicles (SVs; Fig 3A and B) and epididymis (Fig 3E and F) exhibited intense EGFP expression and X-gal staining, whereas the testis exhibited neither LacZ nor EGFP expression (Fig 3E and F). In the prostate, the ventral prostate (VP) lobes and dorsolateral prostate (DLP) lobes exhibited strong LacZ and EGFP expression (Fig 3C and D) compared to that in the anterior prostate (AP) lobes (Fig 2A and B). Immunostaining of K8 was colocalized with EGFP fluorescence in the epithelial lining of the SV (Fig 3A′), the VP (Fig 3C′) and epididymis (Fig 3E′). In addition, the histological sections revealed X-gal-positive staining in the epithelia of corresponding organs (Fig 3B′, D′, and F′). Notably, patchy EGFP and X-gal signals partly overlapped with K8-expressing luminal cells of the AP (Fig 3A″ and B″), indicative of inefficient expression of EGFP and LacZ in the AP of bigenic mice.

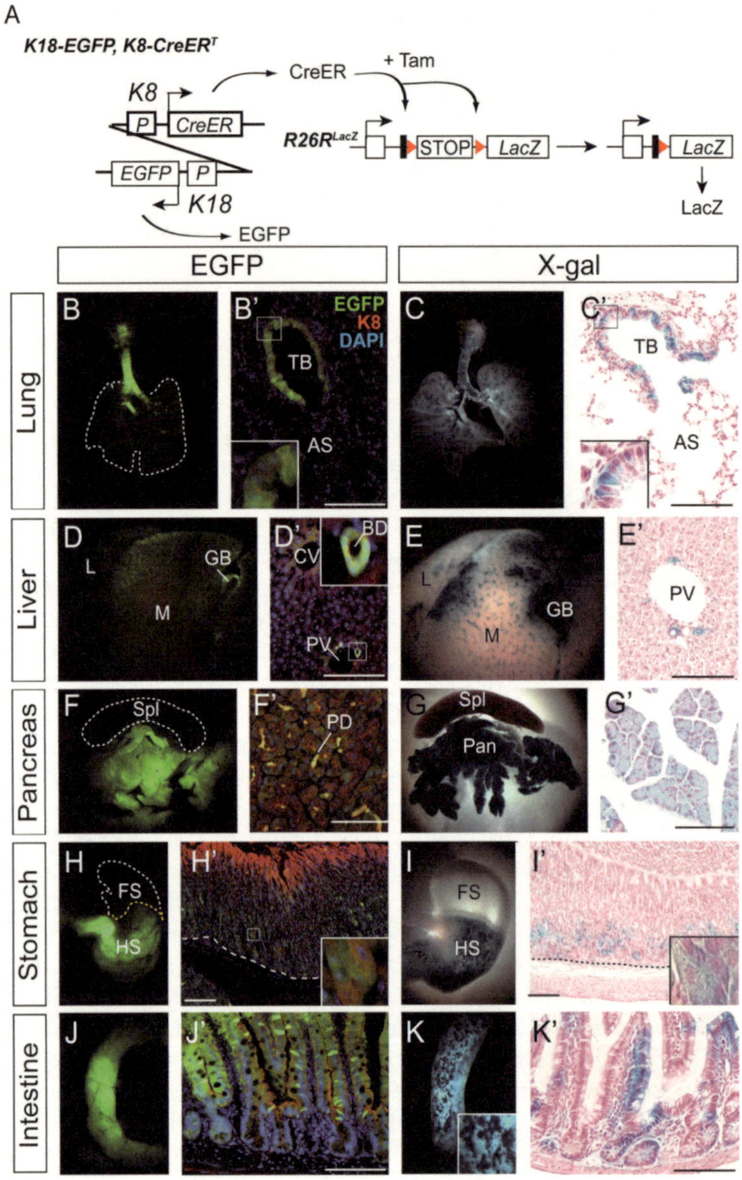

Fig. 2. Evaluation of the visualization marker EGFP and inducible Cre activity of *Tg(K18-EGFP, K8-CreER^T)* mice. (A) Schematic illustration of the genetic tool, *Tg(K18-EGFP, K8-CreER^T)* referred to *K18-EG/K8-CE*, which exhibits EGFP expression under the control of the K18 promoter and inducible Cre activity driven by the K8 promoter, which was evaluated by the Cre reporter allele, *R26R^{lacZ}*, after tamoxifen (Tam) administration. (B-K) Visualization of EGFP and evaluation of Tam-induced Cre-loxP recombination activity in the dissected organs of *K18-EG/K8-CE$^{tg/+}$;R26R$^{LacZ/+}$* mice treated with Tam for 10 days. (B) Whole-mount EGFP expression was visualized in the trachea, bronchus, and bronchiole of the *K18-EG/K8-CE$^{tg/+}$;R26R$^{LacZ/+}$* lung. (B') EGFP and immunofluorescent staining of K8 (red) revealed the colocalization of EGFP and K8 in the bronchiole columnar epithelium but not

in the AS. DAPI staining was used to indicate the nuclei. (C) The presence of LacZ expression was indicated by X-gal-stained epithelial tissues that had similar staining profiles as the EGFP-expressing tissue of the *K18-EG/K8-CE*$^{tg/+}$*;R26R*$^{LacZ/+}$ lung in (B). (C′) A histological section of the X-gal-stained lung was counterstained with Nuclear Fast Red to detect X-gal-stained epithelial cells. Insets in (B′) and (C′), high magnification of the epithelium of the terminal bronchiole (TB); (D) Intense EGFP expression was visualized as branching portal tracts in the *K18-EG/K8CE*$^{tg/+}$*;R26R*$^{LacZ/+}$ liver. GB, gallbladder; L, left liver lobe; M, medial liver lobe; (D′) EGFP and K8 expression was strongly detected in bile ducts (BDs) residing close to the portal vein (PV) and weakly detected in hepatocytes. CV, central vein; (E) Intense X-gal-positive blue patterns were similar to the EGFP expression patterns in the GB and branching portal tracts, but only patchy staining was observed in the liver parenchyma. (E′) Sections of whole-mount X-gal-stained liver exhibited strong blue staining in the BD. (F) and (G) Intense EGFP expression and the presence of LacZ were detected in the pancreas but not in the spleen (Spl). (F′) EGFP and K8 expression as positively detected in the exocrine acini and pancreatic ducts (PDs). (G′) Homogenous blue staining was histologically observed in the pancreatic acini and PDs. (H) and (I) Intense EGFP- and X-gal-positive staining was observed in the hind-stomach (HS), but not in the forestomach (FS). (H′) and (I′) EGFP and LacZ expression were highly localized at the base of the glandular stomach. (J) and (J′) Epithelial cells of the small intestine (jejunum) exhibited a strong EGFP signal. (K) and (K′) Mosaic LacZ activity revealed by X-gal staining in the crypts and upper differentiated epithelium of the jejunum. Scale bar, 100 μm.

In the reproductive tract of our bigenic females, EGFP was detected in the K8-expressing simple epithelium of the oviduct and uterus (Fig 3GG′ and II′). However, mosaic X-gal-positive patterns were observed in the simple epithelium of the oviduct and uterine glands (Fig 3 H′ and J′). Unexpectedly, LacZ and EGFP expression was not detected either grossly (Fig 3 G and H) or microscopically (Fig 3G′ and H′) in the ovarian surface epithelium (OSE; data not shown), which was thought to be the K8/K18-expressing cell type. The lack of EGFP and inducible LacZ expression in the OSE of bigenic mice indicated that the cis-regulatory elements within the K8-K18 intergenic sequence are unable to drive EGFP and CreER^{T} expression in the OSE.

2.2 Temporally controlled fate mapping to evaluate epithelial turnover in the mammary luminal epithelium and intestinal epithelium

In the adult stage, epithelial cell turnover is required to ensure the long-term maintenance of epithelial tissue homeostasis, which may be dysregulated during tumorigenesis. The process for epithelial renewal through generating new cells, differentiation, and migration from their stem/progenitors and niche varies among different epithelial tissues (Blanpain, Horsley and Fuchs 2007). As our *K18-EG/K8-CE*$^{tg/+}$*;R26R*$^{LacZ/+}$ mice were administered Tam by intraperitoneal injection at 6 weeks of age, we could monitor LacZ expression in various epithelial organs at different time points to determine whether inducible Cre activity occurred in higher hierarchical K8-expressing stem/progenitors to continuously give rise to their descendants. If the inducible Cre activity occurred in the stem/progenitors, then permanent LacZ activity could be detected in their descendants during cell turnover. In contrast, if the Tam-induced LacZ-expressing cells are terminally differentiated cells, then the LacZ-positive cells may be replaced by newly generated cells in which the *lox*P-flanked stop cassette of the *R26R* allele is not excised, indicating that these cells arise from K8-independent epithelial progenitors.

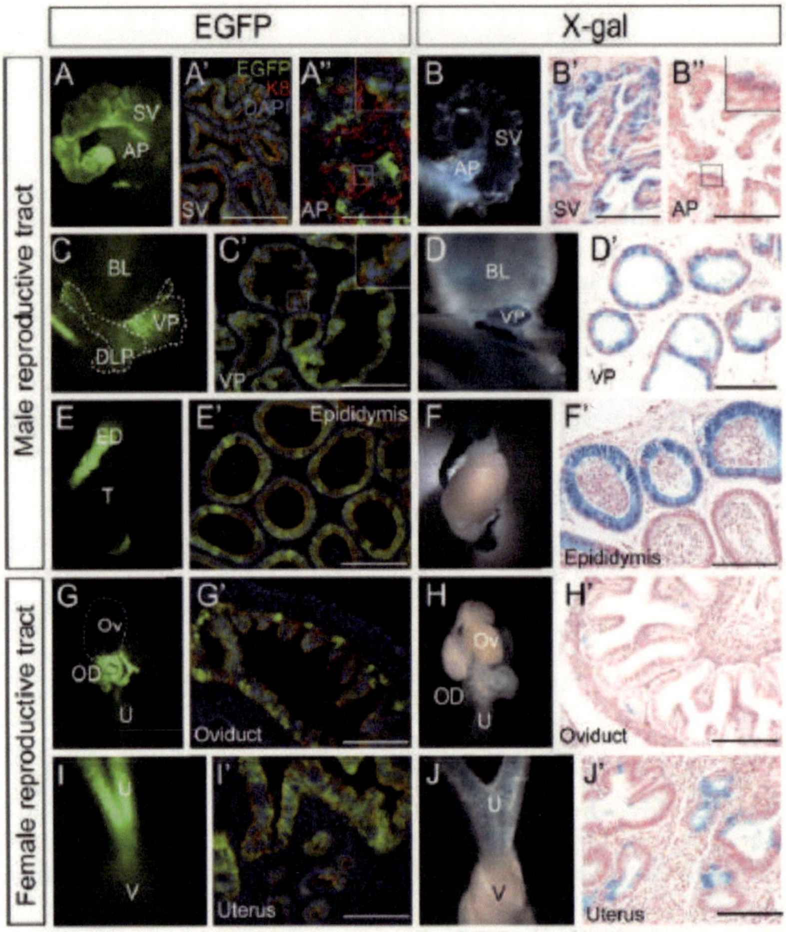

Fig. 3. EGFP visualization and evaluation of Tam-induced Cre activity in the reproductive organs of $K18\text{-}EG/K8\text{-}CE^{tg/+};R26R^{LacZ/+}$ mice treated with Tam for 10 days. (A) and (B) The seminal vesicle (SV) exhibits greater EGFP and LacZ expression than the anterior prostate (AP). (A′) and (B′) Histological sections revealed an intensive EGFP signal (green) coexpressed with K8- (red) and X-gal-stained LacZ-expressing epithelia. (A′′) and (B′′) Histological sections revealed a weak mosaic EGFP signal (green) coexpressed with K8 (red) and few X-gal-stained cells, indicative of poor inducible Cre activity in the AP. (C) and (D) Whole-mount EGFP and LacZ were present in the bladder and prostate [ventral prostate (VP) and dorsolateral prostate (DLP)]. (C′) and (D′) Sections revealed intense EGFP and K8 coexpressing cells and X-gal-stained epithelia in the VP. (E) and (F) Intense EGFP- and X-gal-positive staining was clearly detected in the epididymis but not in the testis. (E′) and (F′) Histological sections of the epididymis exhibited an intense EGFP signal (green) coexpressed with K8 and LacZ activity. (G-J) In the female reproductive tract, an intense EGFP signal was observed in the oviduct (OD) and uterus (U), whereas X-gal staining was more strongly detected in the uterus. (G′-J′) Sections exhibited EGFP and K8 coexpression in the epithelia of the oviduct (G′) and uterus (I′), whereas mosaic X-gal-stained epithelia were observed in the corresponding organs (H′) and (J′). Scale bar, 100 μm.

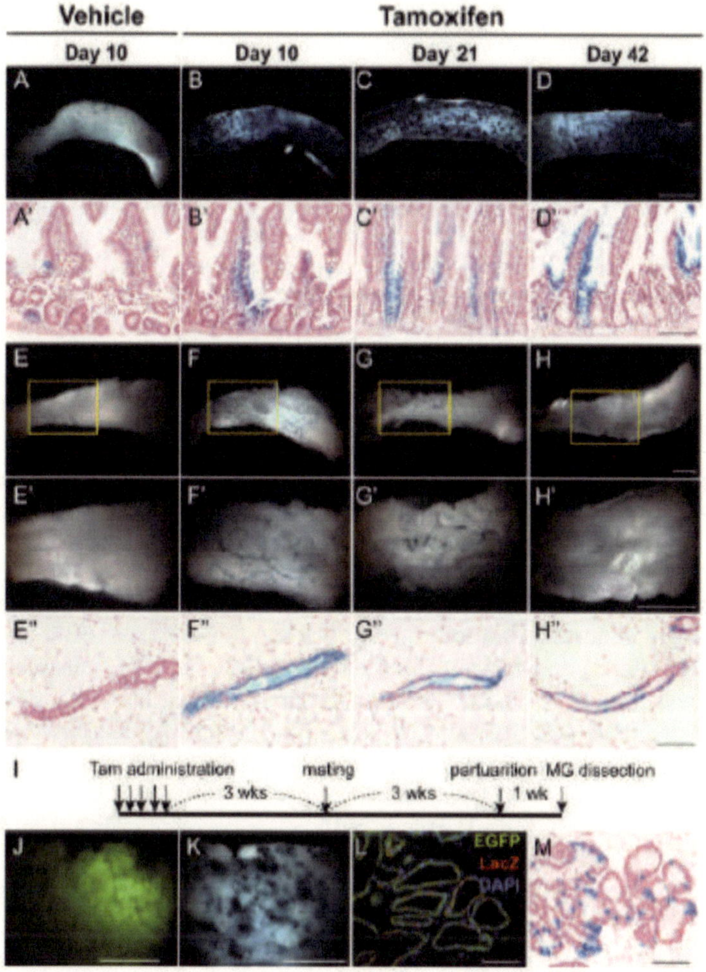

Fig. 4. Intestinal and mammary epithelial turnover monitored by LacZ activity in *K18-EG/K8-CE*$^{tg/+}$;*R26R*$^{LacZ/+}$ mice. (A) Partial X-gal staining was detected in the intestines (jejunum) of the B line-derived *K18-EG/K8-CE*$^{tg/+}$;*R26R*$^{LacZ/+}$ mice in the absence of Tam administration (vehicle treatment) after 10 days. (B-D) After Tam administration for 10, 21, and 42 days, intense X-gal staining patterns were clearly detected in the *K18-EG/K8-CE*$^{tg/+}$;*R26R*$^{LacZ/+}$ intestines. (A′-D′) Histological sections of the aforementioned samples were counterstained with Nuclear Fast Red, and they exhibited continuous X-gal-stained epithelial cells that emerged from the lower crypts to the upper absorptive cells in the *K18-EG/K8-CE*$^{tg/+}$;*R26R*$^{LacZ/+}$ mice treated with Tam (B′-D′) for 10-42 days. Conversely, a few X-gal-positive cells were detected in the intestines of vehicle-treated mice, indicating the leaky expression of LacZ. (E-H) Lower and (E′-H′) higher magnification of X-gal-stained fourth mammary fat pads revealed the presence of X-gal-stained branching ducts in *K18-EG/K8-CE*$^{tg/+}$;*R26R*$^{LacZ/+}$ mammary glands after Tam treatment for 10, 21, and 42 days (FF′-HH′), whereas no X-gal-stained cells were detected in the absence of Tam (EE′). (E″-H″) Histological sections of the aforementioned mammary samples were counterstained with Nuclear Fast Red, and they exhibited X-gal-stained luminal epithelia (F″-H″) in a time-

dependent manner in comparison to the staining in the vehicle control. (I) Timeline for the lineage tracing of a lactating mammary gland. The *K18-EG/K8-CE*$^{tg/+}$*;R26R*$^{LacZ/+}$ female was treated with Tam at 6 weeks of age and followed for 3 weeks to set up mating, and then the animal was analyzed at 1 week postparturition. (J-M) The dissected *K18-EG/K8-CE*$^{tg/+}$*;R26R*$^{LacZ/+}$ mammary gland was visualized by EGFP expression (J-L) and LacZ activity (K-M) both grossly and histologically. (L) Lactating alveolar epithelia of mammary glands exhibited uniform EGFP expression and mosaic patchy LacZ expression. Nuclei were counterstained with DAPI. (M) Histology sections were counterstained with Nuclear Fast Red, and they exhibited a mosaic pattern of X-gal-stained epithelial cells in the lactating mammary gland. Scale bars of A-D, E-H, and E'-H', 0.25 cm; Scale bars of E''-H'' and L-M, 100 μm.

Complete epithelial turnover in the intestine requires approximately 5 days [for review, see (van der Flier and Clevers 2009)]. Conversely, the relatively slower turnover rate of mammary epithelial cells is regulated by the estrous cycle, and these cells undergo alveolar morphogenesis during pregnancy and lactation. Thus, we selectively monitored inducible LacZ activity in intestinal and mammary epithelia at 10, 21, and 42 days after Tam administration. In the absence of Tam administration (vehicle control), spotty X-gal signals were detected in the small intestine (Fig 4AA'), which indicated a leakage of inducible CreER^T activity, resulting in rare but detectable levels of LacZ expression. After 10 days of Tam administration, X-gal-stained intestinal epithelia were detected in the cell lineage that emerged from the crypts, differentiated, and migrated upward to the villi (Fig 4BB'). This phenomenon was also observed after 21 and 42 days of induction (Fig 4CC' and DD'), indicating that the K8-expressing epithelia are composed of stem/progenitor cells that have the capability for long-term intestinal maintenance. In contrast, the numbers of X-gal-stained ductal cells in mammary glands gradually reduced after Tam treatment for 21 and 42 days (Fig 4G-G''and H-H'') compared to the number of X-gal-stained cells after 10 days of Tam treatment (Fig 4F). This observation suggests that the Tam-induced LacZ-expressing cells are replaced by newly generated cells from K8-independent epithelial origins, which give rise to LacZ-negative luminal cells that subsequently replace previous LacZ-positive cells to maintain mammary gland homeostasis.

3. Characterization of *Pten*-deficient epithelial tumors

3.1 The tumor latency, tumor spectrum, and tumor incidence of *K18-EG/K8-CE*$^{tg/+}$*; Pten*$^{fx/fx}$ mice

Throughout intensive analyses of inducible Cre activity controlled by the K8 promoter in various epithelial tissues as shown in Section 2, we further monitored epithelial tumors arising from *Pten*-deficient epithelial tissues to clarify the susceptibility of different epithelia to *Pten* loss in multiple organs. Thus, we generated *K18-EG/K8-CE*$^{tg/+}$*;Pten*$^{fx/+}$, *K18-EG/K8-CE*$^{tg/+}$*;Pten*$^{fx/fx}$ (referred to *K8-Pten*$^{fx/+}$ and *K8-Pten*$^{fx/fx}$, respectively), and their littermate controls and induced Cre-*lox*P recombination using Tam to excise exon 5 of *Pten* as illustrated in Fig 5A. All mice were on a mixed B6/129/Balb/c background.

Our results revealed that 92% of *K8-Pten*$^{fx/fx}$ mice (23/25) and 26.3% of *K8-Pten*$^{fx/+}$ mice (5/19) developed various malignant tumors by 60 and 100 weeks after Tam treatment, respectively (Fig 5B). The cumulative cancer-free survival is presented in Fig 5B. The overall mean latency of *Pten*-deficient tumors was approximately 25 weeks. All tumors were primarily analyzed by gross appearance and H&E-stained histology. The malignant tumors that developed in *K8-Pten*$^{fx/fx}$ and *K8-Pten*$^{fx/+}$ mice are summarized in Table 1.

We found that pancreatic ductal cancer (PDAC; 10 mice), cholangiocarcinoma (CC; 4 mice), hepatocellular carcinoma (HCC; 3 mice), and mammary gland tumors (MGTs; 7 females) accounted for the majority of the identified *Pten*-deficient malignancies (Fig 5C; Table 1), which are selectively described in Sections 3.2-3.4. Prostate cancer (two males) and precancerous lesions (prostate intraepithelial neoplasia) were also frequently found in *K8-Pten$^{fx/fx}$* mice (data not shown). Other malignancies arising from the thyroid, lung, stomach, and uterus were occasionally identified in the *K8-Pten$^{fx/fx}$* mice (Table 1). In addition, multiple tumors arising from different organs were observed in *K8-Pten$^{fx/fx}$* mice (eight mice, 32%; three males and five females; Table 1). Moreover, five different epithelial malignancies arising from the thyroid, lung, pancreas, intestine, and breast were found in five *K8-Pten$^{fx/+}$* females. At present, no malignant tumors have been found in *K8-Pten$^{fx/+}$* males, which may be due to the limited animal numbers (n=7); a higher number of *K8-Pten$^{fx/+}$* males might be required for further confirmation.

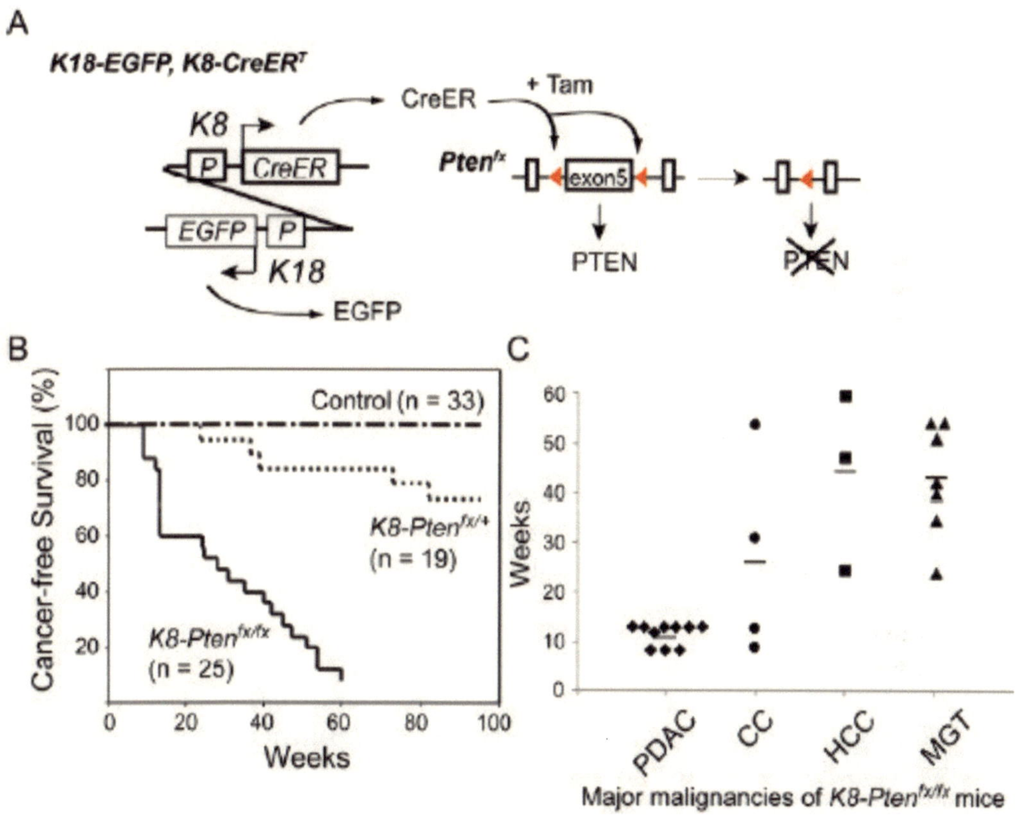

Fig. 5. Analysis of malignant tumors in the *K8-Pten$^{fx/fx}$* and *K8-Pten$^{fx/+}$* mice. (A) Schematic illustration of the genetic tool, *Tg(K18-EGFP, K8-CreER^{T})*, used to conditionally excise the *Pten* floxed allele after Tam administration. (B) Cancer-free survival of control, *K8-Pten$^{fx/+}$*, and *K8-Pten$^{fx/fx}$* mice. (C) Major epithelial malignancies (n≥3) of *K8-Pten$^{fx/fx}$* mice. PDAC, pancreatic ductal cancer; CC, cholangiocarcinoma; HCC, hepatocellular carcinoma; MGT, mammary gland tumor.

	K8-Pten$^{fx/+}$	*K8-Pten*$^{fx/fx}$
Total animal number	19	25
male	7	7
female	12	18
Tumor incidence (%)	5 (26.3)	23 (92.0)
Tumor spectrum (%)		
Follicular thyroid carcinoma	1 (20.0)	1 (3.2)
Lung carcinoma	1 (20.0)	1 (3.2)
Pancreatic ductal adenocarcinoma	1 (20.0)	10 (32.3)
Intra-hepatic cholangiocarcinoma	0	4 (12.9)
Hepatocellular carcinoma	0	3 (9.7)
Gastrointestinal carcinoma	1 (20.0)	2 (6.5)
Prostate carcinoma	0	2 (6.5)
Endometrial carcinoma	0	1 (3.2)
Mammary gland tumor	1 (20.0)	7 (22.6)
Total tumor number	5	31*

*multiple tumors in 3 males and 5 females

Table 1. Malignancies of the *K8-Pten*$^{fx/+}$ and *K8-Pten*$^{fx/fx}$ mice.

3.2 *Pten*-deficient pancreatic malignancies

Among different tumor types, pancreatic malignancies developed approximately 12 weeks before other epithelial lesions, and pancreatic malignancies accounted for the majority of epithelial malignancies in Tam-treated *K8-Pten*$^{fx/fx}$ mice (Fig 5C). Pancreata isolated from control mice (Fig. 6 A-C) and sick *K8-Pten*$^{fx/fx}$ mice (Fig. 6 D-F, G-I, and J-L) were subjected to stereomicroscopy and histology. Grossly, the normal pancreas exhibited vasculature and a white appearance and was a soft organ connected to the caudal lobe of the liver, common bile duct, stomach, duodenum, and spleen (Fig. 6A). In the *Pten*-deficient pancreata, desmoplastic changes and cystic dilation could be identified (Fig. 6 D, G, and J). In addition, the higher EGFP intensity exhibited tubular or patchy patterns in the *K8-Pten*$^{fx/fx}$ mutants (Fig. 6 E, H, and K; arrows) compared to the uniform GFP pattern of the control (Fig. 6B). Microscopically, interlobular ductal hyperplasia (Fig. 6F), acinar-to-ductal metaplasia (Fig. 6I), and PDAC (Fig. 6L) were identified in some *K8-Pten*$^{fx/f}$ mice. In our observations, PDAC progression in *K8-Pten*$^{fx/fx}$ mice is an immediate life-threatening disease as like in humans. In general, our findings were consistent with an earlier report that characterized pancreatic ductal metaplasia and pancreatic cancer initiation in mice in which *Pten* was ablated by *Pdx1-Cre* starting from the developing pancreas specifically (Stanger et al. 2005). Our inducible Cre activity in the K8-expressing cells of the adult mouse pancreas likely includes pancreatic ducts and centroacinal cells in which *Pten* is excised, leading to PDAC.

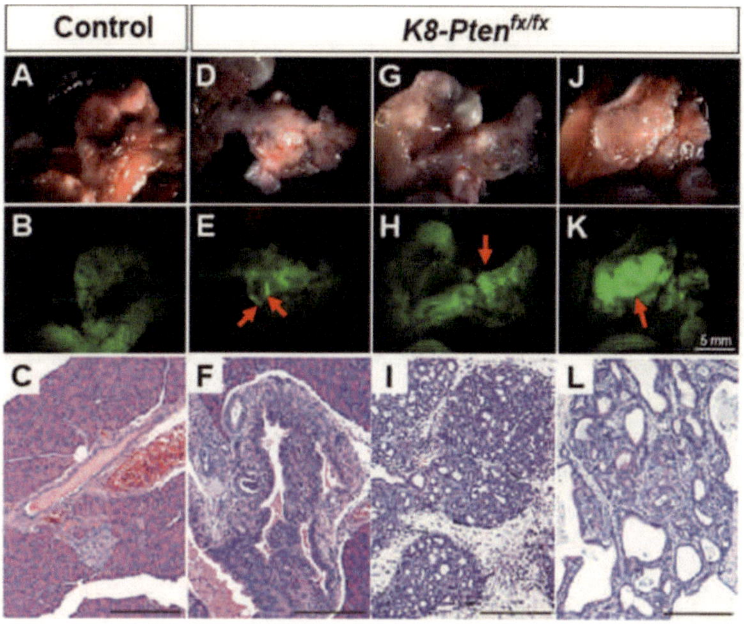

Fig. 6. Pancreatic malignancy of the *K8-Pten$^{fx/fx}$* mice. Age-matched *Tg(K18-EGFP, K8-CreER)* pancreata were used as the control. Gross appearances and EGFP expression in control (A-B) and *K8-Pten$^{fx/fx}$* pancreata (D-E, G-H, and J-K) were observed by stereomicroscopy. H&E-stained histological sections of control pancreata revealed the exocrine acinar gland, pancreatic islet, interlobular duct, and blood vessel (C). Interlobular ductal hyperplasia (F), ductal metaplasia (I), and invasive pancreatic ductal adenocarcinoma (L) were histologically identified in the *K8-Pten$^{fx/fx}$* mice at 9-13 weeks after Tam treatment. Scale bar, 100 μm.

3.3 *Pten*-deficient MGTs

Previously, Li et al used a mammary-specific MMTV-Cre transgenic line to excise the *lox*P-floxed *Pten* critical exon (exon 5) (Li et al. 2002). Some *MMTV-Cre;Pten$^{fx/fx}$* females develop MGTs as early as 2 months of age (Li et al. 2002). In our study, MGT was the most frequent (approximately 38.9%) malignancy in *K8-Pten$^{fx/fx}$* females (7/18 mice). Palpable MGTs were detected at 24-54 weeks (mean latency, 43 weeks) after Tam treatment (Fig 5C), and they were dissected and observed under a stereomicroscope. We found that EGFP-positive branches were clearly revealed in the control mammary gland, although the deeper mammary branches were shielded by thick adipose tissue (Fig 7A). In the *K8-Pten$^{fx/fx}$* mammary solid tumor, higher EGFP intensity was detected in a patchy pattern, which might represent a mass of hyperplastic epithelial cells (Fig 7B). Histologically, the representative *Pten*-deficient MGT was a solid epithelial mass with atypical glandular arrangement (Fig 7D) compared to the normal mammary ducts that were surrounded by adipose tissue (Fig 7C). To determine the effect of induced PTEN loss, we performed immunohistochemistry on the sections of the control and *K8-Pten$^{fx/fx}$* mammary tissues. Our results revealed that PTEN expression could be detected in various cells, including ductal luminal and basal epithelial cells, vascular endothelial cells, and stromal cells, within the control mammary gland (Fig 7E). In contrast, the loss of PTEN was specifically demonstrated in the epithelial tumor cells, but not in the neovascular endothelial cells and stromal cells, of *K8-Pten$^{fx/fx}$* MGTs (Fig 7F).

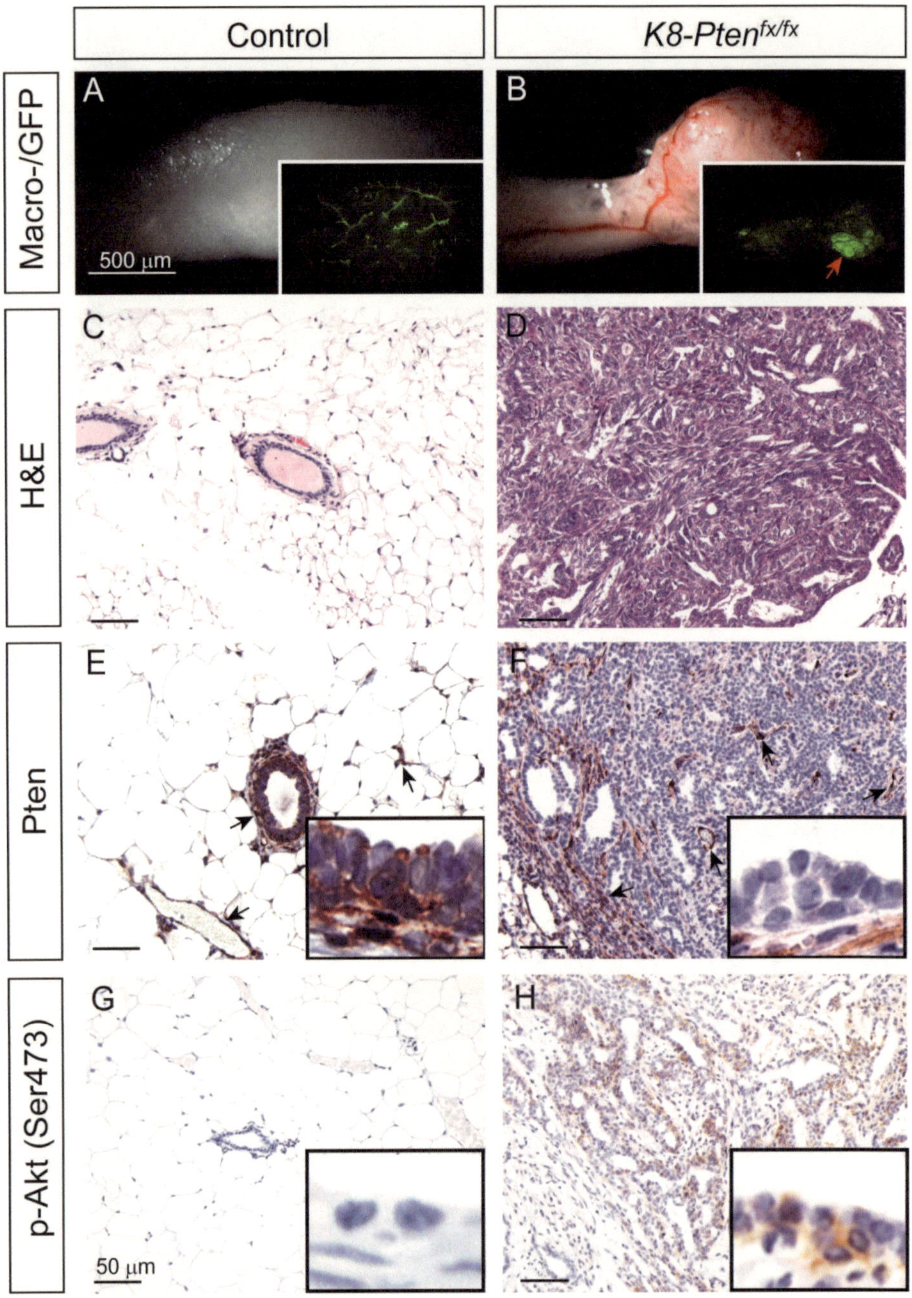

Fig. 7. Mammary tumors of the *K8-Pten*$^{fx/fx}$ females. (A) Mammary fat pad with EGFP-expressing ductal branches (inset) was obtained from a control female (42 weeks after Tam treatment); (B) MGT consisting of an EGFP-expressing tumor mass (inset) was obtained from a *K8-Pten*$^{fx/fx}$ female (42 weeks after Tam treatment); (C) and (D) H&E-stained histological sections of control mammary tissue (C; 54 weeks after Tam treatment) and *K8-Pten*$^{fx/fx}$ MGT (D; 54 weeks after Tam treatment); (E) and (F) PTEN immunohistochemistry

revealed the induced loss of PTEN in a *K8-Pten$^{fx/fx}$* mammary epithelial tumor (F; 54 weeks after Tam treatment), whereas PTEN was expressed in various cell types within age-matched control mammary tissue (arrows; E). Insets, high-power views of the PTEN levels in the control mammary duct (E) and mammary epithelial tumor (F); (G) and (H) Immunohistochemistry of p-Akt(Ser473) revealed cytoplasmic staining of p-Akt in tubular structures infiltrating within a stroma of a *K8-Pten$^{fx/fx}$* MGT (H; 35 weeks after Tam treatment) compared to a negatively stained mammary duct of an age-matched control mouse. Insets, high-power views of the p-Akt(Ser473) levels in the control mammary duct (G) and MGT (H). Scale bar (C-H), 100 μm.

Then, we determined activation of AKT using antibody against phosphorylated AKT, p-Akt(Ser473), and found that AKT phosphorylation appeared in the neoplastic epithelial cells of the *K8-Pten$^{fx/fx}$* MGT (Fig 7H), unlike the controls (Fig 7G).Thus, our data revealed that the mammary luminal epithelium was highly susceptible to *Pten*-deficient mammary tumorigenesis, although it might be replaced by a K8^{+}-independent cell lineage as indicated by Cre reporter (LacZ) activity (Fig. 4E-H).

3.4 *Pten*-deficient HCCs and intrahepatic CCs

Liver-specific *Pten* ablation by albumin (Alb)-Cre has been reported to result in the development of steatohepatitis, metabolic disorders, and HCCs (Horie et al. 2004, Stiles et al. 2004). According to two different reports, the latency of *Pten*-deficient hepatocellular carcinogenesis appears to be required for an extended time. Horie et al reported that *Pten*-deficient HCCs developed in 66% of *Alb-Cre;Pten$^{fx/fx}$* animals at 74-78 weeks of age. Xu et al also found that the incidence of HCCs was 33% by 12-16 months of age (Xu et al. 2006). Interestingly, Xu et al reported that their *Alb-Cre;Pten$^{fx/fx}$* mice developed visible foci of CCs along with HCCs at late onset that were explained by the *Alb-Cre* mice exhibiting Cre activity in both hepatocytes and cholangiocytes (Xu et al. 2006). Moreover, early disease progression and higher penetrance of CCs were demonstrated when the Smad4 conditional allele was introduced into the *Alb-Cre;Pten$^{fx/fx}$* background (Xu et al. 2006).

In our findings, low incidences of HCCs (3/25 mice) and CCs (4/25 mice) were identified in the Tam-treated *K8-Pten$^{fx/fx}$* mice at 9-54 (mean latency, 27 weeks) and 24-60 weeks (mean latency, 44 weeks), respectively (Fig 5C). Our observations indicated a longer period of disease progression for HCCs than for CCs after *Pten* loss was induced. However, the relative susceptibilities of hepatocytes and cholangiocytes to *Pten*-deficient tumorigenesis remain unclear because of the low incidence of both diseases. Moreover, the induced mosaic Cre recombination events in the hepatocytes compared to the uniform and intense reporter (LacZ) activity in the cholangiocytes of bile ducts as shown in Fig 2E should also be considered because differential induction of Cre activity may directly contribute to the differential pace of disease progression initiated in hepatocytes compared to that initiated in cholangiocytes. Nevertheless, we could identify both fatty accumulation in hepatocytes (Fig 8A) and dysplastic/hyperplastic cholangiocytes of the dilated bile ducts (Fig 8B) in the sections of *K8-Pten$^{fx/fx}$* livers at early time points (13 weeks) after Tam treatment. These early events might directly or indirectly lead to HCC (Fig 8D) and CC, which could be identified by K19 expression (Fig 8F), in the Tam-treated *K8-Pten$^{fx/fx}$* mice at late onset.

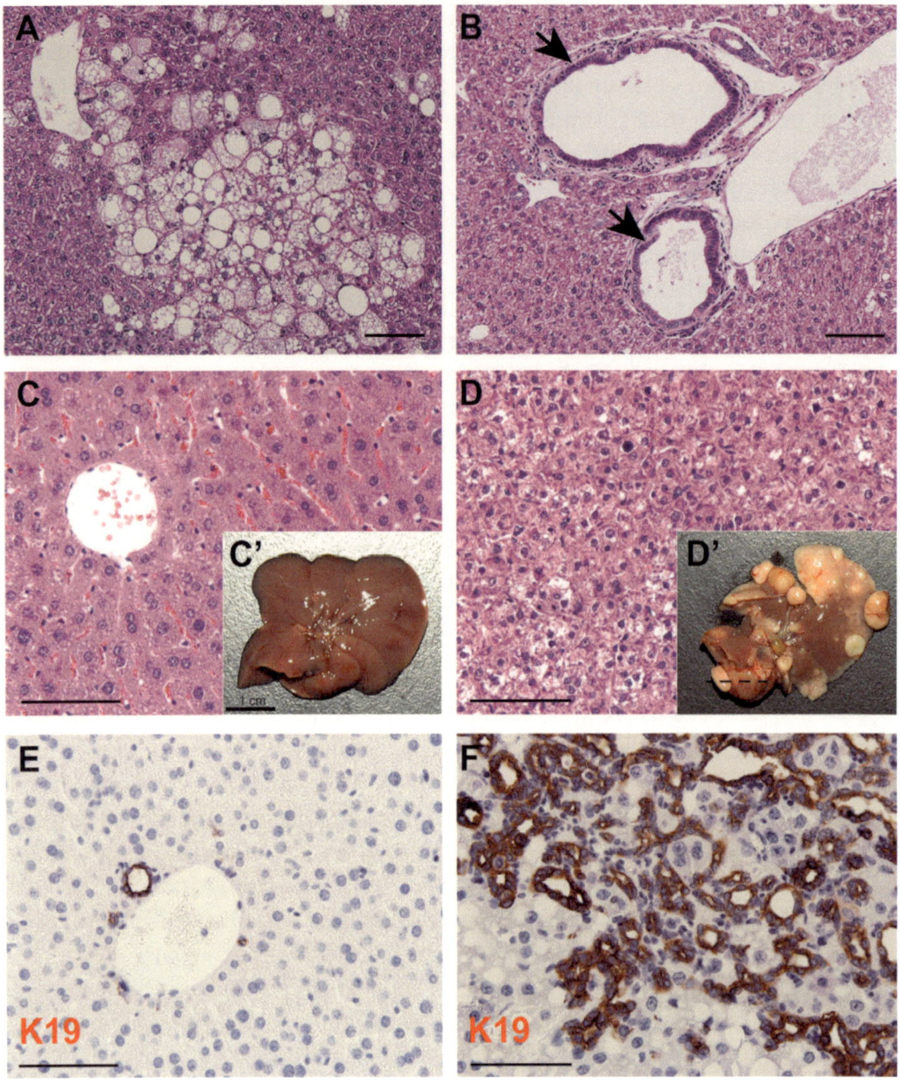

Fig. 8. Liver diseases of the *K8-Pten$^{fx/fx}$* mice. (A) Fatty changes of hepatocytes in a *K8-Pten$^{fx/fx}$* mouse at 13 weeks after Tam treatment; (B) Aberrant dilated bile ducts (arrows) of the portal tract in a *K8-Pten$^{fx/fx}$* mouse at 13 weeks after Tam treatment; (C) H&E-stained section and gross view (C′, inset) of a control liver at 60 weeks after Tam treatment; (D) H&E-stained section and gross view (D′, inset) of a *K8-Pten$^{fx/fx}$* liver at 60 weeks after Tam treatment; (E) and (F) K19 expressed in the control bile ductal cells (E) and in the acinar pattern of a representative *K8-Pten$^{fx/fx}$* CC (31 weeks). Scale bar, 100 μm.

4. Conclusion

In this chapter, we demonstrated that the mouse *K8-K18* intergenic sequence possesses the essential promoters and regulatory elements for controlling the bidirectional expression of *CreER^T* and EGFP across multiple organs. Selectively ablating the tumor suppressor gene

Pten in the epithelial cells of multiple organs in this study provides an entry point to understand epithelial tissue susceptibility to *Pten*-deficient tumorigenesis. Our data reveal that the K8-expressing epithelia of the pancreatic ducts, prostate, and mammary glands are highly susceptible to *Pten*-deficient tumorigenesis. Hepatocytes and cholangiocytes of the liver also possibly undergo tumorigenesis after *Pten* loss, which may evoke a variety of downstream signaling circuits. All *Pten*-deficient malignancies described here are primary tumors that invade locally. Metastasis is rare in our current observation that requires further characterization. In the future, the same approach can possibly be used to establish clinically relevant mouse models to investigate adenocarcinoma initiation and progression by simultaneously creating additional genetic lesions in conjunction with the *K8-Pten*$^{fx/+}$ or *K8-Pten*$^{fx/fx}$ alleles; mice that carry multiple conditional alleles of cancer-related genes can be generated and characterized to understand tumor susceptibility, considering that cancer is a disease of multiple genetic events.

5. Acknowledgment

We thank Yi-Hsuan Chiang, Yu-Lei Chang, Ming-Lun Lee and Wan-Chun Yu for their initial assistance. Authors also thank all members of the laboratories of C.-M. C. (cmchen@ym.edu.tw) and of L.-R. Y. (lryou@ym.edu.tw) for helpful discussion. This work was supported by a grant from the National Health Research Institutes (NHRI-EX99-9901-BI), a grant from the Ministry of Education "Aim for the Top University Plan", grants from the National Science Council (NSC 98-2320-B010-011-MY3, NSC 99-3112-B010-013 (99IR017) to C.M.C. and a technical service was supported by the Taiwan Mouse Clinic (NSC 99-3112-B-001-021).

Note: Methods used in this chapter were described previously (Chen and Behringer 2004, Chen, Chang and Behringer 2004, Chen et al. 2010, Liang et al. 2009, Lu et al. 2007).

6. References

Alessi, D. R., S. R. James, C. P. Downes, A. B. Holmes, P. R. Gaffney, C. B. Reese & P. Cohen (1997) Characterization of a 3-phosphoinositide-dependent protein kinase which phosphorylates and activates protein kinase Balpha. *Curr Biol,* 7, 261-9.

Ali, I. U., L. M. Schriml & M. Dean (1999) Mutational spectra of PTEN/MMAC1 gene: a tumor suppressor with lipid phosphatase activity. *J Natl Cancer Inst,* 91, 1922-32.

Blanpain, C., V. Horsley & E. Fuchs (2007) Epithelial stem cells: turning over new leaves. *Cell,* 128, 445-58.

Brown, E. J., P. A. Beal, C. T. Keith, J. Chen, T. Bum Shin & S. L. Schreiber (1995) Control of p70 S6 kinase by kinase activity of FRAP in vivo. *Nature,* 377, 441-446.

Brunet, A., A. Bonni, M. J. Zigmond, M. Z. Lin, P. Juo, L. S. Hu, M. J. Anderson, K. C. Arden, J. Blenis & M. E. Greenberg (1999) Akt Promotes Cell Survival by Phosphorylating and Inhibiting a Forkhead Transcription Factor. *Cell,* 96, 857-868.

Brunn, G. J., C. C. Hudson, A. Sekuli, J. M. Williams, H. Hosoi, P. J. Houghton, J. C. Lawrence, Jr. & R. T. Abraham. 1997. Phosphorylation of the Translational Repressor PHAS-I by the Mammalian Target of Rapamycin. 99-101.

Carracedo, A. & P. P. Pandolfi (2008) The PTEN-PI3K pathway: of feedbacks and cross-talks. *Oncogene,* 27, 5527-41.

Chen, C. M. & R. R. Behringer (2004) Ovca1 regulates cell proliferation, embryonic development, and tumorigenesis. *Genes Dev,* 18, 320-32.

Chen, C. M., J. L. Chang & R. R. Behringer (2004) Tumor formation in p53 mutant ovaries transplanted into wild-type female hosts. *Oncogene,* 23, 7722-5.

Chen, C. M., H. Y. Wang, L. R. You, R. L. Shang & F. C. Liu (2010) Expression analysis of an evolutionary conserved metallophosphodiesterase gene, Mpped1, in the normal and beta-catenin-deficient malformed dorsal telencephalon. *Dev Dyn,* 239, 1797-806.

Cross, D. A., D. R. Alessi, P. Cohen, M. Andjelkovich & B. A. Hemmings (1995) Inhibition of glycogen synthase kinase-3 by insulin mediated by protein kinase B. *Nature,* 378, 785-9.

Cully, M., H. You, A. J. Levine & T. W. Mak (2006) Beyond PTEN mutations: the PI3K pathway as an integrator of multiple inputs during tumorigenesis. *Nat Rev Cancer,* 6, 184-92.

Datta, S. R., H. Dudek, X. Tao, S. Masters, H. Fu, Y. Gotoh & M. E. Greenberg (1997) Akt Phosphorylation of BAD Couples Survival Signals to the Cell-Intrinsic Death Machinery. *Cell,* 91, 231-241.

Dunlop, E. A. & A. R. Tee (2009) Mammalian target of rapamycin complex 1: Signalling inputs, substrates and feedback mechanisms. *Cellular Signalling,* In Press, Corrected Proof.

Fang, D., D. Hawke, Y. Zheng, Y. Xia, J. Meisenhelder, H. Nika, G. B. Mills, R. Kobayashi, T. Hunter & Z. Lu. 2007. Phosphorylation of beta-Catenin by AKT Promotes beta-Catenin Transcriptional Activity. 11221-11229.

Fujita, N., S. Sato, K. Katayama & T. Tsuruo (2002) Akt-dependent phosphorylation of p27Kip1 promotes binding to 14-3-3 and cytoplasmic localization. *J Biol Chem,* 277, 28706-13.

Hara, K., K. Yonezawa, M. T. Kozlowski, T. Sugimoto, K. Andrabi, Q.-P. Weng, M. Kasuga, I. Nishimoto & J. Avruch. 1997. Regulation of eIF-4E BP1 Phosphorylation by mTOR. 26457-26463.

He, X. C., T. Yin, J. C. Grindley, Q. Tian, T. Sato, W. A. Tao, R. Dirisina, K. S. Porter-Westpfahl, M. Hembree, T. Johnson, L. M. Wiedemann, T. A. Barrett, L. Hood, H. Wu & L. Li (2007) PTEN-deficient intestinal stem cells initiate intestinal polyposis. *Nat Genet,* 39, 189-98.

Horie, Y., A. Suzuki, E. Kataoka, T. Sasaki, K. Hamada, J. Sasaki, K. Mizuno, G. Hasegawa, H. Kishimoto, M. Iizuka, M. Naito, K. Enomoto, S. Watanabe, T. W. Mak & T. Nakano (2004) Hepatocyte-specific Pten deficiency results in steatohepatitis and hepatocellular carcinomas. *J Clin Invest,* 113, 1774-83.

Inoki, K., Y. Li, T. Zhu, J. Wu & K.-L. Guan (2002) TSC2 is phosphorylated and inhibited by Akt and suppresses mTOR signalling. *Nat Cell Biol,* 4, 648-657.

Kishimoto, H., K. Hamada, M. Saunders, S. Backman, T. Sasaki, T. Nakano, T. W. Mak & A. Suzuki (2003) Physiological functions of Pten in mouse tissues. *Cell Struct Funct,* 28, 11-21.

Lesche, R., M. Groszer, J. Gao, Y. Wang, A. Messing, H. Sun, X. Liu & H. Wu (2002) Cre/loxP-mediated inactivation of the murine Pten tumor suppressor gene. *Genesis,* 32, 148-9.

Li, D. M. & H. Sun (1997) TEP1, encoded by a candidate tumor suppressor locus, is a novel protein tyrosine phosphatase regulated by transforming growth factor beta. *Cancer Res,* 57, 2124-9.

Li, G., G. W. Robinson, R. Lesche, H. Martinez-Diaz, Z. Jiang, N. Rozengurt, K. U. Wagner, D. C. Wu, T. F. Lane, X. Liu, L. Hennighausen & H. Wu (2002) Conditional loss of PTEN leads to precocious development and neoplasia in the mammary gland. *Development,* 129, 4159-70.

Li, J., C. Yen, D. Liaw, K. Podsypanina, S. Bose, S. I. Wang, J. Puc, C. Miliaresis, L. Rodgers, R. McCombie, S. H. Bigner, B. C. Giovanella, M. Ittmann, B. Tycko, H. Hibshoosh, M. H. Wigler & R. Parsons (1997) PTEN, a putative protein tyrosine phosphatase gene mutated in human brain, breast, and prostate cancer. *Science,* 275, 1943-7.

Liang, C.-C., L. R. You, J.-L. Chang, T.-F. Tsai & C.-M. Chen (2009) Transgenic mice exhibiting inducible and spontaneous Cre activities driven by a bovine keratin 5 promoter that can be used for the conditional analysis of basal epithelial cells in multiple organs. *J Biomed. Sci.,* 16, 2.

Lu, T.-L., J.-L. Chang, C.-C. Liang, L.-R. You & C.-M. Chen (2007) Tumor Spectrum, Tumor Latency and Tumor Incidence of the Pten-Deficient Mice. *PLoS ONE,* 2, e1237.

Manning, B. D. & L. C. Cantley (2007) AKT/PKB signaling: navigating downstream. *Cell,* 129, 1261-74.

Manning, B. D., A. R. Tee, M. N. Logsdon, J. Blenis & L. C. Cantley (2002) Identification of the Tuberous Sclerosis Complex-2 Tumor Suppressor Gene Product Tuberin as a Target of the Phosphoinositide 3-Kinase/Akt Pathway. *Molecular Cell,* 10, 151-162.

Mayo, L. D. & D. B. Donner (2001) A phosphatidylinositol 3-kinase/Akt pathway promotes translocation of Mdm2 from the cytoplasm to the nucleus. *Proc Natl Acad Sci U S A,* 98, 11598-603.

Peso, L. d., M. Gonzalez-Garcia, C. Page, R. Herrera & G. Nunez. 1997. Interleukin-3-Induced Phosphorylation of BAD Through the Protein Kinase Akt. 687-689.

Sarbassov, D. D., S. M. Ali, D. H. Kim, D. A. Guertin, R. R. Latek, H. Erdjument-Bromage, P. Tempst & D. M. Sabatini (2004) Rictor, a novel binding partner of mTOR, defines a rapamycin-insensitive and raptor-independent pathway that regulates the cytoskeleton. *Curr Biol,* 14, 1296-302.

Sarbassov, D. D., D. A. Guertin, S. M. Ali & D. M. Sabatini (2005) Phosphorylation and regulation of Akt/PKB by the rictor-mTOR complex. *Science,* 307, 1098-101.

Soriano, P. (1999) Generalized lacZ expression with the ROSA26 Cre reporter strain. *Nat Genet,* 21, 70-1.

Stambolic, V., A. Suzuki, J. L. de la Pompa, G. M. Brothers, C. Mirtsos, T. Sasaki, J. Ruland, J. M. Penninger, D. P. Siderovski & T. W. Mak (1998) Negative regulation of PKB/Akt-dependent cell survival by the tumor suppressor PTEN. *Cell,* 95, 29-39.

Stanger, B. Z., B. Stiles, G. Y. Lauwers, N. Bardeesy, M. Mendoza, Y. Wang, A. Greenwood, K. H. Cheng, M. McLaughlin, D. Brown, R. A. Depinho, H. Wu, D. A. Melton & Y. Dor (2005) Pten constrains centroacinar cell expansion and malignant transformation in the pancreas. *Cancer Cell,* 8, 185-95.

Steck, P. A., M. A. Pershouse, S. A. Jasser, W. K. Yung, H. Lin, A. H. Ligon, L. A. Langford, M. L. Baumgard, T. Hattier, T. Davis, C. Frye, R. Hu, B. Swedlund, D. H. Teng & S. V. Tavtigian (1997) Identification of a candidate tumour suppressor gene, MMAC1, at chromosome 10q23.3 that is mutated in multiple advanced cancers. *Nat Genet,* 15, 356-62.

Stiles, B., Y. Wang, A. Stahl, S. Bassilian, W. P. Lee, Y. J. Kim, R. Sherwin, S. Devaskar, R. Lesche, M. A. Magnuson & H. Wu (2004) Liver-specific deletion of negative regulator Pten results in fatty liver and insulin hypersensitivity [corrected]. *Proc Natl Acad Sci U S A,* 101, 2082-7.

van der Flier, L. G. & H. Clevers (2009) Stem cells, self-renewal, and differentiation in the intestinal epithelium. *Annu Rev Physiol,* 71, 241-60.

Wu, X., K. Senechal, M. S. Neshat, Y. E. Whang & C. L. Sawyers (1998) The PTEN/MMAC1 tumor suppressor phosphatase functions as a negative regulator of the phosphoinositide 3-kinase/Akt pathway. *Proc Natl Acad Sci U S A,* 95, 15587-91.

Xu, X., S. Kobayashi, W. Qiao, C. Li, C. Xiao, S. Radaeva, B. Stiles, R. H. Wang, N. Ohara, T. Yoshino, D. LeRoith, M. S. Torbenson, G. J. Gores, H. Wu, B. Gao & C. X. Deng (2006) Induction of intrahepatic cholangiocellular carcinoma by liver-specific disruption of Smad4 and Pten in mice. *J Clin Invest,* 116, 1843-52.

Zhou, B. P., Y. Liao, W. Xia, B. Spohn, M.-H. Lee & M.-C. Hung (2001a) Cytoplasmic localization of p21Cip1/WAF1 by Akt-induced phosphorylation in HER-2/neu-overexpressing cells. *Nat Cell Biol,* 3, 245-252.

Zhou, B. P., Y. Liao, W. Xia, Y. Zou, B. Spohn & M. C. Hung (2001b) HER-2/neu induces p53 ubiquitination via Akt-mediated MDM2 phosphorylation. *Nat Cell Biol,* 3, 973-82.

3

Identification of Tumor Suppressor Genes via Cell Fusion and Chromosomal Transfer

Hong Lok Lung, Arthur Kwok Leung Cheung, Josephine Mun Yee Ko, Yue Cheng and Maria Li Lung
Department of Clinical Oncology and Center for Cancer Research, The University of Hong Kong, Hong Kong

1. Introduction

Loss of DNA or chromosomal deletion was frequently reported in different sporadic tumors, suggesting that those lost regions may contain putative tumor suppressor genes (TSGs). To map and isolate candidate genes from vast randomly lost areas, functional and complementary evidence is usually needed to define these areas to critical regions (CR). This is particularly important when one is dealing with sporadic cancers where clearly defined familial predisposition is present but high cancer risk families are not available for position cloning. A numerous studies have revealed extensive DNA deletions in nasopharyngeal carcinoma (NPC) and esophageal squamous cell carcinoma (ESCC). To identify candidate genes from these cancers, we used cell fusion and microcell-mediated chromosome transfer (MMCT) to introduce the whole chromosome or a chromosome fragment, into NPC and ESCC cell lines. Combined with other molecular approaches, we have successfully identified a number of novel TSGs on various human chromosomes.

The nasopharynx is located behind the nasal cavity in the upper part of the pharynx (Fig. 1). NPC is a type of malignancy which arises from the epithelial cells in the nasopharynx. NPC is an unique cancer, which is commonly found in, Southeast Asia, North Africa, Middle East, and Arctic regions, but rare in most parts of the world (Jeyakumar et al 2006, Wei et al 2005). The esophagus is a tube, which is about 25 cm long, for the food passage from mouth to stomach (Fig. 2). Esophageal cancer (EC) is classified into two major histologic subtypes: squamous cell carcinoma and adenocarcinoma (Daly et al 2000). Esophageal adenocarcinoma (EAC) arises from the cells of glands responsible for producing mucous in the esophageal wall. The majority of the cases (>80%) are ESCC in Hong Kong, while EAC shows a climbing incidence in Western countries. EC varies greatly in geographical distribution; high-risk areas include north-central China in Henan and Shanxi (Holmes et al 2007, Qi et al 2005, Wu et al 2006).

2. Chromosome transfer in tumor studies

2.1 Somatic cell fusion and tumor suppression

The theory for specific chromosomes contributing to tumor suppression was originally proven by somatic cell genetics (Harris et al 1969). In their study, Harris and colleagues fused the mouse tumorigenic cells with non-tumorigenic cells to form a hybrid cell; some hybrid cells maintained the phenotypes of the parental cell lines and did not form tumors in the tumorigenicity assay. This suggests that non-tumorigenic cells contain genes, which are dominant and capable of suppressing the tumorigenic cell growth. The tumor suppression was further observed in human cell fusion experiments (Stanbridge, 1976 and 1992). The unstable tumorigenic hybrids showed loss of the selected chromosomes, resulting in the reemergence of its tumorigenicity properties. These findings suggested that some chromosomes may contain special regions, which can inhibit tumor formation, and thus provided the basis for further development of monochromosome transfer approaches to study the role of a particular chromosome in tumor development. These earlier experiments led to the hypothesis that the human genome might contain a group of genes suppressing tumor growth.

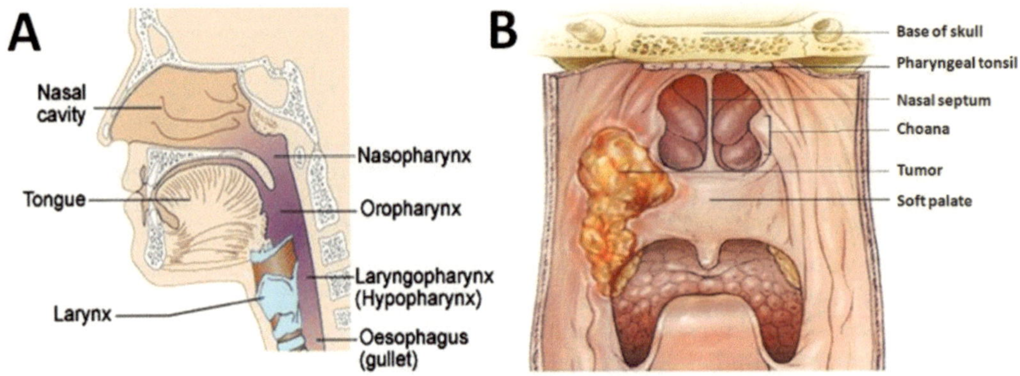

Adapted from Cancer Research UK and American Society of Clinical Oncology

Fig. 1. (A) Anatomy of human nasopharynx. (B) Location of nasopharyngeal carcinoma.

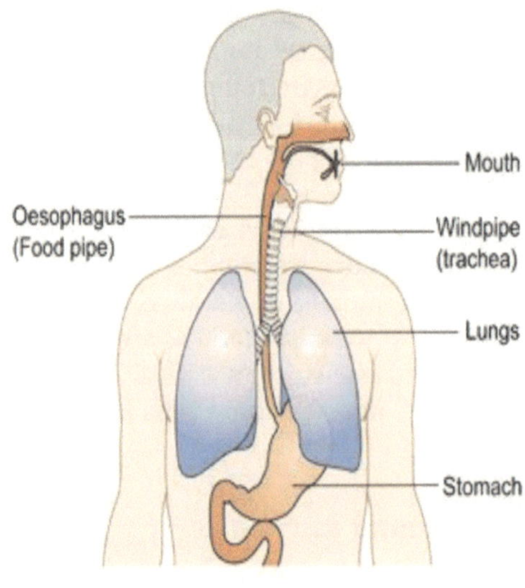

Adapted from Cancer Research UK

Fig. 2. Anatomy of human esophagus.

2.2 MMCT

The microcell-mediated chromosome transfer (MMCT) technique is a functional approach to investigate the tumor suppressive role of a specific chromosome or chromosome fragment in recipient cells. By using this approach, a single human chromosome is transferred into cancer cell lines. Transfers of exogenous chromosomes are tested for their functional ability to complement existing defects present in cancer cells. In this approach, a microcell donor, which contains a human chromosome of interest, is used as a donor to transfer the selected chromosome into tumor cells. Microcells, presumably with one chromosome within a nuclear envelope and plasma membrane, are generated after disruption of the cytoskeleton of the donor cells. The microcells are then fused to a malignant cancer cell line to establish stable microcell hybrids (MCHs) (Anderson et al 1993, Fournier et al 1977a, Stanbridge 1992). DNA genotyping and fluorescence in situ hybridization (FISH) are used for verification of a successful transfer. An in vivo nude mouse assay is then used to assess the tumorigenic potential of MCHs (Cheng et al 1998, Cheng et al 2000, Cheng et al 2002, Cheng et al 2003, Cheng et al 2004, Cheung et al 2009, Lung et al 2008a).

2.3 Advantages of MMCT approach in TSG studies

For the identification of TSGs contributing to the human cancers, initial efforts used the positional cloning of target regions defined by linkage analysis of pedigrees in hereditary cancer studies. The successful finding of the retinoblastoma gene, RB, is a good example (Friend et al 1986). However, the vast majority of the human cancers develop sporadically and involve numerous multiple gross deletions of chromosomal regions known as loss of heterozygosity (LOH). MMCT is a functional complementation approach useful for the identification of recessive-acting TSGs in sporadic cancers (Murakami 2002). Gene transfer approaches into human cancer cells may involve whole cell fusion, microcell fusion for intact or fragmented chromosomes, spheroplast fusion of yeast artificial chromosome (YAC), lipofection of bacteriophage P1, P1-derived artificial chromosome (PAC), bacterial artificial chromosome (BAC), or plasmids carrying the target genes, etc (Table 1) (Murakami 2002).

One of the advantages of the MMCT method is the transfer of a single copy of a chromosome allows strict control of dosage effect. If the transfer method is based on lipofection, it is impossible to control the copy number of DNA integrations into the genome. Compared to other commonly used artificial over-expression systems, the genes transferred by MMCT are expressed under the control of their endogenous promoters and enhancers and are regulated in their native environment. Thus, MMCT provides an ideal method for studying gene expression closely mimicking physiological levels and regulation controls under its native environment. Although the gene transfer by lipofection is convenient, the biological significance of functional studies of genes by the introduction of an expression vector should be carefully evaluated because the ectopic expression level of genes are not always equivalent to that found in the normal or tumor tissues, but are actually extraordinarily high in transfectants. An important issue to be addressed in the functional study of TSGs is whether the growth suppression resulting from exogenous gene over-expression by artificial procedures is a non-specific cytotoxic or cytostatic effect rather than a specific effect due to the expression of the gene itself.

In the second step of the functional complementation cloning of TSGs, the *in vivo* tumorigenicity assay in the immunologically deficient mice is an indicator of the malignant phenotype of cancer cells. The nude mouse tumorigenicity assay allows us to identify genes that fit the ultimate definition of a TSG, which requires functional evidence for the suppression of the malignant phenotype of cancer cells. The functional identification of TSGs in nude mouse assay can exclude the non-specific cytotoxic or cytostatic effects introduced by artificial gene expression. It also identifies a new category of molecules that are not cytotoxic *in vitro*, but are involved in the signaling cascades in different biological processes that hallmark cancer development such as the cell adhesion and sustained angiogenesis, inflammatory responses, evading immune destruction, and the tumor microenvironment.

Vector	Method	Length of the insert	No of genes	Promoter	Position effect	DNA copy number	References
Cell	Whole cell fusion	3 Gb	~30,000	Endogenous	-	2	(Murayama et al 1965) (Harris et al 1969)
Chromosome	Microcell fusion	~ 150 Mb	~1,500	Endogenous	-	1	(Fournier et al 1977b) (Weissman et al 1987) (Koi et al 1989)
Chromosomal fragment	γ-Irradiation + microcell fusion	2-20 Mb	20-200	Endogenous	-	1	(Dowdy et al 1990, Koi et al 1993), (Murakami et al 1995)
YAC	Spheroplast fusion	100-1600 kb	1-20	Endogenous	+ < -	1	(Pavan et al 1990b) (Pachnis et al 1990, Wada et al 1994), (Murakami et al 1998b)
Fragmented YAC	Homologous recombination + Spheroplast fusion	100-500 kb	1-10	Endogenous	+ / -	1	(Pavan et al 1990a), (Murakami et al 1998a)
P1, PAC, BAC	Lipofection	80-200 kb	<10	Endogenous	+ > -	>1-10	(Todd et al 1996)
Plasmid	Lipofection etc.	<5 kb (cDNA)	1	Artificial	+	>1-10	Numerous report

Adapted from Murakami (2002).

Table 1. Gene transfer methods into mammalian cells.

3. How to identify a TSG from a pool of genes?

3.1 MMCT

An intact single chromosome can be introduced into the recipient cell line using MMCT techniques. The establishment of mouse donor cells with a single copy of human chromosome is described previously (Fournier and Ruddle 1977a, Saxon et al 1985, Anderson and Stanbridge 1993). Figure 3 briefly outlines the procedures of MMCT. Donor cells were seeded on day 1 and incubated with 0.04 to 0.1 μg/ml colcemid for 48 to 56 hours to arrest cells in metaphase. Recipient cells were seeded on day 2 with the cell confluence reaching 80-90% the next day. Enucleation of the donor cells was achieved by centrifugation at 13,000 rpm for 65 to 70 min at 34°C with 10 μg/ml cytochalasin B (Sigma, MO, USA). The heterogeneous microcell mixture was then filtered through successive polycarbonate filters of 8/5/3 μm pore sizes (Whatman, Middlesex, UK) to remove large microcells and other cell debris. Microcells were pelleted by centrifugation and resuspended thoroughly in 1 ml DMEM containing 50 μg/ml phytohemagglutinin-p (PHA-P). The recipients were rinsed in PBS once and the microcell/PHA-P suspension was added to the recipient cells and incubated for 20-40 min. Microcells were fused to the recipient cell with 1-2 ml ice-cold PEG-1000. The treated cells were rinsed with PBS four times and fed with medium. The selection medium [hypoxanthine, aminopterin, and thymidine (HAT) + G418] was added on day five. After about three-four weeks selection, only the recipient cells harboring the transferred chromosome containing the neomycin gene on the exogenously transferred chromosome survive; potential hybrids were picked and expanded for further analysis.

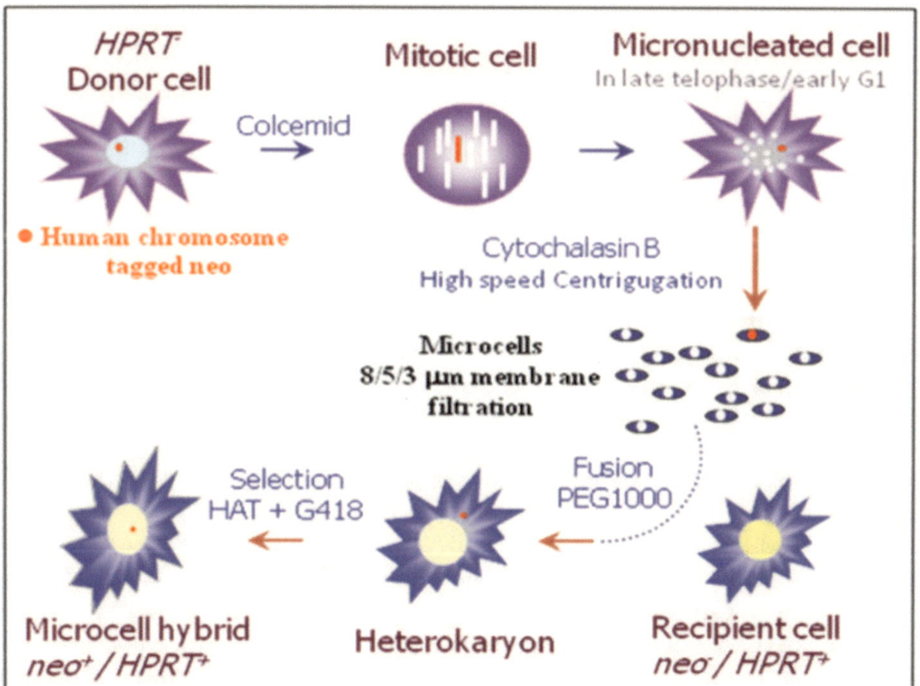

Fig. 3. Schematic diagram of MMCT.

3.2 Confirmation of successful chromosome transfer

The MCHs were subjected to DNA extraction and confirmation for the absence of mouse DNA contamination by DNA slot blot hybridization. Then the MCHs were subjected to microsatellite typing and fluorescence *in situ* hybridization (FISH). For microsatellite analysis, PCR products of microsatellite markers that amplified fragments with various numbers of repeat units are separated by gel or capillary electrophoresis. Microsatellite typing is a fast, simple, and reliable method to identify whether the donor allele has been transferred into the recipient cancer cell line. The high heterozygosity rate of microsatellite markers is used to demonstrate hybrid patterns in MCHs versus the recipient and donor cells to verify successful transfer of the donor human genetic materials into the human cancer cell line at the molecular level after MMCT.

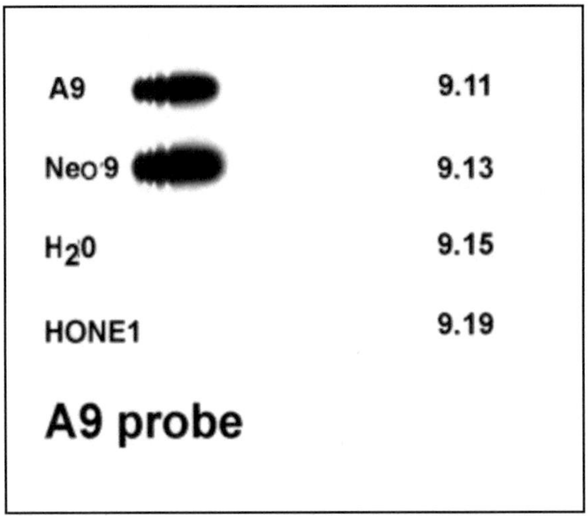

Fig. 4. DNA Slot blot analysis of chromosome 9 MCHs. The DNA of mouse A9 cells was used as a probe. The A9 and donor Neo 9 cells were used as positive controls for presence of mouse DNA, while the recipient cell line, HONE1 was used as a negative control for absence of mouse DNA. All MCHs was found to have no mouse DNA contamination.

3.2.1 DNA slot blot hybridization

The contamination of mouse DNA in MCHs was excluded by slot blot hybridization (Fig. 4). Five micrograms of genomic DNA of recipient cell lines, HONE1, microcell donor, MCHs, and A9 in 6X SSC (0.9 M NaCl and 90 mM Na Citrate, pH 7.4) were transferred onto a HybondTM N nylon membrane (Amersham Biosciences, Uppsala, Sweden) with a BIO-DOT® SF slot blot apparatus (BioRad, CA, USA). The samples on the membrane were denatured for 10 min with a denaturing solution (1.5 M NaCl and 0.5 M NaOH) and then neutralized in 1 M NaCl and 0.5 M Tris-Cl, pH 7 for 5 min. The membrane was dried and cross-linked by UV on an UV transilluminator (Stratagene, CA, USA). A Gene ImagesTM AlkPhos DirectTM Labelling and Detection System (Amersham Biosciences, Uppsala, Sweden) was used according to manufacturer's protocol. In brief, a total of 100 ng of A9 DNA was denatured by heat for 5 min. The probe was labeled by covalently linking to alkaline phosphatase by incubating at 37°C for 30 min with crosslinker solution and reaction buffer. The blot was prehybridized with 0.125 ml/cm2 hybridization buffer containing 12%

w/v urea, 0.5 M NaCl and 4% blocking reagent at 55°C for at least 15 min. The labeled probe was added into hybridization buffer and hybridized to the membrane containing samples at 55°C overnight. The blot was then washed twice with 55°C primary washing buffer (2 M Urea, 0.1% w/v SDS, 50 mM Na phosphate pH 7, 150 mM NaCl, 1 mM $MgCl_2$, 0.2% w/v blocking reagent) for 10 min with gentle agitation. The blot was then washed twice with secondary wash buffer (50 mM Tris-Cl, 100 mM NaCl, 2 mM $MgCl_2$, pH 10) at room temperature for 5 min. A chemiluminescent signal was generated by adding 40 μl/cm^2 CDP-Star detection reagent (Amersham Biosciences, Uppsala, Sweden) and detected on X-ray film.

3.2.2 Microsatellite typing

Microsatellite typing was used in genomic analysis in this study (Fig. 5). The polymorphic markers, showing a high heterozygosity frequency, were used. PCR was performed to amplify genomic regions of particular markers. PCR reactions were carried out with 100 ng of DNA template, 1X PCR buffer, 2.5 mM $MgCl_2$, 200 μM dNTP, 0.1 unit of AmpliTaq Gold DNA polymerase (Applied Biosystems, CA, USA), 0.3 μM of each fluorescence-labeled primer. PCR products were injected into semi-automated ABI PRISMTM 3100 Genetic Analyzer (Applied Biosystems, CA, USA) for capillary electrophoresis and analysis by Genotyper software. All markers were labeled with 6-FAM/VIC/NED fluorescence dye and have annealing temperatures of 55°C.

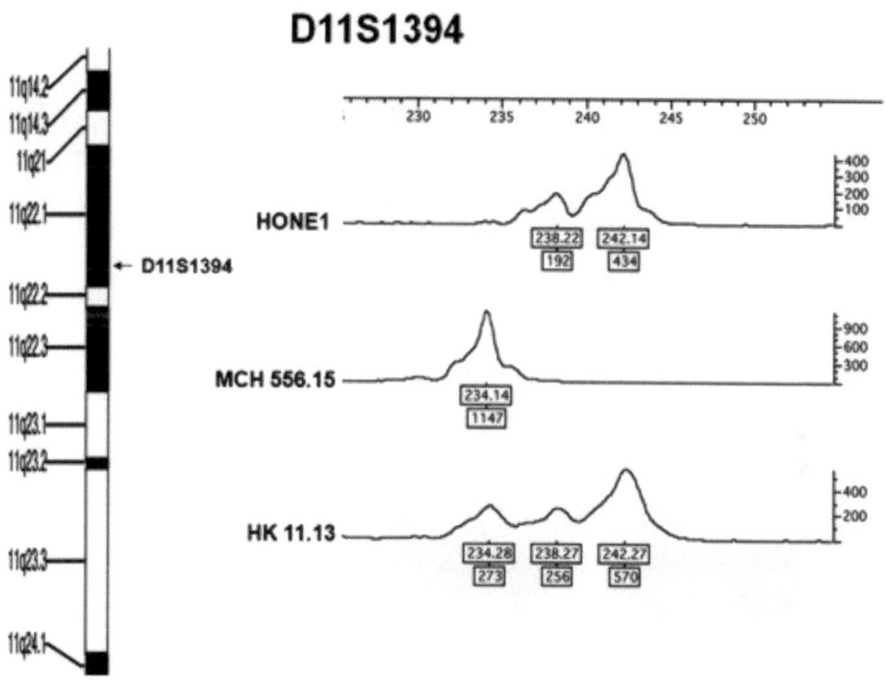

Fig. 5. PCR microsatellite typing of a representative donor, recipient, and hybrid cell line. The recipient HONE1, donor MCH556.15, and MCH HK11.13 cell lines were analyzed with the D11S1394 primers. The combined peak patterns of the hybrid cell line show successful transfer of chromosome 11 in recipient cells.

3.2.3 Whole chromosome painting FISH

The confirmation of the presence of an extra copy of intact human chromosome in the hybrids was performed by whole chromosome painting FISH analysis. To obtain metaphase cells, logarithmic growth phase cells were treated with 0.05 μg/ml colcemid for 4-6 hours. After harvesting the cells by centrifugation at 4000 rpm for 5 min, they were subjected to hypotonic treatment (0.075 M KCl) for no more than 25 min at 37°C. Cells were fixed with methanol/acetic acid (3:1) overnight and then dropped onto glass slides. The whole chromosome paint (WCP) probes were used and they are a mixture of DNA sequences specific to a particular chromosome that are directly labeled with one of the Vysis™ fluorophores. The slides were denatured at 73°C for 5 min [70% (v/v) formamide, 2 X SSC (pH7), 0.1 mM EDTA]. Slides were dehydrated for 1 min in 70%, 85%, and 100% ethanol successively. Probes were hybridized to the slides in LSI/WCP® hybridization buffer at 37°C in dark for overnight. The slide was washed at 73°C in washing solution I (0.4 X SSC, 0.3% NP40) for no more than 2 min, followed by washing with washing solution II (2 X SSC, 0.1% NP40), and counterstained with DAPI. Fluorescence signals were captured on an Olympus BX51 fluorescence microscope with the Spot software.

3.3 *In vivo* nude mouse tumorigenicity assay and establishment of tumor segregants (TSs)

After successful chromosome transfer, MCHs containing an exogenous chromosome were obtained and the tumorigenicity assay was then performed. The tumorigenicity of the each NPC/ESCC cell line was investigated by subcutaneous injection of 1 X 10^7 cells into 6-8 week old female athymic BALB/c *nu/nu* mice. This assay has been repeatedly and successfully used for assessing the degree of tumor suppression in MCH populations (Goyette et al 1992, Saxon et al 1985, Weissman et al 1987). For each tested cell line, at least six sites were injected on three mice (two sites per animal). The animals were monitored regularly for tumor formation and palpable nodules were measured weekly using calipers. After a long period of incubation in the nude mice (>12 weeks), if notable tumors formed, they were surgically removed aseptically and then washed with PBS, followed by mincing the tissues as small as possible in a petri dish. The minced tissue was covered with 5 ml medium and left without any disturbance for at least three days. Medium was withdrawn and 10 ml of fresh medium was added. The cells were then harvested and were the TSs/revertants used in further analysis with their matched MCHs.

3.4 TS analysis

The TSs show a restoration of tumorigenicity in the tumorigenicity assay by elimination of critical regions (CRs) associated with tumor suppression (Cheng et al 2002, Cheung et al 2009). Loss of donor genetic materials detected by microsatellite typing (see Section 3.2.2) was considered significant, when the intensity of the donor to recipient allele ratio in a TS versus its corresponding MCH parental cell line, was equal to or less than 0.8. The significance of these losses was simultaneously verified by bacterial artificial chromosome (BAC) FISH. Furthermore, the differential gene expression profiling between the tumor-suppressive MCH cell lines versus their derived TSs and the highly tumorigenic recipient cell line was revealed by oligo microarray analysis. The BAC FISH and oligo microarray analyses will be discussed in detail.

3.4.1 Bacterial artificial chromosome (BAC) FISH

The BAC DNA probes were prepared by labeling the isolated BAC DNAs by nick translation. In brief, BAC clones were incubated in 5 ml LB medium containing 12.5 µg/ml chloramphenicol at 37°C overnight. Bacterial cells were pelleted down and resuspended in 200 µl of ice-cold alkaline lysis solution I. Four hundred microliters of freshly prepared alkaline lysis solution II were added, mixed by gentle inversion several times, and placed on ice for no more than 5 minutes. A total of 300 µl of ice-cold solution III was added, and the mixture was put on ice for 5 minutes, followed by centrifugation at maximum speed for five minutes at 4°C. Supernatant was transferred into a fresh 1.5 ml tube containing 900 µl of isopropanol at room temperature and mixed by gentle inversion. The precipitated DNA was collected by centrifugation at maximum speed for five minutes at 4°C; supernatant was discarded and the pellet was rinsed with 1 ml of 75% ethanol. The tube was centrifuged for 5 min at room temperature and ethanol was removed. The DNA pellet was air-dried and dissolved in 50 µl TE.

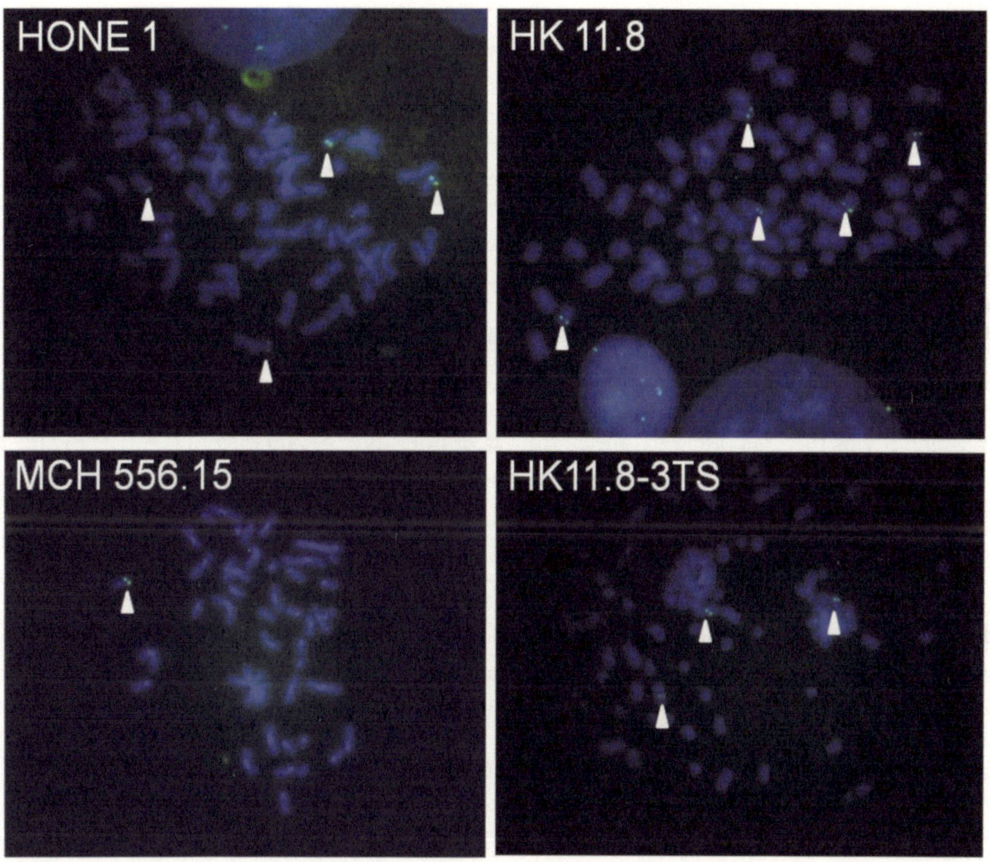

Fig. 6. FISH analysis with BAC CTB-12N1 probe in recipient HONE1 cells, chromosome 11 donor MCH556.15 cells, hybrid HK11.8 cells, and tumor revertant HK11.8-3TS cells. Thirty metaphases on average were observed for each cell line. Four copies of the BAC probe are observed in HONE1 cells, one in the donor cell line, 5 in the hybrid HK11.8 and 3 in the HK11.8-3TS. Arrows (▲) indicate BAC hybridization.

A total of 500 ng of BAC DNA was labeled with 10 µM SpectrumGreen/Orange TM-dUTP (Vysis, IL, USA), nick translation buffer (Vysis, IL, USA), 10 µl nick translation enzyme (Vysis, IL, USA) at 14°C for 16 hours and stopped at 70°C for 10 minutes. The probe was precipitated with 1 µg of COT-1 DNA (Invitrogen, CA, USA) and 2 µg salmon sperm DNA (Invitrogen, CA, USA), 4 µl water, 0.1 volume of 2 M sodium acetate, 2.5 volumes 100% ethanol and centrifuged at maximum speed for 30 min at 4°C. The supernatant was removed. The pellet was air-dried and resuspended in 3 µl water and 7 µl LSI/WCP hybridization buffer. Procedures for the hybridization and detection were the same as that used for the whole chromosome painting FISH. Representative BAC FISH results are shown in Figure 6.

3.4.2 Oligonucleotide microarray

In order to investigate the differentially expressed genes of the tumor-suppressive MCHs versus their matched tumorigenic TSs, oligonucleotide microarray analysis was performed; a TSG is presumably up-regulated in MCHs and down-regulated in TSs (Robertson et al 1997). Therefore, genes with that expression profile are potential TSGs in NPC. This method can also help to identify candidate genes that are downstream of the functional pathways. The 19K or 28K oligonucleotides were spotted on glass slides using a custom-built microarray spotter at the Genome Institute of Singapore. The incorporation of Cy3 and Cy5 to cDNAs, competitive hybridizations, and processing of array images were performed as described (Lin et al 2004).

In brief, a total of 20 µg of total RNA was mixed with 1 µg oligo dT and denatured at 65°C for 5 min. Reverse transcription was done by using 1X first strand buffer, 4 µl of 0.1 M DTT, 2 µl 20X low dT/aa-dUTP mix (1 M dATP, 1 M dGTP, 1 M dCTP, 200 mM dTTP, and 800 mM amminoallyl dUTP), 100 unit of RNase OUT inhibitor (Invitrogen, CA, USA), and 400 units of SuperScript II reverse transcriptase (Invitrogen, CA, USA) and incubated at 42°C for 60 min. Another 200 units of SuperScript II reverse transcriptase was added to the mixture and then it was incubated at 42°C for 60 min. Five microliter of 500 mM EDTA (pH 8) and 10 µl of 1M NaOH were added to the reaction mixture and incubated at 65°C for 45 min, followed by adding 25 µl of 1 M Tris-Cl (pH 7.5) and 400 µl ddH_2O and purified on a YM-30 column (Millipore, MA, USA). One microliter of 500 mM $NaHCO_3$ (pH 9) and fluorescent dye, Cy3 or Cy5 (GE Health Care Life Sciences, NJ, USA), were added to 9 µl of the cDNA for dye incorporation at room temperature for 1 hour.

The chips, which contain synthesized 60-mers of 19K or 28K oligonucleotides, were prehybridized by using DIG Easy Hyb (Roche Diagnostics, Basel, Switzerland) at 42°C for one hour. Four microliter of 4 M hydroxylamine (Sigma, MO, USA) was added to the labeled cDNA at room temperature for 15 min. Thirty-five microliter of 100 mM NaOAc (pH 5.2) was added and mixed with the paired sample labeled with Cy3 and Cy5. The reaction mixtures were purified on YM-30 columns, containing 40 µg of herring sperm DNA (Invitrogen, CA, USA) and 22 µl DIG Easy Hyb were added, followed by denaturing at 65°C for 5 min. The cDNA probe was hybridized onto slides and incubated in the MAUI hybridization chamber (BioMicro Systems, UT, USA) at 42°C for 16 hours. After hybridization, slides were washed with 2X SSC + 0.1% SDS for 30 s, 1X SSC for 30 s and 0.2X SSC for 30 s and 0.05X SSC for 5 s. The slides were then scanned with GenePix 3100 microarray scanner and analyzed by GenePix Pro 4.0 and 5.0 software (Axon Instruments, CA, USA). The results were uploaded to the database from Genome Institute of Singapore

(GIS MAdb, http://gismadb.gis.a-star.edu.sg). The hierarchical clustering was performed by CLUSTER program and the results were viewed by the TREE VIEW program (M. Eisen; http://rana.lbl.gov/EisenSoftware.htm). Stringency was set so that only data sets with expression ratios higher than 1.4 in hybrids/recipient cells and ratios less than 0.6 in hybrids/TSs for both duplicates were selected for further studies.

3.5 Methylation study of candidate tumor suppressor genes

Promoter hypermethylation is a major mechanism for silencing TSG expression. Promoter hypermethylation only occurs at cytosine (C), which is located on the 5′ end of guanine (G) of promoter CpG islands. Addition of a methyl group to cytosine by methyltransferase blocks the binding of the activator or inhibitor to the promoter sequence and consequently there is transcriptional silencing of the gene. By using 5-aza-2′-deoxycytidine, which can demethylate the methyl groups in the CpG islands, gene expression can be restored. Using this approach, methylation status of genes of interest may be elucidated. Besides using the 5-aza-2"-deoxycytidine, bisulfite genomic sequencing (BGS) and methylation-specific PCR (MSP) are other important methods used to analyze promoter hypermethylation. In the bisulfite treatment, the genomic DNAs are modified. All of the unmethylated cytosines are converted to uracils, while the methylated cytosines remain unchanged. By analyzing the promoter sequences and using sequence-specific primers, the promoter hypermethylation status can be determined.

3.5.1 Bisulfite treatment

Genomic DNA was treated with sodium metabisulfite to analyze the promoter hypermethylation status. Two micrograms of DNA were dissolved in 10 µl of water, followed by adding 1.1 µl of 3N NaOH and incubation at 37°C for 15 min. Then 104 µl of urea/metabisulfite solution (6.24 M urea and 2 M sodium metabisulfite; Sigma, MO, USA), 6 µl of 10 mM hydroquinone (Sigma, MO, USA) and 100 µl of mineral oil were added into the mixture and incubated at 55°C for no more than 15 hours. The mixture was then purified by QIAquick PCR purification Kit (Qiagen, CA, USA) according to the manufacturer's protocol and eluted with 200 µl elution buffer. The purified DNA was denatured in 23 µl of 3N NaOH at 37°C for 15 min. The DNA was precipitated by adding 2 µl of tRNA (10 µg/µl; USB, OH, USA), 50 µl of 10 M ammonium acetate, and 500 µl of 100% ethanol, and stored at -20°C for 30 min. The mixture was centrifuged at 12K rpm at 4°C for 20 min; the supernatant was removed. The DNA pellet was washed with 500 µl of 70% ethanol and centrifuged at full speed at 4°C for 20 min. The DNA pellet was air-dried and dissolved in 100 µl of 10 mM Tris-Cl (pH 8.5) solution.

3.5.2 Bisulfite genomic sequencing (BGS) and methylation-specific PCR (MSP)

BGS and MSP PCR reactions were carried out with 5 µl of bisulfite-treated DNA template, 1X PCR buffer, 2.5 mM $MgCl_2$, 200 µM dNTP, 0.1 unit of AmpliTaq Gold DNA polymerase (Applied Biosystems, CA, USA), 0.3 µM of primers. For the BGS, PCR products were then cloned into the TA cloning pMD18T Simple vector (TaKaRa Biotechnology, Dalian, China) and transformed into competent cells. Mini-preparation was performed to extract the plasmid DNA. For each examined cell line, five individual clones were checked to confirm the promoter hypermethylation status. The plasmids were then sequenced by using pMD18T7 forward and reverse sequencing primers and BigDye 3.1 terminator. Signals were detected using an ABI PRISMTM 3100 Genetic Analyzer (Applied Biosystems, CA, USA). The bisulfite sequencing and MSP primers were designed by the MethPrimer (www.urogene.org/methprimer) guide (Li et al 2002).

3.5.3 5-Aza-2'-deoxycytidine treatment

The re-expression of the candidate genes silenced by promoter hypermethylation was investigated using a demethylation reagent. Cells were treated with 5 µM 5-aza-2'-deoxycytidine (Sigma, MO, USA) for five days; freshly diluted drug was changed daily. After 5 days treatment, the cells were harvested for RNA extraction.

3.6 Other functional assays we use to study the tumor suppressive phenotypes

In order to examine the tumor suppressive phenotypes of NPC and EC cells expressing a candidate TSG, various functional assays were performed according to the major hallmarks of cancer (Hanahan et al 2011). Simple proliferation, cell cycle, colony formation, and soft agar assays are routinely performed to assess the inhibitory effects of the transgenes on cell growth ability in normal culture conditions, the change of cell cycle status, the ability of colony formation from a single cells, and the cell growth potential in an the anchorage-independent environment. In addition, the migration, invasion, and angiogenic properties of the tumor suppressive transfectants were also examined. Some of those functional assays will be discussed in detail.

3.6.1 Three-dimensional matrigel culture

Matrigel contains a gelatinous protein mixture of extracellular matrix proteins such as laminin and collagen, which recapitulates the natural environment of tumor cells for better investigation of the functional impact of a candidate TSG. We aim to see whether there is any change in the numbers, sizes, and morphologies of colonies of transfectants with the transgenes versus the vector-alone, when grown in matrigel. In brief, matrigel basement membrane matrix (BD Biosciences, San Jose, CA, USA) was thawed on ice and 100 µl was coated as a bottom layer onto each well of a 24-well cluster plate. Subsequently, a total of 5000 cells resuspended in 0.5 ml growth medium was seeded on top of this bottom matrigel layer. After 2 weeks, images were captured using an inverted light microscope (Nikon TMS, Ontario, Canada) at 20X magnification.

3.6.2 Cell migration and invasion assays

The cell migration and invasion abilities of cells were determined using a micropore chamber assay (BD Biosciences, San Jose, CA, USA). The chamber used for migration study consists of an 8 µm pore size PET membrane at the bottom of the insert, while the chamber used for invasion study is a migration chamber coated with a thin layer of matrigel basement matrix. The migration and invasion abilities of each clone were determined by the number of cells passing through the membrane and the matrigel basement matrix, respectively.

3.6.3 HUVEC tube formation assay

The tube formation assay is an *in vitro* angiogenesis assay to assess the tube formation ability of vascular endothelial cells. Briefly, the Human Umbilical Vein Endothelial Cell

(HUVEC) was cultured in collagen pre-coated TC dishes. The conditioned medium of each cell line was collected by incubating the cells with DMEM/RPMI serum-free medium for 24 hours. The 96-well plate pre-coated with 50 µl growth factor-reduced Matrigel (BD Bioscience, San Jose, CA, USA) per well was used. A total of 4 x 10^4 HUVEC cells resuspended in 100 µl conditioned media supplemented with 1% serum were seeded in each well. The HUVEC cells were then incubated at 37°C for 6 hours to allow the formation of tube-like structures. The tubes formed were captured under microscopy and the total tube length formed by each sample was measured by Spot software (Diagnostic Instruments Inc, Sterling Heights, MI, USA).

3.6.4 Matrigel plug angiogenesis study

In vivo angiogenesis study was performed by matrigel plug angiogenesis analysis. A total of 5 x 10^6 cells mixed with 50 µl DMEM and 250 µl ice-cold matrigel was injected into nude mice subcutaneously to allow gel plug formation. Each sample was injected into one flank of five female athymic nude mice. The matrigel mixed with the cells polymerizes to form a solid gel plug, which allows cell growth and blood vessel formation. After inoculation for 7 days, the matrigel plug was excised, fixed with formalin, embedded in paraffin, sectioned, and mounted onto slides. The slides were stained with hematoxylin and eosin (H&E) for histological observation. The blood vessels formed were stained with monoclonal antibody. The slide was scanned and the signal was quantified by ImageScope v10 software (Aperio, Vista, CA, USA).

3.6.5 Human angiogenesis antibody array

The angiogenesis-related proteins excreted from the TSGs versus the vector-alone transfectants were detected by the human angiogenesis antibody array (RayBiotech, Norcross, GA, USA). The array included two membranes pre-coated with 43 angiogenesis cytokine antibodies. The conditioned media were obtained as described in Section 3.6.3. After blocking and complete washing, the membranes were hybridized with biotin-conjugated antibody at room temperature for 2 hours, followed by hybridizing with HRP-conjugated streptavidin at room temperature for 2 hours. The membranes were then washed again and hybridized with the detection buffer. The signals were exposed to a X-ray film and quantified by Quantity One® software (Biorad, Hercules, CA, USA).

4. Examples of candidate TSGs studied via MMCT and other functional approaches

The technique of microcell fusion to transfer single normal chromosomes was used as a functional assay for the TSG activity (Goyette et al 1992, Saxon et al 1986, Weissman et al 1987). This has been particularly useful in confirming TSG functions associated with specific chromosomes, where the mapping location is suspected, but no candidate TSG has been cloned. In addition, by transferring chromosomes possessing interstitial deletions, it has been possible to map the location of TSGs more precisely (Dowdy et al 1991).

The analysis of tumor biopsy specimens, xenografts, and derived cell lines have identified an extensive chromosomal alterations in human genome, including those derived from chromosomes 1, 3, 9, 11, 12, 13, 14, 16, and 17 (Huang et al 1989, Mitelman et al 1983), Consistent with Knudson's "two-hit" theory, studies of chromosomal loss or deletion may provide useful clues for identification of critical genes involved in inherited cancers. However, it should be appreciated that the limitations of deletion or loss studies in sporadic cases may miss critical regions for several reasons. First, the minimally deleted regions may be obscured when all of the genome shows some degree of LOH, which is common in many sporadic tumors. Second, vast evidence has shown that some TSGs, notably *p16* are silenced or imprinted by epigenetic events such as methylation, irrespective of their LOH status in tumors. Third, LOH was studied in primary tumors with karyotypic complexity, gene dosage changes, and contamination by normal cells. Finally, although LOH is commonly detected in practically all types of human cancers, neither LOH nor CGH (comparative genomic hybridization) studies provide functional evidence. To map novel TSGs, functional and complementary approaches are needed for distinguishing a critical region from extensive randomly lost areas. Chromosome 3 was the first chromosome used for the functional studies of tumor suppression in NPC. In this study we used a series of intact and deleted copies of human chromosome 3 derived from normal cells, with discrete interstitial deletions in the *p* arm, for transfer into the tumorigenic NPC HONE1 cell line. By using the MMCT approach, we successfully transferred these chromosome 3 fragments into HONE1 cells and localized a tumor suppressive region on this chromosome. Comparison of the tumorigenic potential of the MCHs containing these exogenous chromosome 3 fragments identified chromosome 3p21.3 as the first tumor suppressive region in NPC (Cheng et al 1998). This area was subsequently confirmed to harbor several TSGs associated with the development of NPC and other common cancers (Lerman and Minna 2000, Lo *et al* 2001, Yau *et al* 2006, Hesson *et al* 2007). Using these functional approaches, we also investigated known and candidate TSGs in other chromosomes, including chromosomes 9, 11, 13, 14 and 17. These chromosomes contain important TSGs, such as *p16, RB* and *p53* and a number of newly-identified TSGs. However, we only introduce a few of examples of these studies in this chapter due to the space limitation. (Cheng *et al*, 2000, 2002, 2003 and 2004, Ko et al 2005 and 2008, Lung *et al* 2008a and 2008b, Cheung *et al* 2009, Lo *et al* 2007 and 2010)

4.1 Chromosome 3: *ADAMTS9*

In a subsequent study, an intact and two truncated human chromosomes 3 obtained from the same panel of chromosome 3 donor cells, were transferred into the highly tumorigenic ESCC SLMT-1 cell line. Similarly, the ability of these transferred chromosomes to functionally complement defects in the ESCC cell line was assessed by examining the impact of this transfer on tumorigenic potential in nude mice. PCR-microsatellite and BAC FISH analyses were used to narrow down and identify the CR associated specifically with tumor suppression. A 1.61 Mb CR located between markers D3S1600 and D3S1285 was found to be necessary for the tumorigenic suppression of ESCC. These findings further suggest that the CR present in the exogenous chromosomes contains functional tumor suppressive elements. In the study, we identified a candidate TSG, *ADAMTS9*, and one non-coding RNA, ENST351926 mapping to 3p14.2, which are located in the chromosome 3 CR of ESCC. The expression of *ADAMTS9* in tumor suppressive MCHs was confirmed by reverse transcription (RT)–PCR. The positive expression of the gene was observed in all tumor suppressive MCHs, but was not found in tumorigenic MCHs and TSs, strongly suggesting that *ADAMTS9* plays an important role in tumor suppression. The pseudogene is located upstream of the *ADAMTS9* promoter region and whether it can serve as a riboregulator or gene expression regulator remains to be determined (Lo et al 2007).

4.1.1 *ADAMTS9 (A disintegrin-like and metalloprotease with thrombospondin type 1 motif 9)*

As described, using a functional genomic mapping approach, we identified a CR for tumor suppression at 3p14.2 and discovered the important role of A Disintegrin-like And Metalloprotease with ThromboSpondin type 1 motif 9 (ADAMTS9), a gene previously mapped to this region (Clark et al 2000) in ESCC (Holmes and Vaughan 2007). ADAMTS9 encodes a member of a large family of 19 metalloproteases involved in maturation of precursor proteins, extracellular matrix remodeling, cell migration, and inhibition of angiogenesis (Apte 2004, Porter et al 2005). Although the related matrix metalloproteases and ADAM proteases have been clearly implicated in tumor progression and angiogenesis, the role of ADAMTS proteases in cancer is less clearly defined. ADAMTS1 was first identified as an anti-angiogenic molecule (Vazquez et al 1999), and shown to have anti-tumor effects. Recently, methylation studies identified another family member ADAMTS18 as crucial in several human cancers including NPC and ESCC (Jin et al 2007).

As mentioned in the previous section, *ADAMTS9* was identified as one of the differentially expressed genes in these non-tumorigenic MCHs and their matched TS cell lines in our previous study (Lo et al 2007). It was suggested that ADAMTS9 is associated with tumor suppression in human esophageal cancer. Promoter hypermethylation contributes to ADAMTS9 gene silencing in ESCC (Lo et al 2007, Lung et al 2008b). However, the functional impact of ADAMTS9 on cancer development had not been explored. In the follow-up study, we evaluated the hypothesized anti-angiogenic and tumor suppressive functions of ADAMTS9 in ESCC, by stringent tumorigenicity and matrigel plug angiogenesis assays (Lo et al 2010). ADAMTS9 activation suppressed tumor formation in nude mice. In vivo angiogenesis assays revealed a reduction in microvessel numbers in gel plugs injected with tumor-suppressive cell transfectants. Similarly, conditioned media from cell transfectants dramatically reduced the tube-forming capacity of HUVECs. By using the angiogenesis antibody array, we found that these activities were associated with a reduction in expression levels of the pro-angiogenic factors, *MMP9* and *VEGFA*, which were consistently reduced in *ADAMTS9* transfectants. Based on the deletion patterns of the *ADAMTS9* transcripts in tumors and a TS derived from the tumorigenic transfectants, we speculate that the tumor-suppressive activity of *ADAMTS9* in ESCC was associated with the thrombospondin (TSP) domains in the C-terminal region of the gene. Taken together, our data strongly suggest that *ADAMTS9* plays a critical role in the "angiogenic switch" and transforms in the ESCC cell lines from a pro-angiogenic to a non-angiogenic phenotype.

4.2 Chromosome 9: *ENG, DEC1*

The transfer of chromosome 9 containing an interstitial deletion at 9p21 (where the well-known TSG, *p16* is located) to NPC HONE1 cell line did not result in tumor suppression in the nude mouse assay, but *p16* cDNA suppressed growth of HONE1 cells *in vitro* assay. It suggests that *p16* gene plays an important role in this cancer (Cheng et al., 2000). The similar transfer of chromosome 9 into SLMT1 provided the first functional tumor suppressive evidence in ESCC (Yang et al 2005). The result suggested that gene(s) other than p16 on chromosome 9 is (are) important for ESCC tumorigenesis. The ESCC chromosome 9 MCHs exhibited a delayed latency period in tumor formation compared with that of the parental SLMT1 cells. The delay in tumor growth kinetics was hypothesized to be associated with the loss or inactivation of wild type alleles from the exogenous transferred donor chromosome 9. Detailed microsatellite marker-PCR deletion mapping analysis of the tumor suppressive chromosome 9 MCHs and their corresponding derived TSs delineated that the critical regions that may harbor candidate TSGs to a 2.4 Mb region at 9q33-q34 around D9S112.

4.2.1 *ENG (Endoglin)*

The MMCT-identified CR at 9q32-34 is a gene-rich region. *ENG (Endoglin)*, mapping to 9q33-q34.1, is a component of the transforming growth factor beta (TGF-β) receptor complex and is involved in tumor angiogenesis by modulating the biological effect of TGF-β. Significant down-regulation of *ENG* was detected at frequencies of 87.5% in 16 ESCC cell lines, 39.1% directly in 23 ESCC tumor specimens from Hong Kong, and 33.4% in 18 ESCC tumor specimens from the high-risk ESCC region of Henan, China. Both epigenetic methylation and allelic loss appear to contribute to *ENG* down-regulation in ESCC tumors. Subsequent functional studies with restoration of *ENG* in an ESCC cell line demonstrated that *ENG* plays a critical role in ESCC carcinogenesis. Colony formation efficiency was significantly reduced by over-expression of *ENG*. In addition, significantly smaller colonies of *ENG* stable transfectants were formed in Matrigel culture. Significant suppression of invasion efficiency and tumorigenicity were also observed, when comparing the *ENG* stable transfectants with the vector-alone transfectants. No report had yet verified the functional role of *ENG* in ESCC tumor cells. This study provides evidence supporting *ENG*, as a cell invasion and tumor-suppressing gene in ESCC. *ENG* may be functionally involved in TGF-β signaling. Down-regulation of *ENG* in esophageal cancer in this study may provoke cancer progression through blocking the tumor suppression of the TGF-β signaling cascade. For the functional impact of *ENG* in cell migration, *ENG* may suppress cancer cell motility by a TGF-β-dependent mechanism involving activation of the type I TGF-β receptor and Smad1, as reported in the study of prostate cancer cells (Craft et al 2007). In endothelial cells, high endoglin expression stimulates the type I activin receptor-like kinases (ALK1) pathway and indirectly inhibits ALK5 signaling for endothelial cell proliferation and migration, thus promoting the state of angiogenesis. *ENG* may act differently in cancer cell versus endothelial cells. *ENG* may suppress cancer cell proliferation in the pre-malignant stage; meanwhile, its expression could promote angiogenesis facilitating the cancer progression in the late malignant stage. The mechanism of ENG in suppressing ECSC tumor requires further study (Wong et al 2008).

4.2.2 *DEC1 (Deleted in Esophageal Cancer 1)*

DEC1 (*Deleted in Esophageal Cancer 1*) is in the vicinity of the CR at 9q32-34 and is down-regulated frequently in ESCC cell lines and tumor tissues (Leung et al 2008). The DEC1 protein localizes to both the cytoplasm and nucleus. The vesicular pattern of DEC1 in the cytoplasm appears to localize at the Golgi and Golgi-endoplasmic reticulum intermediate compartment. DEC1 is clinically important as the tissue microarray (TMA) study suggested an association of DEC1 expression with lymph node metastasis, early onset ESCC, and familial status (Wong et al 2011b). DEC1 stably transfected clones provided functional evidence for cell growth inhibition in vitro and significant delay in tumor growth in vivo (Yang et al., 2005). DEC1 stable clones showed significantly fewer colony numbers as compared to the vector-alone control. Restoration of DEC1 expression also negatively affected anchorage-independent growth properties of an ESCC cell line (Leung et al 2008). Using cDNA microarray analysis to reveal the differential expression profiling between tumor suppressive *DEC1* clones versus the vector-alone transfectant, *DUSP6* (*dual-specificity phosphatase 6*) was identified as one of the downstream targets of *DEC1*, as it is up-regulated in *DEC1* stable transfectants, C4 and C9, compared to vector-alone stable transfectants. It is expected that in clinical specimens, the higher expression of *DEC1* associates with higher expression of *DUSP6*. This association was observed in tumor tissues in younger aged ESCC patients group. This association was only significant in these two groups, which was limited by the number of available samples (only 26 normal counterpart tissues and 74 tumor tissues). Subsequent functional study of *DUSP* also indicated that *DUSP6* plays a crucial role for ESCC carcinogenesis by inhibiting cell invasion and impairing the epithelial-mesenchymal transition (EMT)-associated phenotype (Wong et al 2011a).

4.3 Chromosome 13: *THSD1*

Chromosome 13q deletions are frequent events in several human cancers, including ESCC (Hu et al 2000, Pack et al 1999), nasopharyngeal (Tsang et al 1999) and lung (Tamura et al 1997) cancers. Molecular evidence of gross deletions which implicate the existence of TSGs came from numerous LOH and CGH studies. Our group has pioneered the identification of the TSGs on chromosome 13 by the functional complementation approach in both NPC and ESCC (Cheng et al 2004, Ko et al 2008). The transfer of intact chromosome 13 in HONE1 cells identified a critical region essential for the viability and growth of NPC MCHs at chromosome 13q12, but it was not RB gene (Cheng et al 2004). By the microsatellite deletion mapping, D13S893 at 13q12, a minimally deleted region of 0.7 Mb, was found to be non-randomly eliminated in the six chromosome 13 MCHs bounded by markers D13S1287 and D13S260. The growth suppressive activity involved at least one novel growth control gene for NPC tumorigenesis. Our subsequent study employed the same MMCT technique in an ESCC model with the ESCC cell line, SLMT1. The transfer of an intact chromosome 13 into this highly tumorigenic recipient cell line conferred tumor suppressive activity, and identified critical regions at 13q12.3, 13q14.11, and 13q14.3. Of interest, a 0.373 Mb at the critical region 2 (CR2), mapped to 13q12.3 and was co-localized to the same CR identified in the NPC model system in our chromosome 13 transfer study (Cheng et al 2004, Ko et al 2008).

4.3.1 *THSD1 (Thrombospondin type I domain-containing 1)*

The ESCC functional studies implicate the importance of chromosome 13q14 in tumor suppression; TS microsatellite-deletion mapping analysis localized two CRs (CR3 at D13S263 and CR4 at D13S133) at chromosomal region 13q14, which are frequently eliminated (Ko et al 2008). Differential gene expression profiles of a reference immortalized normal esophageal epithelial cell line, three tumor-suppressing MCHs, and their tumorigenic parental SLMT1 cell line were revealed by cDNA oligonucleotide microarray analysis. Nine 13q14 candidates genes, including *RB1*, were identified to show down-regulation in SLMT-1 as compared to NE1, the immortalized normal esophageal epithelial cell line, and the MCHs. *RB1* is a well-known TSG mapped to 13q14, but our Western blot analysis indicated that the active form of RB was not increased in the tumor suppressive MCHs (data not shown). The data suggested that novel candidate TSG(s) other than *RB1* should be involved in the observed tumor suppression. RT-PCR was performed for *KIAA0853, ESD, CHC1L, PHF11, RFP2, FLJ11712, THSD1*, and *C13orf9*. Real-time PCR results validated the frequent down-regulation of *THSD1* and *PHF11* in ESCC cell lines. *THSD1* is located between *FLJ11712* and *C13orf9* within 13q14.3, but only specific loss of *THSD1* expression in all cancer cell lines was detected. Since *THSD1* showed a more prominent loss than that of *PHF11*, it was the first target chosen for further functional characterization. Epigenetic silencing and LOH were the mechanisms responsible, at least in part, for the loss of *THSD1* expression in ESCC tumorigenesis. The wild type *THSD1* transfection in SLMT1 resulted in significant reduction of colony formation ability, providing evidence for a growth suppressive role of *THSD1* in ESCC tumorigenesis.

The function of *THSD1* is unknown. It encodes a transmembrane molecule containing a thrombospondin type 1 repeat (TSR), which may be involved in cell adhesion and angiogenesis (de Fraipont et al 2001). Interestingly, analysis of the differential expression levels of this gene in previous microarray studies show that high *THSD1* expression positively correlated with a better distant metastasis survival in breast cancer patients. This is consistent with its loss possibly being associated with metastatic tumor spread; studies are needed to evaluate its potential importance as a biomarker for esophageal carcinoma. Further functional studies on *THSD1* are now underway to elucidate its tumor suppressive role.

4.4 Chromosome 14: *LTBP-2*

Chromosome 14 loss is commonly found in different cancers, including esophageal (Ihara et al 2002), renal (Yoshimoto et al 2007), lung (Weir et al 2007), and colon cancers (Mourra et al 2007). In NPC extensive chromosome 14 allelic loss has been reported (Dodd et al 2006, Lo et al 2000, Lung et al 2001, Shao et al 2002). This suggests the importance of chromosome 14 in tumor development. In our earlier NPC study, chromosome 14q11.2-13.1 and 14q32.1 regions were found to associate with tumor suppression. In those chromosome 14 MCHs, non-random eliminations of two CRs were consistently observed and associated with tumor growth in tumorigenicity assays (Cheng et al 2003). In a later study, a new panel of chromosome 14 MCHs with an intact exogenous chromosome 14 was established. The potent ability to suppress tumor growth in the *in vivo* tumorigenicity assay of all intact chromosome 14 MCHs suggests the ability of chromosome 14 to suppress tumor formation in HONE1 cells. This is consistent with chromosome 14 harboring candidate TSGs involved in NPC development (Cheung et al 2009).

An intact chromosome 14 was also transferred into the ESCC SLMT1 cell line. The tumorigenic potential of microcell hybrids containing the transferred chromosome 14 provided functional evidence that tumor-suppressive regions of chromosome 14 are essential for esophageal cancer. TSs emerging in nude mice during the tumorigenicity assay was analyzed by detailed PCR-microsatellite typing and dual-colour BAC FISH to identify critical non-randomly eliminated regions. A 680-kb CR mapped to 14q32.13 and an approximately 2.2-Mb CR mapped to 14q32.33 were delineated. (Ko et al 2005). Microarray differential gene expression profiling of tumor-suppressive chromosome 14 MCH cell lines and their tumorigenic TSs identified *LTBP-2* (*latent transforming growth factor β binding protein 2*) mapped to 14q24 as a candidate TSG important for ESCC (Chan et al 2011).

4.4.1 *LTBP-2 (Latent transforming growth factor β binding protein 2)*

The extracellular matrix (ECM) protein *LTBP-2* (*Latent transforming growth factor β binding protein 2)* encodes a secretary protein that functions as a component of the ECM microfibrils and belongs to the LTBP/fibrillin family (Chan et al 2011). Unlike other members in LTBP family, LTBP-2 does not form complexes with the small latent TGF-βs. Interestingly, in addition to the first reported tumor suppressor role in ESCC, *LTBP-2* is related to congenital glaucoma and rheumatoid arthritis which are eye and bone diseases, respectively. LTBP-2 expression at the mRNA and protein levels was down-regulated in both ESCC cell lines and primary tumors. One of the mechanisms responsible for the down-regulation of *LTBP-2* is via promoter hypermethylation. Restoration of *LTBP-2* in an ESCC cancer cell line resulted in tumor suppression in nude mouse assay, which is partially explained by the significant reduction of colony-forming ability on matrigel 3D culture and anchorage-independent growth *in vitro*. Further *in vitro* functional characterization of *LTBP-2* demonstrated its inhibitory role in angiogenesis, migration, and invasion of cancer cells. An angiogenesis protein array analysis of conditioned medium from *LTBP-2* stable clone revealed the change in expressions of different cytokines, including GM-CSF, RANTES, VEGF, uPAR, I-309, MMP-1, Angiopoietin-1, and MCP-1, which in turn induce a less favorable microenvironment for angiogenesis and tumor growth. ESCC is a deadly disease and patients are usually diagnosed at late stage. In many late stage tumors, the TGF-β signaling pathway is involved in the activation of EMT program, which is responsible for cancer cell traits promoting malignancy. In contrast, TGF-β is well-known to be anti-proliferative. Interestingly, an inverse correlation of high LTBP-2 and survival in advanced ESCC stage was detected by IHC staining of primary ESCC tissues. LTBP-2 may indirectly regulate TGF-β by competing with LTBP-1 for fibrillin-1 binding site (Hirani et al 2007).

5. Conclusions

In this book chapter, we focus on using MMCT, as a functional approach to identify candidate TSGs. The monochromosome transfers of selected chromosomes into the NPC and ESCC cell lines, HONE1 and SLMT1, were performed to determine whether tumor suppressing activities for NPC and ESCC mapped to chromosomes 3, 9, 11, 13, 14 and 17, as described in our previous reports. While all these experiments have been performed in the two NPC and SLMT1 cell lines HONE1 and SLMT1, it should be appreciated there are a few of well-established and well-characterized NPC and ESCC cell lines available for this kind of study. Not surprisingly, identification of TSGs or regions in these cell lines was subsequently confirmed to be important in other NPC and ESCC cell lines as well as primary tumors. By using the MMCT approach, we successfully identified several CRs associated with tumor suppression in the HONE1/SLMT1 cell line systems. These candidate TSGs mapping to these regions were subsequently studied for their role in tumor suppression assays. We discovered that *ADAMTS9* at 3p14.2, *ENG* and *DEC1* at 9q33-q34, are genes mapped into CRs, and important for tumor suppression in ESCC. Gene expression profiling of the 19K and 28K oligonucleotide microarrays, including tumor-suppressive MCH and tumorigenic TS cell lines, was utilized to identify candidate genes (*THSD1* and *LTBP-2*) within the critical tumor suppressive regions. It is clear now that many genes contribute to the development of these two important cancers.

6. Acknowledgements

We would like to acknowledge the financial support from the Research Grants Council and the University Research Council of the Hong Kong Special Administrative Region, People's

Republic of China. We would also like to acknowledge our local and international collaborators for their cell lines, clinical tissues, TSG constructs, reagents, technologies, and valuable advice. In particular, Eric Stanbridge's contributions to the MMCT and Edison Liu's supply of oligonucleotide arrays, were invaluable for these studies.

7. References

Anderson MJ and Stanbridge EJ (1993). Tumor suppressor genes studied by cell hybridization and chromosome transfer. *Faseb J* 7: 826-833.

Apte SS (2004). A disintegrin-like and metalloprotease (reprolysin type) with thrombospondin type 1 motifs: the ADAMTS family. *Int J Biochem Cell Biol* 36: 981-985.

Chan SH, Yee Ko JM, Chan KW, Chan YP, Tao Q, Hyytiainen M, Keski-Oja J, Law S, Srivastava G, Tang J, Tsao SW, Chen H, Stanbridge EJ and Lung ML (2011). The ECM protein LTBP-2 is a suppressor of esophageal squamous cell carcinoma tumor formation but higher tumor expression associates with poor patient outcome. *Int J Cancer* 129: 565-573.

Cheng Y, Poulos NE, Lung ML, Hampton G, Ou B, Lerman MI and Stanbridge EJ (1998). Functional evidence for a nasopharyngeal carcinoma tumor suppressor gene that maps at chromosome 3p21.3. *Proc Natl Acad Sci U S A* 95: 3042-3047.

Cheng Y, Stanbridge EJ, Kong H, Bengtsson U, Lerman MI and Lung ML (2000). A functional investigation of tumor suppressor gene activities in a nasopharyngeal carcinoma cell line HONE1 using a monochromosome transfer approach. *Genes Chromosomes Cancer* 28: 82-91.

Cheng Y, Chakrabarti R, Garcia-Barcelo M, Ha TJ, Srivatsan ES, Stanbridge EJ and Lung ML (2002). Mapping of nasopharyngeal carcinoma tumor-suppressive activity to a 1.8-megabase region of chromosome band 11q13. *Genes Chromosomes Cancer* 34: 97-103.

Cheng Y, Ko JM, Lung HL, Lo PH, Stanbridge EJ and Lung ML (2003). Monochromosome transfer provides functional evidence for growth-suppressive genes on chromosome 14 in nasopharyngeal carcinoma. *Genes Chromosomes Cancer* 37: 359-368.

Cheng Y, Lung HL, Wong PS, Hao DC, Man CS, Stanbridge EJ and Lung ML (2004). Chromosome 13q12 region critical for the viability and growth of nasopharyngeal carcinoma hybrids. *Int J Cancer* 109: 357-362.

Cheung AK, Lung HL, Ko JM, Cheng Y, Stanbridge EJ, Zabarovsky ER, Nicholls JM, Chua D, Tsao SW, Guan XY and Lung ML (2009). Chromosome 14 transfer and functional studies identify a candidate tumor suppressor gene, mirror image polydactyly 1, in nasopharyngeal carcinoma. *Proc Natl Acad Sci U S A* 106: 14478-14483.

Clark ME, Kelner GS, Turbeville LA, Boyer A, Arden KC and Maki RA (2000). ADAMTS9, a novel member of the ADAM-TS/ metallospondin gene family. *Genomics* 67: 343-350.

Craft CS, Romero D, Vary CP and Bergan RC (2007). Endoglin inhibits prostate cancer motility via activation of the ALK2-Smad1 pathway. *Oncogene* 26: 7240-7250.

Daly JM, Fry WA, Little AG, Winchester DP, McKee RF, Stewart AK and Fremgen AM (2000). Esophageal cancer: results of an American College of Surgeons Patient Care Evaluation Study. *J Am Coll Surg* 190: 562-572; discussion 572-563.

de Fraipont F, Nicholson AC, Feige JJ and Van Meir EG (2001). Thrombospondins and tumor angiogenesis. *Trends Mol Med* 7: 401-407.

Dodd LE, Sengupta S, Chen IH, den Boon JA, Cheng YJ, Westra W, Newton MA, Mittl BF, McShane L, Chen CJ, Ahlquist P and Hildesheim A (2006). Genes involved in DNA repair and nitrosamine metabolism and those located on chromosome 14q32 are dysregulated in nasopharyngeal carcinoma. *Cancer Epidemiol Biomarkers Prev* 15: 2216-2225.

Dowdy SF, Scanlon DJ, Fasching CL, Casey G and Stanbridge EJ (1990). Irradiation microcell-mediated chromosome transfer (XMMCT): the generation of specific chromosomal arm deletions. *Genes Chromosomes Cancer* 2: 318-327.

Dowdy SF, Fasching CL, Araujo D, Lai KM, Livanos E, Weissman BE and Stanbridge EJ (1991). Suppression of tumorigenicity in Wilms tumor by the p15.5-p14 region of chromosome 11. *Science* 254: 293-295.

Fournier RE and Ruddle FH (1977a). Stable association of the human transgenome and host murine chromosomes demonstrated with trispecific microcell hybrids. *Proc Natl Acad Sci U S A* 74: 3937-3941.

Fournier RE and Ruddle FH (1977b). Microcell-mediated transfer of murine chromosomes into mouse, Chinese hamster, and human somatic cells. *Proc Natl Acad Sci U S A* 74: 319-323.

Friend SH, Bernards R, Rogelj S, Weinberg RA, Rapaport JM, Albert DM and Dryja TP (1986). A human DNA segment with properties of the gene that predisposes to retinoblastoma and osteosarcoma. *Nature* 323: 643-646.

Goyette MC, Cho K, Fasching CL, Levy DB, Kinzler KW, Paraskeva C, Vogelstein B and Stanbridge EJ (1992). Progression of colorectal cancer is associated with multiple tumor suppressor gene defects but inhibition of tumorigenicity is accomplished by correction of any single defect via chromosome transfer. *Mol Cell Biol* 12: 1387-1395.

Hanahan D and Weinberg RA (2011). Hallmarks of cancer: the next generation. *Cell* 144: 646-674.

Harris H, Miller OJ, Klein G, Worst P and Tachibana T (1969). Suppression of malignancy by cell fusion. *Nature* 223: 363-368.

Hesson LB, Cooper WN and Latif F (2007). Evaluation of the 3p21.3 tumor-suppressor gene cluster. *Oncogene* 26:7283-7301

Hirani R, Hanssen E and Gibson MA (2007). LTBP-2 specifically interacts with the amino-terminal region of fibrillin-1 and competes with LTBP-1 for binding to this microfibrillar protein. *Matrix Biol* 26: 213-223.

Holmes RS and Vaughan TL (2007). Epidemiology and pathogenesis of esophageal cancer. *Semin Radiat Oncol* 17: 2-9.

Hu N, Roth MJ, Polymeropolous M, Tang ZZ, Emmert-Buck MR, Wang QH, Goldstein AM, Feng SS, Dawsey SM, Ding T, Zhuang ZP, Han XY, Ried T, Giffen C and Taylor PR (2000). Identification of novel regions of allelic loss from a genomewide scan of esophageal squamous-cell carcinoma in a high-risk Chinese population. *Genes Chromosomes Cancer* 27: 217-228.

Huang DP, Ho JH, Chan WK, Lau WH and Lui M (1989). Cytogenetics of undifferentiated nasopharyngeal carcinoma xenografts from southern Chinese. *Int J Cancer* 43: 936-939.

Ihara Y, Kato Y, Bando T, Yamagishi F, Minamimura T, Sakamoto T, Tsukada K and Isobe M (2002). Allelic imbalance of 14q32 in esophageal carcinoma. *Cancer Genet Cytogenet* 135: 177-181.

Jeyakumar A, Brickman TM and Doerr T (2006). Review of nasopharyngeal carcinoma. *Ear Nose Throat J* 85: 168-170, 172-163, 184.

Jin H, Wang X, Ying J, Wong AH, Li H, Lee KY, Srivastava G, Chan AT, Yeo W, Ma BB, Putti TC, Lung ML, Shen ZY, Xu LY, Langford C and Tao Q (2007). Epigenetic identification of ADAMTS18 as a novel 16q23.1 tumor suppressor frequently silenced in esophageal, nasopharyngeal and multiple other carcinomas. *Oncogene* 26: 7490-7498.

Ko JM, Yau WL, Chan PL, Lung HL, Yang L, Lo PH, Tang JC, Srivastava G, Stanbridge EJ and Lung ML (2005). Functional evidence of decreased tumorigenicity associated with monochromosome transfer of chromosome 14 in esophageal cancer and the mapping of tumor-suppressive regions to 14q32. *Genes Chromosomes Cancer* 43: 284-293.

Ko JM, Chan PL, Yau WL, Chan HK, Chan KC, Yu ZY, Kwong FM, Miller LD, Liu ET, Yang LC, Lo PH, Stanbridge EJ, Tang JC, Srivastava G, Tsao SW, Law S and Lung ML (2008). Monochromosome transfer and microarray analysis identify a critical tumor-suppressive region mapping to chromosome 13q14 and THSD1 in esophageal carcinoma. *Mol Cancer Res* 6: 592-603.

Koi M, Morita H, Yamada H, Satoh H, Barrett JC and Oshimura M (1989). Normal human chromosome 11 suppresses tumorigenicity of human cervical tumor cell line SiHa. *Mol Carcinog* 2: 12-21.

Koi M, Johnson LA, Kalikin LM, Little PF, Nakamura Y and Feinberg AP (1993). Tumor cell growth arrest caused by subchromosomal transferable DNA fragments from chromosome 11. *Science* 260: 361-364.

Lerman MI, Minna JD (2000). The 630-kb lung cancer homozygous deletion region on human chromosome 3p21.3: identification and evaluation of the resident candidate tumor suppressor genes. The International Lung Cancer Chromosome 3p21.3 Tumor Suppressor Gene Consortium. *Cancer Res.* 60:6116-6133.

Leung AC, Wong VC, Yang LC, Chan PL, Daigo Y, Nakamura Y, Qi RZ, Miller LD, Liu ET, Wang LD, Li JL, Law S, Tsao SW and Lung ML (2008). Frequent decreased expression of candidate tumor suppressor gene, DEC1, and its anchorage-independent growth properties and impact on global gene expression in esophageal carcinoma. *Int J Cancer* 122: 587-594.

Li LC and Dahiya R (2002). MethPrimer: designing primers for methylation PCRs. *Bioinformatics* 18: 1427-1431.

Lin CY, Strom A, Vega VB, Kong SL, Yeo AL, Thomsen JS, Chan WC, Doray B, Bangarusamy DK, Ramasamy A, Vergara LA, Tang S, Chong A, Bajic VB, Miller LD, Gustafsson JA and Liu ET (2004). Discovery of estrogen receptor alpha target genes and response elements in breast tumor cells. *Genome Biol* 5: R66.

Lo KW, Teo PM, Hui AB, To KF, Tsang YS, Chan SY, Mak KF, Lee JC and Huang DP (2000). High resolution allelotype of microdissected primary nasopharyngeal carcinoma. *Cancer Res* 60: 3348-3353.

Lo KW, Kwong J, Hui AB, Chan SY, To KF, Chan AS, Chow LS, Teo PM, Johnson PJ, Huang DP (2001). High frequency of promoter hypermethylation of RASSF1A in nasopharyngeal carcinoma. Cancer Res. 61:3877-3881.

Lo PH, Leung AC, Kwok CY, Cheung WS, Ko JM, Yang LC, Law S, Wang LD, Li J, Stanbridge EJ, Srivastava G, Tang JC, Tsao SW and Lung ML (2007). Identification of a tumor suppressive critical region mapping to 3p14.2 in esophageal squamous cell carcinoma and studies of a candidate tumor suppressor gene, ADAMTS9. *Oncogene* 26: 148-157.

Lo PH, Lung HL, Cheung AK, Apte SS, Chan KW, Kwong FM, Ko JM, Cheng Y, Law S, Srivastava G, Zabarovsky ER, Tsao SW, Tang JC, Stanbridge EJ and Lung ML (2010). Extracellular protease ADAMTS9 suppresses esophageal and nasopharyngeal carcinoma tumor formation by inhibiting angiogenesis. *Cancer Res* 70: 5567-5576.

Lung HL, Lo CC, Wong CC, Cheung AK, Cheong KF, Wong N, Kwong FM, Chan KC, Law EW, Tsao SW, Chua D, Sham JS, Cheng Y, Stanbridge EJ, Robertson GP and Lung ML (2008a). Identification of tumor suppressive activity by irradiation microcell-mediated chromosome transfer and involvement of alpha B-crystallin in nasopharyngeal carcinoma. *Int J Cancer* 122: 1288-1296.

Lung HL, Lo PH, Xie D, Apte SS, Cheung AK, Cheng Y, Law EW, Chua D, Zeng YX, Tsao SW, Stanbridge EJ and Lung ML (2008b). Characterization of a novel epigenetically-silenced, growth-suppressive gene, ADAMTS9, and its association with lymph node metastases in nasopharyngeal carcinoma. *Int J Cancer* 123: 401-408.

Lung ML, Choi CV, Kong H, Yuen PW, Kwong D, Sham J and Wei WI (2001). Microsatellite allelotyping of chinese nasopharyngeal carcinomas. *Anticancer Res* 21: 3081-3084.

Mitelman F, Mark-Vendel E, Mineur A, Giovanella B and Klein G (1983). A 3q+ marker chromosome in EBV-carrying nasopharyngeal carcinomas. *Int J Cancer* 32: 651-655.

Mourra N, Zeitoun G, Buecher B, Finetti P, Lagarde A, Adelaide J, Birnbaum D, Thomas G and Olschwang S (2007). High frequency of chromosome 14 deletion in early-onset colon cancer. *Dis Colon Rectum* 50: 1881-1886.

Murakami Y, Nobukuni T, Tamura K, Maruyama T, Sekiya T, Arai Y, Gomyou H, Tanigami A, Ohki M, Cabin D, Frischmeyer P, Hunt P and Reeves RH (1998a). Localization of tumor suppressor activity important in nonsmall cell lung carcinoma on chromosome 11q. *Proc Natl Acad Sci U S A* 95: 8153-8158.

Murakami Y and Sekiya T (1998b). Accumulation of genetic alterations and their significance in each primary human cancer and cell line. *Mutat Res* 400: 421-437.

Murakami Y (2002). Functional cloning of a tumor suppressor gene, TSLC1, in human non-small cell lung cancer. *Oncogene* 21: 6936-6948.

Murakami YS, Brothman AR, Leach RJ and White RL (1995). Suppression of malignant phenotype in a human prostate cancer cell line by fragments of normal chromosomal region 17q. *Cancer Res* 55: 3389-3394.

Murayama F and Okada Y (1965). Effect of calcium on the cell fusion reaction caused by HVJ. *Biken J* 8: 103-105.

Pachnis V, Pevny L, Rothstein R and Costantini F (1990). Transfer of a yeast artificial chromosome carrying human DNA from Saccharomyces cerevisiae into mammalian cells. *Proc Natl Acad Sci U S A* 87: 5109-5113.

Pack SD, Karkera JD, Zhuang Z, Pak ED, Balan KV, Hwu P, Park WS, Pham T, Ault DO, Glaser M, Liotta L, Detera-Wadleigh SD and Wadleigh RG (1999). Molecular cytogenetic fingerprinting of esophageal squamous cell carcinoma by comparative genomic hybridization reveals a consistent pattern of chromosomal alterations. *Genes Chromosomes Cancer* 25: 160-168.

Pavan WJ, Hieter P and Reeves RH (1990a). Generation of deletion derivatives by targeted transformation of human-derived yeast artificial chromosomes. *Proc Natl Acad Sci U S A* 87: 1300-1304.

Pavan WJ, Hieter P and Reeves RH (1990b). Modification and transfer into an embryonal carcinoma cell line of a 360-kilobase human-derived yeast artificial chromosome. *Mol Cell Biol* 10: 4163-4169.

Porter S, Clark IM, Kevorkian L and Edwards DR (2005). The ADAMTS metalloproteinases. *Biochem J* 386: 15-27.

Qi Y, Chiu JF, Wang L, Kwong DL and He QY (2005). Comparative proteomic analysis of esophageal squamous cell carcinoma. *Proteomics* 5: 2960-2971.

Robertson GP, Hufford A and Lugo TG (1997). A panel of transferable fragments of human chromosome 11q. *Cytogenet Cell Genet* 79: 53-59.

Saxon PJ, Srivatsan ES, Leipzig GV, Sameshima JH and Stanbridge EJ (1985). Selective transfer of individual human chromosomes to recipient cells. *Mol Cell Biol* 5: 140-146.

Saxon PJ, Srivatsan ES and Stanbridge EJ (1986). Introduction of human chromosome 11 via microcell transfer controls tumorigenic expression of HeLa cells. *EMBO J* 5: 3461-3466.

Shao J, Li Y, Wu Q, Liang X, Yu X, Huang L, Hou J, Huang X, Ernberg I, Hu LF and Zeng Y (2002). High frequency loss of heterozygosity on the long arms of chromosomes 13 and 14 in nasopharyngeal carcinoma in Southern China. *Chin Med J (Engl)* 115: 571-575.

Stanbridge EJ (1976). Suppression of malignancy in human cells. *Nature* 260: 17-20.

Stanbridge EJ (1992). Functional evidence for human tumour suppressor genes: chromosome and molecular genetic studies. *Cancer Surv* 12: 5-24.

Tamura K, Zhang X, Murakami Y, Hirohashi S, Xu HJ, Hu SX, Benedict WF and Sekiya T (1997). Deletion of three distinct regions on chromosome 13q in human non-small-cell lung cancer. *Int J Cancer* 74: 45-49.

Todd MC, Xiang RH, Garcia DK, Kerbacher KE, Moore SL, Hensel CH, Liu P, Siciliano MJ, Kok K, van den Berg A, Veldhuis P, Buys CH, Killary AM and Naylor SL (1996). An 80 Kb P1 clone from chromosome 3p21.3 suppresses tumor growth in vivo. *Oncogene* 13: 2387-2396.

Tsang YS, Lo KW, Leung SF, Choi PH, Fong Y, Lee JC and Huang DP (1999). Two distinct regions of deletion on chromosome 13q in primary nasopharyngeal carcinoma. *Int J Cancer* 83: 305-308.

Vazquez F, Hastings G, Ortega MA, Lane TF, Oikemus S, Lombardo M and Iruela-Arispe ML (1999). METH-1, a human ortholog of ADAMTS-1, and METH-2 are members of a new family of proteins with angio-inhibitory activity. *J Biol Chem* 274: 23349-23357.

Wada M, Ihara Y, Tatsuka M, Mitsui H, Kohno K, Kuwano M and Schlessinger D (1994). HPRT yeast artificial chromosome transfer into human cells by four methods and an involvement of homologous recombination. *Biochem Biophys Res Commun* 200: 1693-1700.

Wei WI and Sham JS (2005). Nasopharyngeal carcinoma. *Lancet* 365: 2041-2054.

Weir BA, Woo MS, Getz G, Perner S, Ding L, Beroukhim R, Lin WM, Province MA, Kraja A, Johnson LA, Shah K, Sato M, Thomas RK, Barletta JA, Borecki IB, Broderick S, Chang AC, Chiang DY, Chirieac LR, Cho J, Fujii Y, Gazdar AF, Giordano T, Greulich H, Hanna M, Johnson BE, Kris MG, Lash A, Lin L, Lindeman N, Mardis ER, McPherson JD, Minna JD, Morgan MB, Nadel M, Orringer MB, Osborne JR, Ozenberger B, Ramos AH, Robinson J, Roth JA, Rusch V, Sasaki H, Shepherd F, Sougnez C, Spitz MR, Tsao MS, Twomey D, Verhaak RG, Weinstock GM, Wheeler DA, Winckler W, Yoshizawa A, Yu S, Zakowski MF, Zhang Q, Beer DG, Wistuba, II, Watson MA, Garraway LA, Ladanyi M, Travis WD, Pao W, Rubin MA, Gabriel SB, Gibbs RA, Varmus HE, Wilson RK, Lander ES and Meyerson M (2007). Characterizing the cancer genome in lung adenocarcinoma. *Nature* 450: 893-898.

Weissman BE, Saxon PJ, Pasquale SR, Jones GR, Geiser AG and Stanbridge EJ (1987). Introduction of a normal human chromosome 11 into a Wilms' tumor cell line controls its tumorigenic expression. *Science* 236: 175-180.

Wong VC, Chan PL, Bernabeu C, Law S, Wang LD, Li JL, Tsao SW, Srivastava G and Lung ML (2008). Identification of an invasion and tumor-suppressing gene, Endoglin (ENG), silenced by both epigenetic inactivation and allelic loss in esophageal squamous cell carcinoma. *Int J Cancer* 123: 2816-2823.

Wong VC, Chen H, Ko JM, Chan KW, Chan YP, Law S, Chua D, Kwong DL, Lung HL, Srivastava G, Tang JC, Tsao SW, Zabarovsky ER, Stanbridge EJ and Lung ML (2011a). Tumor suppressor dual-specificity phosphatase 6 (DUSP6) impairs cell invasion and epithelial-mesenchymal transition (EMT)-associated phenotype. *Int J Cancer.*

Wong VC, Ko JM, Qi RZ, Li PJ, Wang LD, Li JL, Chan YP, Chan KW, Stanbridge EJ and Lung ML (2011b). Abrogated expression of DEC1 during oesophageal squamous cell carcinoma progression is age- and family history-related and significantly associated with lymph node metastasis. *Br J Cancer* 104: 841-849.

Wu X, Chen VW, Ruiz B, Andrews P, Su LJ and Correa P (2006). Incidence of esophageal and gastric carcinomas among American Asians/Pacific Islanders, whites, and blacks: subsite and histology differences. *Cancer* 106: 683-692.

Yang L, Leung AC, Ko JM, Lo PH, Tang JC, Srivastava G, Oshimura M, Stanbridge EJ, Daigo Y, Nakamura Y, Tang CM, Lau KW, Law S and Lung ML (2005). Tumor suppressive role of a 2.4 Mb 9q33-q34 critical region and DEC1 in esophageal squamous cell carcinoma. *Oncogene* 24: 697-705.

Yau WL, Lung HL, Zabarovsky ER, Lerman MI, Sham JS, Chua DT, Tsao SW, Stanbridge EJ, Lung ML (2006). Functional studies of the chromosome 3p21.3 candidate tumor suppressor gene BLU/ZMYND10 in nasopharyngeal carcinoma. *Int J Cancer* 119:2821-2826.

Yoshimoto T, Matsuura K, Karnan S, Tagawa H, Nakada C, Tanigawa M, Tsukamoto Y, Uchida T, Kashima K, Akizuki S, Takeuchi I, Sato F, Mimata H, Seto M and Moriyama M (2007). High-resolution analysis of DNA copy number alterations and gene expression in renal clear cell carcinoma. *J Pathol* 213: 392-401.

4

TP53 Gene Polymorphisms in Cancer Risk: The Modulating Effect of Ageing, Ethnicity and *TP53* Somatic Abnormalities

Evgeny V. Denisov[1], Nadezhda V. Cherdyntseva[1], Nicolay V. Litviakov[1], Elena A. Malinovskaya[1], Natalya N. Babyshkina[1], Valentina A. Belyavskaya[2] and Mikhail I. Voevoda[3]

[1]Cancer Research Institute, Siberian Branch of Russian Academy of Medical Sciences, Tomsk, [2]Research Center of Virology and Biotechnology VECTOR, Koltsovo, [3]Institute of Internal Medicine, Siberian Branch of Russian Academy of Medical Sciences, Novosibirsk, Russian Federation

1. Introduction

The multi-talented "guardian of the genome" p53 is fundamental to preventing tumor development through the regulation of important cellular processes such as cell cycle arrest and senescence, DNA replication and repair, apoptosis, metabolism, antioxidant defense, and autophagy, among others. (Chumakov, 2007; Green and Kroemer, 2009; McCarthy, 2011; Olovnikov et al., 2009; Vousden and Prives, 2009; Vousden and Ryan, 2009). p53 protein is encoded by the *TP53* gene (OMIM no. 191170), the structure of which is extremely variable in both healthy and diseased subjects, particularly in cancer, because of multiple germinal and somatic variations (Olivier et al., 2010; Whibley et al., 2009). Currently, approximately 85 polymorphisms and 27580 somatic mutations are known in the *TP53* gene (Petitjean et al., 2007b). In addition, the *TP53* gene, as a classic tumor suppressor, undergoes a loss of heterozygosity (LOH) and hypo- or hypermethylation (Brosh and Rotter, 2009; Sidhu et al., 2005; Soussi, 2007). From all polymorphisms found in the *TP53* gene, three - rs1042522, rs17878362, and rs1625895 - are well studied in terms of functional characterization, distribution in human populations and association with cancer risk. During the last 15 years, the predisposing value of these *TP53* polymorphic variants has been estimated in relation to many human cancers; however, the data are inconsistent.

It is not surprising that cancer risk is a consequence of the interaction between constitutional genetics and environmental exposure. The combination of genetic background (gene-gene interactions) and environmental endo- and exogenous factors varies among individuals of different ethnical groups and might explain the distinct tumor susceptibility. Cancer is an extremely complicated phenotype and, together with the incomplete penetrance of the inherited tumor risk alleles, interaction with environmental risk factors could substantially alter hereditary susceptibility (Perez-Losada et al., 2011). Nutritional aspects, reproductive factors, and alcohol, smoking, and radiation along with other exposures may considerably influence the genetic background via genotoxic effects or the activation/inhibition of major pathways and modify cancer susceptibility. This statement is especially true of *TP53*, the functionality of which has inducible character and depends on environmental exposure. Additionally, cancer arises as a result of the stepwise accumulation of genetic mutations, chromosomal aberrations and epigenetic alterations (Hanahan and Weinberg, 2011; Marshall, 1991). Thus, *TP53* polymorphisms may define the sequence of mutational events, as previously demonstrated (Denisov et al., 2011; Hrstka et al., 2009; Litviakov et al., 2010; Whibley et al., 2009). Even more importantly, the manifestation of functional roles of *TP53* polymorphisms is tissue- and age-specific, meaning that their effect on p53-controlled processes may vary between cell types and age groups (Azzam et al., 2011; Bonafe et al., 2004; Salvioli et al., 2005). Based on the above reasoning, a simultaneous account of *TP53* polymorphisms and their tissue- and age-specific effects, along with ethnicity-specific genetic background and environmental exposure, may reveal how *TP53* germline variations modify cancer risk. In this review, we focus on the recent findings regarding *TP53* polymorphisms, rs1042522, rs17878362, and rs1625895, their functional role and association with cancer risk, their relationships with environmental exposure and somatic aberrations in tumors, as well as discuss some hypotheses explaining the present contradictions in the biological role of *TP53* variations in cancer.

2. Functional *TP53* polymorphisms and cancer risk

2.1 *TP53* polymorphisms: The functional value

The *TP53* rs1042522 (Ex4+119C>G: C and G alleles) polymorphism displays substitution of C to G in codon 72 of exon 4 of the *TP53* gene, changing the amino acid from proline (Pro) to arginine (Arg) in the proline-rich domain of p53 protein (Harris et al., 1986). p53 forms p53Pro and p52Arg are characterized by molecular differences in protein structure (Table 1); however, the data are contradictory and inconclusive (Naldi et al., 2010; Ozeki et al., 2011; Thomas et al., 1999). In addition, there is no final opinion concerning the influence of *TP53* rs1042522 polymorphism on the p53 mRNA level (Nikbahkt Dastjerdi, 2011; Ribeiro et al., 1997; Siddique et al., 2005; Wang et al., 1999). Further, it is beyond any doubt that p53Pro and p53Arg differ in their capability to regulate p53-dependent cell processes (Table 1). Many thousands of years ago, precisely such p53 functional differentiation was the reason for dramatic changes in the proportion of rs1042522 alleles from equatorial areas to northern latitudes (Beckman et al., 1994; Sjalander et al., 1996). In particular, the rs1042522 C allele is the ancestral form with ~60-95% frequency in African populations, whereas the G allele arose some 30,000 to 50,000 years ago and increased in percentage as populations migrated farther north, where its allele frequency reached 75-85% (Hirshfield et al., 2010; Jeong et al., 2010). The most likely components of evolutionary selection pressure fixing *TP53* alleles into these geographic regions are implantation and reproduction, as well as sunburn resistance (Hirshfield et al., 2010; Hu et al., 2011; Jeong et al., 2010), the antithetic regulation of which has been demonstrated for p53 rs1042522 protein forms (Table 1). Specifically, the rs1042522 G allele exhibits 2-fold higher transcriptional activity toward the *LIF* gene, which encodes a cytokine that is required for optimal implantation and reproduction, compared with the C allele (Feng et al., 2011; Jeong et al., 2010; Kang et al., 2009).

	p53 protein forms						Ref.
	rs1042522		rs17878362		rs1625895		
	G	C	A1	A2	G	A	
p53 protein structure	Identical		Altered topology of G-quadruplexes in intron 3		-	-	(Marcel et al., 2011; Naldi et al., 2010; Ozeki et al., 2011; Thomas et al., 1999)
	Different						
p53 mRNA level	High	Low	High	Low	-	-	(Gemignani et al., 2004; Nikbahkt Dastjerdi, 2011; Ribeiro et al., 1997; Siddique et al., 2005)
	Identical						
Capability to							
transactivation	Low	High	-	-	-	-	(Frank et al., 2011; Thomas et al., 1999)
cell cycle arrest	Low	High	-	-	-	-	(Frank et al., 2011; Pim and Banks, 2004)
senescence induction	Low	High	-	-	-	-	(Frank et al., 2011; Salvioli et al., 2005)
DNA repair	Low	High	High	Low	High	Low	(Siddique and Sabapathy, 2006; Wu et al., 2002)
genomic stability maintenance	Low	High	-	-	High	Low	(Litviakov et al., 2010; Qiu et al., 2008; Schwartz et al., 2011; Siddique and Sabapathy, 2006)
apoptosis activation							
in extrinsic pathway	Low	High	High	Low	High	Low	(Bendesky et al., 2007; Biros et al., 2002; Bonafe et al., 2002; Dumont et al., 2003; Pim and Banks, 2004; Schneider-Stock et al., 2004b; Siddique and Sabapathy, 2006; Wu et al., 2002)
in intrinsic pathway	High	Low					
suppression of transformed cell growth	High	Low	-	-	-	-	(Thomas et al., 1999)
survival in hypoxia	High	Low	-	-	-	-	(Sansone et al., 2007; Vannini et al., 2008)
induction of cell death in hypoxia	Low	High	-	-	-	-	

cell-cell adhesion activation	High	Low	-	-	-	-	(Jeong et al., 2010)
reproduction	High	Low	-	-	-	-	(Feng et al., 2011; Jeong et al., 2010; Kang et al., 2009; Kay et al., 2006)
degradation mediated by							
E6 oncoprotein	High	Low	-	-	-	-	(Storey et al., 1998)
MDM2 ubiquitin ligase	High	Low	-	-	-	-	(Dumont et al., 2003; Ozeki et al., 2011)
	Low	High					
sunburn	High	Low	-	-	-	-	(McGregor et al., 2002; Pezeshki et al., 2006)

Table 1. Structural and functional characteristics of p53 proteins encoded by *TP53* (rs1042522, rs17878362 and rs1625895) polymorphisms.

Moreover, the C allele was found to be increased in women with recurrent implantation failure and individuals undergoing *in vitro* fertilization (IVF), and is a risk factor for implantation failure after IVF (Kang et al., 2009; Kay et al., 2006). Interestingly, the frequency of the G allele has been positively correlated with low winter temperatures (Shi et al., 2009). In this respect, northern populations living in cold climates and having a high percentage of G alleles could be at an advantage due to a reduced risk of implantation failure (Feng et al., 2011; Hu et al., 2011). Additionally, it is critical to note that the geographic distribution of rs1042522 alleles is also linked with the capacity of p53 to regulate pigmentation and sunburn resistance through the activation of tyrosinase, the rate-limiting enzyme for melanin synthesis, and by induction of transcription of the melanogenic cytokine pro-opiomelanocortin (Hirshfield et al., 2010; Khlgatian et al., 2002; Murase et al., 2009). Accordingly, one may reasonably suppose that the p53-dependent stimulation of pigmentation could be a protective mechanism from UV light for light-skinned populations. Previously, a significant positive association between the G allele and susceptibility to sunburn was demonstrated (McGregor et al., 2002; Pezeshki et al., 2006), whereas the C allele was most prevalent in dark-skinned races originating from areas with high ambient UV levels (McGregor et al., 2002).

It should not be forgotten that one of the main functions of *TP53* is the maintenance of genomic stability through the removal of genetically aberrant cells and the suppression of tumor development. Different abilities concerning induction cell cycle arrest, DNA repair, and senescence, the activation of apoptosis and the suppression of transformed cell growth, and survival in hypoxia have been observed for the p53 protein encoded by alleles with *TP53* rs1042522 polymorphism (Table 1). As compared to p53Arg, p53Pro protein (C allele) is the best transactivation molecule (Frank et al., 2011; Thomas et al., 1999) and displays a high capability to block the cell cycle (Frank et al., 2011; Pim and Banks, 2004), induce DNA repair (Siddique and Sabapathy, 2006), remove micronuclei (Siddique and Sabapathy, 2006) and chromosome aberrations (Litviakov et al., 2010; Schwartz et al., 2011), and stimulate cell senescence (Frank et al., 2011; Salvioli et al., 2005) and cell death in hypoxic environments via activation/inhibition of p53-target genes such as *p21, p53R2, p48, GADD45, PAI-1* and the hypoxia response genes. In contrast, p53Arg protein induces apoptosis markedly better and with faster kinetics than p53Pro but mainly through intrinsic pathways and a significant ability to activate the *DR-4, NOXA, PUMA, PIG-3,* and *PERP* genes, localize to the mitochondria and release cytochrome C into the cytosol (Dumont et al., 2003; Jeong et al., 2010; Pim and Banks, 2004; Thomas et al., 1999; Zhu et al., 2010). However, the strongly pronounced apoptotic ability of p53Arg does not protect against the process of carcinogenesis (Zhu et al., 2010). Likewise, p53Arg is more efficient than p53Pro in the suppression of transformed cell growth by the E7 and EJ-ras oncogenes and survival in hypoxia (Thomas et al., 1999; Vannini et al., 2008). Curiously, tumors of the head and neck losing the C and bearing the G allele show a lack of co-expression of Fas/FasL and high expression of Bcl2 proteins, and, as a consequence, markedly reduced apoptosis (Schneider-Stock et al., 2004b). Simply stated, p53Pro protein seems to be the best inductor of apoptosis in the extrinsic pathway. This also results from the fact that p53Pro, but not p53Arg, along with NF-kB, transactivates caspase 4/11, an important component of the extrinsic pathway in apoptosis induction (Azzam et al., 2011; Frank et al., 2011). Aside from the above-mentioned data, it was recently established that the *TP53* rs1042522 polymorphism impacts the apoptotic function of p53 in a tissue-specific manner. Specifically, p53Pro protein more effectively activates programmed cell death in thymus (Frank et al., 2011), whereas in the small intestine, apoptosis is significantly higher in G-expressing cells (Azzam et al., 2011; Zhu et al., 2010). Interestingly, in the spleen, there was no difference in the induction of apoptosis between rs1042522 variants (Azzam et al., 2011). Taken together, the tumor-suppressing function of p53 is considerably modified by *TP53* rs1042522 polymorphism, while the effect of p53 allelic variants on tumor growth, mainly manifested in apoptosis regulation, depends on the genetic and tissue-specific background.

p53 is a multifaceted and multifunctional molecule with implications in a majority of cell processes. There is growing evidence that p53 is involved in regulation of the epithelial-mesenchymal transition (EMT) and cell phenotype, as well as cell migration and invasion (Muller et al., 2011). Breast and lung cancers with p53 mutations exhibit stem cell-like transcriptional patterns and are depleted in terms of the activity of differentiation genes (Mizuno et al., 2010). Furthermore, a loss of p53 leads to decreased expression of microRNA miR-200c, stimulated expression of EMT and stemness markers, and the development of high tumor grades in a cohort of breast tumors (Chang et al., 2011). Interestingly, p53 mutants with gain of novel function enhanced the efficiency of the reprogramming process compared with p53 deficiency (Sarig et al., 2010). As recently published by Jeong et al. (Jeong et al., 2010), *TP53* rs1042522 polymorphism may modify cell-cell adhesion, particularly through the high capability of p53Arg protein to induce expression of the *PERP* gene (Table 1). Additionally, p53Arg possesses the best ability to activate *CHMP4C,* a member of the EMT family of genes.

In comparison with *TP53* rs1042522 polymorphism, rs17878362 and rs1625895 variations are poorly characterized in terms of structural and functional properties. However, the current data are sufficiently convincing of significant influence on p53 activity. The *TP53* rs17878362 polymorphism consists of a 16 bp duplication in intron 3 (PIN3: A1, non-duplicated allele and A2, duplicated allele). In a series of previous studies, it was demonstrated that the presence of the rs17878362 minor allele (A2) results in decreasing p53 mRNA levels, intensity of DNA repair and apoptosis processes (Table 1) (Gemignani et al., 2004; Wu et al.,

2002). In addition, there is an opinion that *TP53* rs17878362 polymorphism may alter the topology of G-quadruplexes in intron 3, regulating the alternative splicing of intron 2, thus modulating the patterns of expression of transcripts encoding either p53 or its N-terminally truncated isoform, Δ40p53 (Marcel et al., 2011). With respect to rs1625895 (IVS6+62A>G: A and G alleles), this polymorphism displays an A>G transversion and, according to literature data, is responsible for changes in the induction of DNA repair and apoptosis and the maintenance of genomic stability (Table 1) (Qiu et al., 2008; Wu et al., 2002). It should be pointed out that *TP53* rs1625895 and rs17878362 polymorphisms are in perfect linkage disequilibrium with rs1042522 (Sjalander et al., 1995; Weston et al., 1997) and, most likely, these intronic variations control the alternative splicing and mRNA level of p53Arg and p53Pro proteins. Consequently, it would be logical to take into account the *TP53* linkage disequilibrium box in disease pathogenesis studies.

2.2 *TP53* polymorphisms: The cancer predisposing value

Owing to the importance of p53 in tumor suppression, *TP53* rs1042522, rs17878362, and rs1625895 polymorphisms altering p53 functionality might affect cancer risk (Whibley et al., 2009). The results of the consortium works and last meta-analyses, demonstrating the predisposing value of *TP53* germline variations in different types of human cancer, are overviewed in Table 2. It should be immediately noticed that in a majority of cancers, the data are inconclusive, and further studies are needed to clarify the associations. In addition, there are certain annoying mistakes in some meta-analyses, which result in entirely noncredible data, and it would be valuable to provide a new, more accurate estimation of association of *TP53* polymorphisms with cancer risk (Economopoulos and Sergentanis, 2010; Lu et al., 2011a; Lu et al., 2011b; Lu et al., 2011c; Sergentanis and Economopoulos, 2010a, 2011). However, in spite of the present disagreements and methodological flaws, association tendencies for some cancer localizations are clear (Table 2). Simply stated, the rs1042522 C allele is associated with increased susceptibility to cancers, including of the lung (Dai et al., 2009; Francisco et al., 2010; Li et al., 2009; Yan et al., 2009), head and neck (Francisco et al., 2010), thyroid (Francisco et al., 2010), esophagus (Wang et al., 2010a; Zhao et al., 2010), pancreas (Liu et al., 2011), liver (Chen et al., 2011; Francisco et al., 2010), gallbladder (Liu et al., 2011), nasopharynx (Zhuo et al., 2009b), and cervix (Francisco et al., 2010; Klug et al., 2009). No significant contribution of *TP53* rs1042522 polymorphism to oral cancer has been reported (Zhuo et al., 2009c). A high heterogeneity of results was observed in breast (He et al., 2011; Hu et al., 2010b; Lu et al., 2011b; Ma et al., 2011; Peng et al., 2011; Sergentanis and Economopoulos, 2010b; The Breast Cancer Association Consortium, 2006; Zhang et al., 2010b; Zhuo et al., 2009a), colon and rectum (Dahabreh et al., 2010; Economopoulos and Sergentanis, 2010; Economopoulos et al., 2010; Liu et al., 2011; Tang et al., 2010; Wang et al., 2010b) cancers. Though still not quite clear, cancer of the ovary (Schildkraut et al., 2009; Zhang et al., 2008), endometrium (Francisco et al., 2010; Jiang et al., 2010b), stomach (Francisco et al., 2010; Gao et al., 2009; Liu et al., 2011), bladder (Jiang et al., 2010a; Li et al., 2010), prostate (Zhang et al., 2010a; Zhang et al., 2011b; Zhu et al., 2011), and skin (Francisco et al., 2010; Jiang et al., 2011) appear to be affected. As for the rs17878362 polymorphism, a clear association of the A2 allele with a high risk of breast cancer (He et al., 2011; Hu et al., 2010a; Hu et al., 2010b; Zhang et al., 2011a) and a lack of involvement in lung (Hu et al., 2010a), ovary (Schildkraut et al., 2009), colon and rectum (Hu et al., 2010a) cancer susceptibility has been demonstrated. Interestingly, Peng et al. (Peng et al., 2011) did not show a dependence of breast cancer development on rs17878362 germline variation. For the

rs1625895 polymorphism, no association with breast (He et al., 2011; Hu et al., 2010b) or ovary (Schildkraut et al., 2009) cancers has been presented in the available literature.
Cancer is a heterogeneous polygenic disorder with a well-established gene environment playing an important role in disease etiology (Hanahan and Weinberg, 2011; Perez-Losada et al., 2011). The significant heterogeneity of the associative value of *TP53* polymorphisms, especially rs1042522 variation, among human cancers is most likely explained by specific p53 inducible functionality essentially depending on ethnicity-related genetic background and environmental exposure, tissue and age specificity (Azzam et al., 2011; Chung et al., 2010; Donehower, 2006; Francisco et al., 2010; van Heemst et al., 2005). The complex of lifestyle endo- and exogenous factors of each ethnic group, the proportion of which increases with age, may dramatically modulate the contribution of *TP53* polymorphisms to cancer risk through, for example, genotoxic effects and epigenetic modifications of the *TP53* gene structure. Exogenous modifiable factors, such as alcohol, smoking and betel or areca quid chewing, and radiation and chemical poisoning, together with endogenous estrogen metabolites and other secreted chemicals, have been found to be involved in DNA damage and epigenetic alterations (De Bont and van Larebeke, 2004; Hsu et al., 2010; Seviour and Lin, 2010). In this case, *TP53* functionally different polymorphisms serving as background for origin of *TP53* abnormalities, such as mutations and a loss of heterozygosity (LOH), promote neoplastic transformation by switching off p53-dependent control of genomic stability and further accumulation of genetic damage (Denisov et al., 2011). As a classic tumor suppressor, *TP53* inactivation seems to underlie Knudson's "two-hit" model supposing that two mutations or "hits" (point mutation and loss of allele, producing LOH) are required to inactivate genes and cause cancer or promote disease progression (Knudson, 1971); however, there are tumors that are exceptions to this rule (Donehower and Lozano, 2009; Thiagalingam et al., 2002). Nevertheless, the simultaneous presence of mutations and LOH in the *TP53* gene is a widespread phenomenon in human cancer, suggesting that one inactivation is not sufficient to completely inactivate p53 (Baker et al., 1990; Nigro et al., 1989).

Cancers	rs1042522	rs17878362	rs1625895	Ref.
Breast	no	no	-	(Ma et al., 2011; Peng et al., 2011; The Breast Cancer Association Consortium, 2006; Zhuo et al., 2009a)
	C↓, Mediterraneans	A2↑	no	(Hu et al., 2010a; Hu et al., 2010b)
	G↑	-	-	(Lu et al., 2011b; Sergentanis and Economopoulos, 2010b; Zhang et al., 2010b)
	G↑, Indians	A2↑	no	(He et al., 2011)
	no	A2↑	-	(Zhang et al., 2011a)
Lung, head and neck, thyroid	C↑	no	-	(Dai et al., 2009; Francisco et al., 2010; Hu et al., 2010a; Li et al., 2009; Truong et al., 2010; Yan et al., 2009)

Gynecologic				
Ovary	no	no	no	(Schildkraut et al., 2009)
	C↓	-	-	(Zhang et al., 2008)
Cervix	G↑*	-	-	(Klug et al., 2009)
	C↓	-	-	(Francisco et al., 2010)
Endometrium	no	-	-	(Jiang et al., 2010b)
	C↑	-	-	(Francisco et al., 2010)
Digestive tract				
Oral cavity	no	-	-	(Zhuo et al., 2009c)
Stomach	C↑	-	-	(Francisco et al., 2010; Liu et al., 2011)
	C↑, diffuse type, Asians	-	-	(Gao et al., 2009)
	C↓, intestinal type, Caucasians			
Esophagus, pancreas, liver, gallbladder	C↑	-	-	(Chen et al., 2011; Francisco et al., 2010; Liu et al., 2011; Wang et al., 2010a; Zhao et al., 2010)
Colon and rectum	no	no	-	(Economopoulos and Sergentanis, 2010; Hu et al., 2010a; Tang et al., 2010; Wang et al., 2010b)
	C↓, Caucasians (tendency)†	-	-	(Economopoulos et al., 2010)
	C↓*	-	-	(Dahabreh et al., 2010)
	C↑	-	-	(Liu et al., 2011)
Total group without oral cavity	C↑, Asians	-	-	(Liu et al., 2011)
Bladder	G↑, Caucasians	-	-	(Li et al., 2010)
	G↓, Asians	-	-	(Jiang et al., 2010a)
Nasopharynx	G↓, C↑	-	-	(Zhuo et al., 2009b)
Prostate	no	-	-	(Zhu et al., 2011)
	G↑, Caucasians	-	-	(Zhang et al., 2010a)
	C↓‡	-	-	(Zhang et al., 2011b)
Skin	no	-	-	(Jiang et al., 2011)
	C↓	-	-	(Francisco et al., 2010)

↑allele increases cancer risk. ↓allele decreases cancer risk.
*only in non-epidemiological studies and studies, where controls were not in Hardy–Weinberg equilibrium and polymorphism analysis was determined from tumor tissue. †in studies where controls did not deviate from the Hardy-Weinberg equilibrium. ‡in population-based control subjects.

Table 2. The association of *TP53* gene polymorphisms with human cancers (data from the consortium works and the last meta-analyses).

2.3 *TP53* polymorphisms: The background for *TP53* abnormalities

TP53 gene mutations, represented by specific single monoallelic missense aberrations, are "universal" genetic abnormalities in human tumors, with a frequency varying from 10 to close to 100% (Brosh and Rotter, 2009; Olivier et al., 2010; Rivlin et al., 2011). *TP53* mutants display a loss of transactivation capability via conformational changes in p53 protein structure, as well as gain-of-function effects through the activation of multidrug resistance genes (*ABCB1, ABCC1, ABCG1,* and *MVP*), growth factor receptor genes (*EGFR, bFGF,* and *VEGF*), oncogenes (*c-Myc, c-Fos,* and *Ras*) or via the inhibition of paralogs p63 and p73, which are responsible for the induction of apoptosis (Brosh and Rotter, 2009; Olivier et al., 2010; Oren and Rotter, 2010). Due to tumor-promoting effects, *TP53* mutations have been shown to contribute to poor prognosis and therapeutic effectiveness in a majority of cancers (Brosh and Rotter, 2009; Olivier et al., 2010; Petitjean et al., 2007a). Despite the high *TP53* mutability, there is data concerning the presence of alternative inactivation pathways through the methylation of CG repeats in the *TP53* gene (Almeida et al., 2009; Amatya et al., 2005; Kang et al., 2001; Sidhu et al., 2005). Although the promoter region of *TP53* does not contain a classic CpG island, the methylation of one or two CG sites may result in significant inhibitory effects in gene expression (Sidhu et al., 2005). As for the LOH in the region of the *TP53* gene (17p13.1) or allelic imbalance (AI) as currently, the abnormality is detected in a majority of tumors leading to cancer progression and poor prognosis (Ellsworth et al., 2005; Frohling and Dohner, 2008; Lee et al., 2006; Tsuda, 2009; Willman and Hromas, 2010).

At present, it is not known which of these inactivation hits occurs first; however, the initial step by way of LOH is expected to create prerequisites for mutations in retained *TP53* alleles through a significant increase in genomic instability caused by the dramatic reduction of p53 functionality. In contrast, point mutations and methylation do not always result in inactivation or alteration of the activity of the corresponding protein. Information concerning the simultaneous occurrence of LOH and mutations in the *TP53* gene is well represented in association with rs1042522 alleles (Table 3). However, it was quite recently shown that rs17878362 and rs1625895 germline variations are also associated with *TP53* somatic abnormalities in tumor cells (Denisov et al., 2011; Marcel et al., 2009), although the data are not numerous enough and require further confirmation. Several studies reported that LOH more often occurs at the C allele than at the G allele in tumor cells of rs1042522 heterozygous cancer patients. This phenomenon is typical for cancers of the breast (Bonafe et al., 2003; Denisov et al., 2009; Denisov et al., 2011; Wegman et al., 2009), lung (Nelson et al., 2005; Papadakis et al., 2002), head and neck (Marin et al., 2000; Mitra et al., 2007), colon and rectum (Schneider-Stock et al., 2004a), renal pelvis, ureter and bladder (Furihata et al., 2002), oral cavity (Hsieh et al., 2005), vulva (Brooks et al., 2000; Marin et al., 2000), liver (Anzola et al., 2003), skin (Marin et al., 2000; McGregor et al., 2002), esophagus (Kawaguchi et al., 2000), and cervix (Pegoraro et al., 2002). However, the early studies on renal, bladder and oral cancer models did not show any differences in the preference of LOH at the rs1042522 alleles (Oka et al., 1991; Tandle et al., 2001). An interesting situation is that two reports involving ovary cancer have demonstrated contradictory results concerning preferential loss of the rs1042522 alleles in tumor (Buller et al., 1997; Wang et al., 2004); however, in a study by Wang et al. (Wang et al., 2004), the differences did not reach statistical significance. In a majority of cancers with a loss of the C allele, *TP53* gene mutations are significantly more frequent displayed in the retained G variant. Interestingly, persons with the GG and GC genotype in blood also have an increased frequency of *TP53* somatic mutations (Table 3).

Cancers	Preferential loss		Preferential mutation		Ref.
	G	C	G	C	
Breast	yes	no	no	no	(Kyndi et al., 2006)
	no	yes	-	-	(Bonafe et al., 2003)
	-	-	yes	no	(Langerod et al., 2002)
	no	yes	yes	no	(Wegman et al., 2009)
	no	yes	yes	no	(Denisov et al., 2009; Denisov et al., 2011)
Head and neck	no	yes	yes	no	(Mitra et al., 2007)
	no	yes	yes	no	(Marin et al., 2000)
Renal pelvis, ureter and bladder	no	no	-	-	(Oka et al., 1991)
	no	yes	yes	no	(Furihata et al., 2002)
Oral cavity	no	yes†	yes	no	(Hsieh et al., 2005)
	no	no	-	-	(Tandle et al., 2001)
Colon and rectum	no	yes	yes	no	(Schneider-Stock et al., 2004a)
	-	-	yes	no	(Godai et al., 2009)
Stomach	-	-	no	no	(Belyavskaya et al., 2006)
Vulva	no	yes	yes	no	(Brooks et al., 2000)
	no	yes	yes	no	(Marin et al., 2000)
Skin	no	yes	yes	no	
	-	-	no	yes	(Almquist et al., 2011)
	no	yes	no	no	(McGregor et al., 2002)
Liver (hepatitis C virus)	no	yes	-	-	(Anzola et al., 2003)
Esophagus (HPV)	no	yes	-	-	(Kawaguchi et al., 2000)
Cervix (HPV)	no	yes	-	-	(Pegoraro et al., 2002)
Ovary	no	yes	no	yes	(Buller et al., 1997)
- advanced cancer	yes	no	no	yes	(Wang et al., 2004)
Lung					
- non-small cell cancer	-	-	no	yes	(Hu et al., 2005; Mechanic et al., 2005; Szymanowska et al., 2006)
	-	-	yes	no	(Lind et al., 2007)
	no	yes	yes	no	(Nelson et al., 2005)
- advanced cancer	no	yes	-	-	(Papadakis et al., 2002)
Total group of human cancers at the background of radiation	no	yes	-	-	[own unpublished data]

†C allele is preferentially lost in oral squamous cell carcinomas associated with cigarette smoking and areca quid chewing, while the frequency of G allele loss is increased with alcohol drinking.

Table 3. The preferential loss and mutation of *TP53* rs1042522 alleles in human cancer.

Selective loss of the rs1042522 C allele and retention and mutation of the G variant seems to be a unique phenomenon, of which the molecular mechanism, point of origin and biological significance remain unclear. As opposed to hereditary cancer, the origin of which occurs in Knudson's "two-hit" model, in sporadic tumors, the question of whether the mutation or LOH arises first is not resolved, likely due to the high variability of inactivation modes among target (tumor suppressor) genes in cancer development (Thiagalingam et al., 2002; Wilentz et al., 2001). Thus, one may suppose that the LOH and mutations arise in any alleles and in any order but not simultaneously in the two allelic variants because the chances of this "scenario" are very low. Accordingly, in *TP53* rs1042522 heterozygous carriers, the following groups of cells are theoretically possible: with LOH at both the C and G alleles and mutations in both the C and G alleles (Fig. 1). It is most likely that any variations from monoallelic inactivation hits may provoke neoplastic transformation because a 50% reduction in *TP53* gene dosage, protein expression and activity is sufficient to promote tumorigenesis (Donehower and Lozano, 2009); however, loss of the chromosome region underlying LOH is always more dramatic than point mutation. The selective advantage will be displayed for the two groups of cells lacking the C allele and having a mutation in the G variant because of the uncontrolled proliferation caused by the withdrawal of cell cycle checking and the high survival capacity in hypoxia and conditions of chemotherapy provoked by the preferential activation of hypoxia and multidrug resistance genes by p53Arg and inactivation of p73 protein, an important determinant of cellular sensitivity to anticancer agents (Bergamaschi et al., 2003; Sansone et al., 2007; Siddique and Sabapathy, 2006; Vannini et al., 2008). The dramatically increased genomic instability in these cells will most likely result in the second inactivation hit by mutation of the retained G allele in one clone and loss of the C variant in the other. Thus, any of these variants will lead to formation of a cell clone lacking the C allele and having the mutated G variant, the presence of which has been reported in a majority of human cancers (see above). As opposed to single monoallelic inactivation sufficient for tumorigenesis, biallelic switching of p53 activity may accelerate tumors to invade and metastasize. Taken together, the "two-hit" model of *TP53* somatic abnormalities was suggested to explain the regular occurrence of loss of the rs1042522 C allele and mutation of the G variant in human tumors.

The biological value of *TP53* somatic abnormalities in the rs1042522 polymorphic region is well investigated in relation to tumor onset and progression. Nonetheless, there are difficulties in determining the specific interrelationship between certain rs1042522 inactivation hits and tumor development, perhaps due to tissue-specific manifestation of *TP53* allelic variants (Azzam et al., 2011). In particular, the positive contribution of loss of the C allele to short disease-free and overall survival, as well as tumor spreading, has been established in breast and colorectal cancers (Bonafe et al., 2003; Schneider-Stock et al., 2004a). Interestingly, inactivation of the C allele, already having mutations, has been associated with short survival and a worse outcome in patients with lung, ovarian and colorectal neoplasias (Godai et al., 2009; Nelson et al., 2005; Wang et al., 2004). In contrast, patients lacking the G variant in breast tumors possessed early tumor onset and more recurrence and short disease-free survival (Kyndi et al., 2006; Wegman et al., 2009). In addition, it should be pointed out that preferential loss of the C allele in human tumors may imply a protective effect of this variant regarding cancer development (Denisov et al., 2010; Denisov et al., 2011); however, the current disagreements between meta-analyses (Table 2) and studies reporting rs1042522 allelic loss in tumors (Table 3) allow us to consider this statement as not quite truthful. Likely, further studies are needed to clarify the above-mentioned hypothesis.

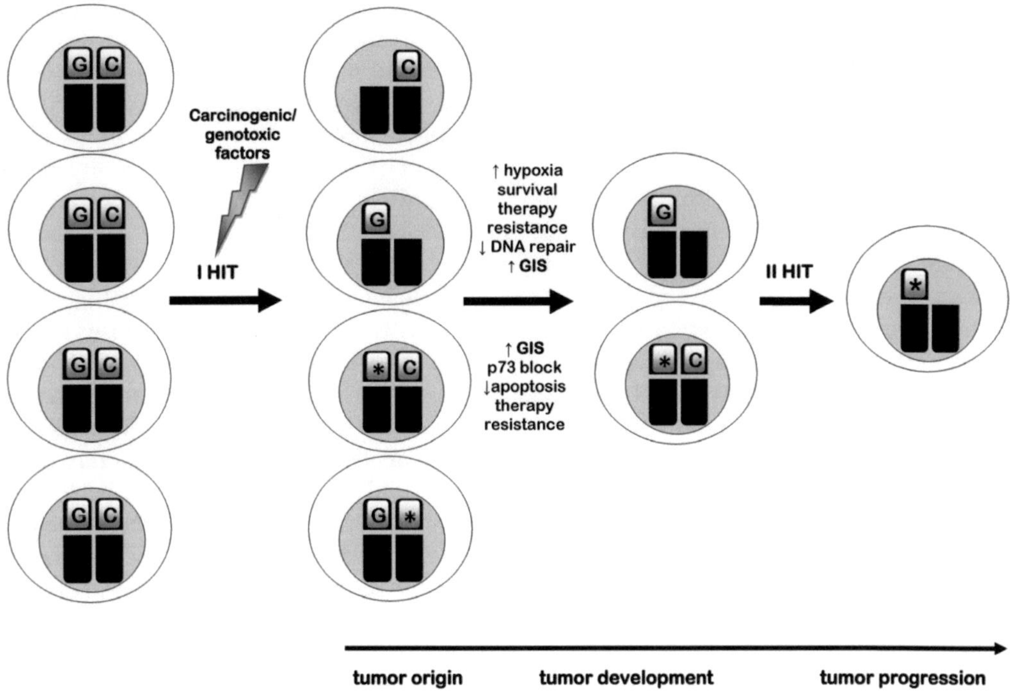

Fig. 1. The "two-hit" model of regular occurrence of *TP53* somatic abnormalities depending on the *TP53* rs1042522 polymorphism and environmental exposure. This model describes rs1042522-specific origin of *TP53* somatic aberrations in cancer tumors. At the first stage, LOH (indicated as a loss of chromosome arm) and/or mutation (indicated as asterisk on the chromosome arm) arise in any rs1042522 allele and in any order resulting in neoplastic transformation. From all tumor clones, only two ones with loss of the C allele and mutation in the G variant will have selective advantage via high survival capacity in hypoxia and therapy conditions, low ability to DNA repair and apoptosis. The dramatically increased genomic instability (GIS) in these cells will cause second inactivation forming the predominant tumor clone with loss of the C allele and mutation in the retained G variant. It is most likely that complete inactivation of p53 will impart invasive and/or metastatic potential to these cells.

In summary, the cancer predisposing effect of the *TP53* rs1042522 polymorphism through environment-induced regular occurrence of *TP53* somatic abnormalities has been reviewed in the present study. The "two-hit" model was suggested to explain the universal phenomenon for a majority of human tumors, consisting of a preferential loss of the C allele and mutation of the G variant. As reviewed herein, functional differentiation between rs1042522 allelic variants and its tissue specificity underlie selective pressure to maintain cells in which the C allele is lost and the G allele is mutated. Moreover, the inactivation of both the C and G allelic variants, resulting in a dramatic reduction in p53 functionality, may serve as an important background for tumorigenesis, as explained by the results of a study series on the association of *TP53* abnormalities in the rs1042522 polymorphic region with tumor onset and aggressiveness (Bonafe et al., 2003; Godai et al., 2009; Kyndi et al., 2006; Nelson et al., 2005; Schneider-Stock et al., 2004a; Wang et al., 2004; Wegman et al., 2009).

2.4 *TP53* polymorphisms: The cancer predisposing effect and aging

p53 is emerging as an important player in the regulation of senescence and longevity with pronounced antagonistic pleiotropy (Campisi, 2005; Donehower, 2006; Vigneron and Vousden, 2010). By suppressing cancers early in life, p53 is clearly a longevity assurance gene. However, there is some evidence that p53 might accelerate aging and reduce longevity late in life (Donehower, 2006). Results have shown that the genotype distribution of *TP53* polymorphisms, mainly the rs1042522 germline variation, in both healthy persons and cancer patients, is also consistent with antagonistic pleiotropy. As early as 1999, Bonafe et al. (Bonafe et al., 1999) demonstrated a slightly increased percentage of rs1042522 C carriers among Italian centenarians. Later, this research team reported that the presence of only major genotypes for rs1042522, rs17878362, and rs1625895, absence of the GSTT1 deletion, and the simultaneous occurrence of the *TP53* genotypes with minor alleles and the GSTT1 deletion, were much more frequent in young subjects than in centenarians (Gaspari et al., 2003). However, our data did not confirm this fact, likely due to the small study sample (Belyavskaya et al., 2005). Based on the observations, it is most likely that the reason for disagreement can be explained by the different genetic backgrounds modifying the age-specific functionality of *TP53* polymorphisms (Belyavskaya et al., 2005). With respect to cancer, an age-specific dependence of cancer risk has been reported for *TP53* polymorphisms (Cherdyntseva et al., 2010; Chung et al., 2010; Gervas et al., 2007; Perel'muter et al., 2008). In this aspect, it is of note that some contradictions in the above-mentioned meta-analyses could be due to age-related effects of *TP53* germline variations. For example, breast cancer is one of a few diseases for which *TP53* rs1042522 polymorphism raises many questions (He et al., 2011; Hu et al., 2010b; Lu et al., 2011b; Ma et al., 2011; Peng et al., 2011; Sergentanis and Economopoulos, 2010b; The Breast Cancer Association Consortium, 2006; Zhang et al., 2010b; Zhuo et al., 2009a). According to our data, the C allele contributes to high breast cancer risk in the premenopausal period (Cherdyntseva et al., 2011), whereas a combination of rs1042522, rs17878362, and rs1625895 major genotypes often occurs in postmenopausal BC (Perel'muter et al., 2008). Therefore, a more accurate meta-analysis that takes into account age specificity is required to clarify the associations between rs1042522 and breast cancer risk. Interestingly, an age-associated change in the *TP53* genotype distribution was also observed for lung cancer: the elderly (60-79 yr) affected subjects were characterized by an increased frequency of *TP53* major genotypes, whereas a high proportion of heterozygous genotype combinations was frequently detected in mature (40-59 yr) patients (Cherdyntseva et al., 2010; Gervas et al., 2007). These data not only agreed with recent meta-analyses (Dai et al., 2009; Francisco et al., 2010; Li et al., 2009; Yan et al., 2009) but also suggest that age might be an important modifier of the association between *TP53* rs1042522 polymorphism and lung cancer risk. With regard to rs17878362 and rs1625895 germline variations, the alteration in frequency of their genotypes is most likely linked to the regulation of *TP53* gene dosage particularly that which results in an increase in expression of the rs1042522 G allele, as already mentioned previously. Curiously enough, a high percentage of rs1042522 GG genotype was displayed in elderly patients with both breast and lung cancer. It is possible that apoptosis preferentially activated by p53Arg protein can lead to tissue atrophy, organ degeneration and cancer-related aging phenotypes (Campisi, 2005; Rodier et al., 2007). Moreover, it is known that the effect of *TP53* rs1042522 polymorphism becomes evident as the age of individuals increases (Bonafe et al., 2004; Salvioli et al., 2005). In particular, cells isolated from centenarians and sexagenarians, GG carriers, undergo oxidative stress-induced apoptosis to a higher extent than cells obtained from C carriers (Bonafe et al., 2004). Additionally, individuals that live a long time with the C allele display slower cell cycle kinetics and an increased propensity to undergo cell senescence than age-matched persons not expressing the C variant (Salvioli et al., 2005). These findings result from the preferential induction of p21, cyclin-dependent kinase inhibitor 1, and, likely, age-dependent activation of PAI-1, plasminogen activator inhibitor 1, by p53Pro protein (Salvioli et al., 2005; Testa et al., 2009).

Notwithstanding the age-specific effect of *TP53* polymorphisms on cancer risk, interesting findings concerning their influence on longevity have been provided by Van Heemst et al. (van Heemst et al., 2005). Elderly patients, carriers of the CC genotype, display a 41% increased survival despite a 2.54-fold high cancer mortality. Interestingly, some have suggested that the increased longevity of individuals with the CC genotype may be due to a generally increased robustness after a diagnosis of cancer or other life-threatening diseases, perhaps via an age-dependent capability of p53Pro to stimulate the expression of PAI-1 (Bojesen and Nordestgaard, 2008; Orsted et al., 2007; Testa et al., 2009).

p53 is a central node in the molecular network of safeguarding the integrity of the genome. p53 activation can immediately result in alterations in the expression of more than a thousand genes (Kannan et al., 2011). However, the fate of p53 is also under the rigorous control of other molecular players. Quite recently, based on the results of an association study and epistatic interaction analysis, the age- and estrogen receptor-specific interplay between *TP53* and *FGFR2* has been demonstrated in breast cancer (Cherdyntseva et al., 2011). It was found that combinations of *FGFR2* rs1219648 minor and *TP53* rs1042522, rs17878362, and rs1625895 major genotypes were associated with a high risk of BC, particularly in the postmenopausal period. In contrast, combinations of the *FGFR2* and *TP53* major genotypes had a protective effect against BC, especially in premenopausal women. Of note, all observations were ER-dependent. A possible explanation arises from evidence that FGFR2, upregulated by estrogens through the rs1219648 (G allele)-formed estrogen receptor site, may result in p53 inactivation via the induction of MDM2 ubiquitin ligase (Cherdyntseva et al., 2011). Importantly, the presence of the minor rs1219648 allele may lead to elevated *FGFR2* expression in tumor cells by itself (Meyer et al., 2008). Another point of view is based on a molecular network consisting of the preferential activation of apoptosis and cancer-related aging phenotype by p53Arg protein and the further induction of *FGFR2* expression leading to the transactivation of cancer genes and increased proliferation. The above-mentioned reasoning allows us once again to conclude that the p53-associated cellular defense system that controls cancer suppression directly depends on age-related features of the human organism, and this phenomenon should be taken into account in future association studies.

2.5 *TP53* polymorphisms: The cancer predisposing effect and ethnicity

The *TP53* polymorphism distribution dramatically changes across the globe (Beckman et al., 1994; Sjalander et al., 1996), indicating selective pressure to fix *TP53* alleles in certain geographic areas. As noted in previous sections of this review, the functionally different p53 polymorphic proteins have the advantage of depending on specific environmental conditions (Hirshfield et al., 2010; Hu et al., 2011; Jeong et al., 2010). In addition, manifestation of the cancer predisposing effects of *TP53* polymorphisms may also be altered between the different ethnic groups (Weston et al., 1997). In the literature, there is a significant amount of evidence that *TP53* polymorphisms (rs1042522, rs17878362, and rs1625895) differently influence cancer risk depending on ethnic components. For instance, *TP53* rs1042522 polymorphism has a protective value against breast cancer in inhabitants of the Mediterranean area (Hu et al., 2010b), but a predisposing effect in Indians (He et al., 2011). In addition, Sergentanis and Economopoulos (Sergentanis and Economopoulos, 2010b) showed an enhancement of the association between the C allele and cancer, both breast cancer and lung cancer, with increasing latitude. Similar ethnicity-specific contribution of *TP53* rs1042522 germline variation is also typical for other human cancers (Table 2) (Economopoulos et al., 2010; Gao et al., 2009; Jiang et al., 2010a; Li et al., 2010; Liu et al., 2011; Zhang et al., 2010a). Interestingly enough, the allelic expression of human genes, like allele frequency, was found to differ between ethnic groups (Spielman et al., 2007). Siddique et al. showed that the expression of *TP53* rs1042522 alleles is selectively regulated in different ethnic populations: healthy Asian heterozygote individuals preferentially express the C allele, whereas Caucasians express the G allele. Conversely, approximately 75% of Chinese heterozygote patients with breast cancer predominantly express the G allele (Siddique et al., 2005). Although the potential reason for this phenomenon could be preferential loss of the C allele in breast tumors of heterozygous patients, as mentioned above, the data of Siddique et al. may indirectly confirm a predisposing role of the G allele in breast cancer development, as shown in some meta-analyses (He et al., 2011; Lu et al., 2011b; Sergentanis and Economopoulos, 2010b; Zhang et al., 2010b). In addition, our research team first showed the high risk potential of the G allele and trend toward the protective value of the C variant in relation to breast cancer development in Mongolian ethnic groups (Tuvans, Altaians, Khakases, and Buryats) living in the Siberia region of Russia (Pisareva et al., in press). It is of note that our earlier data demonstrated significantly lower breast cancer incidence in these ethnic groups in comparison with Caucasians living in the same region (Pisareva et al., 2007). Moreover, it is known that Caucasians are approximately 2-fold more prone to breast cancer than Asians (Siddique et al., 2005). As evident from the above, there is a specific selective pressure against high breast cancer incidence in people of Asian ethnicity, and a possible explanation for this might be the functional impact of the *TP53* rs1042522 polymorphism, of which the C allele is overrepresented in these populations. As indicated previously, the *TP53* rs1042522 polymorphism has a significant effect on the origin of *TP53* somatic abnormalities, especially mutations, and, thus, may predispose one to cancer. Race-specific differences in the frequency of *TP53* alterations have been shown between colorectal patients of Afro-American and Caucasian origin, with the prevalence of mutations in the former, which were rs1042522 CC carriers. Surprisingly, the African American CC genotype was associated with a high risk of lymph node metastasis and increased mortality (Katkoori et al., 2009). Although the above evidence is small in number and needs further approval, calculation of the ethnic component is essential to perform accurate and qualitatively correct association studies.

In summary, a disparity between different ethnicities (races) in various cancer incidences and outcomes depends on genetic differences affecting the biology of malignancy. Moreover, recent evidence indicates ethnic differences in toxicity from certain anticancer treatments as well their effectiveness, which apparently contributes to survival (Mahdi et al., 2011; Soo et al., 2011). This might be explained by the diversity in genotype variants, gene expression levels and epigenetic alterations providing different race/ethnicity-specific functional pathways. p53 is a key player contributing to the defense against cancer and has been shown to be involved in tumor progression and the response to cytostatic drugs via the regulation of metabolism and repair of DNA damage induced by chemotherapy. Therefore, the analysis of *TP53* rs1042522 polymorphism together with other deciding factors may help to understand racial differences in cancer aggressiveness and clinical outcomes, which could increase treatment efficacy.

3. Conclusions

p53 (*TP53* gene) is a key tumor suppressor that balances the need for cell proliferation against the need for cancer suppression, thereby maintaining genomic integrity. Polymorphisms in the *TP53* gene significantly modify p53 functionality, thereby affecting the mechanisms of cancer prevention. Despite the substantial progress in molecular genetics and the understanding of tumorigenesis mechanisms in recent years, the value of *TP53* polymorphisms is not entirely clear in relation to a predisposition to or protection from cancer risk. In the present review, we focused on available information concerning the functional role of *TP53* polymorphisms and data from consortium works and the latest meta-analyses demonstrating their effect on cancer risk. We supposed that the disagreements and ambiguities in these studies are linked to the changeable nature of *TP53* polymorphism manifestation dependent on environmental exposure, mainly age features and ethnic components of the analyzed individuals. In our opinion, the possible variations of the impact of *TP53* polymorphisms on cancer susceptibility, mainly for rs1042522, might be presented as a complex gene-environmental mechanism realized through a regular occurrence of *TP53* somatic abnormalities and selective pressure against certain *TP53* alleles. Overall, the environment-specific character of *TP53* polymorphisms has been reviewed to demonstrate potential cancer risk-modifying factors, which should be taken into account to avoid unclear and ambiguous results in future association studies.

4. References

Almeida, L.O., Custodio, A.C., Pinto, G.R., Santos, M.J., Almeida, J.R., Clara, C.A., Rey, J.A. & Casartelli, C. (2009). Polymorphisms and DNA methylation of gene *TP53* associated with extra-axial brain tumors. *Genet Mol Res*, Vol.8, No.1, pp. 8-18, (February 2009), ISSN 1676-5680

Almquist, L.M., Karagas, M.R., Christensen, B.C., Welsh, M.M., Perry, A.E., Storm, C.A. & Nelson, H.H. (2011). The role of *TP53* and MDM2 polymorphisms in *TP53* mutagenesis and risk of non-melanoma skin cancer. *Carcinogenesis*, Vol.32, No.3, pp. 327-330, (December 2010), ISSN 1460-2180

Amatya, V.J., Naumann, U., Weller, M. & Ohgaki, H. (2005). *TP53* promoter methylation in human gliomas. *Acta Neuropathol*, Vol.110, No.2, pp. 178-184, (Jule 2005), ISSN 0001-6322

Anzola, M., Cuevas, N., Lopez-Martinez, M., Saiz, A., Burgos, J.J. & de Pancorbo, M.M. (2003). Frequent loss of p53 codon 72 Pro variant in hepatitis C virus-positive carriers with hepatocellular carcinoma. *Cancer Lett*, Vol.193, No.2, pp. 199-205, (April 2003), ISSN 0304-3835

Azzam, G.A., Frank, A.K., Hollstein, M. & Murphy, M.E. (2011). Tissue-specific apoptotic effects of the p53 codon 72 polymorphism in a mouse model. *Cell Cycle*, Vol.10, No.9, pp. 1352-1355, (May 2011), ISSN 1551-4005

Baker, S.J., Preisinger, A.C., Jessup, J.M., Paraskeva, C., Markowitz, S., Willson, J.K., Hamilton, S. & Vogelstein, B. (1990). p53 gene mutations occur in combination with 17p allelic deletions as late events in colorectal tumorigenesis. *Cancer Res*, Vol.50, No.23, pp. 7717-7722, (December 1990), ISSN 0008-5472

Beckman, G., Birgander, R., Sjalander, A., Saha, N., Holmberg, P.A., Kivela, A. & Beckman, L. (1994). Is p53 polymorphism maintained by natural selection? *Hum Hered*, Vol.44, No.5, pp. 266-270, (September 1994), ISSN 0001-5652

Belyavskaya, V.A., Smetannikova, N.A., Maksimov, V.N., Smetannikova, M.A., Bolotnova, T.V., Ustinov, S.N., Shabalin, A.V. & Voevoda, M.I. (2005). The search for "Longevity" and "Non-longevity" genes: the role of polymorphism of some keys genes of immunological homeostasis in development of pathology reducing lifespan. *Molecular Medicine (Russian)*, Vol.3, pp. 55-60

Belyavskaya, V.A., Vardosanidze, V.K., Smirnova, O.Y., Karakin, E.I., Savkin, I.V., Gervas, P.A., Cherdyntseva, N.V. & Voevoda, M.I. (2006). Genetic status of p53 in stomach cancer: somatic mutations and polymorphism of codon 72. *Bull Exp Biol Med*, Vol.141, No.2, pp. 243-246, (September 2006), ISSN 0007-4888

Bendesky, A., Rosales, A., Salazar, A.M., Sordo, M., Peniche, J. & Ostrosky-Wegman, P. (2007). p53 codon 72 polymorphism, DNA damage and repair, and risk of non-melanoma skin cancer. *Mutat Res*, Vol.619, No.1-2, pp. 38-44, (April 2007), ISSN 0027-5107

Bergamaschi, D., Gasco, M., Hiller, L., Sullivan, A., Syed, N., Trigiante, G., Yulug, I., Merlano, M., Numico, G., Comino, A., Attard, M., Reelfs, O., Gusterson, B., Bell, A.K., Heath, V., Tavassoli, M., Farrell, P.J., Smith, P., Lu, X. & Crook, T. (2003). p53 polymorphism influences response in cancer chemotherapy via modulation of p73-dependent apoptosis. *Cancer Cell*, Vol.3, No.4, pp. 387-402, (May 2003), ISSN 1535-6108

Biros, E., Kohut, A., Biros, I., Kalina, I., Bogyiova, E. & Stubna, J. (2002). A link between the p53 germ line polymorphisms and white blood cells apoptosis in lung cancer patients. *Lung Cancer*, Vol.35, No.3, pp. 231-235, (February 2002), ISSN 0169-5002

Bojesen, S.E. & Nordestgaard, B.G. (2008). The common germline Arg72Pro polymorphism of p53 and increased longevity in humans. *Cell Cycle*, Vol.7, No.2, pp. 158-163, (February 2008), ISSN 1551-4005

Bonafe, M., Olivieri, F., Mari, D., Baggio, G., Mattace, R., Berardelli, M., Sansoni, P., De Benedictis, G., De Luca, M., March egiani, F., Cavallone, L., Cardelli, M., Giovagnetti, S., Ferrucci, L., Amadio, L., Lisa, R., Tucci, M.G., Troiano, L., Pini, G., Gueresi, P., Morellini, M., Sorbi, S., Passeri, G., Barbi, C., Valensin, S., Monti, D., Deiana, L., Pes, G.M., Carru, C. & Franceschi, C. (1999). P53 codon 72 polymorphism and longevity: additional data on centenarians from continental Italy and Sardinia. *Am J Hum Genet*, Vol.65, No.6, pp. 1782-1785, (December 1999), ISSN 0002-9297

Bonafe, M., Salvioli, S., Barbi, C., Mishto, M., Trapassi, C., Gemelli, C., Storci, G., Olivieri, F., Monti, D. & Franceschi, C. (2002). p53 codon 72 genotype affects apoptosis by cytosine arabinoside in blood leukocytes. *Biochem Biophys Res Commun*, Vol.299, No.4, pp. 539-541, (December 2002), ISSN 0006-291X

Bonafe, M., Ceccarelli, C., Farabegoli, F., Santini, D., Taffurelli, M., Barbi, C., Marzi, E., Trapassi, C., Storci, G., Olivieri, F. & Franceschi, C. (2003). Retention of the p53 codon 72 arginine allele is associated with a reduction of disease-free and overall survival in arginine/proline heterozygous breast cancer patients. *Clin Cancer Res*, Vol.9, No.13, pp. 4860-4864, (October 2003), ISSN 1078-0432

Bonafe, M., Salvioli, S., Barbi, C., Trapassi, C., Tocco, F., Storci, G., Invidia, L., Vannini, I., Rossi, M., Marzi, E., Mishto, M., Capri, M., Olivieri, F., Antonicelli, R., Memo, M., Uberti, D., Nacmias, B., Sorbi, S., Monti, D. & Franceschi, C. (2004). The different apoptotic potential of the p53 codon 72 alleles increases with age and modulates in vivo ischaemia-induced cell death. *Cell Death Differ*, Vol.11, No.9, pp. 962-973, (May 2004), ISSN 1350-9047

Brooks, L.A., Tidy, J.A., Gusterson, B., Hiller, L., O'Nions, J., Gasco, M., Marin, M.C., Farrell, P.J., Kaelin, W.G., Jr. & Crook, T. (2000). Preferential retention of codon 72 arginine p53 in squamous cell carcinomas of the vulva occurs in cancers positive and negative for human papillomavirus. *Cancer Res*, Vol.60, No.24, pp. 6875-6877, (December 2000), ISSN 0008-5472

Brosh, R. & Rotter, V. (2009). When mutants gain new powers: news from the mutant p53 field. *Nat Rev Cancer*, Vol.9, No.10, pp. 701-713, (August 2009), ISSN 1474-1768

Buller, R.E., Sood, A., Fullenkamp, C., Sorosky, J., Powills, K. & Anderson, B. (1997). The influence of the p53 codon 72 polymorphism on ovarian carcinogenesis and prognosis. *Cancer Gene Ther*, Vol.4, No.4, pp. 239-245, (Jule 1997), ISSN 0929-1903

Campisi, J. (2005). Senescent cells, tumor suppression, and organismal aging: good citizens, bad neighbors. *Cell*, Vol.120, No.4, pp. 513-522, (March 2005), ISSN 0092-8674

Chang, C.J., Chao, C.H., Xia, W., Yang, J.Y., Xiong, Y., Li, C.W., Yu, W.H., Rehman, S.K., Hsu, J.L., Lee, H.H., Liu, M., Chen, C.T., Yu, D. & Hung, M.C. (2011). p53 regulates epithelial-mesenchymal transition and stem cell properties through modulating miRNAs. *Nat Cell Biol*, Vol.13, No.3, pp. 317-323, (February 2011), ISSN 1476-4679

Chen, X., Liu, F., Li, B., Wei, Y.G., Yan, L.N. & Wen, T.F. (2011). p53 codon 72 polymorphism and liver cancer susceptibility: a meta-analysis of epidemiologic studies. *World J Gastroenterol*, Vol.17, No.9, pp. 1211-1218, (March 2011), ISSN 1007-9327

Cherdyntseva, N., Gervas, P., Litvyakov, N., Stakcheeva, M., Ponomaryeva, A., Dobrodeev, A., Denisov, E., Belyavskaya, V. & Choinzonov, E. (2010). Age-related function of tumor suppressor gene *TP53*: contribution to cancer risk and progression. *Exp Oncol*, Vol.32, No.3, pp. 205-208, (September 2010), ISSN 1812-9269

Cherdyntseva, N.V., Denisov, E.V., Litviakov, N.V., Maksimov, V.N., Malinovskaya, E.A., Babyshkina, N.N., Slonimskaya, E.M., Voevoda, M.I. & Choinzonov, E.L. (2011). Crosstalk between the *FGFR2* and *TP53* genes in breast cancer: data from an association study and epistatic interaction analysis. *DNA Cell Biol* (August 2011), DOI: 10.1089/dna.2011.1351, ISSN 1044-5498

Chumakov, P.M. (2007). Versatile functions of p53 protein in multicellular organisms. *Biochemistry (Mosc)*, Vol.72, No.13, pp. 1399-1421, (February 2008), ISSN 0006-2979

Chung, W.H., Dao, R.L., Chen, L.K. & Hung, S.I. (2010). The role of genetic variants in human longevity. *Ageing Res Rev*, Vol.9, Suppl.1, pp. S67-78, (August 2010), ISSN 1872-9649

Dahabreh, I.J., Linardou, H., Bouzika, P., Varvarigou, V. & Murray, S. (2010). *TP53* Arg72Pro polymorphism and colorectal cancer risk: a systematic review and meta-analysis. *Cancer Epidemiol Biomarkers Prev*, Vol.19, No.7, pp. 1840-1847, (Jule 2010), ISSN 1538-7755

Dai, S., Mao, C., Jiang, L., Wang, G. & Cheng, H. (2009). P53 polymorphism and lung cancer susceptibility: a pooled analysis of 32 case-control studies. *Hum Genet*, Vol.125, No.5-6, pp. 633-638, (April 2009), ISSN 1432-1203

De Bont, R. & van Larebeke, N. (2004). Endogenous DNA damage in humans: a review of quantitative data. *Mutagenesis*, Vol.19, No.3, pp. 169-185, (May 2004), ISSN 0267-8357

Denisov, E.V., Cherdyntseva, N.V., Litvyakov, N.V., Slonimskaya, E.M., Malinovskaya, E.A., Voevoda, M.I., Belyavskaya, V.A. & Stegniy, V.N. (2009). *TP53* mutations and Arg72Pro polymorphism in breast cancers. *Cancer Genet Cytogenet*, Vol.192, No.2. pp. 93-95, (Jule 2009), ISSN 1873-4456

Denisov, E.V., Litviakov, N.V., Goncharik, O.O., Karpov, A.B., Takhauov, R.M. & Cherdyntseva, N.V. (2010). Genetic testing of cancer predisposition and progression: analysis of gene variations in tumor is required, *Proceedings of 35th ESMO Congress*, pp. viii348-viii349, Milan, Italy, October 8-12, 2010.

Denisov, E.V., Sukhanovskaya, T.V., Dultseva, T.S., Malinovskaya, E.A., Litviakov, N.V., Slonimskaya, E.M., Choinzonov, E.L. & Cherdyntseva, N.V. (2011). Coordination of *TP53* abnormalities in breast cancer: data from analysis of *TP53* polymorphisms, loss of heterozygosity, methylation and mutations.*Genet Test Mol Biomarkers* (August 2011), DOI: 10.1089/gtmb.2011.0038, ISSN 1945-0257

Donehower, L. (2006). p53, longevity assurance and longevity suppression. *Drug Discovery Today: Disease Mechanisms*, Vol.3, No.1, pp. 33-39, (Spring 2006)

Donehower, L.A. & Lozano, G. (2009). 20 years studying p53 functions in genetically engineered mice. *Nat Rev Cancer*, Vol.9, No.11, pp. 831-841, (September 2009), ISSN 1474-1768

Dumont, P., Leu, J.I., Della Pietra, A.C., 3rd, George, D.L. & Murphy, M. (2003). The codon 72 polymorphic variants of p53 have markedly different apoptotic potential. *Nat Genet*, Vol.33, No.3, pp. 357-365, (February 2003), ISSN 1061-4036

Economopoulos, K.P. & Sergentanis, T.N. (2010). Methodological remarks concerning the recent meta-analysis on p53 codon 72 polymorphism and colorectal cancer risk. *Eur J Surg Oncol*, Vol.36, No.12, pp. 1225-1226; author reply 1227-1228, (October 2010), ISSN 1532-2157

Economopoulos, K.P., Sergentanis, T.N., Zagouri, F. & Zografos, G.C. (2010). Association between p53 Arg72Pro polymorphism and colorectal cancer risk: a meta-analysis. *Onkologie*, Vol.33, No.12, pp. 666-674, (December 2010), ISSN 1423-0240

Ellsworth, R.E., Ellsworth, D.L., Neatrour, D.M., Deyarmin, B., Lubert, S.M., Sarachine, M.J., Brown, P., Hooke, J.A. & Shriver, C.D. (2005). Allelic imbalance in primary breast carcinomas and metastatic tumors of the axillary lymph nodes. *Mol Cancer Res*, Vol.3, No.2, pp. 71-77, (March 2005), ISSN 1541-7786

Feng, Z., Zhang, C., Kang, H.J., Sun, Y., Wang, H., Naqvi, A., Frank, A.K., Rosenwaks, Z., Murphy, M.E., Levine, A.J. & Hu, W. (2011). Regulation of female reproduction by p53 and its family members. *FASEB J*, Vol.25, No.7, pp. 2245-2255, (March 2011), ISSN 1530-6860

Francisco, G., Menezes, P.R., Eluf-Neto, J. & Chammas, R. (2010). Arg72Pro *TP53* polymorphism and cancer susceptibility: A comprehensive meta-analysis of 302 case-control studies. *Int J Cancer*, Vol.129, No.4, pp. 920-930, (August 2010), ISSN 1097-0215

Frank, A.K., Leu, J.I., Zhou, Y., Devarajan, K., Nedelko, T., Klein-Szanto, A., Hollstein, M. & Murphy, M.E. (2011). The codon 72 polymorphism of p53 regulates interaction with NF-{kappa}b and transactivation of genes involved in immunity and inflammation. *Mol Cell Biol*, Vol.31, No.6, pp. 1201-1213, (January 2011), ISSN 1098-5549

Frohling, S. & Dohner, H. (2008). Chromosomal abnormalities in cancer. *N Engl J Med*, Vol.359, No.7, pp. 722-734, (August 2008), ISSN 1533-4406

Furihata, M., Takeuchi, T., Matsumoto, M., Kurabayashi, A., Ohtsuki, Y., Terao, N., Kuwahara, M. & Shuin, T. (2002). p53 mutation arising in Arg72 allele in the tumorigenesis and development of carcinoma of the urinary tract. *Clin Cancer Res*, Vol.8, No.5, pp. 1192-1195, (May 2002), ISSN 1078-0432

Gao, L., Nieters, A. & Brenner, H. (2009). Cell proliferation-related genetic polymorphisms and gastric cancer risk: systematic review and meta-analysis. *Eur J Hum Genet*, Vol.17, No.12, pp. 1658-1667, (June 2009), ISSN 1476-5438

Gaspari, L., Pedotti, P., Bonafe, M., Franceschi, C., Marinelli, D., Mari, D., Garte, S. & Taioli, E. (2003). Metabolic gene polymorphisms and p53 mutations in healthy centenarians and younger controls. *Biomarkers*, Vol.8, No.6, pp. 522-528, (June 2004), ISSN 1354-750X

Gemignani, F., Moreno, V., Landi, S., Moullan, N., Chabrier, A., Gutierrez-Enriquez, S., Hall, J., Guino, E., Peinado, M.A., Capella, G. & Canzian, F. (2004). A *TP53* polymorphism is associated with increased risk of colorectal cancer and with reduced levels of *TP53* mRNA. *Oncogene*, Vol.23, No.10, pp. 1954-1956, (December 2003), ISSN 0950-9232

Gervas, P.A., Cherdyntseva, N.V., Belyavskaya, V.A., Vasileva, M.V., Dobrodeev, A.Y., Rudyk, Y.N., Miller, S.V., Tuzikov, S.A. & Voevoda, M.I. (2007). Polymorphism of p53 gene-oncosupressor: age-specific features in the risk of lung cancer development. *Siberian Journal of Oncology (Russian)*, Vol.2, No.22, pp. 49-54

Godai, T.I., Suda, T., Sugano, N., Tsuchida, K., Shiozawa, M., Sekiguchi, H., Sekiyama, A., Yoshihara, M., Matsukuma, S., Sakuma, Y., Tsuchiya, E., Kameda, Y., Akaike, M. & Miyagi, Y. (2009). Identification of colorectal cancer patients with tumors carrying the *TP53* mutation on the codon 72 proline allele that benefited most from 5-fluorouracil (5-FU) based postoperative chemotherapy. *BMC Cancer*, Vol.9, pp. 420, (December 2009), ISSN 1471-2407

Green, D.R. & Kroemer, G. (2009). Cytoplasmic functions of the tumour suppressor p53. *Nature*, Vol.458, No.7242, pp. 1127-1130, (May 2009), ISSN 1476-4687

Hanahan, D. & Weinberg, R.A. (2011). Hallmarks of cancer: the next generation. *Cell*, Vol.144, No.5, pp. 646-674, (March 2011), ISSN 1097-4172

Harris, N., Brill, E., Shohat, O., Prokocimer, M., Wolf, D., Arai, N. & Rotter, V. (1986). Molecular basis for heterogeneity of the human p53 protein. *Mol Cell Biol*, Vol.6, No.12, pp. 4650-4656, (December 1986), ISSN 0270-7306

He, X.F., Su, J., Zhang, Y., Huang, X., Liu, Y., Ding, D.P., Wang, W. & Arparkorn, K. (2011). Association between the p53 polymorphisms and breast cancer risk: meta-analysis based on case-control study. *Breast Cancer Res Treat,* (May 2011), DOI: 10.1007/s10549-011-1583-2, ISSN 1573-7217

Hirshfield, K.M., Rebbeck, T.R. & Levine, A.J. (2010). Germline mutations and polymorphisms in the origins of cancers in women. *J Oncol,* Vol.2010, pp. 297671, (January 2010), ISSN 1687-8469

Hrstka, R., Coates, P.J. & Vojtesek, B. (2009). Polymorphisms in p53 and the p53 pathway: roles in cancer susceptibility and response to treatment. *J Cell Mol Med,* Vol.13, No.3, pp. 440-453, (April 2009), ISSN 1582-4934

Hsieh, L.L., Huang, T.H., Chen, I.H., Liao, C.T., Wang, H.M., Lai, C.H., Liou, S.H., Chang, J.T. & Cheng, A.J. (2005). p53 polymorphisms associated with mutations in and loss of heterozygosity of the p53 gene in male oral squamous cell carcinomas in Taiwan. *Br J Cancer,* Vol.92, No.1, pp. 30-35, (December 2004), ISSN 0007-0920

Hsu, P.Y., Hsu, H.K., Singer, G.A., Yan, P.S., Rodriguez, B.A., Liu, J.C., Weng, Y.I., Deatherage, D.E., Chen, Z., Pereira, J.S., Lopez, R., Russo, J., Wang, Q., Lamartiniere, C.A., Nephew, K.P. & Huang, T.H. (2010). Estrogen-mediated epigenetic repression of large chromosomal regions through DNA looping. *Genome Res,* Vol.20, No.6, pp. 733-744, (May 2010), ISSN 1549-5469

Hu, W., Zheng, T. & Wang, J. (2011). Regulation of fertility by the p53 family members. *Genes & Cancer,* (April 2011), Vol.2, No.4, pp.420-430, ISSN 1947-6019

Hu, Y., McDermott, M.P. & Ahrendt, S.A. (2005). The p53 codon 72 proline allele is associated with p53 gene mutations in non-small cell lung cancer. *Clin Cancer Res,* Vol.11, No.7, pp. 2502-2509, (April 2005), ISSN 1078-0432

Hu, Z., Li, X., Qu, X., He, Y., Ring, B.Z., Song, E. & Su, L. (2010a). Intron 3 16 bp duplication polymorphism of *TP53* contributes to cancer susceptibility: a meta-analysis. *Carcinogenesis,* Vol.31, No.4, pp. 643-647, (January 2010), ISSN 1460-2180

Hu, Z., Li, X., Yuan, R., Ring, B.Z. & Su, L. (2010b). Three common *TP53* polymorphisms in susceptibility to breast cancer, evidence from meta-analysis. *Breast Cancer Res Treat,* Vol.120, No.3, pp. 705-714, (August 2009), ISSN 1573-7217

Jeong, B.S., Hu, W., Belyi, V., Rabadan, R. & Levine, A.J. (2010). Differential levels of transcription of p53-regulated genes by the arginine/proline polymorphism: p53 with arginine at codon 72 favors apoptosis. *FASEB J,* Vol.24, No.5, pp. 1347-1353, (December 2009), ISSN 1530-6860

Jiang, D.K., Ren, W.H., Yao, L., Wang, W.Z., Peng, B. & Yu, L. (2010a). Meta-analysis of association between *TP53* Arg72Pro polymorphism and bladder cancer risk. *Urology,* Vol.76, No.3, pp. 761-767, (Jule 2010), ISSN 1527-9995

Jiang, D.K., Yao, L., Ren, W.H., Wang, W.Z., Peng, B. & Yu, L. (2010b). *TP53* Arg72Pro polymorphism and endometrial cancer risk: a meta-analysis. *Med Oncol,* (June 2010), DOI: 10.1007/s12032-010-9597-x, ISSN 1559-131X

Jiang, D.K., Wang, W.Z., Ren, W.H., Yao, L., Peng, B. & Yu, L. (2011). *TP53* Arg72Pro polymorphism and skin cancer risk: a meta-analysis. *J Invest Dermatol,* Vol.131, No.1, pp. 220-228, (September 2010), ISSN 1523-1747

Kang, H.J., Feng, Z., Sun, Y., Atwal, G., Murphy, M.E., Rebbeck, T.R., Rosenwaks, Z., Levine, A.J. & Hu, W. (2009). Single-nucleotide polymorphisms in the p53 pathway regulate fertility in humans. *Proc Natl Acad Sci U S A*, Vol.106, No.24, pp. 9761-9766, (May 2009), ISSN 1091-6490

Kang, J.H., Kim, S.J., Noh, D.Y., Park, I.A., Choe, K.J., Yoo, O.J. & Kang, H.S. (2001). Methylation in the p53 promoter is a supplementary route to breast carcinogenesis: correlation between CpG methylation in the p53 promoter and the mutation of the p53 gene in the progression from ductal carcinoma in situ to invasive ductal carcinoma. *Lab Invest*, Vol.81, No.4, pp. 573-579, (April 2001), ISSN 0023-6837

Kannan, K., Rechavi, G. & Givol, D. (2011). p53's Dilemma in Transcription: Analysis by Microarrays, In: *p53*, A. Ayed & T.Hupp, (Ed.), 216, Springer-Verlag, ISBN 978-1-4419-8230-8, New-York, USA

Katkoori, V.R., Jia, X., Shanmugam, C., Wan, W., Meleth, S., Bumpers, H., Grizzle, W.E. & Manne, U. (2009). Prognostic significance of p53 codon 72 polymorphism differs with race in colorectal adenocarcinoma. *Clin Cancer Res*, Vol.15, No.7, pp. 2406-2416, (April 2009), ISSN 1078-0432

Kawaguchi, H., Ohno, S., Araki, K., Miyazaki, M., Saeki, H., Watanabe, M., Tanaka, S. & Sugimachi, K. (2000). p53 polymorphism in human papillomavirus-associated esophageal cancer. *Cancer Res*, Vol.60, No.11, pp. 2753-2755, (June 2000), ISSN 0008-5472

Kay, C., Jeyendran, R.S. & Coulam, C.B. (2006). p53 tumour suppressor gene polymorphism is associated with recurrent implantation failure. *Reprod Biomed Online*, Vol.13, No.4, pp. 492-496, (September 2006), ISSN 1472-6483

Khlgatian, M.K., Hadshiew, I.M., Asawanonda, P., Yaar, M., Eller, M.S., Fujita, M., Norris, D.A. & Gilchrest, B.A. (2002). Tyrosinase gene expression is regulated by p53. *J Invest Dermatol*, Vol.118, No.1, pp. 126-132, (February 2002), ISSN 0022-202X

Klug, S.J., Ressing, M., Koenig, J., Abba, M.C., Agorastos, T., Brenna, S.M., Ciotti, M., Das, B.R., Del Mistro, A., Dybikowska, A., Giuliano, A.R., Gudleviciene, Z., Gyllensten, U., Haws, A.L., Helland, A., Herrington, C.S., Hildesheim, A., Humbey, O., Jee, S.H., Kim, J.W., Madeleine, M.M., Menczer, J., Ngan, H.Y., Nishikawa, A., Niwa, Y., Pegoraro, R., Pillai, M.R., Ranzani, G., Rezza, G., Rosenthal, A.N., Roychoudhury, S., Saranath, D., Schmitt, V.M., Sengupta, S., Settheetham-Ishida, W., Shirasawa, H., Snijders, P.J., Stoler, M.H., Suarez-Rincon, A.E., Szarka, K., Tachezy, R., Ueda, M., van der Zee, A.G., von Knebel Doeberitz, M., Wu, M.T., Yamashita, T., Zehbe, I. & Blettner, M. (2009). *TP53* codon 72 polymorphism and cervical cancer: a pooled analysis of individual data from 49 studies. *Lancet Oncol*, Vol.10, No.8, pp. 772-784, (Jule 2009), ISSN 1474-5488

Knudson, A.G., Jr. (1971). Mutation and cancer: statistical study of retinoblastoma. *Proc Natl Acad Sci U S A*, Vol.68, No.4, pp. 820-823, (April 1971), ISSN 0027-8424

Kyndi, M., Alsner, J., Hansen, L.L., Sorensen, F.B. & Overgaard, J. (2006). LOH rather than genotypes of *TP53* codon 72 is associated with disease-free survival in primary breast cancer. *Acta Oncol*, Vol.45, No.5, pp. 602-609, (Jule 2006), ISSN 0284-186X

Langerod, A., Bukholm, I.R., Bregard, A., Lonning, P.E., Andersen, T.I., Rognum, T.O., Meling, G.I., Lothe, R.A. & Borresen-Dale, A.L. (2002). The *TP53* codon 72 polymorphism May affect the function of *TP53* mutations in breast carcinomas but not in colorectal carcinomas. *Cancer Epidemiol Biomarkers Prev*, Vol.11, No.12, pp. 1684-1688, (December 2002), ISSN 1055-9965

Lee, S.H., Kim, S.R., Park, C.H., Cho, S.J. & Choi, Y.H. (2006). Loss of heterozygosity of chromosome 17p13 and p53 expression in invasive ductal carcinomas. *J Breast Cancer*, Vol.9, No.4, pp. 309-316, (November 2006)

Li, D.B., Wei, X., Jiang, L.H., Wang, Y. & Xu, F. (2010). Meta-analysis of epidemiological studies of association of P53 codon 72 polymorphism with bladder cancer. *Genet Mol Res*, Vol.9, No.3, pp. 1599-1605, (August 2010), ISSN 1676-5680

Li, Y., Qiu, L.X., Shen, X.K., Lv, X.J., Qian, X.P. & Song, Y. (2009). A meta-analysis of *TP53* codon 72 polymorphism and lung cancer risk: evidence from 15,857 subjects. *Lung Cancer*, Vol.66, No.1, pp. 15-21, (January 2009), ISSN 1872-8332

Lind, H., Ekstrom, P.O., Ryberg, D., Skaug, V., Andreassen, T., Stangeland, L., Haugen, A. & Zienolddiny, S. (2007). Frequency of *TP53* mutations in relation to Arg72Pro genotypes in non small cell lung cancer. *Cancer Epidemiol Biomarkers Prev*, Vol.16, No.10, pp. 2077-2081, (October 2007), ISSN 1055-9965

Litviakov, N., Denisov, E., Takhauov, R., Karpov, A., Skobel'skaja, E., Vasil'eva, E., Goncharik, O., Ageeva, A., Mamonova, N. & Mezheritskiy, S. (2010). Association between *TP53* gene ARG72PRO polymorphism and chromosome aberrations in human cancers. *Molecular Carcinogenesis*, Vol.49, No.6, pp. 521-524, (June 2010), ISSN 1098-2744

Liu, L., Wang, K., Zhu, Z.M. & Shao, J.H. (2011). Associations between P53 Arg72Pro and development of digestive tract cancers: a meta-analysis. *Arch Med Res*, Vol.42, No.1, pp. 60-69, (March 2011), ISSN 1873-5487

Lu, P.H., Chen, M.B., Wei, M.X., Jiang, Z.Y. & Li, C. (2011a). A small number of subjects do not always indicate that they are minor variants data for inclusion in a pooled analysis. *Breast Cancer Res Treat*, Vol.126, No.1, pp. 249-252, (November 2010), ISSN 1573-7217

Lu, P.H., Tao, G.Q., Liu, X., Li, C. & Wei, M.X. (2011b). No significant association results obtained from significant association evidence: the ongoing uncertainty of *TP53* codon 72 polymorphism and breast cancer risk. *Breast Cancer Res Treat*, Vol.125, No.2, pp. 601-603, (October 2010), ISSN 1573-7217

Lu, P.H., Wei, M.X., Li, C., Shen, W. & Chen, M.B. (2011c). Need for clarification of data in a recent meta-analysis about *TP53* codon 72 polymorphism and cancer susceptibility. *Carcinogenesis*, Vol.32, No.3, pp. 443, (December 2010), ISSN 1460-2180

Ma, Y., Yang, J., Liu, Z., Zhang, P., Yang, Z., Wang, Y. & Qin, H. (2011). No significant association between the *TP53* codon 72 polymorphism and breast cancer risk: a meta-analysis of 21 studies involving 24,063 subjects. *Breast Cancer Res Treat*, Vol.125, No.1, pp. 201-205, (May 2010), ISSN 1573-7217

Mahdi, H., Kumar, S., Hanna, R.K., Munkarah, A.R., Lockhart, D., Morris, R.T., Tamimi, H., Swensen, R.E. & Doherty, M. (2011). Disparities in treatment and survival between African American and White women with vaginal cancer. *Gynecol Oncol*, Vol.122, No.1, pp. 38-41, (April 2011), ISSN 1095-6859

Marcel, V., Palmero, E.I., Falagan-Lotsch, P., Martel-Planche, G., Ashton-Prolla, P., Olivier, M., Brentani, R.R., Hainaut, P. & Achatz, M.I. (2009). *TP53* PIN3 and MDM2 SNP309 polymorphisms as genetic modifiers in the Li-Fraumeni syndrome: impact on age at first diagnosis. *J Med Genet*, Vol.46, No.11, pp. 766-772, (June 2009), ISSN 1468-6244

Marcel, V., Tran, P.L., Sagne, C., Martel-Planche, G., Vaslin, L., Teulade-Fichou, M.P., Hall, J., Mergny, J.L., Hainaut, P. & Van Dyck, E. (2011). G-quadruplex structures in *TP53* intron 3: role in alternative splicing and in production of p53 mRNA isoforms. *Carcinogenesis*, Vol.32, No.3, pp. 271-278, (November 2010), ISSN 1460-2180

Marin, M.C., Jost, C.A., Brooks, L.A., Irwin, M.S., O'Nions, J., Tidy, J.A., James, N., McGregor, J.M., Harwood, C.A., Yulug, I.G., Vousden, K.H., Allday, M.J., Gusterson, B., Ikawa, S., Hinds, P.W., Crook, T. & Kaelin, W.G., Jr. (2000). A common polymorphism acts as an intragenic modifier of mutant p53 behaviour. *Nat Genet*, Vol.25, No.1, pp. 47-54, (May 2000), ISSN 1061-4036

Marshall, C.J. (1991). Tumor suppressor genes. *Cell*, Vol.64, No.2, pp. 313-326, (January 1991), ISSN 0092-8674

McCarthy, N. (2011). Tumour suppressors: Selective justice. *Nat Rev Cancer*, Vol.11, No.1, pp. 4, (January 2011), ISSN 1474-1768

McGregor, J.M., Harwood, C.A., Brooks, L., Fisher, S.A., Kelly, D.A., O'Nions, J., Young, A.R., Surentheran, T., Breuer, J., Millard, T.P., Lewis, C.M., Leigh, I.M., Storey, A. & Crook, T. (2002). Relationship between p53 codon 72 polymorphism and susceptibility to sunburn and skin cancer. *J Invest Dermatol*, Vol.119, No.1, pp. 84-90, (August 2002), ISSN 0022-202X

Mechanic, L.E., Marrogi, A.J., Welsh, J.A., Bowman, E.D., Khan, M.A., Enewold, L., Zheng, Y.L., Chanock, S., Shields, P.G. & Harris, C.C. (2005). Polymorphisms in XPD and *TP53* and mutation in human lung cancer. *Carcinogenesis*, Vol.26, No.3, pp. 597-604, (November 2004), ISSN 0143-3334

Meyer, K.B., Maia, A.T., O'Reilly, M., Teschendorff, A.E., Chin, S.F., Caldas, C. & Ponder, B.A. (2008). Allele-specific up-regulation of *FGFR2* increases susceptibility to breast cancer. *PLoS Biol*, Vol.6, No.5, pp. e108, (May 2008), ISSN 1545-7885

Mitra, S., Banerjee, S., Misra, C., Singh, R.K., Roy, A., Sengupta, A., Panda, C.K. & Roychoudhury, S. (2007). Interplay between human papilloma virus infection and p53 gene alterations in head and neck squamous cell carcinoma of an Indian patient population. *J Clin Pathol*, Vol.60, No.9, pp. 1040-1047, (November 2006), ISSN 0021-9746

Mizuno, H., Spike, B.T., Wahl, G.M. & Levine, A.J. (2010). Inactivation of p53 in breast cancers correlates with stem cell transcriptional signatures. *Proc Natl Acad Sci U S A*, Vol.107, No.52, pp. 22745-22750, (December 2010), ISSN 1091-6490

Muller, P.A., Vousden, K.H. & Norman, J.C. (2011). p53 and its mutants in tumor cell migration and invasion. *J Cell Biol*, Vol.192, No.2, pp. 209-218, (January 2011), ISSN 1540-8140

Murase, D., Hachiya, A., Amano, Y., Ohuchi, A., Kitahara, T. & Takema, Y. (2009). The essential role of p53 in hyperpigmentation of the skin via regulation of paracrine melanogenic cytokine receptor signaling. *J Biol Chem*, Vol.284, No.7, pp. 4343-4353, (December 2008), ISSN 0021-9258

Naldi, M., Pistolozzi, M., Bertucci, C., De Simone, A., Altilia, S., Pierini, M., Franceschi, C., Salvioli, S. & Andrisano, V. (2010). Structural characterization of p53 isoforms due to the polymorphism at codon 72 by mass spectrometry and circular dichroism. *J Pharm Biomed Anal*, Vol.53, No.2, pp. 200-206, (April 2010), ISSN 1873-264X

Nelson, H.H., Wilkojmen, M., Marsit, C.J. & Kelsey, K.T. (2005). *TP53* mutation, allelism and survival in non-small cell lung cancer. *Carcinogenesis*, Vol.26, No.10, pp. 1770-1773, (May 2005), ISSN 0143-3334

Nigro, J.M., Baker, S.J., Preisinger, A.C., Jessup, J.M., Hostetter, R., Cleary, K., Bigner, S.H., Davidson, N., Baylin, S., Devilee, P. & et al. (1989). Mutations in the p53 gene occur in diverse human tumour types. *Nature*, Vol.342, No.6250, pp. 705-708, (December 1989), ISSN 0028-0836

Nikbahkt Dastjerdi, M. (2011). *TP53* codon 72 polymorphism and p53 protein expression in colorectal cancer specimens in isfahan. *Acta Med Iran*, Vol.49, No.2, pp. 71-77, (May 2011), ISSN 1735-9694

Nordgard, S.H., Alnaes, G.I., Hihn, B., Lingjaerde, O.C., Liestol, K., Tsalenko, A., Sorlie, T., Lonning, P.E., Borresen-Dale, A.L. & Kristensen, V.N. (2008). Pathway based analysis of SNPs with relevance to 5-FU therapy: relation to intratumoral mRNA expression and survival. *Int J Cancer*, Vol.123, No.3, pp. 577-585, (May 2008), ISSN 1097-0215

Oka, K., Ishikawa, J., Bruner, J.M., Takahashi, R. & Saya, H. (1991). Detection of loss of heterozygosity in the p53 gene in renal cell carcinoma and bladder cancer using the polymerase chain reaction. *Mol Carcinog*, Vol.4, No.1, pp. 10-13, (January 1991), ISSN 0899-1987

Olivier, M., Hollstein, M. & Hainaut, P. (2010). *TP53* mutations in human cancers: origins, consequences, and clinical use. *Cold Spring Harb Perspect Biol*, Vol.2, No.1, pp. a001008, (February 2010), ISSN 1943-0264

Olovnikov, I.A., Kravchenko, J.E. & Chumakov, P.M. (2009). Homeostatic functions of the p53 tumor suppressor: regulation of energy metabolism and antioxidant defense. *Semin Cancer Biol*, Vol.19, No.1, pp. 32-41, (December 2008), ISSN 1096-3650

Oren, M. & Rotter, V. (2010). Mutant p53 gain-of-function in cancer. *Cold Spring Harb Perspect Biol*, Vol.2, No.2, pp. a001107, (February 2010), ISSN 1943-0264

Orsted, D.D., Bojesen, S.E., Tybjaerg-Hansen, A. & Nordestgaard, B.G. (2007). Tumor suppressor p53 Arg72Pro polymorphism and longevity, cancer survival, and risk of cancer in the general population. *J Exp Med*, Vol.204, No.6, pp. 1295-1301, (May 2007), ISSN 0022-1007

Ozeki, C., Sawai, Y., Shibata, T., Kohno, T., Okamoto, K., Yokota, J., Tashiro, F., Tanuma, S., Sakai, R., Kawase, T., Kitabayashi, I., Taya, Y. & Ohki, R. (2011). Cancer Susceptibility Polymorphism of p53 at Codon 72 Affects Phosphorylation and Degradation of p53 Protein. *J Biol Chem*, Vol.286, No.20, pp. 18251-18260, (April 2011), ISSN 1083-351X

Papadakis, E.D., Soulitzis, N. & Spandidos, D.A. (2002). Association of p53 codon 72 polymorphism with advanced lung cancer: the Arg allele is preferentially retained in tumours arising in Arg/Pro germline heterozygotes. *Br J Cancer*, Vol.87, No.9, pp. 1013-1018, (November 2002), ISSN 0007-0920

Pegoraro, R.J., Rom, L., Lanning, P.A., Moodley, M., Naiker, S. & Moodley, J. (2002). P53 codon 72 polymorphism and human papillomavirus type in relation to cervical cancer in South African women. *Int J Gynecol Cancer*, Vol.12, No.4, pp. 383-388, (Jule 2002), ISSN 1048-891X

Peng, S., Lu, B., Ruan, W., Zhu, Y., Sheng, H. & Lai, M. (2011). Genetic polymorphisms and breast cancer risk: evidence from meta-analyses, pooled analyses, and genome-wide association studies. *Breast Cancer Res Treat*, Vol.127, No.2, pp. 309-324, (March 2011), ISSN 1573-7217

Perel'muter, V.M., Zav'ialova, M.V., Vtorushin, S.V., Slonimskaia, E.M., Kritskaia, N.G., Garbukov, E., Litviakov, N.V., Stakheeva, M.N., Babyshkina, N.N., Malinovskaia, E.A., Denisov, E.V., Grigor'eva, E.S., Nazarenko, M.S., Sennikov, S.V., Goreva, E.P., Kozlov, V.A., Voevoda, M.I., Maksimov, V.N., Beliavskaia, V.A. & Cherdyntseva, N.V. (2008). Genetic and clinical and pathological characteristics of breast cancer in premenopausal and postmenopausal women. *Adv Gerontol (Russian)*, Vol.21, No.4, pp. 643-653, (January 2008), ISSN 1561-9125

Perez-Losada, J., Castellanos-Martin, A. & Mao, J.H. (2011). Cancer evolution and individual susceptibility. *Integr Biol (Camb)*, Vol.3, No.4, pp. 316-328, (January 2011), ISSN 1757-9708

Petitjean, A., Achatz, M., Borresen-Dale, A., Hainaut, P. & Olivier, M. (2007a). *TP53* mutations in human cancers: functional selection and impact on cancer prognosis and outcomes. *Oncogene*, Vol.26, No.15, pp. 2157-2165, (April 2007), ISSN 0950-9232

Petitjean, A., Mathe, E., Kato, S., Ishioka, C., Tavtigian, S.V., Hainaut, P. & Olivier, M. (2007b). Impact of mutant p53 functional properties on *TP53* mutation patterns and tumor phenotype: lessons from recent developments in the IARC *TP53* database. *Hum Mutat*, Vol.28, No.6, pp. 622-629, (February 2007), ISSN 1098-1004

Pezeshki, A., Sari-Aslani, F., Ghaderi, A. & Doroudchi, M. (2006). p53 codon 72 polymorphism in basal cell carcinoma of the skin. *Pathol Oncol Res*, Vol.12, No.1, pp. 29-33, (March 2006), ISSN 1219-4956

Pim, D. & Banks, L. (2004). p53 polymorphic variants at codon 72 exert different effects on cell cycle progression. *Int J Cancer*, Vol.108, No.2, pp. 196-199, (November 2003), ISSN 0020-7136

Pisareva, L.F., Odintsova, I.N., Ivanov, P.M. & Nikolaeva, T.I. (2007). The breast cancer incidence in aboriginal and alien population of Sakha Republic. *Siberian Journal of Oncology (Russian)*, Vol.3, pp. 69-72

Pisareva, L.F., Odintsova, I.N., Ananina, O.A., Malinovskaia, E.A., Stukanov, S.L., Panferova, E.V., Shivit-ool, A.A., Choinzonov, E.L. & Cherdyntseva, N.V. (in press). Breast cancer incidence in Caucasian and Mongolian populations living in Siberia and Far East region of Russian Federation. *Zdravookhranenie Rossiiskoi Federatsii (Russian)*

Qiu, Y.L., Wang, W., Wang, T., Liu, J., Sun, P., Qian, J., Jin, L. & Xia, Z.L. (2008). Genetic polymorphisms, messenger RNA expression of p53, p21, and CCND1, and possible links with chromosomal aberrations in Chinese vinyl chloride-exposed workers. *Cancer Epidemiol Biomarkers Prev*, Vol.17, No.10, pp. 2578-2584, (October 2008), ISSN 1055-9965

Ribeiro, J.C., Barnetson, A.R., Fisher, R.J., Mameghan, H. & Russell, P.J. (1997). Relationship between radiation response and p53 status in human bladder cancer cells. *Int J Radiat Biol*, Vol.72, No.1, pp. 11-20, (Jule 1997), ISSN 0955-3002

Rivlin, N., Brosh, R., Oren, M. & Rotter, V. (2011). Mutations in the p53 Tumor Suppressor Gene: Important Milestones at the Various Steps of Tumorigenesis. *Genes & Cancer*, (April 2011), Vol.2, No.4, pp.466-474, ISSN 1947-6027

Rodier, F., Campisi, J. & Bhaumik, D. (2007). Two faces of p53: aging and tumor suppression. *Nucleic Acids Res*, Vol.35, No.22, pp. 7475-7484, (October 2007), ISSN 1362-4962

Salvioli, S., Bonafe, M., Barbi, C., Storci, G., Trapassi, C., Tocco, F., Gravina, S., Rossi, M., Tiberi, L., Mondello, C., Monti, D. & Franceschi, C. (2005). p53 codon 72 alleles influence the response to anticancer drugs in cells from aged people by regulating the cell cycle inhibitor p21WAF1. *Cell Cycle*, Vol.4, No.9, pp. 1264-1271, (August 2005), ISSN 1551-4005

Sansone, P., Storci, G., Pandolfi, S., Montanaro, L., Chieco, P. & Bonafe, M. (2007). The p53 codon 72 proline allele is endowed with enhanced cell-death inducing potential in cancer cells exposed to hypoxia. *Br J Cancer*, Vol.96, No.8, pp. 1302-1308, (April 2007), ISSN 0007-0920

Sarig, R., Rivlin, N., Brosh, R., Bornstein, C., Kamer, I., Ezra, O., Molchadsky, A., Goldfinger, N., Brenner, O. & Rotter, V. (2010). Mutant p53 facilitates somatic cell reprogramming and augments the malignant potential of reprogrammed cells. *J Exp Med*, Vol.207, No.10, pp. 2127-2140, (August 2010), ISSN 1540-9538

Schildkraut, J.M., Goode, E.L., Clyde, M.A., Iversen, E.S., Moorman, P.G., Berchuck, A., Marks, J.R., Lissowska, J., Brinton, L., Peplonska, B., Cunningham, J.M., Vierkant, R.A., Rider, D.N., Chenevix-Trench, G., Webb, P.M., Beesley, J., Chen, X., Phelan, C., Sutphen, R., Sellers, T.A., Pearce, L., Wu, A.H., Van Den Berg, D., Conti, D., Elund, C.K., Anderson, R., Goodman, M.T., Lurie, G., Carney, M.E., Thompson, P.J., Gayther, S.A., Ramus, S.J., Jacobs, I., Kruger Kjaer, S., Hogdall, E., Blaakaer, J., Hogdall, C., Easton, D.F., Song, H., Pharoah, P.D., Whittemore, A.S., McGuire, V., Quaye, L., Anton-Culver, H., Ziogas, A., Terry, K.L., Cramer, D.W., Hankinson, S.E., Tworoger, S.S., Calingaert, B., Chanock, S., Sherman, M. & Garcia-Closas, M. (2009). Single nucleotide polymorphisms in the *TP53* region and susceptibility to invasive epithelial ovarian cancer. *Cancer Res*, Vol.69, No.6, pp. 2349-2357, (March 2009), ISSN 1538-7445

Schneider-Stock, R., Boltze, C., Peters, B., Szibor, R., Landt, O., Meyer, F. & Roessner, A. (2004a). Selective loss of codon 72 proline p53 and frequent mutational inactivation of the retained arginine allele in colorectal cancer. *Neoplasia*, Vol.6, No.5, pp. 529-535, (November 2004), ISSN 1522-8002

Schneider-Stock, R., Mawrin, C., Motsch, C., Boltze, C., Peters, B., Hartig, R., Buhtz, P., Giers, A., Rohrbeck, A., Freigang, B. & Roessner, A. (2004b). Retention of the arginine allele in codon 72 of the p53 gene correlates with poor apoptosis in head and neck cancer. *Am J Pathol*, Vol.164, No.4, pp. 1233-1241, (March 2004), ISSN 0002-9440

Schwartz, J.L., Plotnik, D., Slovic, J., Li, T., Racelis, M., Deeg, H.J. & Friedman, D.L. (2011). *TP53* codon-72 polymorphisms identify different radiation sensitivities to g2-chromosome breakage in human lymphoblast cells. *Environ Mol Mutagen*, Vol.52, No.1, pp. 77-80, (November 2010), ISSN 1098-2280

Sergentanis, T.N. & Economopoulos, K.P. (2010a). Eligible and not eligible studies in the recent meta-analysis about p53 polymorphism and breast cancer risk. *Breast Cancer Res Treat*, Vol.120, No.1, pp. 261-262, (September 2009), ISSN 1573-7217

Sergentanis, T.N. & Economopoulos, K.P. (2010b). Latitude May modify the effect of *TP53* codon 72 polymorphism on cancer risk. *Cancer*, Vol.116, No.14, pp. 3523, (June 2010), ISSN 0008-543X

Sergentanis, T.N. & Economopoulos, K.P. (2011). Re: Jiang et al.: Meta-analysis of association between *TP53* Arg72Pro polymorphism and bladder cancer risk (Urology 2010;76:765). *Urology*, Vol.77, No.1, pp. 259-260, (January 2011), ISSN 1527-9995

Seviour, E.G. & Lin, S.Y. (2010). The DNA damage response: Balancing the scale between cancer and ageing. *Aging (Albany NY)*, Vol.2, No.12, pp. 900-907, (December 2010), ISSN 1945-4589

Shi, H., Tan, S.J., Zhong, H., Hu, W., Levine, A., Xiao, C.J., Peng, Y., Qi, X.B., Shou, W.H., Ma, R.L., Li, Y., Su, B. & Lu, X. (2009). Winter temperature and UV are tightly linked to genetic changes in the p53 tumor suppressor pathway in Eastern Asia. *Am J Hum Genet*, Vol.84, No.4, pp. 534-541, (April 2009), ISSN 1537-6605

Siddique, M. & Sabapathy, K. (2006). Trp53-dependent DNA-repair is affected by the codon 72 polymorphism. *Oncogene*, Vol.25, No.25, pp. 3489-3500, (February 2006), ISSN 0950-9232

Siddique, M.M., Balram, C., Fiszer-Maliszewska, L., Aggarwal, A., Tan, A., Tan, P., Soo, K.C. & Sabapathy, K. (2005). Evidence for selective expression of the p53 codon 72 polymorphs: implications in cancer development. *Cancer Epidemiol Biomarkers Prev*, Vol.14, No.9, pp. 2245-2252, (September 2005), ISSN 1055-9965

Sidhu, S., Martin, E., Gicquel, C., Melki, J., Clark, S.J., Campbell, P., Magarey, C.J., Schulte, K.M., Roher, H.D., Delbridge, L. & Robinson, B.G. (2005). Mutation and methylation analysis of *TP53* in adrenal carcinogenesis. *Eur J Surg Oncol*, Vol.31, No.5, pp. 549-554, (June 2005), ISSN 0748-7983

Sjalander, A., Birgander, R., Kivela, A. & Beckman, G. (1995). p53 polymorphisms and haplotypes in different ethnic groups. *Hum Hered*, Vol.45, No.3, pp. 144-149, (May 1995), ISSN 0001-5652

Sjalander, A., Birgander, R., Saha, N., Beckman, L. & Beckman, G. (1996). p53 polymorphisms and haplotypes show distinct differences between major ethnic groups. *Hum Hered*, Vol.46, No.1, pp. 41-48, (January 1996), ISSN 0001-5652

Soo, R.A., Loh, M., Mok, T.S., Ou, S.H., Cho, B.C., Yeo, W.L., Tenen, D.G. & Soong, R. (2011). Ethnic differences in survival outcome in patients with advanced stage non-small cell lung cancer: results of a meta-analysis of randomized controlled trials. *J Thorac Oncol*, Vol.6, No.6, pp. 1030-1038, (May 2011), ISSN 1556-1380

Soussi, T. (2007). p53 alterations in human cancer: more questions than answers. *Oncogene*, Vol.26, No.15, pp. 2145-2156, (April 2007), ISSN 0950-9232

Spielman, R.S., Bastone, L.A., Burdick, J.T., Morley, M., Ewens, W.J. & Cheung, V.G. (2007). Common genetic variants account for differences in gene expression among ethnic groups. *Nat Genet*, Vol.39, No.2, pp. 226-231, (January 2007), ISSN 1061-4036

Storey, A., Thomas, M., Kalita, A., Harwood, C., Gardiol, D., Mantovani, F., Breuer, J., Leigh, I.M., Matlashewski, G. & Banks, L. (1998). Role of a p53 polymorphism in the development of human papillomavirus-associated cancer. *Nature*, Vol.393, No.6682, pp. 229-234, (June 1998), ISSN 0028-0836

Szymanowska, A., Jassem, E., Dziadziuszko, R., Borg, A., Limon, J., Kobierska-Gulida, G., Rzyman, W. & Jassem, J. (2006). Increased risk of non-small cell lung cancer and frequency of somatic *TP53* gene mutations in Pro72 carriers of *TP53* Arg72Pro polymorphism. *Lung Cancer*, Vol.52, No.1, pp. 9-14, (February 2006), ISSN 0169-5002

Tandle, A.T., Sanghvi, V. & Saranath, D. (2001). Determination of p53 genotypes in oral cancer patients from India. *Br J Cancer*, Vol.84, No.6, pp. 739-742, (March 2001), ISSN 0007-0920

Tang, N.P., Wu, Y.M., Wang, B. & Ma, J. (2010). Systematic review and meta-analysis of the association between P53 codon 72 polymorphism and colorectal cancer. *Eur J Surg Oncol*, Vol.36, No.5, pp. 431-438, (April 2010), ISSN 1532-2157

Testa, R., Bonfigli, A.R., Salvioli, S., Invidia, L., Pierini, M., Sirolla, C., Marra, M., Testa, I., Fazioli, F., Recchioni, R., March eselli, F., Olivieri, F., Lanari, L. & Franceschi, C. (2009). The Pro/Pro genotype of the p53 codon 72 polymorphism modulates PAI-1 plasma levels in ageing. *Mech Ageing Dev*, Vol.130, No.8, pp. 497-500, (June 2009), ISSN 1872-6216

The Breast Cancer Association Consortium. (2006). Commonly studied single-nucleotide polymorphisms and breast cancer: results from the Breast Cancer Association Consortium. *J Natl Cancer Inst*, Vol.98, No.19, pp. 1382-1396, (October 2006), ISSN 1460-2105

Thiagalingam, S., Foy, R.L., Cheng, K.H., Lee, H.J., Thiagalingam, A. & Ponte, J.F. (2002). Loss of heterozygosity as a predictor to map tumor suppressor genes in cancer: molecular basis of its occurrence. *Curr Opin Oncol*, Vol.14, No.1, pp. 65-72, (January 2002), ISSN 1040-8746

Thomas, M., Kalita, A., Labrecque, S., Pim, D., Banks, L. & Matlashewski, G. (1999). Two polymorphic variants of wild-type p53 differ biochemically and biologically. *Mol Cell Biol*, Vol.19, No.2, pp. 1092-1100, (February 1999), ISSN 0270-7306

Truong, T., Sauter, W., McKay, J.D., Hosgood, H.D., 3rd, Gallagher, C., Amos, C.I., Spitz, M., Muscat, J., Lazarus, P., Illig, T., Wichmann, H.E., Bickeboller, H., Risch, A., Dienemann, H., Zhang, Z.F., Naeim, B.P., Yang, P., Zienolddiny, S., Haugen, A., Le March and, L., Hong, Y.C., Kim, J.H., Duell, E.J., Andrew, A.S., Kiyohara, C., Shen, H., Matsuo, K., Suzuki, T., Seow, A., Ng, D.P., Lan, Q., Zaridze, D., Szeszenia-Dabrowska, N., Lissowska, J., Rudnai, P., Fabianova, E., Constantinescu, V., Bencko, V., Foretova, L., Janout, V., Caporaso, N.E., Albanes, D., Thun, M., Landi, M.T., Trubicka, J., Lener, M., Lubinski, J., Wang, Y., Chabrier, A., Boffetta, P., Brennan, P. & Hung, R.J. (2010). International Lung Cancer Consortium: coordinated association study of 10 potential lung cancer susceptibility variants. *Carcinogenesis*, Vol.31, No.4, pp. 625-633, (January 2010), ISSN 1460-2180

Tsuda, H. (2009). Gene and chromosomal alterations in sporadic breast cancer: correlation with histopathological features and implications for genesis and progression. *Breast Cancer*, Vol.16, No.3, pp. 186-201, (May 2009), ISSN 1880-4233

van Heemst, D., Mooijaart, S.P., Beekman, M., Schreuder, J., de Craen, A.J., Brandt, B.W., Slagboom, P.E. & Westendorp, R.G. (2005). Variation in the human *TP53* gene affects old age survival and cancer mortality. *Exp Gerontol*, Vol.40, No.1-2, pp. 11-15, (March 2005), ISSN 0531-5565

Vannini, I., Zoli, W., Tesei, A., Rosetti, M., Sansone, P., Storci, G., Passardi, A., Massa, I., Ricci, M., Gusolfino, D., Fabbri, F., Ulivi, P., Brigliadori, G., Amadori, D. & Bonafe, M. (2008). Role of p53 codon 72 arginine allele in cell survival in vitro and in the clinical outcome of patients with advanced breast cancer. *Tumour Biol*, Vol.29, No.3, pp. 145-151, (Jule 2008), ISSN 1423-0380

Vigneron, A. & Vousden, K.H. (2010). p53, ROS and senescence in the control of aging. *Aging (Albany NY)*, Vol.2, No.8, pp. 471-474, (August 2010), ISSN 1945-4589

Vousden, K.H. & Prives, C. (2009). Blinded by the light: The growing complexity of p53. *Cell*, Vol.137, No.3, pp. 413-431, (May 2009), ISSN 1097-4172

Vousden, K.H. & Ryan, K.M. (2009). p53 and metabolism. *Nat Rev Cancer*, Vol.9, No.10, pp. 691-700, (September 2009), ISSN 1474-1768

Wang, B., Wang, D., Zhang, D., Li, A., Liu, D., Liu, H. & Jin, H. (2010a). Pro variant of *TP53* Arg72Pro contributes to esophageal squamous cell carcinoma risk: evidence from a meta-analysis. *Eur J Cancer Prev*, Vol.19, No.4, pp. 299-307, (April 2010), ISSN 1473-5709

Wang, J.J., Zheng, Y., Sun, L., Wang, L., Yu, P.B., Dong, J.H., Zhang, L., Xu, J., Shi, W. & Ren, Y.C. (2010b). *TP53* codon 72 polymorphism and colorectal cancer susceptibility: a meta-analysis. *Mol Biol Rep*, (December 2010), DOI: 10.1007/s11033-010-0619-8, ISSN 1573-4978

Wang, Y., Kringen, P., Kristensen, G.B., Holm, R., Baekelandt, M.M., Olivier, M., Skomedal, H., Hainaut, P., Trope, C.G., Abeler, V.M., Nesland, J.M., Borresen-Dale, A.L. & Helland, A. (2004). Effect of the codon 72 polymorphism (c.215G>C, p.Arg72Pro) in combination with somatic sequence variants in the *TP53* gene on survival in patients with advanced ovarian carcinoma. *Hum Mutat*, Vol.24, No.1, pp. 21-34, (June 2004), ISSN 1098-1004

Wang, Y.C., Chen, C.Y., Chen, S.K., Chang, Y.Y. & Lin, P. (1999). p53 codon 72 polymorphism in Taiwanese lung cancer patients: association with lung cancer susceptibility and prognosis. *Clin Cancer Res*, Vol.5, No.1, pp. 129-134, (January 1999), ISSN 1078-0432

Wegman, P.P., Marcus, N.J., Malakkaran, B.P. & Wingren, S. (2009). Biological significance of allele specific loss of the p53 gene in breast carcinomas. *Breast Cancer Res Treat*, Vol.118, No.1, pp. 15-20, (October 2008), ISSN 1573-7217

Weston, A., Pan, C.F., Ksieski, H.B., Wallenstein, S., Berkowitz, G.S., Tartter, P.I., Bleiweiss, I.J., Brower, S.T., Senie, R.T. & Wolff, M.S. (1997). p53 haplotype determination in breast cancer. *Cancer Epidemiol Biomarkers Prev*, Vol.6, No.2, pp. 105-112, (February 1997), ISSN 1055-9965

Whibley, C., Pharoah, P.D. & Hollstein, M. (2009). p53 polymorphisms: cancer implications. *Nat Rev Cancer*, Vol.9, No.2, pp. 95-107, (January 2009), ISSN 1474-1768

Wilentz, R.E., Argani, P. & Hruban, R.H. (2001). Loss of heterozygosity or intragenic mutation, which comes first? *Am J Pathol*, Vol.158, No.5, pp. 1561-1563, (May 2001), ISSN 0002-9440

Willman, C.L. & Hromas, R.A. (2010). Genomic alterations and chromosomal aberrations in human cancer, In: *Holland Frei Cancer Medicine*, W.K. Hong et al., (Ed.), 104-132, People's Medical Publishing House-USA, ISBN 1607950146, Shelton, USA

Wu, X., Zhao, H., Amos, C.I., Shete, S., Makan, N., Hong, W.K., Kadlubar, F.F. & Spitz, M.R. (2002). p53 genotypes and haplotypes associated with lung cancer susceptibility and ethnicity. *J Natl Cancer Inst*, Vol.94, No.9, pp. 681-690, (May 2002), ISSN 0027-8874

Yan, L., Zhang, D., Chen, C., Mao, Y., Xie, Y., Li, Y., Huang, Y. & Han, B. (2009). *TP53* Arg72Pro polymorphism and lung cancer risk: a meta-analysis. *Int J Cancer*, Vol.125, No.12, pp. 2903-2911, (Jule 2009), ISSN 1097-0215

Zhang, B., Beeghly-Fadiel, A., Long, J. & Zheng, W. (2011a). Genetic variants associated with breast-cancer risk: comprehensive research synopsis, meta-analysis, and epidemiological evidence. *Lancet Oncol*, Vol.12, No.5, pp. 477-488, (April 2011), ISSN 1474-5488

Zhang, J., Zhuo, W.L., Zheng, Y. & Zhang, Y.S. (2010a). Polymorphisms of *TP53* codon 72 with prostate carcinoma risk: a meta-analysis. *Med Oncol*, Vol.27, No.2, pp. 540-546, (June 2009), ISSN 1559-131X

Zhang, L., Shao, N., Yu, Q., Hua, L., Mi, Y. & Feng, N. (2011b). Association between p53 Pro72Arg polymorphism and prostate cancer risk: a meta-analysis. *Journal of Biomedical Research*, Vol.25, No.1, pp. 25-32, (January 2011)

Zhang, Z., Fu, G., Wang, M., Tong, N., Wang, S. & Zhang, Z. (2008). P53 codon 72 polymorphism and ovarian cancer risk: a meta-analysis. *Journal of Nanjing Medical University*, Vol.22, No.5, pp. 279-285, (September 2008)

Zhang, Z., Wang, M., Wu, D., Tong, N. & Tian, Y. (2010b). P53 codon 72 polymorphism contributes to breast cancer risk: a meta-analysis based on 39 case-control studies. *Breast Cancer Res Treat*, Vol.120, No.2, pp. 509-517, (Jule 2009), ISSN 1573-7217

Zhao, Y., Wang, F., Shan, S., Qiu, X., Li, X., Jiao, F., Wang, J. & Du, Y. (2010). Genetic polymorphism of p53, but not GSTP1, is association with susceptibility to esophageal cancer risk - a meta-analysis. *Int J Med Sci*, Vol.7, No.5, pp. 300-308, (September 2010), ISSN 1449-1907

Zhu, F., Dolle, M.E., Berton, T.R., Kuiper, R.V., Capps, C., Espejo, A., McArthur, M.J., Bedford, M.T., van Steeg, H., de Vries, A. & Johnson, D.G. (2010). Mouse models for the p53 R72P polymorphism mimic human phenotypes. *Cancer Res*, Vol.70, No.14, pp. 5851-5859, (Jule 2010), ISSN 1538-7445

Zhu, Y., Wang, J., He, Q. & Zhang, J.Q. (2011). Association of p53 codon 72 polymorphism with prostate cancer: a meta-analysis. *Mol Biol Rep*, Vol.38, No.3, pp. 1603-1607, (September 2010), ISSN 1573-4978

Zhuo, W., Zhang, Y., Xiang, Z., Cai, L. & Chen, Z. (2009a). Polymorphisms of *TP53* codon 72 with breast carcinoma risk: evidence from 12226 cases and 10782 controls. *J Exp Clin Cancer Res*, Vol.28, pp. 115, (August 2009), ISSN 1756-9966

Zhuo, X.L., Cai, L., Xiang, Z.L., Zhuo, W.L., Wang, Y. & Zhang, X.Y. (2009b). *TP53* codon 72 polymorphism contributes to nasopharyngeal cancer susceptibility: a meta-analysis. *Arch Med Res*, Vol.40, No.4, pp. 299-305, (Jule 2009), ISSN 1873-5487

Zhuo, X.L., Li, Q., Zhou, Y., Cai, L., Xiang, Z.L., Yuan, W. & Zhang, X.Y. (2009c). Study on *TP53* codon 72 polymorphisms with oral carcinoma susceptibility. *Arch Med Res*, Vol.40, No.7, pp. 625-634, (January 2010), ISSN 1873-5487

5

Epigenetics and Tumor Suppressor Genes

MingZhou Guo, XueFeng Liu and WeiMin Zhang
Department of Gastroenterology & Hepatology, Chinese PLA General Hospital
China

1. Introduction

Genes which protect cells from malignant transformation were referred to as tumor suppressor genes (TSGs). Since the first description of TSG, *Rb* (retinoblastoma susceptibility gene), a myriad of genes have been identified as TSGs. These TSGs play critical roles in cell cycle control, apoptosis, DNA damage detection and repair, adhesion, metastasis, senescence, and carcinogen detoxification. Loss function of TSGs may cause uncontrolled cell growth and cancer. TSGs may be inactivated by different mechanisms during carcinogenesis. In addition to genetic changes, epigenetic aberration plays an important role in inactivation of TSGs. Epigenetics is described as heritable changes in gene expression that do not involve a change in the DNA sequence (Berger et al., 2009). DNA methylation and histone modification are two predominant epigenetic changes. More recently, non-coding RNAs were regarded as new epigenetic regulation tools. The purpose of this chapter is to describe the effects of epigenetic modification on TSGs.

2. Epigenetic changes during carcinogenesis

Initially, cancer was thought to be driven by a series of genetic changes. Epigenetics is now recognized as more important player in the initiation and progression of cancers (Rodríguez-Paredes & Esteller, 2011). DNA methylation at the cytosine residue of the CpG dinucleotides is one of the best-studied epigenetic changes (Bird, 2002; M.M. Suzuki & Bird, 2008). In normal cells, CpG loci are methylated scatteringly across the genome. By contrast, short CpG-rich DNA regions, called 'CpG islands', are normally unmethylated. These 'CpG islands' are preferentially located in the promoter region of about 60% of human genes. Global DNA hypomethylation was the first epigenetic alteration found in human cancer (Feinberg & Vogelstein, 1983). Hypomethylation may lead to deleterious consequences, including genome instability, activation of transposable elements, or loss of genomic imprinting (Esteller, 2008). However, promoter-specific hypermethylation was regarded as the major epigenetic change of cancer, which is associated with TSGs silencing (Herman & Baylin, 2003).

Histone modification is another kind of epigenetic changes. Histones are subject to a wide range of post-transcriptional modifications in their N-terminal tails, including acetylation, methylation, phosphorylation, ubiquitination, SUMOylation and ADP-ribosylation (Kouzarides, 2007; Campos & Reinberg, 2009). It has been proposed that distinct histone modifications form different 'histone codes' (Strahl & Allis, 2000). Generally, histone acetylation is associated with transcriptional activation, while the role of histone methylation in gene expression relies on the specific residue and methylation state. One of the common hallmarks of human cancer is global loss of monoacetylation of lysine (K) 16 and trimethylation of lysine 20 on histone H4 (H4K16ac and H4K20me3) along with hypomethylation in repetitive DNA sequences (Fraga et al., 2005). Conversely, loss of acetylation of H3K9 and H4K16 (H3K9ac and H4K16ac) as well as trimethylation of H3K4 (H3K4me3) and gain of trimethylation of H3K27 (H3K27me3) and dimethylation of H3K9 (H3K9me2) occur at the promoters of TSGs and contribute to tumorigenesis by silencing of these critical genes (Figure 1) (Esteller, 2007a). In brief, aberrant 'epigenomes' marked by global DNA hypomethylation, promoter-specific hypermethylation, and abnormal histone modifications are main epigenetic changes in cancer. Since silencing of TSGs caused by CpG island hypermethylation and repressive histone modification is the common epigenetic event in human cancers, the following discussion will focus on the epigenetic silencing of TSGs during tumorigenesis.

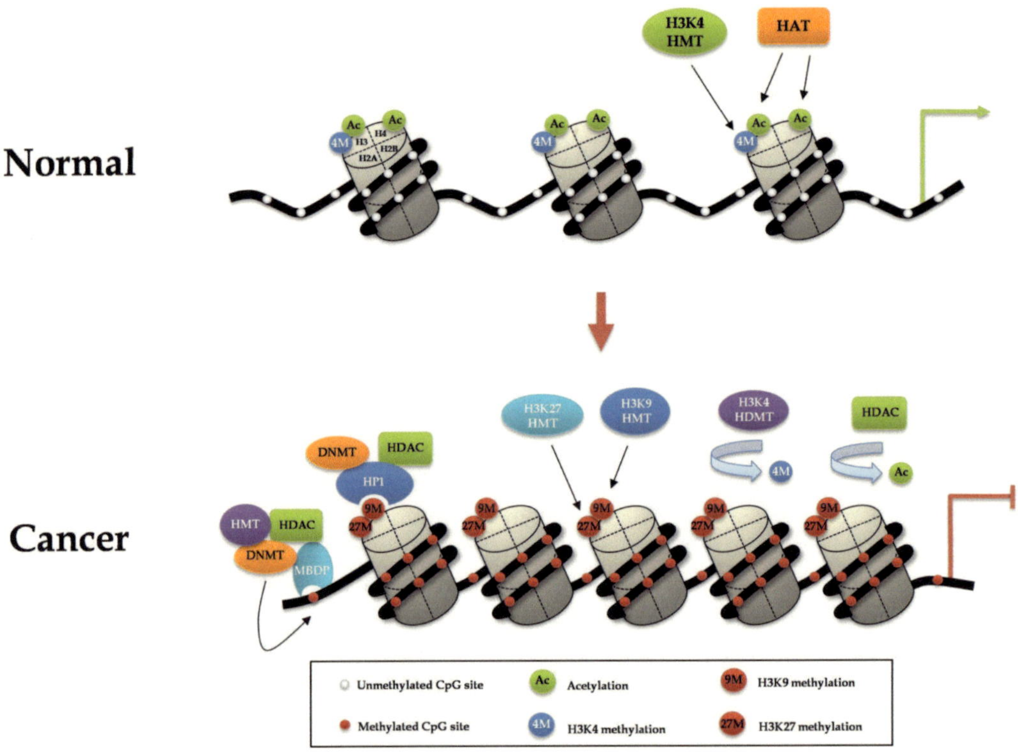

Fig. 1. Mechanisms of TSGs silencing by epigenetic changes during carcinogenesis.

In normal cells, promoter region is unmethylated and possesses active histone modifications (e.g., H3K4me and acetylation of H3 and H4). Transcription of TSGs was activated. In cancer cells, the promoter region is densely methylated, active histone modifications were lost and inactive histone modifications were induced (e.g., hypoacetylation of histones H3 and H4, loss of H3K4me3, and gain of H3K9me and H3K27me3). MBDPs bind to methylated DNA. HDACs and HMTs were recruited. Transcription of TSGs was inactivated.

3. DNA methylation of TSGs

3.1 DNA methyltransferase

DNA methylation is catalyzed by DNA methyltransferases (DNMTs), which add methyl groups to the cytosine of CpG dinucleotides. Three main DNMTs have been identified. DNMT1 maintains the existing methylation patterns following DNA replication, whereas DNMT3A and DNMT3B are responsible for *de novo* methylation patterns (Bird, 2002; M.M. Suzuki & Bird, 2008). Overexpresion of DNMTs has been observed in cancers, which contributes to CpG island hypermethylation of TSGs and concomitant silencing of gene expression (Robert et al., 2002; Nosho et al., 2009). Although DNMTs have been classified as maintenance or *de novo* methyltransferases, all three DNMTs participate in both *de novo* and maintenance methylation, and cooperate to silence TSGs in human cancer (Rhee et al., 2000; G.D. Kim et al., 2002; Rhee et al., 2002). More recently, three independent groups revealed that somatic mutations in DNMT3A occur in acute myeloid leukemia (AML), and lead to some gene expression and methylation changes (Shah & Licht, 2011). The other DNMTs, including DNMT3L and DNMT2, were reported recently. DNMT3L appears to be required for the methylation of imprinted genes in germ cells, and interacts with DNMT3a and 3b in *de novo* methyltransferase activity (Chen et al., 2005). But the biological function of DNMT2 remains unclear, its strong binding to DNA suggests that it may mark specific sequences in the genome (Dong et al., 2001).

3.2 Hypermethylation of TSGs in cancer

Promoter region hypermethylation is accepted as the mechanism of inactivation of TSGs in human cancers. The initial finding of CpG island hypermethylation of *Rb* in human cancer (Greger et al., 1989) was followed by the discovery of other TSGs undergoing methylation-associated inactivation, such as *VHL* (von Hippel-Lindau tumor suppressor), *p16INK4a* (cyclin-dependent kinase inhibitor 2A [CDKN2A]), *BRCA1* (breast-cancer susceptibility gene 1), and *hMLH1* (mutL homolog-1) (Esteller, 2002, 2008). These methylated TSGs are distributed in all cellular pathways relevant to tumor development, such as cell cycle regulation, DNA repair, apoptosis, transcriptional regulation, carcinogen-metabolism and drug resistance, angiogenesis, metastasis and cell-adherence (Esteller, 2002, 2008).
Hypermethylation of TSGs occurs at any time during carcinogenesis, especially in the early stages of the neoplastic process, which may facilitate cells to obtain further genetic lesions (Feinberg et al., 2006). One example is hypermethylation of DNA repair gene *MGMT* (O6-methylguanine-DNA methyltransferase) in the early phase of tumorigenesis, which results in the accumulation of genetic mutations that arise from the defects in DNA repair (Esteller et al., 2001a; Kuester et al., 2009). In addition, silencing of TSGs by promoter hypermethylation also let neoplastic cells addict to a particular oncogenic pathway, such as loss of *SFRP* (secreted frizzled-related proteins) expression in early stage of colon cancer activating the Wnt pathway (Baylin & Ohm, 2006). Furthermore, hypermethylation-induced silencing of transcription factors, such as *GATA-4* and *GATA-5* in colorectal and gastric cancers (Akiyama et al., 2003) as well as in esophageal cancer (Guo et al., 2006a), can also lead to inactivation of their downstream targets. Importantly, the increasing atypia observed at the histologic level is associated with the increasing number of methylated CpG islands at gene promoter regions. Our previous study suggested that the accumulation of DNA methylation was happened during esophagus carcinogenesis (Guo et al., 2006b).

The patterns of aberrant methylation of TSGs may represent different tumor types (Costello et al., 2000; Paz et al., 2003). Hypermethytion of *GSTP1* (glutathione S-transferase-π) was found in 80–90% of prostate cancers but hardly in other tumor types (Lee et al., 1994; Esteller et al., 1998; Cairns et al., 2001). Another finding indicated that *CDX2* (caudal related homeobox gene) methylation is a feature of squamous esophageal cancer (Guo et al., 2007). Tumor-type specific hypermethylation occurs not only in sporadic tumor but also in inherited cancer syndromes (Esteller et al., 2001b), where hypermethylation serves as the second hit in the Knudson's two-hit model for TSG inactivation (Grady et al., 2000). But some TSGs, such as *BRCA2, hMSH2, hMSH3, hMSH6, p19INK4d, CHK1, CHK2, MTAP* and *NKX3.1*, are rarely methylated in caner (Esteller, 2007b). The mechanism of tumor-type specific methylation remains unclear. Several hypotheses have been proposed to explain this phenomenon: (1) in certain tumor type hypermethylation might occur at particular genes which confer a selective clonal advantage; (2) there are common sequence motifs in the hypermethylated promoters of TSGs (Esteller, 2007b); (3) selective DNA methylation can be directed by other chromatin players, such as Polycomb proteins, pinpointing 'methylable' islands (Schlesinger et al., 2006; Esteller, 2007b).

3.3 Mechanisms of TSGs silencing by DNA methylation

It was proposed as one of the mechanisms that DNA methylation may directly block the specific binding sites of transcription factors (Comb & Goodman, 1990; Deng et al., 2001). Another more acceptable mechanism is that methyl-CpG-binding proteins (MBDPs) recognize m5CpG sequences and silence transcription. There are five well-known MBDPs which were regarded as important "translators" between DNA methylation and transcriptional silencing, including MeCP2, MBD1, MBD2, MBD3 and MBD4 (Lopez-Serra & Esteller, 2008). MBDPs bind to methylated DNA, and then histone modification enzymes were recruited to establish silenced chromatin model (Nan et al., 1998; Fuks et al., 2003).

4. Regulation of TSGs by histone modifications

Hypermethylation of TSGs in human cancer was extensively studied. But limited researches were performed on the regulation of gene expression by histone modifications. One of the main reasons is lacking rapid and comprehensive methods to analyze the histone modifications (Esteller, 2007a; Taby & Issa, 2010). Importantly, the effective histone modifications were discovered during the past decade, especially histone acetylation and methylation on TSGs regulation.

4.1 Histone acetylation

Histone acetylation occurs mainly at lysine residues of the H3 and H4, and makes RNA polymerase and transcription factors easier to access the promoter region. Therefore, in general, the acetylation of histone lysines is associated with euchromatin and transcriptional activation of gene expression, whereas the deacetylated residues are associated with heterochromatin and transcriptional gene silencing. Histone acetyltransferases (HATs) and deacetylases (HDACs) are, respectively, responsible for the addition and removal of acetyl groups from lysine residues. The precise balance between HATs and HDACs determines the status of histone acetylation (Ellis et al., 2009; Taby & Issa, 2010). In cancer cells, disruption of the balance between HATs and HDACs contributes to transcriptional inactivation of

TSGs. The typical example of gene silencing by this mechanism is the inactivation of cyclin-dependent kinase inhibitor *p21WAF1* by hypoacetylation in the absence of CpG-island hypermethylation (Richon et al., 2000). Interestingly, some TSGs with CpG island hypermethylation, can also be re-expressed through inhibition of SIRT1 (a class III HDAC), which increases H4K16 and H3K9 acetylation at promoters without affecting the hypermethylation status (Pruitt et al., 2006). Furthermore, in addition to regulation of TSGs at transcriptional level, HATs/HDACs influence the activity of TSGs by post-translational modifications (Glozak et al., 2005). For example, p53 is subjected to extensive acetylation mediated by HATs such as Tip60 (Sykes et al., 2006) and p300 (Gu & Roeder, 1997) and can be deacetylated by HDACs like SIRT1 (Yi & Luo, 2010). The aberrant histone acetylation of TSGs during carcinogenesis may result from the alteration in HATs/HDACs. Inactivation of HAT activity through gene mutation (e.g., missense mutations of p300) or viral oncoproteins (e.g., the inactivation of p300 by E1A and SV40) has been reported in both hematological and solid tumors, whereas misdirection of HAT activities as a result of chromosomal translocations (e.g., mixed lineage leukemia protein [MLL]-CBP [MLL-CBP]) has been implicated in the onset and progression of acute leukemia (Ellis et al., 2009). On the other hand, overexpression of HDACs in solid tumors (Song et al., 2005) and aberrant recruitment them to specific promoters through interaction with proto-oncogenes in leukemias (Ellis et al., 2009) have also been reported.

4.2 Histone methylation

Similar to histone acetylation, histone methylation is dynamically regulated by the opposing activities of histone methyltransferases (HMTs) and histone demethylases (HDMTs), such as KDM1/LSD1 and the Jumonji domain-containing protein (JMJD) family. Methylation takes place on both lysine and arginine residues, and has different degrees, known as mono-, di-, and tri-methylation. In most instances, methylation at H3K9, H3K27 and H3K20 is associated with transcriptional repression, whereas methylation of H3K4, H3K36 and H3K79 is associated with transcriptional activation (Ellis et al., 2009; Taby & Issa, 2010). The shifting of balance between HMTs and HDMTs in cancer also causes the silencing of TSGs. For instance, the H3K27me3-specific HMT EZH2 (enhancer of zeste homolog 2), catalytic subunit of PRC2 (Polycomb-repressive complex 2), is overexpressed in a broad range of hematopoietic and solid tumors, including prostate, breast, colon, skin and lung cancer (Tsang & Cheng, 2011). Mechanistically, the overabundance of EZH2 in cancer leads to transcriptional silencing of TSGs, such as *RUNX3* and *DAB2IP* through trimethylation of H3H27 (Fujii et al., 2008; Min et al., 2010). Conversely, the H3K27me3 repressive mark is demethylated by UTX/JMJD3 proteins, which belongs to JMJD family (Agger et al., 2007). Loss-of-function mutations of UTX in human cancers suggest UTX as a tumor suppressor gene (Van Haaften et al., 2009). This mutation could increase H3K27me3 level, and inactive *Rb* (Herz et al., 2010; J.K. Wang et al., 2010). The altered expression profiles of other histone methylation-modifying enzymes or abnormal targeting of these enzymes also contribute to inactivation of TSGs, such as downregulation of *BRCA1* in breast cancer cells caused by overexpression of PLU-1 (a member of JMJD family responsible for demethylation of H3K4) (Yamane et al., 2007). Finally, it is worth to be mentioned that the histone methylation-modifying enzymes also directly target non-histone proteins (Lan & Shi, 2009). Similar to the case of acetylation, p53 activity can be regulated by methylation or demethylation through HMTs or HDMTs (Huang et al., 2007, 2010).

5. Regulation of TSGs by interplay between DNA methylation and histone modifications

In addition to the independent effect, DNA methylation and histone modifications may interact with each other to reorganize chromatin structure and gene expression (Cedar & Bergman, 2009; Murr, 2010). Promoter region hypermethylation of TSGs is associated with histone modifications in cancer cells (e.g., hypoacetylation of histone H3 and H4, loss of H3K4me3, and gain of H3K9me and H3K27me3) (Esteller, 2008) (Figure 1). These connections might be carried out by the direct interaction of DNA methylation machinery and histone modification enzymes (Cedar & Bergman, 2009). However, the question of which epigenetic change is the initial event still remains controversial. Emerging evidence indicates that histone modifications may induce DNA methylation. For example, H3K9me2 may be necessary for DNA methylation in some TSGs, such as *p16INK4a* (Bachman et al., 2003). In this model, H3K9me2 can serve as a binding site for heterochromatin protein 1 (HP1), and thus generating a local heterochromatin by interacting with DNMTs and HDACs (Smallwood et al., 2007). On the other hand, DNA methylation machinery may recruit histone modification enzymes as well. The dynamic epigenetic silencing of *GSTP1* in prostate cancers is one of the good examples. It was reported that CpG island methylation of *GSTP1* played a critical role in deacetylation of H3K9 and concomitant methylation of H3K9 (Stirzaker et al., 2004). The link of DNA methylation and histone modifications might be mediated by MBDPs, which could recruit the HDACs and HMTs to the promoter methylated target genes (Nan et al., 1998; Fuks et al., 2003; Stirzaker et al., 2004). Furthermore, DNMTs themselves are associated with histone modification enzymes, such as HDACs (Fuks et al., 2000), and G9a (Estève et al., 2006).

6. Regulation of epigenetic modification machinery by TSGs

The roles of epigenetic modifications in regulation of TSGs expression are widely accepted. As transcription factors, some TSGs may be involved in regulation of the epigenetic modification machinery. p53, one of the most well-documented TSGs, has been reported to regulate histone modification. HATs, such as p300/CBP and TRRAP, are recruited to target gene depended on binding of p53 to promoter, and thus induces gene expression (Barlev et al., 2001; Vrba et al., 2008). At the same time, p53 may cause repression of a subset target genes, such as *MAP4*, *AFP* and *Nanog* through recruiting SIN3A-HDAC (Murphy et al., 1999; Lin et al., 2004; Nguyen et al., 2005). More recently, Zeng et al showed that p53 recruit both HDAC and PcG to *ARF* locus to repress its expression by a negative feedback manner during normal cell growth (Zeng et al., 2011). Similar example was reported in RB protein. RB-mediated transcriptional repression was induced through the association with a variety of chromatin modification and remodeling enzymes, including DNMTs, HDACs, HMTs (Luo et al., 1998; Robertson et al., 2000; Kotake et al., 2007) and Brg1/Brm (Dunaief et al., 1994; Strober et al., 1996). The other examples, such as maspin was also known to direct epigenetic regulation. Maspin was regarded as an endogenous inhibitor of HDAC1 (Li et al., 2006). It is noticeable that the interaction of TSGs and histone modification enzymes may produce different outcomes. TSGs and histone modification enzymes may regulate each other, which may be determined upon different cellar states.

7. Non-coding RNAs enter epigenetic world

Non-coding RNAs (ncRNAs) are functional RNA molecules that do not code for proteins. Based on size, they are divided into different classes: long ncRNAs (lncRNAs), Piwi-interacting RNAs (piRNAs), small interfering RNAs (siRNAs), microRNAs (miRNAs), etc (Brosnan & Voinnet, 2009). NcRNAs can regulate gene expression through a diversity of mechanisms. Recently, a handful of studies have implicated ncRNAs in a variety of disease states, especially in cancer. Many ncRNAs, such as miRNAs and lncRNAs could play the similar roles as TSGs, and also function as oncogens that in turn regulate the expressions of TSGs in transcriptional and post-transcriptional level.

7.1 Interplay between MiRNAs and epigenetic machinery

MiRNAs are small ncRNAs with 19~22nt, which regulate gene expression via translational inhibition or mRNA degradation in a sequence-specific manner. MiRNAs could function as TSGs or oncogenes in cancer. In the last few years, increasing evidence has indicated that a substantial number of miRNA genes with tumor suppression functions are associated with CpG islands and silenced by epigenetic alterations in cancers. Indeed, miR-127 was found to be embedded in a CpG island region and epigenetically silenced by both promoter hypermethylation and histone modifications in cancer cells, and could be reactivated following treatment with combination of DNA demethylating agent and HDAC inhibitor (Saito et al., 2006). miR-9-1 was also found to be hypermethylated and consequently down-regulated in breast cancer (Lehmann et al., 2008) as well as the hypermethylation of clustered miR-34b and miR-34c in colon cancer (Toyota et al., 2008). Intriguingly, miRNAs are not only epigenetically regulated but also act as chromatin modifiers to regulate the gene expression (Valeri et al., 2009). Fabbri et al reported the first evidence that miR-29s (miR-29a, -29b, -29c) directly target DNMT3a and DNMT3b (Fabbri et al., 2007). After miR-29s treatment, the epigenetically silenced TSGs like *p15INK4b* and *ESR1* were re-expressed comparably to use of DNMT inhibitors (Fabbri et al., 2007; Garzon et al., 2009). Similarly, HMTs are also targets of miRNAs. Studies have shown that miR-101 exerts its tumor suppressive properties by targeting the EZH2 (Varambally et al., 2008; Friedman et al., 2009).

7.2 LncRNA: A new player in epigenetics

LncRNAs are emerging as new players in human cancers with potential roles in both oncogenic and tumor suppressive pathways, and the most fascinating thing is that they could play crucial roles in epigenetic modifications. Notably, evidence has suggested that lncRNAs can mediate epigenetic changes by recruiting chromatin remodeling complexes to specific genomic loci (Mercer et al., 2009). For example, *ANRIL*, a antisense to the *INK4n/ARF/INK4a* promoter, interacts with PRC1 component CBX7 to repress the transcription of *INK4n/ARF/INK4a* locus (Yap et al., 2010). On the other hand, lncRNAs could function as TSGs and modulate the epigenetic machinery by interaction with other proteins. In response to DNA damage, ncRNAs transcribed from the 5' regulatory region of *CCND1*, binds to and activate TLS, which inhibits CBP/p300 histone acetyltransferase activities leading to repression of *CCND1* transcription (X. Wang et al., 2008).

8. Screening candidate TSGs by epigenetic strategies

TSGs are generally silenced by CpG island hypermethylation and repressive histone modifications. So, epigenetic signatures may be applied to screen tumor suppressor. It is important to isolate epigenetically silenced genes in cancer. To this end, many procedures were reported. For example, by comparation of genes expression level before and after 5-aza-2′-deoxycytidine (5-aza-CdR) treatment, Suzuki et al isolated hypermethylation silenced genes *SFRPs* in colonic cancer cell lines and further analyzed their tumor suppressor function (H. Suzuki et al., 2002). Similarly, Gery et al employed microarray analysis to identify genes reactivated in lung cancer after combined treatment with 5-aza-CdR and SAHA. In this screen, *Per1* was identified as a candidate tumor suppressor in lung cancer, and DNA hypermethylation and histone H3 acetylation are potential mechanisms for silencing *Per1* (Gery et al., 2007). For the promoter CpG island hypermathylation detection, anti-mC immunological techniques, HPLC-TLC, HPCE, ERMA, bisulphite sequencing, MSP, MSP-ISH and DNA methylation mircroarray were employed (Laird, 2003). ChIP, ChIP coupled with microarray hybridization (ChIP-chip), ChIP coupled with next-generation DNA sequencing (ChIP-seq), mass spectrometry (Rasoulpour et al., 2011) were used to determine the regional or global repressive histone modifications (deacetylation of specific H3 and H4 lysine or methylation of H4K9/27 even the combination).

9. Clinical application

Understanding of how epigenetic alterations contribute to TSGs regulation would facilitate its transformation and clinical application. Based on the characters of stability, variability and reversibility, epigenetic modifications have potentials as both cancer biomarkers for detection, prognosis, and therapy prediction, and drug targets for cancer therapy (Mulero-Navarro & Esteller, 2008).

9.1 Epigenetic biomarkers

As described previously, each tumor type may be represented by a different methylation pattern. Promoter region Hypermethylation usually occurred in the early stage of carcinogenesis. Therefore it is possible to detect early lesions by examination of TSGs methylation. Previous study has shown that *HIN-1* (high in normal-1) methylation is an early event of human esophageal cancer (Guo et al., 2008). TSGs methylation can also be the predictors of tumor prognosis. For example, methylation of the promoter region of *p16INK4a*, *CDH13* (H-cadherin gene), *RASSF1A* (Ras association domain family 1 gene) and *APC* (adenomatous polyposis coli gene) in patients with stage I NSCLC treated with surgery is associated with increased risk of early recurrence (Brock et al., 2008). In addition, DNA methylation may serve as chemotherapy predictor. The representative methylation markers to predict drug-responsiveness are *MGMT* (Esteller et al., 2000), *hMLH1* (Plumb et al., 2000), *WRN* (the Werner syndrome–associated gene) (Agrelo et al., 2006), *IGFBP-3* (insulin-like growth factor–binding protein-3) (Ibanez et al., 2010), or *BRCA1* (Veeck et al., 2010) (Table 1).

9.2 Epigenetic agents

Unlike genetic mutations, epigenetic silenced TSGs can be awakened by drugs. Many epigenetic drugs have been discovered to rescue the functions of TSGs by reversing aberrant epigenetic changes. US Food and Drug Administration (FDA) have approved four epigenetic drugs for cancer therapy. Two DNMT inhibitors, 5-aza-CR (vidaza) and 5-aza-CdR (decitabine), were used in the treatment of myelodysplastic syndromes and leukemia, while two HDAC inhibitors, vorinostat (suberoylanilide hydroxamic acid [SAHA]) and romidepsin (FK-228), were applied in cutaneous T cell lymphoma (Rodríguez-Paredes &

Esteller, 2011). These drugs can be administrated in combination or independent manner. Despite promising results, epigenetic related therapy still remains challenge. Similar with epigenetic changes in TSGs, ncRNAs pattern in cancer may serve as diagnosis, prognosis and chemosensitivity marker and therapeutic target.

Hypermethylated TSGs	Gene Function	Representative Cancer Type	Ref.	Potential Clinical Application
GSTP1	Conjugation to glutathione	Prostate cancer	(Lee et al., 1994)	Detection
GATA-4/-5	Transcription factor	esophageal cancer	(Guo et al., 2006a)	
APC	Wnt signaling	Colorectal cancer; breast cancer	(Mulero-Navarro & Esteller, 2008)	
CDX2	Homeobox transcription factor	Squamous esophageal cancer	(Guo et al., 2007)	
p16INK4a	Cyclin-dependent kinase inhibitor	Colorectal cancer	(Esteller et al., 2001c)	Prognosis
SFRP1	Antagonists of Wnt signaling	Breast cancer	(Veeck et al., 2006)	
DAPK	Pro-apoptotic	NSCLC	(Tang et al., 2000)	
EMP3	myelin-related gene	glioma and neuroblastoma	(Alaminos et al., 2005)	
CDH1	E cadherin, cell adhesion	NSCLC	(D. S. Kim et al., 2007)	
CDH13	H cadherin, cell adhesion	NSCLC	(D. S. Kim et al., 2007)	
MGMT	DNA repair of 06–alkyl-guanine	gliomas	(Esteller et al., 2000)	Chemosensitivity
hMLH1	DNA mismatch repair	Ovarian and colon cancer	(Plumb et al., 2000)	
BRCA1	DNA repair, transcription	Breast cancers	(Veeck et al., 2010)	
WRN	DNA repair	Colorectal cancer	(Agrelo et al., 2006)	
IGFBP-3	Growth-factor-binding protein	NSCLC	(Ibanez et al., 2010	

CDH1 (E cadherin), EMP3 (epithelial membrane protein 3), DAPK (death-associated protein kinase).

Table 1. Representative epigenetic markers in cancer.

10. Conclusion

Aberrant epigenetic changes play important roles in human carcinogenesis. Major epigenetic changes include DNA methylation, aberrant histone modification and alterations of noncoding RNA patterns. The expression of TSGs was regulated by epigenetic modification. Epigenetic silencing of TSGs by promoter region hypermethylation in combination with repressive histone modifications was recognized as a common feature of various human cancers. Undoubtedly, understanding of the inactivation of TSGs is of fundamental importance in exploration of the pathogenesis and progression of cancer, and thus facilitating to yield attractive cancer biomarkers and therapeutic targets. The pivotal roles of ncRNAs in the development of cancer have refreshed the complicated epigenetic network, which provides a possibility on developing ncRNAs mediated diagnostics, prognostics and therapeutics. It is possible, in the near future, to find novel cancer-specific biomarkers and gene-specific drugs with low cytotoxicity.

11. References

Agger, K., Cloos, PA., Christensen, J., Pasini, D., Rose, S., Rappsilber, J., Issaeva, I., Canaani, E., Salcini, AE. & Helin, K. (2007). UTX and JMJD3 are histone H3K27 demethylases involved in HOX gene regulation and development. *Nature,* Vol.449, No.7163, pp.731-734, 0028-0836.

Agrelo, R., Cheng, WH., Setien, F., Ropero, S., Espada, J., Fraga, MF., Herranz, M., Paz, MF., Sanchez-Cespedes, M., Artiga, MJ., Guerrero, D., Castells, A., von Kobbe, C., Bohr, VA. & Esteller, M. (2006). Epigenetic inactivation of the premature aging Werner syndrome gene in human cancer. *Proceedings of the National Academy of Sciences of the United States of America,* Vol.103, No.23, pp.8822-8827.

Akiyama, Y., Watkins, N., Suzuki, H., Jair, KW., Van Engeland, M., Esteller, M., Sakai, H., Ren, CY., Yuasa, Y., Herman, JG. & Baylin, SB. (2003). GATA-4 and GATA-5 transcription factor genes and potential downstream antitumor target genes are epigenetically silenced in colorectal and gastric cancer. *Molecular and Cellular Biology,* Vol.23, No.23, pp.8429-8439,0270-7306.

Alaminos, M., Dávalos, V., Ropero, S., Setién, F., Paz, MF., Herranz, M., Fraga, MF., Mora, J., Cheung, NK., Gerald, WL. & Esteller, M. (2005). EMP3, a myelin-related gene located in the critical 19q13. 3 region, is epigenetically silenced and exhibits features of a candidate tumor suppressor in glioma and neuroblastoma. *Cancer Research,* Vol.65, No.7, pp.2565-2571,0008-5472.

Bachman, KE., Park, BH., Rhee, I., Rajagopalan, H., Herman, JG., Baylin, SB., Kinzler, KW. & Vogelstein, B. (2003). Histone modifications and silencing prior to DNA methylation of a tumor suppressor gene. *Cancer Cell,* Vol.3, No.1, pp.89-95,1535-6108.

Barlev, NA., Liu, L., Chehab, NH., Mansfield, K., Harris, KG., Halazonetis, TD. & Berger, SL. (2001). Acetylation of p53 activates transcription through recruitment of coactivators/histone acetyltransferases. *Molecular Cell,* Vol.8, No.6, pp.1243-1254,1097-2765.

Baylin, SB. & Ohm, JE. (2006). Epigenetic gene silencing in cancer - a mechanism for early oncogenic pathway addiction? *Nature Reviews Cancer,* Vol.6, No.2, pp.107-116,1474-175X.

Berger, SL., Kouzarides, T., Shiekhattar, R. & Shilatifard, A. (2009). An operational definition of epigenetics. *Genes & Development*, Vol.23, No.7, pp.781-783,1549-5477

Bird, A. (2002). DNA methylation patterns and epigenetic memory. *Genes & Development*, Vol.16, No.1, pp.6-21,0890-9369.

Brock, MV., Hooker, CM., Ota-Machida, E., Han, Y., Guo, M., Ames, S., Glöckner, S., Piantadosi, S., Gabrielson, E., Pridham, G., Pelosky, K., Belinsky, SA., Yang, SC., Baylin, SB. & Herman, JG. (2008). DNA methylation markers and early recurrence in stage I lung cancer. *The New England Journal of Medicine*, Vol.358, No.11, pp.1118-1128,1533-4406.

Brosnan, CA. & Voinnet, O. (2009). The long and the short of noncoding RNAs. *Current Opinion in Cell Biology*, Vol.21, No.3, pp.416-425,1879-0410

Cairns, P., Esteller, M., Herman, JG., Schoenberg, M., Jeronimo, C., Sanchez-Cespedes, M., Chow, NH., Grasso, M., Wu, L., Westra, WB. & Sidransky, D. (2001). Molecular detection of prostate cancer in urine by GSTP1 hypermethylation. *Clinical Cancer Research*, Vol.7, No.9, pp.2727-2730,1078-0432

Campos, EI. & Reinberg, D. (2009). Histones: annotating chromatin. *Annual Review of Genetics*, Vol.43, No.1, pp.559-599,0066-4197.

Cedar, H. & Bergman, Y. (2009). Linking DNA methylation and histone modification: patterns and paradigms. *Nature Reviews Genetics*, Vol.10, No.5, pp.295-304,1471-0056.

Chen, ZX., Mann, JR., Hsieh, CL., Riggs, AD. & Chédin F. (2005). Physical and functional interactions between the human DNMT3L protein and members of the de novo methyltransferase family. *Journal of Cellular Biochemistry*, Vol.95, No.5, pp.902-917,0730-2312

Comb, M. & Goodman, HM. (1990). CpG methylation inhibits proenkephalin gene expression and binding of the transcription factor AP-2. *Nucleic Acids Research*, Vol.18, No.13, pp.3975-3982,0305-1048.

Costello, JF., Frühwald, MC., Smiraglia, DJ., Rush, LJ., Robertson, GP., Gao, X., Wright, FA., Feramisco, JD., Peltomäki, P., Lang, JC., Schuller, DE., Yu, L., Bloomfield, CD., Caligiuri, MA., Yates, A., Nishikawa, R., Su Huang, H., Petrelli, NJ., Zhang, X., O'Dorisio, MS., Held, WA., Cavenee, WK. & Plass C. (2000). Aberrant CpG-island methylation has non-random and tumour-type-specific patterns. *Nature Genetics*, Vol.24, No.2, pp.132-138.

Deng, G., Chen, A., Pong, E. & Kim, YS. (2001). Methylation in hMLH1 promoter interferes with its binding to transcription factor CBF and inhibits gene expression. *Oncogene*, Vol.20, No.48, pp.7120-7127,0950-9232.

Dong, A., Yoder, JA., Zhang, X., Zhou, L., Bestor, TH. & Cheng, X. (2001). Structure of human DNMT2, an enigmatic DNA methyltransferase homolog that displays denaturant-resistant binding to DNA. *Nucleic Acids Research*, Vol.29, No.2, pp.439-448,1362-4962

Dunaief, JL., Strober, BE., Guha, S., Khavari, PA., Alin, K., Luban, J., Begemann, M., Crabtree, GR. & Goff, SP. (1994). The retinoblastoma protein and BRG1 form a complex and cooperate to induce cell cycle arrest. *Cell*, Vol.79, No.1, pp.119-130,0092-8674.

Ellis, L., Atadja, PW. & Johnstone, RW. (2009). Epigenetics in cancer: targeting chromatin modifications. *Molecular Cancer Therapeutics*, Vol.8, No.6, pp.1409-1420,1535-7163.

Estève, PO., Chin, HG., Smallwood, A., Feehery, GR., Gangisetty, O., Karpf, AR., Carey, MF. & Pradhan, S. (2006). Direct interaction between DNMT1 and G9a coordinates DNA and histone methylation during replication. *Genes & Development*, Vol.20, No.22, pp.3089-3103,0890-9369.

Esteller, M., Corn, PG., Urena, JM., Gabrielson, E., Baylin, SB. & Herman, JG. (1998). Inactivation of glutathione S-transferase P1 gene by promoter hypermethylation in human neoplasia. *Cancer Research*, Vol.58, No.20, pp.4515-4518,0008-5472.

Esteller, M., Garcia-Foncillas, J., Andion, E., Goodman, SN., Hidalgo, OF., Vanaclocha, V., Baylin, SB. & Herman, JG. (2000). Inactivation of the DNA-repair gene MGMT and the clinical response of gliomas to alkylating agents. *New England Journal of Medicine*, Vol.343, No.19, pp.1350-1354,0028-4793.

Esteller, M., Risques, RA., Toyota, M., Capella, G., Moreno, V., Peinado, MA., Baylin, SB. & Herman, JG. (2001a). Promoter hypermethylation of the DNA repair gene O6-methylguanine-DNA methyltransferase is associated with the presence of G: C to A: T transition mutations in p53 in human colorectal tumorigenesis. *Cancer Research*, Vol.61, No.12, pp.4689-4692,0008-5472.

Esteller, M., Fraga, MF., Guo, M., Garcia-Foncillas, J., Hedenfalk, I., Godwin, AK., Trojan, J., Vaurs-Barrière, C., Bignon, YJ., Ramus, S., Benitez, J., Caldes, T., Akiyama, Y., Yuasa, Y., Launonen, V., Canal, MJ., Rodriguez, R., Capella, G., Peinado, MA., Borg, A., Aaltonen, LA., Ponder, BA., Baylin, SB. & Herman JG. (2001b). DNA methylation patterns in hereditary human cancers mimic sporadic tumorigenesis. *Human Molecular Genetics*, Vol.10, No.26, pp.3001-3007,0964-6906.

Esteller, M., Gonzalez, S., Risques, RA., Marcuello, E., Mangues, R., Germa, JR., Herman, JG., Capella, G. & Peinado, MA. (2001c). K-ras and p16 aberrations confer poor prognosis in human colorectal cancer. *Journal of Clinical Oncology*, Vol.19, No.2, pp.299-304,0732-183X

Esteller, M. (2002). CpG island hypermethylation and tumor suppressor genes: a booming present, a brighter future. *Oncogene*, Vol.21, No.35, pp.5427-5440,0950-9232.

Esteller, M. (2007a). Cancer epigenomics: DNA methylomes and histone-modification maps. *Nature Reviews Genetics*, Vol.8, No.4, pp.286-298,1471-0056.

Esteller, M. (2007b). Epigenetic gene silencing in cancer: the DNA hypermethylome. *Human Molecular Genetics*, Vol.16, No.1, pp.50-59,0964-6906.

Esteller, M. (2008). Epigenetics in cancer. *The New England Journal of Medicine*, Vol.358, No.11, pp.1148-1159.

Fabbri, M., Garzon, R., Cimmino, A., Liu, Z., Zanesi, N., Callegari, E., Liu, S., Alder, H., Costinean, S., Fernandez-Cymering, C., Volinia, S., Guler, G., Morrison, CD., Chan, KK., Marcucci, G., Calin, GA., Huebner, K. & Croce CM. (2007). MicroRNA-29 family reverts aberrant methylation in lung cancer by targeting DNA methyltransferases 3A and 3B. *Proceedings of the National Academy of Sciences of the United States of America*, Vol.104, No.40, pp.15805-15810.

Feinberg, AP. & Vogelstein, B. (1983). Hypomethylation distinguishes genes of some human cancers from their normal counterparts. *Nature*, Vol.301, No.5895, pp.89-92,0028-0836.

Feinberg, AP., Ohlsson, R. & Henikoff, S. (2006). The epigenetic progenitor origin of human cancer. *Nature Reviews Genetics*, Vol.7, No.1, pp.21-33,1471-0056.

Fraga, MF., Ballestar, E., Villar-Garea, A., Boix-Chornet, M., Espada, J., Schotta, G., Bonaldi, T., Haydon, C., Ropero, S., Petrie, K., Iyer, NG., Pérez-Rosado, A., Calvo, E., Lopez, JA., Cano, A., Calasanz, MJ., Colomer, D., Piris, MA., Ahn, N., Imhof, A., Caldas, C., Jenuwein, T. & Esteller, M. (2005). Loss of acetylation at Lys16 and trimethylation at Lys20 of histone H4 is a common hallmark of human cancer. *Nature Genetics*, Vol.37, No.4, pp.391-400.

Friedman, JM., Liang, G., Liu, CC., Wolff, EM., Tsai, YC., Ye, W., Zhou, X. & Jones, PA. (2009). The putative tumor suppressor microRNA-101 modulates the cancer epigenome by repressing the polycomb group protein EZH2. *Cancer Research*, Vol.69, No.6, pp.2623-2629,0008-5472.

Fujii, S., Ito, K., Ito, Y. & Ochiai, A. (2008). Enhancer of zeste homologue 2 (EZH2) down-regulates RUNX3 by increasing histone H3 methylation. *Journal of Biological Chemistry*, Vol.283, No.25, pp.17324-17332,0021-9258.

Fuks, F., Burgers, WA., Brehm, A., Hughes-Davies, L. & Kouzarides, T. (2000). DNA methyltransferase Dnmt1 associates with histone deacetylase activity. *Nature Genetics*, Vol.24, No.1, pp.88-91.

Fuks, F., Hurd, PJ., Wolf, D., Nan, X., Bird, AP. & Kouzarides, T. (2003). The methyl-CpG-binding protein MeCP2 links DNA methylation to histone methylation. *Journal of Biological Chemistry*, Vol.278, No.6, pp.4035-4040,0021-9258.

Garzon, R., Liu, S., Fabbri, M., Liu, Z., Heaphy, CE., Callegari, E., Schwind, S., Pang, J., Yu, J., Muthusamy, N., Havelange, V., Volinia, S., Blum, W., Rush, LJ., Perrotti, D., Andreeff, M., Bloomfield, CD., Byrd, JC., Chan, K., Wu, LC., Croce, CM. & Marcucci G. (2009). MicroRNA-29b induces global DNA hypomethylation and tumor suppressor gene reexpression in acute myeloid leukemia by targeting directly DNMT3A and 3B and indirectly DNMT1. *Blood*, Vol.113, No.25, pp.6411-6418,0006-4971.

Gery, S., Komatsu, N., Kawamata, N., Miller, CW., Desmond, J., Virk, RK., Marchevsky, A., McKenna, R., Taguchi, H. & Koeffler, HP. (2007). Epigenetic silencing of the candidate tumor suppressor gene Per1 in non-small cell lung cancer. *Clinical Cancer Research*, Vol.13, No.5, pp.1399-1404,1078-0432

Glozak, MA., Sengupta, N., Zhang, X. & Seto, E. (2005). Acetylation and deacetylation of non-histone proteins. *Gene*, Vol.363, pp.15-23,0378-1119.

Grady, WM., Willis, J., Guilford, PJ., Dunbier, AK., Toro, TT., Lynch, H., Wiesner, G., Ferguson, K., Eng, C., Park, JG., Kim, SJ. & Markowitz, S. (2000). Methylation of the CDH1 promoter as the second genetic hit in hereditary diffuse gastric cancer. *Nature Genetics*, Vol.26, No.1, pp.16-17.

Greger, V., Passarge, E., Höpping, W., Messmer, E. & Horsthemke, B. (1989). Epigenetic changes may contribute to the formation and spontaneous regression of retinoblastoma. *Human Genetics*, Vol.83, No.2, pp.155-158,0340-6717.

Gu, W. & Roeder, RG. (1997). Activation of p53 sequence-specific DNA binding by acetylation of the p53 C-terminal domain. *Cell*, Vol.90, No.4, pp.595-606,0092-8674.

Guo, M., House, MG., Akiyama, Y., Qi, Y., Capagna, D., Harmon, J., Baylin, SB., Brock, MV. & Herman, JG. (2006a). Hypermethylation of the GATA gene family in esophageal cancer. *International Journal of Cancer* , Vol.119, No.9, pp.2078-2083,0020-7136.

Guo, M., Ren, J., House, MG., Qi, Y., Brock, MV. & Herman, JG. (2006b). Accumulation of promoter methylation suggests epigenetic progression in squamous cell carcinoma of the esophagus. *Clinical Cancer Research*, Vol.12, No.15, pp.4515-4522,1078-0432.

Guo, M., House, MG., Suzuki, H., Ye, Y., Brock, MV., Lu, F., Liu, Z., Rustgi, AK. & Herman, JG. (2007). Epigenetic silencing of CDX2 is a feature of squamous esophageal cancer. *International Journal of Cancer*, Vol.121, No.6, pp.1219-1226,1097-0215.

Guo, M., Ren, J., Brock, MV., Herman, JG. & Carraway, HE. (2008). Promoter methylation of HIN-1 in the progression to esophageal squamous cancer. *Epigenetics*, Vol.3, No.6, pp.336-341,1559-2308.

Herman JG. & Baylin SB. (2003). Gene silencing in cancer in association with promoter hypermethylation. *New England Journal of Medicine*, Vol.349, No.21, pp.2042-2054.

Herz, HM., Madden, LD., Chen, Z., Bolduc, C., Buff, E., Gupta, R., Davuluri, R., Shilatifard, A., Hariharan, IK. & Bergmann, A. (2010). The H3K27me3 demethylase dUTX is a suppressor of notch-and Rb-dependent tumors in Drosophila. *Molecular and Cellular Biology*, Vol.30, No.10, pp.2485-2497,0270-7306.

Huang, J., Sengupta, R., Espejo, AB., Lee, MG., Dorsey, JA., Richter, M., Opravil, S., Shiekhattar, R., Bedford, MT., Jenuwein, T. & Berger,SL. (2007). p53 is regulated by the lysine demethylase LSD1. *Nature*, Vol.449, No.7158, pp.105-108,0028-0836.

Huang, J., Dorsey, J., Chuikov, S., Zhang, X., Jenuwein, T., Reinberg, D. & Berger, SL. (2010). G9a and Glp methylate lysine 373 in the tumor suppressor p53. *Journal of Biological Chemistry*, Vol.285, No.13, pp.9636-9641,0021-9258.

Ibanez de Caceres, I., Cortes-Sempere M., Moratilla, C., Machado-Pinilla, R., Rodriguez-Fanjul, V., Manguán-García, C., Cejas, P., López-Ríos, F., Paz-Ares, L., de CastroCarpeño, J., Nistal, M., Belda-Iniesta, C. & Perona, R. (2010). IGFBP-3 hypermethylation-derived deficiency mediates cisplatin resistance in non-small-cell lung cancer. *Oncogene*, Vol.29, No.11, pp.1681-1690,0950-9232.

Kim, DS., Kim, MJ., Lee, JY., Kim, YZ., Kim, EJ. & Park, JY. (2007). Aberrant methylation of E-cadherin and H-cadherin genes in nonsmall cell lung cancer and its relation to clinicopathologic features. *Cancer*, Vol.110, No.12, pp.2785-2792,0008-543X .

Kim, GD., Ni, J., Kelesoglu, N., Roberts, RJ. & Pradhan, S. (2002). Co-operation and communication between the human maintenance and de novo DNA (cytosine-5) methyltransferases. *The EMBO Journal*, Vol.21, No.15, pp.4183-4195.

Kotake, Y., Cao, R., Viatour, P., Sage, J., Zhang, Y. & Xiong, Y. (2007). pRB family proteins are required for H3K27 trimethylation and Polycomb repression complexes binding to and silencing p16INK4a tumor suppressor gene. *Genes & Development*, Vol.21, No.1, pp.49-54,0890-9369.

Kouzarides, T. (2007). Chromatin modifications and their function. *Cell*, Vol.128, No.4, pp.693-705,0092-8674.

Kuester, D., El-Rifai, W., Peng, D., Ruemmele, P., Kroeckel, I., Peters, B., Moskaluk, CA., Stolte, M., Mönkemüller, K., Meyer, F., Schulz, HU., Hartmann, A., Roessner, A. & Schneider-Stock, R. (2009). Silencing of MGMT expression by promoter hypermethylation in the metaplasia-dysplasia-carcinoma sequence of Barrett's esophagus. *Cancer Letters*, Vol.275, No.1, pp.117-126,0304-3835.

Laird, PW. (2003). The power and the promise of DNA methylation markers. *Nature Reviews Cancer*, Vol.3, No.4, pp.253-266,1474-175X.

Lan, F. & Shi, Y. (2009). Epigenetic regulation: methylation of histone and non-histone proteins. *Science in China Series C: Life Sciences*, Vol.52, No.4, pp.311-322,1006-9305.

Lee, WH., Morton, RA., Epstein, JI., Brooks, JD., Campbell, PA., Bova, GS., Hsieh, WS., Isaacs, WB. & Nelson, WG. (1994). Cytidine methylation of regulatory sequences near the pi-class glutathione S-transferase gene accompanies human prostatic carcinogenesis. *Proceedings of the National Academy of Sciences of the United States of America*, Vol.91, No.24, pp.11733-11737.

Lehmann, U., Hasemeier, B., Christgen, M., Müller, M., Römermann, D., Länger, F. & Kreipe, H. (2008). Epigenetic inactivation of microRNA gene has-mir-9-1 in human breast cancer. *The Journal of Pathology*, Vol.214, No.1, pp.17-24,1096-9896.

Li, X., Yin, S., Meng, Y., Sakr, W. & Sheng, S. (2006). Endogenous inhibition of histone deacetylase 1 by tumor-suppressive maspin. *Cancer Research*, Vol.66, No.18, pp.9323-9329,0008-5472.

Lin, T., Chao, C., Saito, S., Mazur, SJ., Murphy, ME., Appella, E. & Xu, Y. (2004). p53 induces differentiation of mouse embryonic stem cells by suppressing Nanog expression. *Nature Cell Biology*, Vol.7, No.2, pp.165-171,1465-7392.

Lopez-Serra, L. & Esteller, M. (2008). Proteins that bind methylated DNA and human cancer: reading the wrong words. *British Journal of Cancer*, Vol.98, No.12, pp.1881-1885,0007-0920.

Luo, RX., Postigo, AA. & Dean, DC. (1998). Rb interacts with histone deacetylase to repress transcription. *Cell*, Vol.92, No.4, pp.463-473,0092-8674.

Mercer, TR., Dinger, ME. & Mattick, JS. (2009). Long non-coding RNAs: insights into functions. *Nature Reviews Genetics*, Vol.10, No.3, pp.155-159,1471-0056.

Min, J., Zaslavsky, A., Fedele, G., McLaughlin, SK., Reczek, EE., De Raedt, T., Guney, I., Strochlic, DE., Macconaill, LE., Beroukhim, R., Bronson, RT., Ryeom, S., Hahn, WC., Loda, M. & Cichowski, K. (2010). An oncogene-tumor suppressor cascade drives metastatic prostate cancer by coordinately activating Ras and nuclear factor-kappaB. *Nature Medicine*, Vol.16, No.3, pp.286-294,1546-170X.

Mulero-Navarro, S. & Esteller, M. (2008). Epigenetic biomarkers for human cancer: the time is now. *Critical Reviews in Oncology/Hematology*, Vol.68, No.1, pp.1-11,1040-8428.

Murphy, M., Ahn, J., Walker, KK., Hoffman, WH., Evans, RM., Levine, AJ. & George, DL. (1999). Transcriptional repression by wild-type p53 utilizes histone deacetylases, mediated by interaction with mSin3a. *Genes & Development*, Vol.13, No.19, pp.2490-2501,0890-9369.

Murr, R. (2010). Interplay between different epigenetic modifications and mechanisms. *Advances in Genetics*, Vol.70, No.10, pp.101-141,0065-2660.

Nan, X., Ng, HH., Johnson, CA., Laherty, CD., Turner, BM., Eisenman, RN. & Bird, A. (1998). Transcriptional repression by the methyl-CpG-binding protein MeCP2 involves a histone deacetylase complex. *Nature*, Vol.393, No.6683, pp.386-389,0028-0836.

Nguyen, TT., Cho, K., Stratton, SA. & Barton, MC. (2005). Transcription factor interactions and chromatin modifications associated with p53-mediated, developmental repression of the alpha-fetoprotein gene. *Molecular and Cellular Biology*, Vol.25, No.6, pp.2147-2157,0270-7306.

Nosho, K., Shima, K., Irahara, N., Kure, S., Baba, Y., Kirkner, GJ., Chen, L., Gokhale, S., Hazra, A., Spiegelman, D., Giovannucci, EL., Jaenisch, R., Fuchs, CS. & Ogino, S. (2009). DNMT3B expression might contribute to CpG island methylator phenotype in colorectal cancer. *Clinical Cancer Research*, Vol.15, No.11, pp.3663-3671,1078-0432.

Paz, MF., Fraga, MF., Avila, S., Guo, M., Pollan, M., Herman, JG. & Esteller, M. (2003). A systematic profile of DNA methylation in human cancer cell lines. *Cancer Research*, Vol.63, No.5, pp.1114-1121,0008-5472.

Plumb, JA., Strathdee, G., Sludden, J., Kaye, SB. & Brown, R. (2000). Reversal of drug resistance in human tumor xenografts by 2'-deoxy-5-azacytidine-induced demethylation of the hMLH1 gene promoter. *Cancer Research*, Vol.60, No.21, pp.6039-6044,0008-5472

Pruitt, K., Zinn, RL., Ohm, JE., McGarvey, KM., Kang, SH., Watkins, DN., Herman, JG. & Baylin, SB. (2006). Inhibition of SIRT1 reactivates silenced cancer genes without loss of promoter DNA hypermethylation. *PLoS Genetics*, Vol.2, No.3, pp.e40.

Rasoulpour, RJ., LeBaron, MJ., Ellis-Hutchings, RG., Klapacz, J. & Gollapudi, BB. (2011). Epigenetic screening in product safety assessment: are we there yet? *Toxicology Mechanisms and Methods*, Vol.21, No.4, pp.298-311,1537-6516.

Rhee, I., Jair, KW., Yen, RW., Lengauer, C., Herman, JG., Kinzler, KW., Vogelstein, B., Baylin, SB. & Schuebel, KE. (2000). CpG methylation is maintained in human cancer cells lacking DNMT1. *Nature*, Vol.404, No.6781, pp.1003-1007,0028-0836.

Rhee, I., Bachman, KE., Park, BH., Jair, KW., Yen, RW., Schuebel, KE., Cui, H., Feinberg, AP., Lengauer, C., Kinzler, KW., Baylin SB. & Vogelstein B. (2002). DNMT1 and DNMT3b cooperate to silence genes in human cancer cells. *Nature*, Vol.416, No.6880, pp.552-556,0028-0836.

Richon, VM., Sandhoff, TW., Rifkind, RA. & Marks, PA. (2000). Histone deacetylase inhibitor selectively induces p21WAF1 expression and gene-associated histone acetylation. *Proceedings of the National Academy of Sciences of the United States of America*, Vol.97, No.18, pp.10014-10019.

Robert, MF., Morin, S., Beaulieu, N., Gauthier, F., Chute, IC., Barsalou, A. & MacLeod, AR. (2002). DNMT1 is required to maintain CpG methylation and aberrant gene silencing in human cancer cells. *Nature Genetics*, Vol.33, No.1, pp.61-65.

Robertson, KD., Ait-Si-Ali, S., Yokochi, T., Wade, PA., Jones, PL. & Wolffe, AP. (2000). DNMT1 forms a complex with Rb, E2F1 and HDAC1 and represses transcription from E2F-responsive promoters. *Nature Genetics*, Vol.25, No.3, pp.338-342.

Rodríguez-Paredes, M. & Esteller, M. (2011). Cancer epigenetics reaches mainstream oncology. *Nature Medicine*, Vol.17, No.3, pp.330-339,1078-8956.

Saito, Y., Liang, G., Egger, G., Friedman, JM., Chuang, JC., Coetzee, GA. & Jones, PA. (2006). Specific activation of microRNA-127 with downregulation of the proto-oncogene BCL6 by chromatin-modifying drugs in human cancer cells. *Cancer Cell*, Vol.9, No.6, pp.435-443,1535-6108.

Schlesinger, Y., Straussman, R., Keshet, I., Farkash, S., Hecht, M., Zimmerman, J., Eden, E., Yakhini, Z., Ben-Shushan, E., Reubinoff, BE., Bergman, Y., Simon I. & Cedar H. (2006). Polycomb-mediated methylation on Lys27 of histone H3 pre-marks genes for de novo methylation in cancer. *Nature Genetics*, Vol.39, No.2, pp.232-236,1061-4036.

Shah, MY. & Licht, JD. (2011). DNMT3A mutations in acute myeloid leukemia. *Nature Genetics*, Vol.43, No.4, pp.289-290,1546-1718.

Smallwood, A., Estève, PO., Pradhan, S. & Carey, M. (2007). Functional cooperation between HP1 and DNMT1 mediates gene silencing. *Genes & Development*, Vol.21, No.10, pp.1169-1178,0890-9369.

Song, J., Noh, JH., Lee, JH., Eun, JW., Ahn, YM., Kim, SY., Lee, SH., Park, WS., Yoo, NJ., Lee, JY. & Nam, SW. (2005). Increased expression of histone deacetylase 2 is found in human gastric cancer. *Apmis*, Vol.113, No.4, pp.264-268,1600-0463.

Stirzaker, C., Song, JZ., Davidson, B. & Clark, SJ. (2004). Transcriptional gene silencing promotes DNA hypermethylation through a sequential change in chromatin modifications in cancer cells. *Cancer Research*, Vol.64, No.11, pp.3871-3877,0008-5472.

Strahl, BD. & Allis, CD. (2000). The language of covalent histone modifications. *Nature*, Vol.403, No.6765, pp.41-45.

Strober, BE., Dunaief, JL. & Goff, SP. (1996). Functional interactions between the hBRM/hBRG1 transcriptional activators and the pRB family of proteins. *Molecular and Cellular Biology*, Vol.16, No.4, pp.1576-1583,0270-7306.

Suzuki, H., Gabrielson, E., Chen, W., Anbazhagan, R., van Engeland, M., Weijenberg, MP., Herman, JG. & Baylin, SB. (2002). A genomic screen for genes upregulated by demethylation and histone deacetylase inhibition in human colorectal cancer. *Nature Genetics*, Vol.31, No.2, pp.141-149,1061-4036.

Suzuki, MM. & Bird, A. (2008). DNA methylation landscapes: provocative insights from epigenomics. *Nature Reviews Genetics*, Vol.9, No.6, pp.465-476,1471-0056.

Sykes, SM., Mellert, HS., Holbert, MA., Li, K., Marmorstein, R., Lane, WS. & McMahon, SB. (2006). Acetylation of the p53 DNA-binding domain regulates apoptosis induction. *Molecular Cell*, Vol.24, No.6, pp.841-851,1097-2765.

Taby, R. & Issa, JP. (2010). Cancer epigenetics. *CA: A Cancer Journal for Clinicians*, Vol.60, No.6, pp.376-392.

Tang, X., Khuri, FR., Lee, JJ., Kemp, BL., Liu, D., Hong, WK. & Mao, L. (2000). Hypermethylation of the death-associated protein (DAP) kinase promoter and aggressiveness in stage I non-small-cell lung cancer. *Journal of the National Cancer Institute*, Vol.92, No.18, pp.1511-1516,0027-8874.

Toyota, M., Suzuki, H., Sasaki, Y., Maruyama, R., Imai, K., Shinomura, Y. & Tokino, T. (2008). Epigenetic silencing of microRNA-34b/c and B-cell translocation gene 4 is associated with CpG island methylation in colorectal cancer. *Cancer Research*, Vol.68, No.11, pp.4123-4132,0008-5472.

Tsang, DP. & Cheng, AS. (2011). Epigenetic regulation of signaling pathways in cancer: role of the histone methyltransferase EZH2. *Journal of Gastroenterology and Hepatology*, Vol.26, No.1, pp.19-27.

Valeri, N., Vannini, I., Fanini, F., Calore, F., Adair, B. & Fabbri, M. (2009). Epigenetics, miRNAs, and human cancer: a new chapter in human gene regulation. *Mammalian Genome*, Vol.20, No.9, pp.573-580,0938-8990.

Van Haaften, G., Dalgliesh, GL., Davies, H., Chen, L., Bignell, G., Greenman, C., Edkins, S., Hardy, C., O'Meara, S. & Teague, J. (2009). Somatic mutations of the histone H3K27 demethylase gene UTX in human cancer. *Nature Genetics*, Vol.41, No.5, pp.521-523,1061-4036.

Varambally, S., Cao, Q., Mani, RS., Shankar, S., Wang, X., Ateeq, B., Laxman, B., Cao, X., Jing, X. & Ramnarayanan, K. (2008). Genomic loss of microRNA-101 leads to overexpression of histone methyltransferase EZH2 in cancer. *Science*, Vol.322, No.5908, pp.1695-1699,0036-8075.

Veeck, J., Niederacher, D., An, H., Klopocki, E., Wiesmann, F., Betz, B., Galm, O., Camara, O., Dürst, M., Kristiansen, G., Huszka C., Knüchel R. & Dahl E. (2006). Aberrant methylation of the Wnt antagonist SFRP1 in breast cancer is associated with unfavourable prognosis. *Oncogene*, Vol.25, No.24, pp.3479-3488,0950-9232.

Veeck, J., Ropero, S., Setien, F., Gonzalez-Suarez, E., Osorio, A., Benitez, J., Herman, JG. & Esteller, M. (2010). BRCA1 CpG island hypermethylation predicts sensitivity to poly (adenosine diphosphate)-ribose polymerase inhibitors. *Journal of Clinical Oncology*, Vol.28, No.29, pp.563-564,0732-183X.

Vrba, L., Junk, DJ., Novak, P. & Futscher, BW. (2008). p53 induces distinct epigenetic states at its direct target promoters. *BMC Genomics*, Vol.9, No.1, pp.486,1471-2164.

Wang, JK., Tsai, MC., Poulin, G., Adler, AS., Chen, S., Liu, H., Shi, Y. & Chang, HY. (2010). The histone demethylase UTX enables RB-dependent cell fate control. *Genes & Development*, Vol.24, No.4, pp.327-332,0890-9369.

Wang, X., Arai, S., Song, X., Reichart, D., Du, K., Pascual, G., Tempst, P., Rosenfeld, MG., Glass, CK. & Kurokawa, R. (2008). Induced ncRNAs allosterically modify RNA-binding proteins in cis to inhibit transcription. *Nature*, Vol.454, No.7200, pp.126-130,0028-0836.

Yamane, K., Tateishi, K., Klose, RJ., Fang, J., Fabrizio, LA., Erdjument-Bromage, H., Taylor-Papadimitriou, J., Tempst, P. & Zhang, Y. (2007). PLU-1 is an H3K4 demethylase involved in transcriptional repression and breast cancer cell proliferation. *Molecular Cell*, Vol.25, No.6, pp.801-812,1097-2765.

Yap, KL., Li, S., Muñoz-Cabello, AM., Raguz, S., Zeng, L., Mujtaba, S., Gil, J., Walsh, MJ. & Zhou, MM. (2010). Molecular interplay of the noncoding RNA ANRIL and methylated histone H3 lysine 27 by polycomb CBX7 in transcriptional silencing of INK4a. *Molecular Cell*, Vol.38, No.5, pp.662-674,1097-2765.

Yi, J. & Luo, J. (2010). SIRT1 and p53, effect on cancer, senescence and beyond. *Biochimica et Biophysica Acta (BBA)-Proteins & Proteomics*, Vol.1804, No.8, pp.1684-1689,1570-9639.

Zeng, Y., Kotake, Y., Pei, XH., Smith, MD. & Xiong, Y. (2011). p53 Binds to and Is Required for the Repression of Arf Tumor Suppressor by HDAC and Polycomb. *Cancer Research*, Vol.71, No.7, pp.2781-2792,0008-5472.

6

Therapeutic Targeting of p53-Mediated Apoptosis Pathway in Head and Neck Squamous Cell Carcinomas: Current Progress and Challenges

Solachuddin Jauhari Arief Ichwan[1], Muhammad Taher Bakhtiar[2], Kiyoshi Ohtani[3] and Masa-Aki Ikeda[4]
[1]*Kulliyyah of Dentistry, International Islamic University Malaysia, Kuantan,*
[2]*Kulliyyah of Pharmacy, International Islamic University Malaysia, Kuantan,*
[3]*Department of Bioscience, School of Science and Technology, Kwansei Gakuin University, Sanda-shi, Hyogo,*
[4]*Section of Molecular Craniofacial Embryology, Tokyo Medical and Dental University, Bunkyo-ku, Tokyo,*
[1,2]*Malaysia*
[3,4]*Japan*

1. Introduction

Since its discovery three decades ago, p53 has been one of the most intensively and extensively studied tumor suppressor gene, which is accounted more than fifty eight thousand papers have been published to date. The p53 tumor suppressor protein was initially identified as a cellular protein that interacts with a viral oncoprotein, simian virus 40 (SV40) large T antigen. The p53 cDNA isolated from tumor cells (i.e. mutant p53) exhibited oncogenic activity and was therefore initially recognized as an oncogene (Lane & Crawford, 1979). Nevertheless, the identification of wild-type p53 gene and subsequent functional studies in the late 1980's revealed its real action as a tumor suppressor gene (Finlay at al., 1989).

p53 tumor suppressor plays a critical role in the cellular response to genotoxic stress as a major defense against cancer, by maintaining genome integrity to prevent cells from inappropriate growth and division. Mutation of the p53 gene is known as the most common genetic changes in the development of human cancers. p53 regulates a wide variety of target genes responsible for different cellular outcomes related to its function as a tumor suppressor such as cell cycle arrest, apoptotic cell death, senescence, or DNA repair, depending on the cell type and cellular stress. Given the fact that apoptosis is an evolutionary conserved process through which the organisms remove abnormal cells, and thus represents a fundamental roadblock to tumorigenesis (reviewed in Ichwan 2008), it is not surprising that the role in apoptosis has been the focus for most of the scientists working on p53 in cancer treatment research. Loss of p53-dependent apoptosis caused by p53 mutation is believed to be a critical step for carcinogenesis in majority of human malignancies including Head and Neck

Squamous Cell Carcinoma (HNSCC). (Gleich, 2000; Vousden, 2000). Indeed, targeting the p53 pathway of apoptosis to restore the function of p53 gene lost or functionally inactivated in cancer cells has been pursued in recent years.

HNSCC is the most frequently occurring malignant tumor with poor prognosis resulting in major morbidity and mortality. HNSCC is the eighth most common cancer worldwide (Wang et al., 2009; Jemal et al. 2008) and it is increasing in incidence because it is often poorly understood by society in general and frequently ignored in its early stages. The main treatment of HNSCC is either radiotherapy or radical surgery depend on the location and the size of the tumor, which is often combined with adjuvant chemotherapy. However, those conventional therapies in particular radiotherapy and chemotherapy, are non-selective and can cause damage to normal tissue. Modification of the approaches have improved cure rate in only approximately half of the patients (Ichwan & Ikeda, 2008; Thomas & Grandis, 2009). Recently, dramatic improvements in our knowledge of the molecular and genetic basis of HNSCC combined with advances in technology have resulted in novel molecular therapies for the disease by targeting of specific molecule in cancer therapy to selectively destroys cancer cells including targeting the function of p53 tumor suppressor. This chapter attempts to discuss the current state and challenges of the p53-mediated apoptosis pathway as a target in HNSCC therapy.

2. p53: Its structure and role in apoptosis

The structure and sequence of the p53 corresponds to key features of the protein and are well conserved in all vertebrates (Hainaut & Hollstein, 2000). The human *p53* gene is located on the short arm of chromosome 17 at 17p13.1 (Isobe et al, 1986; McBride et al, 1986). The p53 protein consists of four functional domains: N-terminal transactivation domain, central core (DNA-binding domain, DBD), tetramerization domain and C-terminal regulatory domain (Fig. 1A). The DBD displays sequence-specific activity in binding to the consensus motif whereas C-terminal domain binds DNA nonspecifically (Melero et al, 2011). For its role as transcription factor, before they interact and recognizing by recognizing consensus sequences (DNA binding sites) of its target genes, p53 proteins need to form tetramers (Xu et al, 2011; Melero et al, 2011). Therefore, the protein is organized in two stably folded domains, the tetramerization and DNA-binding domains that are linked and flanked by intrinsically disordered segments (Melero et al, 2011) (Fig. 1B). In addition to p53, there are two other members in the unique protein family named p63 and p73 (Irwin & Kaelin, 2001). Structurally and functionally, all of these three proteins are related to each other. However, p53 seems to be evolving in the higher organisms to prevent tumorigenesis. Compared with the other genes in p53 family, p53 structure is the simplest among them.

p53 acts as a transcription factor and mediates its effect by modulating the expression of its downstream target genes (El-Deiry, 1998; Ko & Prives, 1996). A number of p53-target genes have been identified and their function in the p53-pathway has been established. In the most recent genome- wide analyses, of the *p53* binding suggest that hundreds of genes may be up- or down- regulated by *p53* (Smeenk et al., 2008).

In normal conditions, the amount of p53 protein in the cell is maintained at very low levels, which is tightly controlled by its important negative regulator which also an upstream target, MDM2 (also known as HDM2) (Vousden and Lu, 2002). MDM2 and p53 regulate each other through an autoregulatory feedback loop. The MDM2 activity is also modulated by its structural homologue partner protein called MDMX (also known as MDM4, HDM4, or HDMX). MDM2 forms a heterodimers with MDM2 through C-terminal RING domain interactions (Brown et al, 2009). The MDM2-MDMX complex ubiquitinates p53 and thus targets it for proteasome-mediated degradation. MDM2 also inactivates p53 by both repressing its transcriptional activity (Wiman, 2010; Brown et al, 2009; Vousden & Lane, 2007). Likewise MDM2, MDMX also binds directly to p53 and inhibits its transcriptional activity, however it does not induce p53 degradation. (Bottger 1999 in Shangary 2008). Besides MDM2 and MDM4 complex, ARF tumor suppressor also play a crucial role in preventing p53 from MDM2-induced degradation and stabilizing p53 by interacting with MDM2 (Brown et al, 2009) (Fig. 2).

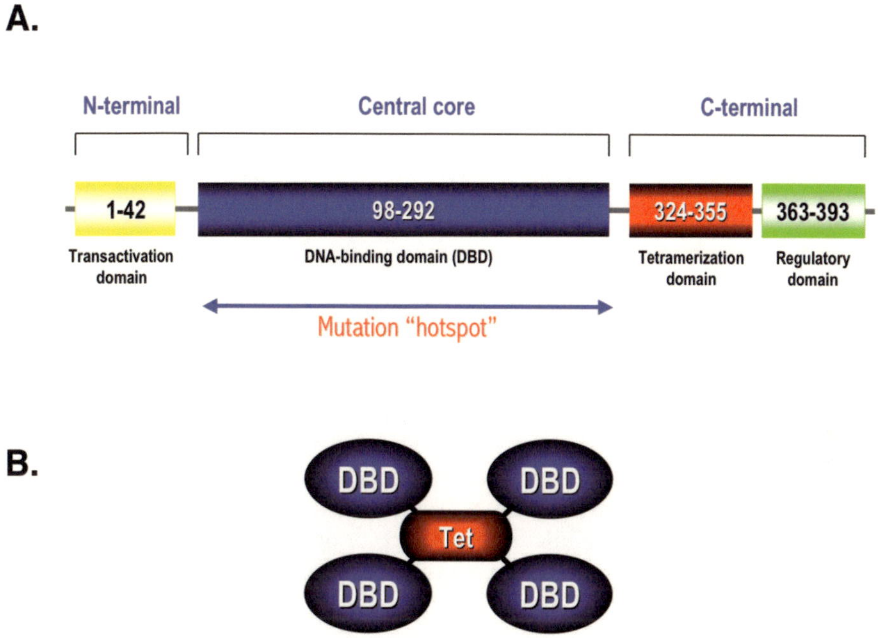

Fig. 1. Schematic representation of: A. Structure of human p53. Note the mutation hotspot is located at DBD. B. Organization of p53 as tetramers.

Upon cellular stresses such as DNA damage, oncogene activation, hypoxia, oxidative stress, mitotic spindle damage and ribonucleotide depletion, p53 is activated, the ability of MDM2 to interact with the p53 expression is diminished, resulting in the stabilization of p53 protein. On the other hand, MDM2 is degraded by ARF, causing release of p53 from the p53-MDM2 complex in the nucleus (Sherr, 2006).

The release of p53 from MDM2-mediated inhibition leads to the stabilization of p53 protein and the activation of its transcription activity, as a consequence of which p53 modulates the expression of its downstream target genes involved in cell cycle arrest, DNA repair, senescence, apoptosis, and inhibition of angiogenesis/metastasis as the final outcomes, Several general factors that influence this decision include p53 expression levels, the type of stress signal, the cell type and the cellular context at the time of exposure to stress (reviewed by Haupt et al., 2003; Balint &Vousden, 2001) (Fig. 2). Nevertheless, the exact criteria and the clear mechanism(s) leading to the choice between these final outcomes still need to be further elucidated.

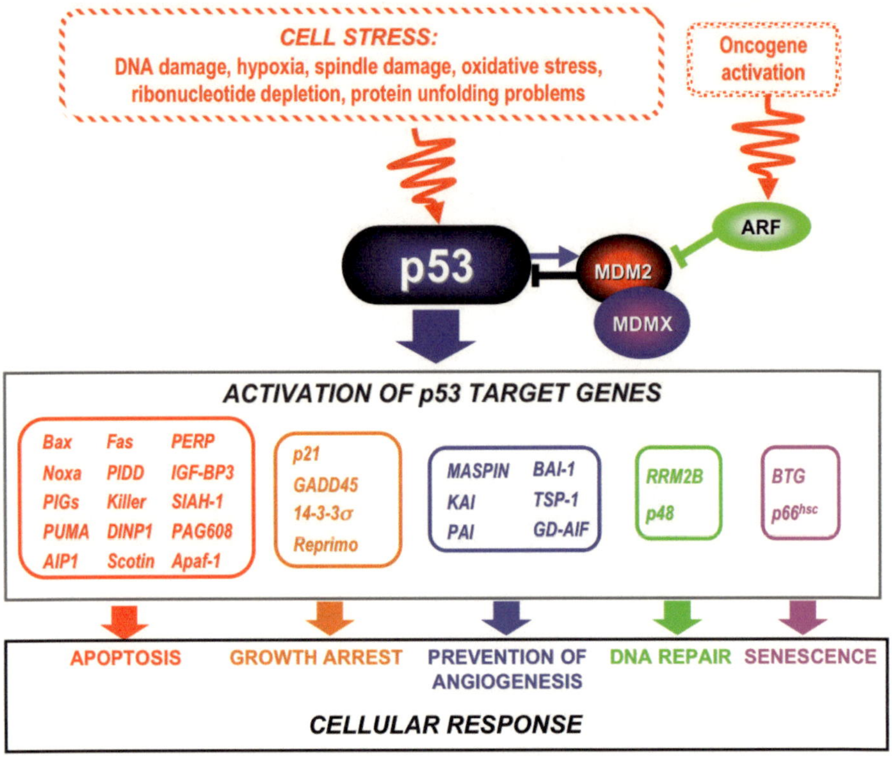

Fig. 2. Cell cycle control by p53. The p53 expression is tightly regulated by MDM2 in a negative feed-back loop manner, whereas MDM2 expression is modulated by MDMX and negatively controlled by ARF. Cellular stresses and/or oncogene activation, disrupts the MDM2-p53 interaction resulting in the stabilization of p53 protein thus modulating the activation of its downstream genes involved in various cellular responses.

p53 triggers apoptosis when cells suffer severe, irreparable damage, whereas it causes cell-cycle arrest when the damage is mild, thereby enabling the cell to fix the damage (Haupt et al., 2003). Depending on the strength of DNA damage, p53 preferentially modulate transcription of either pro-arrest or pro-apoptotic target genes. Upon severe DNA damage, p53 activates expression of multiple target genes whose products execute apoptosis, although evidence indicates that p53 also induces apoptosis in a transcription-independent manner(Gottlieb & Oren, 1998). p53 serves as a regulator of the apoptotic process that can modulate key control points in both the extrinsic (consists of cell surface receptors such as Fas, KILLER) and intrinsic pathways (centers on the mitochondria such as Bax, PUMA, Noxa, p53AIP1, PERP, PIDD) (Fridman & Lowe, 2003). Therefore, p53 apoptotic target genes are enlisted according to their functions in death receptor pathways, mitochondrial machinery and others that play distinct roles in p53-mediated apoptosis (Fridman & Lowe, 2003).

Numerous studies have demonstrated that the stabilization and activation of p53 protein is not only regulated by its interactions with other proteins but also highly governed via complex networks of posttranslational modifications including phosphorylation, ubiquitylation, acetylation, sumoylation, neddylation, ADP-ribosylation, and cytoplasmic sequestration (Vogelstein et al., 2000). The N- and C-terminal regions of p53 is identified where most of these modifications taken place (Bai and Zhu, 2006). Phosphorylation and acetylation have been thought as the major modifications enhancing the transcription activating ability of p53 because these modifications generally result in p53 stabilization and accumulation in the nucleus, where p53 interacts with sequence-specific sites of its target genes (Xu, 2003; Appella et al., 2001). p53 is phosphorylated on a number of serine residues in the N- and C-terminal domains (Bode & Dong, 2003). Phosphorylation of Ser46 following severe DNA-damage has been shown to be critical for inducing p53-mediated apoptosis (Oda et al., 2000). Severe, irreparable DNA damage induces phosphorylation at Ser46, and Ser46 phosphorylated p53 selectively transactivates pro-apoptotic genes, including *p53AIP1* that is critical for p53-mediated apoptotic induction. Ser46 phosphorylation would change the affinity of p53 to its target gene promoters, shifting from pro-arrest genes to pro-apoptotic genes (reviewed in Ichwan & Ikeda, 2008) (Fig. 3). The most recent study using analysis of genome-wide binding profiles of phosphorylated p53 has demonstrated that the extent of Ser46 phosphorylation of p53 bound to DNA is higher than Ser15 phosphorylation in cells directed towards apoptosis and the amount of chromatin-associated p53 phosphorylated at Ser46 is higher on certain apoptosis related target genes (Smeenk et al., 2011).

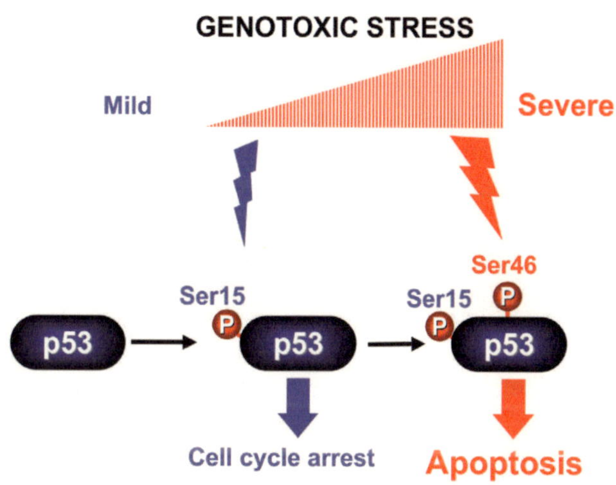

Fig. 3. Phosphorylation of p53 at either Ser15 or Ser46 residue is selectively induced depend on the degree of genotoxic stress (Adopted with modification from Ichwan & Ikeda, 2008).

p53 is also posttranslationally modified through acetylation at Lys370, Lys372, Lys373, Lys381, and Lys382 by p300/CBP and at Lys320 by PCAF (p300/CBP-associated factor). Acetylation augments p53 DNA binding, and to stimulate p53-mediated transactivation of its downstream target genes through the recruitment of coactivators (Ozaki & Nakagawara, 2011). Additionally, acetylation has been suggested to regulate the stability of p53 by inhibiting its ubiquitylation by MDM2. In vivo, acetylation at Lys320, Lys373, and Lys382 is induced by many genotoxic agents such as UV-or Ionizing radiation, hypoxia, oxidative stress, and even depletion of ribonucleotide pools (Bai & Zhu, 2006). p53 can also be deacetylated by HDAC1 (Histone Deacetylase-1) and SIRT1 (Silent mating type information regulation 2 homolog 1). Intrinsic deacetylase activity of human SIRT1 attenuates p53-dependent cell cycle arrest and apoptosis through down-regulation of the p21WAF1 and Bax (Brown et al., 2009).

3. Dysfunctions of p53-mediated apoptotic pathway in HNSCC

Dysfunction of p53 by mutation and/or attenuated expression of the wild-type p53 by oncogenic proteins account in majority of tumor development have been well documented in HNSCC. Loss of heterozygosity 17p and mutations of the p53 have been detected in approximately half of all primary and most of recurrent cases of HNSCC (Nemunaitis et al., 2009; Gasco & Crook, 2003; Osman et al., 2002; Taylor et al., 1999). Studies of HNSCC and cell lines suggested that after mutation of one *TP53* allele, the remaining wild-type allele is deleted and accordingly the mutant phenotype expressed (Nylander et al., 2000 as cited in Yin et al., 1999). Mutations in *p53* gene consist of high proportion of missense mutations, which lead to expression of mutated protein at high levels (reviewed in Goldstein et al., 2011 and Nylander et al., 2000). More than ninety percent of the mutations are found in "hot spots" DBD (Fig 1), which highlighted several residues, such as R175, R282, R273 and the mostly occurred, R248. In HNSCC the main part is found within exons 5–8, but the pattern has been shown to vary between countries and races (Nylander et al., 2000). These mutations involved either in making direct contacts with DNA or support the structure of DNA binding surface. The examples of mutant proteins categorized as "contact" are R248 and R273, while "structural" are R175 and R282 (Joerger & Ferscht, 2010). Structural mutants cause deformation that created internal cavities or surface crevices in the protein scaffold, thus inducing conformational changes in the DNA binding surface (Olivier et al., 2009). Intriguingly, it has also been suggested that instead of the p53 loss-of-function, there are also "gain-of-function" mutants with oncogenic properties; they possess dominant negative activity due to their abilities to prevent wild-type p53 from binding to the promoter of its target genes through formation of a heterotetramer complex (Fig. 4) (Ichwan & Ikeda, 2008). Unfortunately, such mutants are usually has a prolonged half-life (Nylander 2000; Prives & Hall, 1999) and may neutralize the apoptotic activity of exogenous wild-type p53. Defect in Ser46 phosphorylation is also responsible for the acquisition of p53 resistance to p53 gene transfer on HNSCC (Ichwan et al., 2006). Furthermore, specific polymorphic forms at codon 72 "gain-of-function" p53 mutants which encode polymorphic alleles encode either proline (72P) or arginine (72R) have been shown to exhibit significant differences in the biochemical properties of the p53 protein (Murphy, 2006). In HNSCC cells, mutant p53 proteins with 72R are commonly found than 72P (Marin et al., 2000; Brooks et al., 2000). The mutants that harbors 72R allele have also been shown to physically interact with a member of p53 family, p73 and repress its apoptotic activity in cancer cells (Marin et al., 2000).

Accumulating evidences have shown that roughly half of all HNSCC cases still retain normal (wild-type) p53, supporting the idea that HNSCC is not characterized by a single molecular change. In this circumstance, the expression of the wild-type p53 may be inactivated by amplification or overexpression of oncogenic protein including MDM2, MDMX and HPV-E6 (Fig. 4).

Amplified expression of either MDM2 and MDMX, in which both are known as p53 inhibitors would severely degrade the protein, resulting in apoptotic blockade. Indeed, MDM2 is overexpressed in a variety of human cancers in HNSCC and has become a prognostic marker (Valentin-Vega et al., 2007; Huang et al., 2001; Ganly et al., 2000; Matsumura et al., 1996). The G-allele single nucleotide polymorphism at 309 of MDM2 (MDM2 SNP309G) has been shown to be associated with significantly higher levels of the

MDM2 expression (reviewed in Vasquez et al., 2008). MDM2 overexpression also induces centrosome hyperamplification and chromosome in cultured HNSCC cells (Caroll et al., 1999). The scenario may become worse when MDMX are excessively co-expressed as reported in a study in which majority of tumors with amplified MDM2 were also positive for MDMX (Valentin-Vega et al., 2007). Since MDMX potentiates MDM2, overexpression of MDMX may accelerate the p53 degradation and subsequently result in abrogation of p53-mediated apoptotic pathway.

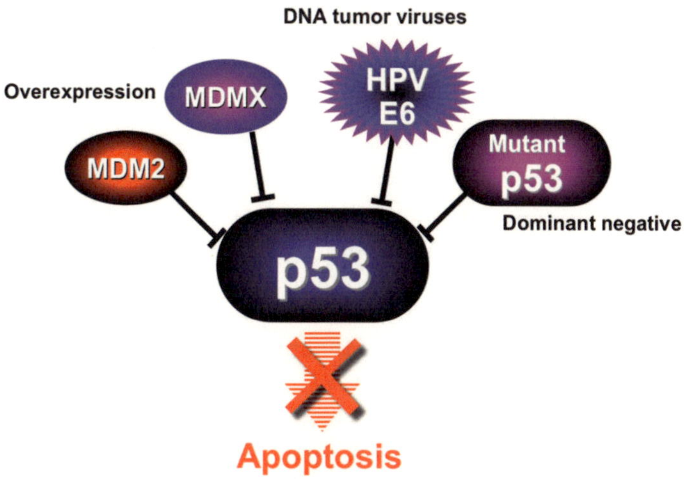

Fig. 4. The pro-apoptotic function of p53 is abrogated in HNSCC by mutation and/or oncogenic proteins MDM2, MDMX, HPV-E6.

HPV-E6 is an oncoprotein encoded by human papillomavirus (HPV), a double-stranded DNA virus that commonly associated with a diverse of human neoplasms such as warts (benign papilloma) as well as malignancy at cervical, vulvar, vaginal, anal, penile, and more recently HNSCC (Chung et al., 2009). More than 100 types of HPV have been identified but the most commonly detected HPV in HNSCC is HPV-16, which has been showed in 90–95% of all HPV positive HNSCC cases, followed by HPV-18, HPV-33, and HPV-33 (reviewed in Perez-Ordonez et al., 2006). The viral genome also encodes another two oncogenic proteins E5 and E7. However the key players involved in tumorigenesis are attributed to E6 and E7. The oncogenic potential of E6 and E7 are due to their ability to induce degradation of the tumor suppressors p53 and pRB respectively (Werness et al., 1990; Dyson et al., 1989). The HPV-E6 binds to and targets p53 for inactivation and degradation by forming a complex with an E3 ubiquitin ligase, E6-associated protein (E6AP)(Chung et al., 2009).

4. Restoration of p53-mediated apoptosis in HNSCC: The challenges and strategies to overcome

Conventional treatment of HNSCC to destroy cancer cells by combination of radiotherapy and chemotherapy is often non-selective because it also destroys normal cells. Moreover, some cancer cells may acquire resistance to chemotherapy (i.e. doxorubicin, cisplatin, etc) and radiation due to the expression some forms of mutant p53 that enhanced tumorigenic potential (Thomas & Grandis, 2009). For the past few years, several novel anticancer therapeutic strategies for restoration of the p53 pathway have been developed such as gene therapy, DNA vaccine, small-molecule inhibitors, antisense molecules, and tumor vaccines (Bayon et al., 2011). In particular, gene therapy, which represents the use of genetic material for therapeutic purposes, has been regarded as a promising therapeutic approach (Vattemi & Claudio, 2009). Several strategies have been developed for HNSCC gene therapy including targeting the function of p53 tumor suppressor gene. Indeed, HNSCC has become the focus of p53-targeted gene therapy and an ideal model for testing the efficacy of gene therapy strategies in a localized area with minimal systemic exposure to the agent (Thomas & Grandis, 2009). The replacement of the mutated gene with wild-type p53 gene transfer (mostly using recombinant adenovirus Ad-p53) has been explored as a popular approach, either as a single anticancer agent or combined with other agents. Various studies have reported that wild-type p53 gene transfer efficiently induces apoptosis in most of cancer cells including HNSCC (reviewed in Ichwan & Ikeda, 2008). Clinically, this approach is usually carried out through local injection of recombinant Ad-p53 into tumors. Several "brand names" of the recombinant adenoviruses have been introduced (Table 1). China became the first country to approve the use of Ad-p53 as a gene therapy agent (Gendicine) for HNSCC treatment. (Pearson at al., 2004). However, the clinical efficacy relies on the bystander effect in the tumor since not all cells will be injected (Brown et al., 2009), thus it may require multiple rounds of treatment. Moreover, some HNSCC cells are found to be resistant to Ad-p53 gene transfer (Ichwan et al., 2006). Although mechanisms underlying the p53 resistance have not been fully understood, it has been reported that certain dominant negative mutant p53 proteins expressed in p53-resistant tumors may interfere the action of exogenous wild-type p53 and inhibition of the mutant p53 protein using mutant specific small interfering RNA (siRNA) simultaneously restored the p53-mediated apoptosis in p53-resistant HNSCC cells (Ichwan et al., 2006). Defect in phosphorylation of p53 protein at Ser46, which is critical for p53-mediated apoptosis, also plays a role for the acquisition of the resistance to p53 gene transfer in HNSCC cells and this resistance can be overcome by introducing p53S46D mutant that mimicks Ser46 phosphorylation (Ichwan et al., 2006). In regard to the potential use of recombinant adenoviruses in HNSCC treatment, specific oncolytic adenoviruses have been designed on the idea that the virus only replicate in cancer cells that lack p53 function. Examples of these oncolytic viruses are ONYX-015, currently under Phase III development in the United States (Vattemi & Claudio, 2006) and H101 that have been commercially approved in China (Crompton & Kirn, 2007).

Reactivating mutant p53 has been considered as an alternative strategy to treat HNSCC carrying mutated p53. Several small molecules have been discovered (Table 1) and all of them are still under early stage of preclinical trial. So far, the are only two reports regarding the utilization of these molecules to induce p53-dependent apoptosis on HNSCC cells. PRIMA-1 and CP-31398 work by protecting p53 mutants from unfolding (Roh et al., 2011). and induce the expression of p53-dependent pro-apoptotic mediators PUMA, Noxa, and Bax thus restoring p53-dependent transcription (Wang et al., 2007; Ho & Li, 2005). WR1065 has been proven as a radioprotector in a Phase III randomized trial (Brizel et al., 2002).

Agent/Molecule	Stage in HNSCC clinical trial	Mechanism of action	Reference
Gendicine	Approved (in China)	Wild-type p53 restoration using recombinant adenovirus encoding p53	Pearson et al., 2004
Advexin	Phase III		Nemunatitis, 2011
SCH 58500	N/A		Vasquez et al., 2008
CDB3	N/A	Mutant p53 reactivation	Vasquez et al., 2008
CP-31398	Preclinical		Roh et al., 2011
Ellipticine	N/A		Vasquez, et al., 2008
WR1065	Phase III		Brizel et al., 2000
PRIMA-1	Preclinical		Roh et al., 2011
MIRA-1	N/A		Vasquez, et al., 2008
Nutlin3	Preclinical	p53 stabilization via inhibition of MDM2-p53 interaction	Roh et al., 2011 Vassilev et al., 2004
M219	N/A		Shangary et al., 2008
RITA	Preclinical		Roh et al., 2011
HL198C	N/A	p53 stabilization via inhibition of MDM2-E3 ligase	Atwal et al., 2007
ONYX-015	Phase III	Oncolytic adenoviruses	Vattemi & Claudio, 2006
H101	Approved (in China)		Crompton & Kirn, 2007

Table 1. Agents that targeting p53-mediated apoptosis.

Different strategies are applied to restore p53-dependent apoptosis in the HNSCC cells that retain wild-type p53 but are not active because of the expression of negative regulatory proteins MDM2, MDMX and HPV-E6. Therefore, diminishing the expression of those p53 inhibitors would be the ultimate choice. To this end, siRNA and specific small molecule inhibitors have been shown to be feasible. Previous studies have shown that siRNA delivery into HPV-E6 positive cancer cells induces rapid apoptosis and restore p53 response (Jiang & Milner 2002; Butz et al., 2003). On the other hand, introduction of siRNA did not induce apoptosis but markedly sensitized the different HPV-E6 expressing cells to the chemotherapy drugs (Koivusalo et al., 2005). siRNA treatment also seems effective to silence MDM2 and MDMX overexpression in some cancer cell lines (Lane et al., 2010; Brown et al., 2009; Zhang et al. 2005). Despite these promising achievements, the delivery of siRNA into the tumor of a patient is an important burden since siRNA is prone to degradation. To accomplish this, antisense oligonucleotide carried in an adenoviral vector could be used instead of siRNA; nonetheless, the clinical efficacy still needs to be confirmed. Recent advancements in research on the p53 pathway has been lead to the discovery of several non-genotoxic small compounds to activate the p53 response (Table 1) that targeting p53-MDM2 complex. Nutlin3 is the first molecule known to mimic p53 binding by interacting with the hydrophobic pocket of MDM2, discovered by a combination of high-throughput screening and computer modeling (Vassilev et al., 2004).

Subsequently, another MDM2 inhibitor MI-219 was discovered (Shangary et al., 2008). Both have been shown to disrupt p53-MDM2 interaction through binding to MDM2 thereby reactivate p53-dependent apoptosis and are currently under Phase I clinical trial. RITA works by binding to p53 thus protecting it from interacting to MDM2 and was shown more effective in inducing apoptosis than the Nutlin3 (Issaeva et al., 2004). HL198C stabilize p53 by inhibiting MDM2 ubiquitin ligase activity (Atwal et al., 2007). Despite their early-stage (most are still in the preclinical trial) of development, the utilization of above-mentioned molecules may emerge as an attractive approach in the p53-based cancer therapy for HNSCC.

5. Conclusion

Dramatic advances in gaining knowledge of the p53 pathway have shift paradigms in cancer therapy. The ability of p53 tumor suppressor gene to induce apoptosis has been targeted as a novel therapeutic strategy for the patients with HNSCC in which aberrant function of p53 is a common event. Several molecular approaches including wild-type p53 gene transfer and non-genotoxic molecules that capable to reactivate the p53-mediated apoptosis pathways in HNSCC have been established. Regardless a number of successful clinical trials, most of the attempts are still in preclinical stage and yet also facing a number of obstacles. Likewise other malignancies, HNSCC is caused by multiple genetic changes therefore p53 novel mechanisms for p53-induced apoptosis will remain challenging. Further intense efforts are still required to achieve a more efficient therapy of HNSCC in the future.

6. Acknowledgment

We thank Dr. Teng Ma from Section Molecular Craniofacial Embryology, Tokyo Medical and Dental University and Ms. Zafirah Liyana from Kulliyyah of Pharmacy International Islamic University Malaysia for providing literature retrieval. We also thank Ms. Wastuti Hidayati Suriyah from Kulliyyah of Pharmacy International Islamic University Malaysia for her kind technical assistance. This work was supported in part by the Research Endowment Fund, International Islamic University Malaysia, Grant No EDW-B 110210499 and EDW-B 0905277.

7. References

Atwal, G. S., Bond, G. L., Metsuyanim, S., Papa, M., Friedman, E., Distelman-Menachem, T., Ben Asher, E., Lancet, D., Ross, D. A., Sninsky, J., White, T. J., Levine, A. J., & Yarden, R. (2007). Haplotype Structure and selection of The MDM2 Oncogene in Humans. Proceedings *of National Academy of Sciences U.S.A.*, 104, pp 4524–4529, ISSN 0027-8424

Bakalkin G, et al. (1995). p53 Binds Single-Stranded DNA Ends Through the C-Terminal Domain and Internal DNA Segments Via The Middle Domain. *Nucleic Acids Research*, 23, pp 362–369, ISSN 0305-1048

Balint, E. E. & Vousden, K. H. (2001). Activation and Activities of the p53 Tumour Suppressor Protein. *British Journal of Cancer,* 85, pp 1813-1823, ISSN 0007-0920

Bargonetti, J., Manfredi, J. J., Chen, X., Marshak, D. R. & Prives, C. (1993). A Proteolytic Fragment from the Central Region of p53 has Marked Sequence-Specific DNA-Binding Activity when Generated from Wild Type but not from Oncogenic Mutant p53 Protein. *Genes and Development,* 7, pp 2565–2574, ISSN 0890-9369

Bayon, R & Wenig, B. L. Targeted Molecular Therapy in Head and Neck Squamous Cell Carcinoma. Downloaded on March 29, 2011, http://emedicine.medscape.com/article/854971-overview

Bode, A. M., & Dong, Z. (2004). Post-translational Modification of p53 in Tumorigenesis. *Nature Reviews Cancer,* 4, pp 793-805, ISSN 1474-175X

Bottger, V., Bottger, A. & Garcia-Echeverria, C., et al. (1999). Comparative Study of the p53 - Mdm2 and p53-MDMX Interfaces. *Oncogene,* 18, pp 189–199, ISSN 0950-9232

Brizel, D. M., Wasserman, T. H., Strnad, V., Rudat, V., Monnier, A., Eschwege, F., Zhang, J., Russell, L., Oster, W., & Sauer, R. (2000). Phase III randomized trial of amifostine as a radioprotector in head and neck cancer. *Journal of Clinical Oncology,* 18, pp 3339-3345, ISSN 0732-183X

Brooks, L. A., Tidy, J. A., Gusterson, B., Hiller, L., O'Nions, J., Gasco, M., Marin, M. C., Farrell, P. J., Kaelin, W. G. Jr., Crook, T. (2000). Preferential Retention of Codon 72 Arginine p53 in Squamous Cell Carcinomas of The Vulva Occurs in Cancers Positive and Negative For Human Papillomavirus. *Cancer Research,* 15, pp 6875-6877, ISSN 0008-5472

Brown, C. J., Lain, S., Verma, C. S., Fersht, A. R. & Lane, D. P. (2009). Awakening Guardian Angels: Drugging the p53 Pathway. *Nature Reviews Cancer,* 9, pp 862-873, ISSN 1474-175X

Butz, K., Ristriani, T., Hengstermann, A., Denk, C., Scheffner, M., & Hoppe-Seyler, F. (2003). siRNA Targeting of The Viral E6 Oncogene Efficiently Kills Human Papillomavirus-Positive Cancer Cells. *Oncogene,* 22, pp 5938–5945, ISSN 0950-9232

Carroll, P. E., Okuda, M., Horn, H. F., Biddinger, P., Stambrook, P. J., Gleich, L. L., Li, Y. Q., Tarapore, P. & Fukasawa, K. (1999). Centrosome Hyperamplifcation in Human Cancer: Chromosome Instability Induced by p53 Mutation and/or MDM2 Overexpression. *Oncogene* ,18, pp 1935-1944, ISSN 0950-9232

Christine, H., Chung & Gillison, M. L. (2009). Human Papillomavirus in Head and Neck Cancer: Its Role in Pathogenesis and Clinical Implications. *Clinical Cancer Research,* 15, pp 6758-6762, ISSN 1078-0432

Crompton, A. M. & Kirn, D. H. (2007). From ONYX-015 to Armed Vaccinia Viruses: the education and evolution of oncolytic virus development. *Current Cancer Drug Targets,* 7 pp 133-139, ISSN 1568-0096

Dyson, N., Howley, P. M., Munger, K. & Harlow, E. (1989). The Human Papilloma Virus- 16 E7 Oncoprotein is able to Bind to the Retinoblastoma Gene Product. *Science,* 243, pp 934-937, ISSN 0036-8075

El-Deiry, W. S. (1998). Regulation of p53 Downstream Genes. *Seminars in Cancer Biology,* 8, pp 345-357, ISSN 1044-579X

Finlay, C. A., Hinds, P. W. & Levine, A. J. (1989). The p53 Proto-oncogene can Act as a Suppressor of Transformation. *Cell,* 57, pp 1083-1093, ISSN 0092-8674

Fridman, J. S., & Lowe, S. W. (2003). Control of Apoptosis by p53. *Oncogene*, 22, pp 9030-9040, ISSN 0950-9232

Ganly, I., Soutar, D. S., Brown, R. & Kaye, S. B. (2000). p53 Alterations in Recurrent Squamous Cell Cancer of the Head and Neck Refractory to Radiotherapy. *British Journal of Cancer*, 82, pp 392–398, ISSN 0007-0920

Gasco, M. & Crook, T. (2003). The p53 Network in Head and Neck Cancer. *Oral Oncology*, 39, pp 222-231, ISSN 1368-8375

Gleich, L. L. (2000). Gene Therapy For Head and Neck Cancer. *Laryngoscope*, 110, pp 708-726, ISSN 0023-852X

Goldstein, I., Marcel, V., Olivier, M., Oren, M., Rotter, V. & Hainaut, P. (2011). Review: Understanding Wild- Type and Mutant p53 Activities in Human Cancer: New Landmarks on The Way to Targeted Therapies. *Cancer Gene Therapy*, 18, pp 2-11, ISSN 0929-1903

Gottlieb, T. M. & Oren, M. (1998). p53 and Apoptosis. *Seminars in Cancer Biology*, 8, pp 359-368, ISSN 1044-579X

Hainaut, P., & Hollstein, M. (2000). p53 and Human Cancer: The First Ten Thousand Mutations. *Advances in Cancer Research*, 77, pp 81-137, ISSN 0065-230X

Harwood, C. A., Yulug, I. G., Vousden, K. H., Allday, M. J., Gusterson, B., Ikawa, S., Hinds, P. W., Crook, T., & Kaelin, W. G. Jr. (2000). A Common Polymorphism Acts as an Intragenic Modifier of Mutant p53 Behaviour. *Nature Genetics*, 25, pp 47-54, ISSN 1061-4036

Haupt S., Berger, M., Goldberg, Z. & Haupt, Y. (2003). Apoptosis – The p53 Network. *Journal of Cell Science*, 116, pp 4077-4085, ISSN 0021-9533

Ho, C. K., & Li, G. (2005). Mutant p53 Melanoma Cell Lines Respond Differently to CP-31398-induced Apoptosis. *British Journal of Dermatology*, 153, pp 900-910, ISSN 0007-0963

Huang, J. S., Ho, T. J., Chiang, C. P., Kok, S. H., Kuo, Y. S. & Kuo, M. Y. (2001). MDM2 Expression in Areca quid Chewing-Associated Oral Squamous Cell Carcinomas in Taiwan. *Journal of Oral Pathology and Medicine*, 30, pp 53-58, ISSN 0904-2512

Ichwan, S. J. A. & Ikeda, M. A. (2008). Defect in Ser46 Phosphorylation of p53 Protein: A Resistance Mechanism against p53 Gene Transfer in Oral Squamous Cell Carcinoma Cells. *Journal of Oral Biosciences*, 50, pp 98-106, ISSN 1349-0079

Ichwan, S. J., Yamada, S., Sumrejkanchanakij, P., Ibrahim-Auerkari, E, Eto, K., & Ikeda, M. A. (2006). Defect in Serine 46 Phosphorylation of p53 Contributes to Acquisition of p53 Resistance in Oral Squamous Cell Carcinoma Cells. *Oncogene*, 25, pp 1216-1224, ISSN 0950-9232

Irwin, M. S., & Kaelin W.G. (2001). p53 Family Update: p73 and p63 Develop Their Own Identities. *Cell Growth and Differentiation, 12*, pp 337-349, ISSN 1044-9523

Irwin, M. S., & Kaelin W.G. (2001). p53 family update: p73 and p63 Develop Their Own Identities. *Cell Growth and Differentiation, 12*, pp 337-349.

Isobe, M., Emanuel, B. S., Givol, D., Oren, M., & Croce, C. M. (1986). Localization of Gene for Human p53 Tumour Antigen to Band 17p13. *Nature*, 320 pp 84–85, ISSN 0028-0836

Jemal, A., Siegel, R., Ward, E., Hao, Y., Xu, J., Murray, T. & Thun, M. J. (2008). Cancer Statistics. *CA: A Cancer Journal for Clinicians*, 58, pp 71–96, ISSN 0007-9235

Jiang, M. & Milner, J. (2002). Selective Silencing of Viral Gene Expression in HPV-Positive Human Cervical Carcinoma Cells Treated With siRNA, a Primer of RNA Interference. *Oncogene,* 21, pp 6041–6048, ISSN 0950-9232

Joerger, A. C., & Fersht, A. R. (2010). The Tumor Suppressor p53: From Structures to Drug Discovery. *Cold Spring Harbor Perspective in Biology,* 2, pp a000919, ISSN 1943-0264

Ko, L. J., Prives, C. (1996). p53: Puzzle and Paradigm. *Genes and Development,* 10, pp 1054-1072, ISSN 0890-9369

Koivusalo, R., Krausz, E., Helenius, H., & Hietanen, S. (2005). Chemotherapy compounds in cervical cancer cells primed by reconstitution of p53 function after short interfering RNA mediated degradation of human papillomavirus 18 E6 mRNA. Opposite Effect of siRNA in Combination With Different Drugs. *Molecular Pharmacology,* 68, pp 372–382, ISSN 0026-895X

Lane, D. P. & Crawford, L. V. (1979). T-Antigen is Bound to a Host Protein in SV40-Transformed Cells. *Nature,* 278, pp 261-263, ISSN 0028-0836

Lane, D. P., Cheok, C. F., & Lain, S. (2010). p53-based Cancer Therapy. *Cold Spring Harbor Perspectives in Biology,* 2, pp a001222.

Marin, M. C., Jost, C. A., Brooks, L. A., Irwin, M. S., O'Nions, J., Tidy, J. A., James, N., McGregor, J. M., Harwood, C. A., Yulug, I. G., Vousden, K. H., Allday, M. J., Gusterson, B., Ikawa, S., Hinds, P. W., Crook, T., Kaelin, W. G. Jr. (2000). A Common Polymorphism Acts As an Intragenic Modifier of Mutant p53 Behaviour. *Nature Genetics,* 25, pp 47-54, ISSN 1061-4036

Matsumura, T., Yoshihama, Y., Kimura, T., Shintani, S. & Alcade, R. E. (1996). p53 and MDM2 Expression in Oral Squamous Cell Carcinoma. *Oncology,* 53, pp 308–312, ISSN 0890-9091

McBride, O. W., Merry, D., & Givol, D. (1986). The Gene for Human p53 Cellular Tumor Antigen is Located on Chromosome 17 Short Arm (17p13). *Proceedings of National Academy of Sciences U.S.A.,* 83, pp 130–134, ISSN 0027-8424

Melero, R., Rajagopalan, S., Lázaro, M., Joerger, A. C., Brandt, T., Veprintsev, D. T., Lasso, G., Gilc, D., Scheres S. H. W., Carazo, J. M., Fersht, A. R. & Valle, M. (2011). Electron Microscopy Studies on the Quaternary Structure of p53 Reveal Different Binding Modes for p53 Tetramers in Complex with DNA. *Proceedings of National Academy of Sciences U.S.A.,* 108, pp 557–562, ISSN 0027-8424

Murphy, M. E. (2006). Polymorphic Variants in The p53 Pathway. *Cell Death and Differentiation,* 13, pp 916-920, ISSN 1350-9047

Nemunaitis, J., & Nemunaitisv J. (2011). Head and neck cancer: response to p53-based therapeutics. *Head and Neck,* 33, pp 131-134.

Nemunaitis, J., Clayman, G., Agarwal, S. S. Hrushesky, W., Wells, J. R., Moore, C., Hamm, J., Yoo, G., Baselga, J., Murphy, B. A., Menander, K. A., Licato, L. L., Chada, S., Gibbons, R. D., Olivier, M., Hainaut, P., Roth, J. A., Sobol, R. E., & Goodwin, W. J. (2009). Squamous Cell Carcinoma of the Head and Neck Biomarkers Predict *p53* Gene Therapy Efficacy in Recurrent. *Clinical Cancer Research,* 15, pp 7719-7725, ISSN 1078-0432

Nylander, K., Dabelsteen, E. & Hall, P. A. (2000). The p53 Molecule and Its Prognostic Role in Squamous Cell Carcinomas of The Head and Neck. *Journal of Oral Pathology and Medicine*, 29, pp 413–425, ISSN 0904-2512

Oda, K., Arakawa, H., Tanaka, T., Matsuda, K., Tanikawa, C., Mori, T., Nishimori, H., Tamai, K., Tokino, T., Nakamura, Y., & Taya, Y. (2000). p53AIP1., a Potential Mediator of p53-Dependent Apoptosis., and its Regulation by Ser-46-Phosphorylated p53. *Cell*, 102, pp 849-862, ISSN 0092-8674

Olivier, M., Hollstein, M. & Hainaut, P. (2009). TP53 Mutations in Human Cancers: Origins, Consequences, and Clinical Use. *Cold Spring Harbor Perspective in Biology*, 2, pp a001008, ISSN 1943-0264

Osman, I., Sherman, E., Singh, B., Venkatraman, E., Zelefsky, M., Bosl, G., Scher, H., Shah, J., Shaha, A., Kraus, D., Cordon-Cardo, C., Pfister, D.G. (2002). Alteration of p53 Pathway in Squamous Cell Carcinoma of the Head and Neck: Impact of Treatment Outcome in Patients Treated with Larynx Preservation Intent. *Journal of Clinical Oncology*, 20, pp 2980–2987, ISSN 0732-183X

Pearson, S., Jia, H., & Kandachi, K. (2004). China Approves First Gene Therapy. *Nature Biotechnology*, 22, pp 3 – 4, ISSN 1087-0156

Perez-Ordonez, B., Beauchemin, M., & Jordan, R. C. K. (2006). Molecular Biology of Squamous Cell Carcinoma of the Head and Neck. *Journal Clinical of Pathology*, 59, pp 445–453, ISSN 0021-9746

Prives, C. & Hall, P. A. (1999). The p53 Pathway. *The Journal of Pathology*, 187, pp 112–126, ISSN 1096-9896

Roh J. L., Kang, S. K., Minn, I., Califano, J. A., Sidransky, D. & Koch, W. M. (2011). p53-Reactivating small Molecules Induce Apoptosis and Enhance Chemotherapeutic Cytotoxicity in Head and Neck Squamous Cell Carcinoma. *Oral Oncology*, 47 pp 8-15, ISSN 1368-8375

Shangary, S. & Wang, S. (2008). Targeting the MDM2-p53 Interaction for Cancer Therapy. *Clinical Cancer Research*, 14, pp 5318–5324, ISSN 1078-0432

Shangary, S., Qin, D., McEachern, D., Liu, M., Miller, R. S., Qiu, S., Nikolovska-Coleska, Z., Ding, K., Wang, G., Chen, J., Bernard, D., Zhang, J., Lu, Y., Gu, Q., Shah, R. B., Pienta, K. J., Ling, X., Kang, S., Guo, M., Sun, Y., Yang, D., & Wang, S. (2008). Temporal Activation of p53 By a Specific MDM2 Inhibitor is Selectively Toxic to Tumors and Leads to Complete Tumor Growth Inhibition. *Proceedings of National Academy of Sciences U.S.A.*, 105, pp 3933–3938, ISSN 0027-8424

Sherr, C. J. (2006). Divorcing ARF and p53: An Unsettled Case. *Nature Reviews Cancer*, 6, pp 663-673, ISSN 1474-175X

Smeenk, L., Heeringen, S. J., Koeppel, M., Gilbert, B. & Janssen-Megens, E., et al. (2011) Role of p53 Serine 46 in p53 Target Gene Regulation. *PLoS ONE* , 6, pp e17574, ISSN 1932-6203

Smeenk, L., van Heeringen, S. J., Koeppel, M., van Driel, M. A., Bartels, S. J. J., Akkers, R. C., Denissov, S., Stunnenberg, H. G., Lohrum, M. (2008). Characterization of Genome-wide p53-binding sites Upon Stress Response. *Nucleic Acids Research, 36*, pp 3639–3654, ISSN 0305-1048

Smeenk, L., van Heeringen, S. J., Koeppel, M., van Driel, M. A., Bartels, S. J. J., Akkers, R. C., Denissov, S., Stunnenberg, H. G., & Lohrum, M. (2008). Characterization of Genome-Wide p53-Binding Sites Upon Stress Response. *Nucleic Acids Research, 36,* pp 3639–3654, ISSN 0305-1048

Taylor, D., Koch, W. M., Zahurak, M., Shah, K., Sidransky, D. & Westra, W. H. (1999). Immunohistochemical Detection of the p53 Protein Accumulation in Head and Neck Cancer: Correlation with p53 Gene Alterations. *Human Pathology,* 30, pp 1221–1225, ISSN 0046-8177

Thomas, S. M. & Grandis, J. R. (2009). The Current State of Head and Neck Cancer Gene Therapy. *Human Gene Therapy,* 20, pp 1565–1575, ISSN 1043-0342

Valentin-Vega, Y. A., Barboza, J. A., Chau, G. P., El-Naggar, A. K. & Lozano, G. (2007). High Levels of the p53 Inhibitor MDM4 in Head and Neck Squamous Carcinomas. *Human Pathology,* 38, pp 1553-1562, ISSN 0046-8177

Vassilev, L. T., Vu, B. T., Graves, B., Carvajal, D., Podlaski, F., Filipovic, Z., Kong, N., Kammlott, U., Lukacs, C., Klein, C., Fotouhi, N., & Liu, E. A. (2004). *In Vivo* Activation of The P53 Pathway by Small-Molecule Antagonists of MDM2. *Science,* 303, 844–848, ISSN 0036-8075

Vattemi, E., & Claudio, P. P. (2006). Adenoviral gene therapy in head and neck cancer. *Drug News and Perspectives,* 19, pp 329-337. ISSN: 0214-0934

Vattemi, E., & Claudio, P. P. (2009). The Feasibility of Gene Therapy in The Treatment of Head and Neck Cancer. *Head and Neck Oncology,* 1, pp 3. ISSN: 1758-3284

Vazquez, A., Bond E. E., Levine, A. J., & Bond, G. L. (2008). The Genetics of the p53 Pathway, Apoptosis and Cancer Therapy. *Nature Reviews Drug Discovery,* 7, pp 979-987, ISSN 1474-1776

Vousden, K. H. & Lane, D. P. (2007). p53 in Health and Disease. *Nature Reviews Molecular Cell Biology,* 8, pp 275–283, ISSN 1471-0072

Vousden, K. H. & Lu, X. (2002). Live or Let Die: The Cell's Response to p53. *Nature Reviews Cancer,* 2, pp 594–604, ISSN 1474-175X

Vousden, K. H. (2000). p53: Death Star. *Cell,* 103, pp 691-694, ISSN 0092-8674

Wang, F., Arun, P., Friedman, J., Chen, Z. & Van Waes, C. (2009). Current and Potential Inflammation Targeted Therapies in Head and Neck Cancer. *Current Opinion in Pharmacology,* 9, pp 389–395, ISSN 1471-4892

Wang, T., Lee, K., Rehman, A., & Daoud, S. S. (2007). PRIMA-1 Induces Apoptosis by Inhibiting JNK Signaling But Promoting the Activation of Bax. *Biochemical and Biophysical Research Communications,* 352, pp 203–212, ISSN 0006-291X

Werness, B. A., Levine A. J. & Howley, P. M. (1990). Association of Human Papillomavirus Types 16 and 18 E6 Proteins with p53. *Science,* 248, pp 76-79, ISSN 0036-8075

Wiman, K. G. (2010). Pharmacological Reactivation of Mutant p53: From Protein Structure to the Cancer Patient. *Oncogene,* 29, pp 4245–4252, ISSN 0950-9232

Xu, J., Reumers, J., Couceiro, J. R., Smet, F. D., Gallardo R., Rudyak, S., Cornelis, A., Rozenski, J., Zwolinska, A., Marine, J. C., Lambrechts, D., Suh, Y. A., Rousseau, F. & Schymkowitz, J. (2011). Gain of Function of Mutant p53 by Coaggregation with Multiple Tumor Suppressors. *Nature Chemical Biology,* 7, pp 285–295, ISSN 1552-4450

Yin, X. Y., Smith, M. L., Whiteside, T. L., Johnson, J. T., Heberman, R. B. & Locker, J. (1993). Abnormalities in the *p53* Gene in Tumors and Cell Lines of Human Squamous Cell Carcinomas of the Head and Neck. *International Journal of Cancer*, 54, pp 322–327, ISSN 0020-7136

Zhang, R., Wang, H., & Agrawal, S. (2005). Novel Antisense Anti-MDM2 Mixed-Backbone Oligonucleotides: Proof of Principle, In Vitro and In Vivo Activities, and Mechanisms. *Current Cancer Drug Targets*, 5, pp 43–49, ISSN 1568-0096

7

Signaling Mechanisms of Transforming Growth Factor-β (TGF-β) in Cancer: TGF-β Induces Apoptosis in Lung Cells by a Smad-Dependent Mechanism

Mi Jung Lim, Tiffany Lin and Sonia B. Jakowlew
National Cancer Institute, Cancer Training Branch,
Bethesda, Maryland,
USA

1. Introduction

1.1 TGF-β ligands, receptors and smads

Transforming Growth Factor-beta (TGF-β), a cytokine that is expressed in a variety of normal tissues, including the lung (Bartram & Spear, 2004; Jakowlew et al., 1995, 1998; Kang et al., 2000; Montuenga et al., 1998), exerts diverse effects on a wide variety of cellular processes, including proliferation, differentiation, and apoptosis (Elliot & Blobe, 2005; Massagué, 1998). More than sixty different TGF-β family members have been identified in various oraganisms, with at least 29 of these proteins being encoded in humans. Among the many proteins in the TGF-β superfamily are four TGF-β ligands, five activins, eight bone morphogenetic proteins (BMP), and 15 growth and differentiation factors (GDF). Three TGF-β isoforms have been identified in humans, including TGF-β1, TGF-β2, and TGF-β3, with each being a homodimeric polypeptide with a molecular weight of 25-kDa. All three TGF-β isoforms are initially synthesized as 55-kDa pro-proteins that consist of an amino-terminal pro-region and a carboxy-terminal mature region (Gentry et al., 1988). The pro-region facilitates necessary dimerization of the pro-proteins for future activity. TGF-β is secreted in a latent, inactive form in which the 12.5-kDa carboxyl-terminal 112 amino acid-long mature form is non-covalently associated with the 80-kDa Latency-Associated Peptide (LAP) amino-terminal remainder (Barcellos-Hoff, 1996; Barcellos-Hoff & Ewan, 2000). The LAP forms a complex with the 12.5-kDa TGF-β to keep it inactive (Arndjelovic et al., 2003; Stander et al., 1999). This complex is referred to as the small latent TGF-β complex. The small latent TGF-β complex may associate with members of the latent TGF-β-binding protein (LTBP) family to form the large latent TGF-β complex (Öklü & Hesketh, 2000). The liberation of TGF-β from the latent complexes is referred to as activation (Annes et al., 2003). The precise steps that are involved in liberation of the bioactive dimer are not completely understood, but may involve cleavage of the LTBP or LAP or both (Hyytiäinen et al., 2004).

Active TGF-β exerts its effects with specific high affinity receptors. In mammals, five TGF-β superfamily type I receptors and seven type II receptors have been identified (Derynck et al.,

2001; Massagué, 2000). The TGF-β type I and type II receptors are structurally related transmembrane glycoproteins that consist of an extracellular N-terminal ligand-binding domain with more than ten cysteine residues that regulate the dimeric structure, a transmembrane region, and a C-terminal serine/threonine kinase domain. The type I receptors, but not type II receptors, have a highly conserved region that is rich in glycine and serine residues, referred to as the GS domain, in the juxtamembrane domain next to the N-terminus of the kinase domain. The GS domain is a target for the type II receptor kinase, and upon its phosphorylation on specific serine and threonine residues, the type I receptor becomes activated (Heldin et al., 1997; Massagué, 2000). Being downstream of the type II receptor, the type I receptor plays an important role in determining the specifity of intracellular signals. The type I and II receptors exist as homodimers at the cell surface in the absence of ligands, but have an inherent heteromeric affinity for each other. Only select combinations of type I and II receptors act as ligand-binding signaling complexes. The molecular basis of the selectivity of the type I-type II receptor interactions remains poorly understood, but the structural complement at the interface may help define the selectivity of the receptor combinations. Most of the TGF-β ligands bind with high affinity to the type I receptor, also known as activin receptor-like kinase (ALK), or to the type II receptor, while others bind efficiently only to heteromeric receptor combinations.

The intracellular signal transduction triggered by the kinase activity of TGF-β involves the phosphorylation of Smad family proteins and in turn, complex changes in the transcriptional regulation of various response genes. The Smad family proteins include Smad 1, 2, 3, 4, 5, 7, and 8. The Smads are divided into three subclasses depending on their structure and function: the receptor-regulated Smads (R-Smads), common-mediator Smad (Co-Smad), and inhibitory Smads (I-Smads). In general, the R-Smads, Smads 2 and 3, function downstream of the TGF-β ligands, while Smads 1, 5, and 8 are downstream of members of the BMP and GDF subfamilies of ligands. Smads 1, 2, 3, 5, and 8 are direct substrates for the TGF-β type I receptor kinase, whereas Co-Smad, Smad 4, participates in Smad complex formation. Smads 6 and 7, the I-Smads, interfere with TGF-β-induced Smad-dependent signal transduction (Park, 2005; Whitman, 1997). Activation of cell surface receptors by ligands leads to phosphorylation of the R-Smads at two serine residues in a SSXS motif at their extreme C-termini. This phosphorylation allows the R-Smads to form both homomeric and heteromeric complexes with Smad4 that accumulate in the nucleus. There, they are directly involved in transcriptional regulation of target genes in cooperation with other transcription factors.

Signaling by TGF-β is mediated by a ligand-induced heteromeric complex of two types of transmembrane serine/threonine kinase receptors designated as TGF-β type I receptor (TGF-β RI) and type II receptor (TGF-β RII). Initial ligand binding to constitutively active TGF-β RII is followed by recruitment of TGF-β RI into the heteromeric complex. Subsequent phosphorylation of TGF-β RI at its GS-domain and activation is mediated by TGF-β RII and leads to activation of TGF-β RI. Upon this activating phosphorylation, TGF-β RI phosphorylates the receptor-activated Smad proteins (R-Smads), Smad2 and Smad3, which form a heteromeric complex with the co-Smad, Smad4, and enter the nucleus. In the nucleus, the Smad complex associates with other transcription factors for transcriptional activation of specific target genes (Massagué and Wotton, 2000; ten Dijke et al., 2000; Wrana and Attisano, 2000).

1.2 Tumor suppressor activity of TGF-β

TGF-β was originally called one of the most potent polypeptide growth inhibitors isolated from natural sources (Moses et al., 1985; Tucker et al., 1984). When it was demonstrated that TGF-β could act as an autocrine negative growth regulator in the several different epithelial cell lines, it was hypothesized that TGF-β may act as an inhibitor of tumor progression, a tumor suppressor (Artega et al., 1990; Glick et al., 1989). The identification and characterization of the intermediates in the TGF-β signaling pathway, comprised of the genes and proteins for the TGF-β receptors and Smads, has increased our understanding of the role of TGF-β as a tumor suppressor. The involvement of the TGF-β signaling pathway in tumor suppression is shown by mutations in the genes that encode the TGF-β receptors and Smad proteins in human tumors.

The gene for TGF-β RII is frequently mutated in colon carcinoma cells from patients with hereditary non-polyposis colorectal cancer that also show microsatellite instability, as well as in gastric cancers and gliomas (Chung et al., 1996; Izumoto et al., 1997; Markowitz et al., 1995). A specific region of adenine nucleotides in the coding region of TGF-β RII is prone to mutation in these patients from germline defects in their capacity for DNA mismatch repair. The nucleotide deletions or additions result in a shortened version of TGF-β RII that cannot participate in signaling transduction (Lu et al., 1996). However, the TGF-β RII gene is not mutated in other types of carcinoma with microsatellite instability, including breast, liver, pancreatic, and endometrial carcinoma (Abe et al., 1996; Kawate et al., 1999; Vincent et al., 1996), while, a somatic frameshift mutation in the polyadenine tract of the TGF-β RII gene does occur in some endometrial cancer patients (Parekh et al., 2002). Missense and inactivating mutations in TGF-β RII have also been detected in colon cancers that do not exhibit microsatellite instability (Grady et al., 1999). Expression of TGF-β RII can be decreased in some cases of carcinoma, including head and neck squamous carcinoma, breast carcinoma, and laryngeal carcinoma (Eisma et al., 1996; Franchi et al., 2001; Gobbi et al., 1999). Re-expression of TGF-β RII in carcinoma cells that have either lost expression of TGF-β RII or show reduced TGF-β RII expression can inhibit the ability to become malignant.

Although less common than in TGF-β RII, mutations in TGF-β RI also occur in patients with a variety of cancers, including ovarian cancers, metastatic breast cancers, T-cell lymphomas, and head and neck cancer metastases (Chen et al., 1998, 2001; Goggins, 1998; Schiemann et al., 1999). Patients with ovarian cancer show a high frequency of mutations of TGF-β RI (Chen et al., 2001), while expression of TGF-β RI is transcriptionally repressed by DNA methylation in cells from patients with gastric cancer (Kang et al., 1999). Over-expression of TGF-β RI in colon carcinoma cells with low levels of TGF-β RI also inhibits tumor progression as with TGF-β RII (Wang et al., 1996). Mutations in TGF-β RI do not appear to be associated with TGF-β RII mutations; such mutations suggest that these TGF-β receptors may function as tumor suppressors.

Decreased TGF-β receptor expression or availability of TGF-β receptors at the cell surface may allow tumor cells to escape the growth inhibitory function of TGF-β (Kim et al., 2000). Expression of the TGF-β receptors in tumor cells may also be reduced by altered levels or activities of transcription factors that are required for expression of TGF-β RII, such as the Ets transcription factor. Hypermethylation of CpG islands in the promoters of TGF-β RI and TGF-β RII or mutations in the TGF-β RII promoter that interfere with transcription factor binding may also result in transcriptional silencing (Amoroso, et al., 1998). Decreased TGF-β RII function results in resistance to the growth inhibitory activity of TGF-β, but other TGF-β responses may not be affected in a similar fashion because they may require different levels of signaling (Chen et al., 1993; Fafeur et al., 1993). The tumor suppressor role of TGF-β RII has been demonstrated by expressing wildtype TGF-β RII in cancer cells that lack a functional TGF-β RII allele (Sun et al., 1994; Wang et al., 1995) or by over-expressing TGF-β RII *in vitro* (Turco et al., 1999). Enhanced expression of TGF-β RII seems to confer growth inhibition, to suppress anchorage independent growth, and to significantly reduce tumor formation in experimental mice compared with parental cells. Over-expression of TGF-β RI or TGF-β RII in transgenic mice also shows enhanced tumor suppressor activity (Cui et al., 1996; Minn et al., 2005), while expression of dominant-negative forms of TGF-β RII increases tumor formation (Böttinger et al., 1997; Go et al., 1999).

Some of the genes for Smad proteins that function as mediators of TGF-β signal transduction also have mutations and deletions that occur in human carcinomas. Mutations in the genes encoding Smad2 and Smad3 are relatively rare and seem to occur only in a limited number of lung and colon carcinomas for Smad2 (Riggens et al., 1996; Uchida et al., 1996), and gastric cancer for Smad3 (Han et al., 2004). In contrast, mutational inactivation of Smad4 (DPC4) is prominent in pancreatic carcer (Hahn et al., 1996). Mutations of Smad4 can be detected in human colorectal cancer, especially in those patients with late stage, metastatic disease (Maitra et al., 2000). This suggests that Smad4 may play a central role in TGF-β-mediated tumor suppression. Inactivation of the genes encoding Smad2 and Smad4 occurs by several means, including deletion of entire chromosome segments, small deletions, and frameshift, nonsense, or missense mutations (Massagué & Wotton, 2000; Massagué et al., 2000). Mutations in Smad4 are detected principally in pancreatic carcinomas, and in colon carcinomas, and in other types of carcinomas, although with less frequency. Inactivation of both alleles of Smad4 and haploinsufficiency of the Smad4 locus may contribute to the progression of pancreatic and gastric cancers (Luttges et al., 2000; Xu et al., 2000). The existence of Smad4 mutations in several juvenile polyposis families further supports the suggestion that Smad4 is a tumor suppressor (Howe, 1998). Inactivating mutations in Smad4 are also observed in conjunction with mutations in TGF-β RI and TGF-β RII (Grady et al., 1999). This suggests that Smad4 also has tumor suppressor activities that are not related to TGF-β signaling. Alterations of Smad signaling, and of phosphorylation of Smad2 in particular, are associated with poor prognosis in human breast carcinomas, colon carcinomas, and head and neck squamous cell carcinomas (Xie et al., 2002, 2003a, 2000b). Loss of Smad3 expression in gastric cancer tissues and cell lines increases susceptibility to tumorigenesis (Han et al., 2004). Introduction of Smad3 into human gastric cancer cells that do not express Smad3 restores responsiveness to TGF-β. In addition, loss of Smad4 expression and/or activity may increase the Ras signaling pathway to result in tumor progression (Iglesias et al., 2004). A protein-based strategy has been used to rapidly identify the most common alterations in the TGF-β signaling pathway by combining measurements of the levels and the state of activation of Smad signaling intermediates with DNA-based diagnostic assays (Yan et al., 2000). A mechanism for TGF-β resistance has been identified in TGF-β refractory squamous cell carcinoma cell lines using this protein-based strategy.

1.3 TGF-β and apoptosis

Another mechanism by which the tumor suppressor activity of TGF-β is mediated is through the process of programmed cell death or apoptosis. Unlike the molecular mechanisms by which TGF-β participates in cell proliferation and differentiation that have been well described, the mechanisms by which TGF-β exerts its apoptotic effects are only poorly understood in comparison. TGF-β-dependent apoptosis is important in the elimination of damaged or abnormal cells from many normal tissues (Schuster and Krieglstein, 2002). For example, TGF-β is implicated to play a role in controlling liver size, and intravenous injection of TGF-β induces apoptosis in normal and regressing liver (Schulte-Hermann et al., 1993). Hepatic over-expression of TGF-β in transgenic mice causes apoptosis, as does treatment of primary hepatocytes with TGF-β. The apoptotic fate of cells after they are treated with TGF-β1 is often determined by cellular context and experimental conditions. For example, TGF-β acts as a death stimulus inducing apoptotic death in fetal hepatocytes and podocytes (Herrera et al., 2001; Schiffer et al., 2001), whereas it elicits pro-survival activity to protect macrophages against apoptosis (Chin et al., 1999; Schlapbach et al., 2000). A regulated balance of cell division and apoptosis is required for normal morphogenesis, and alterations in these processes can lead to neoplastic transformation. Cell cycle progression and the onset of apoptosis have been connected in DNA-damaged cells through the analysis of the activation of the apoptotic cascade in $p21^{Cip1}$-deficient HCT116 colorectal cancer cells (Le et al., 2005; Pardali et al., 2005). DNA damage induces a similar level of p53 activation and proapoptotic Bcl-2 family member PUMA induction in $p21^{Cip1}$-deficient cells compared to wildtype isogenic counterparts. However, only $p21^{Cip1}$-deficient cells show extensive cytochrome C release, mitochondrial membrane depolarization, and caspase activation. When ectopically expressed in $p21^{Cip1}$-deficient cells, $p21^{Cip1}$, $p27^{Kip1}$, and $p16^{Ink4a}$ are all similarly effective at causing cell cycle arrest and inhibiting DNA damage-induced apoptotic events. Application of TGF-β stimulates apoptosis in various epithelial cells. Preliminary findings show that TGF-β induces apoptosis through the regulation of the expression of various pro- and anti-apoptotic molecules, including p53, Bad, Bax, Bik, Bcl-2, and Bcl-XL (Motyl et al., 1998; Saltzman et al., 1998; Sanchez-Capelo, 2005; Teramoto et al., 1998). TGF-β-induced apoptosis can also be mediated by caspases (Brown et al., 1998; Chen and Chang, 1997; Choi et al., 1998; Saltzman et al., 1998). The mitochondrial septin-like protein, Apoptosis-Related Protein in the TGF-β Signaling Pathway (ARTS), enhances cell death induced by TGF-β through activation of caspase 3 (Larisch et al., 2000). In addition, TGF-β-induced apoptosis is associated with the generation of reactive oxygen species (Albright et al., 2003). Antioxidants can block the TGF-β-induced apoptotic process. Resistance to apoptosis is one of the characteristics of cancer cells during progressive tumorigenesis. Apoptosis of human prostate cancer cells that is induced by TGF-β or over-expression of Smad7 is caused by a specific activation of the p38 MAP kinase pathway that may occur in a TGF-β-activated kinase 1 (TAK1) and mitogen-activated protein kinase kinase 3 (MKK3)-dependent manner (Edlund et al., 2003). Members of the Mixed Lineage Kinase 3 (MLK3) family also mediate TGF-β-induced apoptosis in hepatoma cells (Kim et al., 2004). There is also strong evidence that the stress- and cytokine-inducible Growth Arrest and DNA Damage (GADD) inducible gene 45 protein (Mita et al., 2002; Takekawa & Saito, 1998; Takekawa et al., 2002; Yoo et al., 2003) and GADD153 protein (Park et al., 1992), also known as CCAAT/enhancer-binding Homologous Protein (CHOP) (Ron & Habener, 1992), CCAAT/Enhancer-Binding Protein-zeta (C/EBP-ζ) (Hanson, 1998), and DNA Damage Inducible Transcript-3 (DDIT3) (Fornace et al., 1989), function in the p38 Mitogen-Activated Protein Kinase (MAPK) pathway and induce apoptosis (Corazarri et al., 2003). It has also been shown that Smad-dependent expression of GADD45b is responsible for the delayed activation of p38 MAP kinase by TGF-β1 in pancreatic carcinoma cells (Takekawa et al., 2002). Activation of GADD45b by the TGF-β receptor/Smad signaling pathway also mediates the induction of proteoglycan biglycan expression by TGF-β, also with the involvement of mitogen activated protein kinase kinase 6 (MKK6) and p38 MAP kinase

(Mita et al., 2005). The p38 MAP kinase and p160/Rho/ROCK pathways have a role in TGF-β-mediated Smad-dependent growth inhibition of breast cancer cells (Kamaraju & Roberts, 2005). Smad3 contributes in a non-redundant manner to the induction of apoptosis in the mammary gland, but is dispensible for TGF-β effects on proliferation and differentiation in this tissue. TGF-β-induced p160/Rho/ROCK activation is also involved in the inhibition of Cdc25A, with resulting cell cycle arrest. TGF-β also regulates radiation-induced apoptosis and this is reduced in TGF-β1 null mice along with decreased p53 phosphorylation. TGF-β regulates biglycan gene expression through p38 MAP kinase signaling downstream of the Smads that also requires the small GTPase Rac1 (Groth et al., 2005). However, TGF-β-Receptor activated p38 MAP kinase also mediates Smad-independent responses in breast cancer cells (Yu et al., 2002). Non-Smad signal transducers that are under the control of TGF-β provide quantitative regulation of the signaling pathway, and serve as nodes for cross-talk with other signaling pathways, such as Notch, tyrosine kinase, G-protein-coupled receptor kinases, and cytokine receptors (Moustakas & Heldin, 2005). One of the characteristics of cancer cells during progressive tumorigenesis is resistance to apoptosis (Hanahan & Weinberg, 2000). Increasing the sensitivity of tumor cells to anticancer therapy is tightly correlated with the induction of apoptosis by anticancer drugs. Thus, it would be promising for disease treatment, including lung cancer, to activate TGF-β-mediated apoptosis by modulating the function of TGF-β in specific normal and tumor cell types.

1.4 TGF-β and lung

There is accumulating evidence that TGF-β may have a role in lung cancer and in lung disease. For example, elevated levels of TGF-β1 have been shown in plasma and lung tumors of patients with advanced lung cancer, and the prognosis of lung cancer patients who showed positive TGF-β1 was poorer than that of patients who were negative for this growth factor (Kong et al., 1996; Takanami et al., 1997). Lung cancer patients who responded to radiation therapy showed a decrease in circulating TGF-β levels compared to patients with no response or stable disease (Vujaskovic and Groen, 2000). One potential function of TGF-β in lungs and airways is regulation of epithelial cell survival through apoptosis. TGF-β1 treatment of lung bronchial BEAS-2B cells increased apoptosis in cells exhibiting overexpression of Smad2 or Smad 3 (Yanagisawa et al., 1998). TGF-β1 treatment also enhanced Fas-induced apoptosis of alveolar and airway epithelial cells, and Fas-mediated apoptosis of alveolar epithelial cells was reported to be associated with increased expression of TGF-β1 (Hagimoto et al., 2002; Hagimoto et al., 1997).

Besides TGF-β1, interleukin (IL)-6 is a multifunctional cytokine that is produced by a variety of cells during infection, trauma, and immunological challenge (Kishimoto et al., 1995). IL-6 has been shown to mediate many inflammatory processes in the lung (Taga, 1997), and its dysregulated release has been implicated in the pathogenesis of a variety of respiratory conditions, including interstitial lung diseases (Berger, 2002; Bhatia & Moochhala, 2004; Shahar et al., 1996). IL-6 has been reported to have different effects on apoptosis of fibroblasts from normal and fibrotic lungs, with fibrotic lung cells showing enhanced resistance to apoptosis (Moodley et al., 2003) and to induce an increase in expression and activity of cathepsin, a cysteine protease that plays a major role in lysosomal bulk proteolysis, protein processing, matrix degradation, and tissue remodeling in the lung, in A549 lung cells (Gerber et al., 2001). Earlier reports have examined cross-talk between TGF-β and IL-6 in epithelial cells, with TGF-β playing a role in the negative regulation of IL-6 signaling in intestinal epithelial cells (Walia et al., 2003), as well as activating IL-6 expression in prostate cancer cells (Park et al., 2003). In addition, bronchial epithelial 16 cells that are undergoing apoptosis have been shown to produce significantly more TGF-β, but less IL-6, than non-apoptotic cells (Hodge et al., 2002). This suggests that increased production of TGF-β and decreased expression of IL-6 by lung epithelial cells may contribute to the inhibition of proliferation, squamous metaplasia, and reduction of inflammation in lung injury.

Lung cancer is the most lethal type of lung injury/cancer for both men and women. In the United States, in 2007, the most recent year for which statistics are currently available, lung cancer accounted for more deaths than breast, prostate and colon cancer combined, according to the U.S. Cancer Statistics Working Group. In that year, 109,643 men and 93,893 women were diagnosed with lung cancer, and 88,329 men and 70,354 women died from lung cancer. The National Cancer Institute estimates there were 222,520 new cases of lung cancer and 157,300 deaths from lung cancer in 2010. Currently, 85% of lung cancer patients die within 5 years of diagnosis. This reflects the urgent need for improved therapies. Targeting signal transduction pathways that affect therapeutic resistance is one approach to improve patient outcomes. In normal cells, signaling is tightly regulated and begins with the transduction of signals through growth factor receptors or integrins to intracellular kinase enzymes, culminating in the regulation of cellular processes. Precise regulation of processes like cell division and apoptosis is required for normal morphogenesis, and alterations in these processes can lead to cancer. Increasing the sensitivity of tumor cells to anticancer therapy is tightly correlated with induction of apoptosis by anticancer drugs. Thus, it would be promising for disease treatment, including lung cancer, to activate TGF-β-mediated apoptosis by modulating the function of TGF-β in specific normal and tumor cells.

We reported earlier that apoptosis is significantly decreased in the bronchio-alvelolar epithelium of mice that are heterozygous for TGF-β1 (Tang et al., 1998). This is consistent with a role for endogenous TGF-β1 in regulating apoptosis in lung. Here, we examined the ability of immortalized normal lung alveolar type II epithelial C10 cells to respond to TGF-β1 and the functionality of the TGF-β1 signal transduction pathway in these cells. Our findings show that TGF-β1-mediated signaling induces apoptosis in C10 cells by a Smad-dependent mechanism that requires activation of p38 MAPK and inhibition of the AKT pathway induced by IL-6. Furthermore, the GADD family members GADD45b and GADD153 are mediators of p38 MAPK activation in the process of TGF-β1-mediated apoptosis.

2. Materials and methods

2.1 Cell culture and reagents

Previously established non-tumorigenic C10 cells derived from normal mouse lung epithelium were obtained from Dr. A. Malkinson (University of Colorado, Denver, CO). Cells were cultured in CMRL-1066 medium (Invitrogen, San Diego, CA) containing 10% heat-inactivated fetal bovine serum (FBS). Gadd153-deficient and wildtype cells were grown in DMEM with 10% non-heat inactivated FBS (Zinszner et al., 1998). Cells were treated with 5 ng/ml recombinant human TGF-β1 obtained from R&D Systems (Minneapolis, MN) in a vehicle of 4 mM HCl containing 1 ng/ml BSA or vehicle alone. Antibodies against phospho-specific and total p38 MAPK, ERK, JNK and AKT were from Cell Signaling Technologies (Beverly, MA). Antibodies against SMAD7 and GADD153 were from Santa Cruz Biotechnology (Santa Cruz, CA) and anti-hemagglutinin antibodies were from Covance (Berkeley, CA). The MAPK inhibitor SB203580 was from Calbiochem (San Diego, CA).

2.2 Plasmid constructs

The hamster Gadd153 promoter fragments have been described previously (Luethy et al., 1990). The 5′-deletion constructs of the hamster Gadd153 promoter containing fragments -778 to +21, -225 to +21 and -36 to +21 were used to generate a Luciferase assay system in the pGL3-basic vector (Promega, Madison, WI). The 5′-deletion constructs (-165 to +21 and -105 to +21) of the hamster Gadd153 promoter were generated by PCR using the 5′-primers (GGATATCGTCAGTGCCAGCGTGCCG and GGATATCGTCAGTGCCAGCGTGCCG, respectively) and the 3′-primer (ggaagcttgtgtgagactcaggctactg) and subcloned into the pGL3-basic vector. The mouse Gadd153- expressing plasmid was made by RT-PCR amplification using the 5′-primer (CGAAGCTTCCAGAAGGAAGTGCATC) and the 3′-primer (CGGGATCCGGAGAGACAGACAGG). All constructs were verified by DNA sequencing.

2.3 Transient transfection and Luciferase assays

C10 cells were transfected with 1-2 μg/well of DNAs and 1 ng/well of Renilla Luciferase reporter plasmid pRLTK (Promega) to normalize transfection efficiencies using Lipofectamine 2000 (Invitrogen). After 18-24 hours, cells were treated with TGF-β1 or vehicle. After 18 hours, cells were lysed and Luciferase activity was measured using a dual-luciferase reporter assay system (Promega). All assays were performed in duplicate.

2.4 Generation of stable cell lines

C10 cells were transfected with HA-tagged Gadd45b, antisense Gadd45b, Gadd153 or Smad7 expression plasmids. Twenty-four hours after transfection, and every 4 days thereafter, the medium was replaced with fresh selection medium containing neomycin G418 (Invitrogen) at 800-μg/ml for 2 weeks. Neomycin-resistant clones were then individually transferred and expanded. After two additional passages in selection medium, independent clones were cultured in standard medium. As a mock control, the pcDNA3 empty vector was used to transfect C10 cells and selected in the presence of neomycin.

2.5 Western blot analysis

C10 cells were stimulated in the presence or absence of TGF-β1. Freshly collected cells were homogenized in lysis buffer containing 0.05 mM Tris-HCl pH 7.4, 0.25% Na-deoxycholate, 150 mM NaCl and 1 mM EDTA with protease inhibitors. Equal amounts of cell lysates were heated at 70°C for 10 minutes in sample loading buffer, separated by electrophoresis and transferred to membrane filters. Membranes were blocked with 5% nonfat dry milk in TBST buffer containing 50 mM Tris-HCl pH 7.5, 150 mM NaCl and 0.05% Tween 20 for 1 hour at room temperature, washed in TBST and incubated with various primary antibodies overnight at 4°C. Membranes were then incubated with horseradish peroxidase-conjugated secondary antibody for 1 hour at room temperature, washed in TBST buffer and proteins were visualized by enhanced chemiluminescence according to the manufacturer's directions (Pierce, Rockford IL).

2.6 Detection of apoptosis

For DNA fragmentation assays, the Apoptotic DNA Ladder kit (Roche Applied Sciences, Indianapolis, IN) was used according to the manufacturer's directions. Apoptosis was also quantitated by a Cell Death Detection ELISA assay (Roche Applied Sciences). All data points for the Cell Death Detection ELISA assay were determined in triplicate.

2.7 Semi-quantitative and real-time reverse transcription-polymerase chain reaction amplification

Total RNA was isolated from C10 cells using Trizol reagent according to the manufacturer's directions (Invitrogen). Reverse transcription (RT) was performed, followed by amplification by polymerase chain reaction (PCR) with oligonucleotide primers including Gadd45b 5'-primer (gggggattttgcaatcttct) and 3'-primer (cggtgaggcgatcctga), Gadd153 5′-primer (ccagtcagagttctatggc) and 3′-primer (catgcttggtgcaggctgac) and glucose 6-phosphate dehydrogenase (G6PD) 5′-primer (actgcagttccgagacgtgg) and 3′-primer (cagaagaggcagagtatagatggtg). As an internal control, mRNA for glucose-6-phosphate dehydrogenase (G6pd) was also amplified. Relative quantification of the mRNA levels of the target genes was determined using the DDC_T method (Schmittgen et al., 2008). Results were expressed as N-fold difference in treated relative to untreated sample. All assays were performed twice in duplicate in independent PCR amplification reactions.

2.8 Interleukin-6 immunoassay

The levels of IL-6 in the supernatant of cultured cells were quantitated using a mouse Quantikine system (R&D Systems). Each measurement was performed in triplicate and an average value was recorded as pg/ml.

2.9 Statistics

Results were expressed as means ± standard error (S.E.) and the differences between means of treated and control groups were analyzed using the Student's t test for paired data. A value of $p < 0.05$ was considered to be significant.

3. Results

3.1 TGF-β1 mediates apoptosis in mouse lung C10 cells

Mouse lung C10 cells are a stable cell line originally derived from a Balb/c mouse lung explant with characteristics of alveolar type II pneumocytes (Smith et al., 1984). These normal cells are not transformed, are non-tumorigenic, and contain only wildtype K-ras alleles (Malkinson et al., 1997). Here, we examined the responsiveness of TGF-β1 in C10 cells. TGF-β1 addition to C10 cells transiently transfected with Smad2 (ARE)- or Smad3 ((SBE)4)-dependent constructs augmented the transcriptional activity of these constructs by 11-fold and 1.6-fold, respectively (Figure 1A), indicating that C10 cells respond to TGF-β1 and Smad signaling is functional. Dramatic morphological changes characteristic of apoptosis, including large vacuoles, cell shrinkage and cytoplasmic blebbing were observed at 48 hours after TGF-β1 addition (Fig. 1B). Treatment with TGF-β1 also induced a 150- to 200-bp internucleosomal DNA cleavage that produced a DNA fragmentation laddering pattern by 48 hours, and that was also detected by ELISA assay (Figure 1C and 1D).

3.2 TGF-β1 activates p38 MAPK

The MAPK signaling pathway, including p38 MAPK, extracellular signal-regulated kinase (ERK), and c-Jun N-terminal kinase (JNK), has been implicated in many physiological and pathological processes, including apoptosis (Javelaude & Mauviel, 2005; Zavadil & Böttinger, 2005). To study the possible role of the MAPK pathway in TGF-β1-mediated apoptosis in lung cells, C10 cells were treated with exogenous TGF-β1, and activation of p38 MAPK, ERK1/ERK2, and JNK was then also examined using antibodies specific for total and phosphorylated forms of each protein kinase. As shown in Figure 2A, there was a dramatic activation of p38 MAPK that occurred by 48 hours and the timing of activation of p38 MAPK by TGF-β1 coincided with induction of apoptosis by TGF-β1 (Figure 1). Activation of ERK1/ERK2 showed complex patterns of reduction and induction that were only modest. No activation of JNK by TGF-β1 was detected (data not shown).

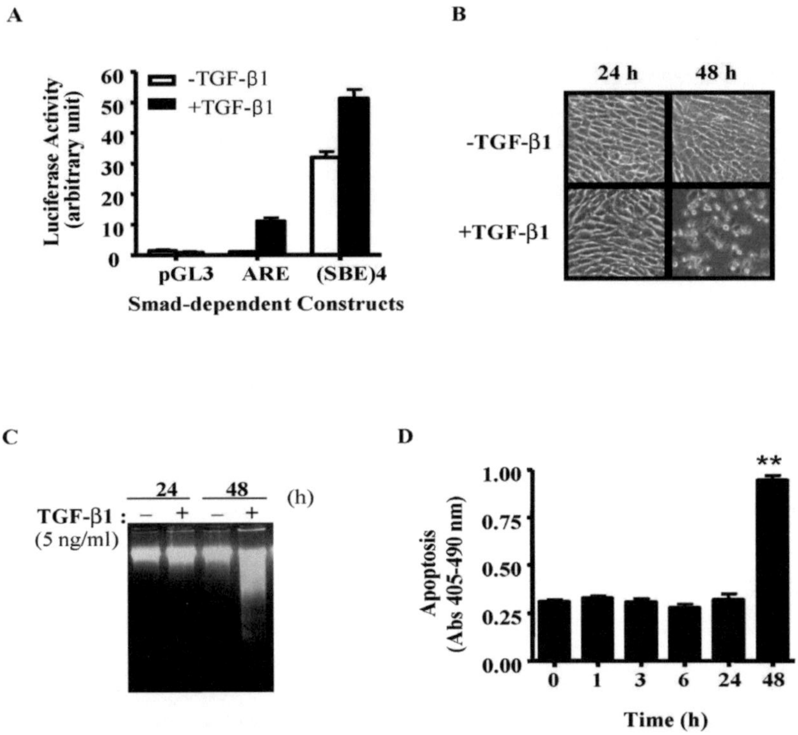

Fig. 1. TGF-β1 induces apoptosis in mouse lung C10 cells.
A, Effect of TGF-β1 on basal ARE-Luc and (SBE)4-Luc transcription in C10 cells. C10 cells were transiently transfected with Smad2(ARE)-Luc, Smad3((SBE)4)-Luc or 3TP-Lux Luciferase reporters and cultured in vehicle (open bars) or TGF-β1 (filled bars) for 18-h. Luciferase activity was normalized to Renilla Luciferase values. The pGL3-basic empty vector control is shown. The results shown are the means standard error (S.E.) of two independent experiments performed in triplicate. B, Morphology of C10 cells by phase contrast microscopy at 24- and 48 hours after addition of TGF-β1. Magnification: 200X. The apoptotic response was determined by examining the DNA fragmentation pattern by C, gel electrophoresis and D, Cell Death Detection ELISA assay at various times after treatment with TGF-β1. **, $p < 0.001$ versus control.

Because of the dramatic activation of p38 MAPK and induction of apoptosis by TGF-β1 in C10 cells, we chose to examine the role of p38 MAPK in this delayed apoptosis with MAPK SB203580, a potent inhibitor of p38 MAPK. Treatment of C10 cells with SB203580 strongly inhibited TGF-β1-induced apoptosis at 48 hours as determined by DNA fragmentation (Figure 2B). Inhibition of TGF-β1-induced apoptosis by SB203580 by 66% at 48 hours was also detected by ELISA assay (Figure 2C). Treatment of C10 cells with SB203580 also abrogated the morphological changes characteristic of apoptosis that were observed after 48 hours (Figure 2D). Our findings suggest that p38 MAPK activation by TGF-β1 is involved in TGF-β1-mediated apoptosis in C10 cells.

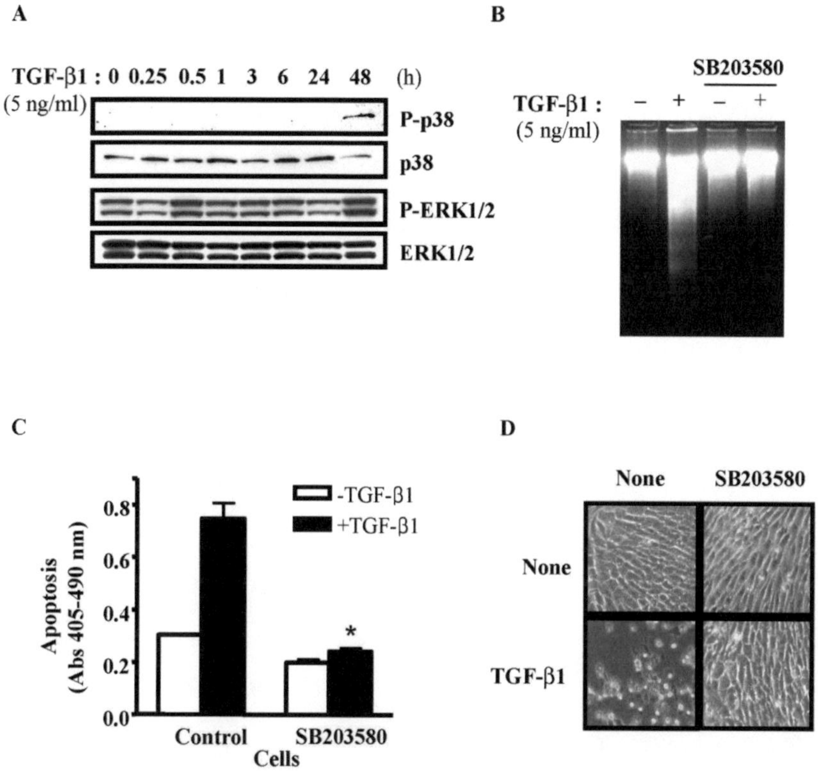

Fig. 2. Activation of p38 MAPK by TGF-β1 results in apoptosis in C10 cells.
A, Time course of phosphorylation of endogenous p38 MAP and ERK kinases after stimulation by TGF-β1. Total cell lysates were prepared from untreated or TGF-β1-treated cells and used for immunoblotting. Phosphorylated (P) and non-phosphorylated forms of p38 MAPK and ERK are indicated in the upper and lower panels, respectively. B-D, Cells were treated with TGF-β1 or vehicle alone in the presence or absence of 10 μM SB203580. The apoptotic response of C10 cells was determined by examining the DNA fragmentation pattern by B, gel electrophoresis and C, ELISA assay. The results shown are the means S.E. of two independent experiments performed in triplicate. *, $p < 0.001$ versus control. D, Morphology of C10 cells by phase contrast microscopy at 48 hours after treatment with TGF-β1 and SB203580. Magnification: 200X.

3.3 TGF-β1 increases Gadd45b mRNA

Since induction of apoptosis by TGF-β1 and activation of p38 MAPK occurred at a late time after addition of TGF-β1 in C10 cells, we considered the possiblity that additional protein mediators may be needed to activate p38 MAPK in response to TGF-β1. Previous studies have suggested the stress- and cytokine-inducible GADD45 family proteins (GADD45a, GADD45b, and GADD45g) function as specific activators of MEKK4, a MAPK kinase upstream in the p38 MAPK pathway (Mita et al., 2002), and induce apoptosis (Takekawa & Saito, 1998). To test the possible involvement of GADD family proteins in TGF-β1-mediated apoptosis in C10 cells, we first examined expression of Gadd mRNA transcripts following treatment with TGF-β1 in these cells. Semi-quantitative and real-time RT-PCR amplification of RNA showed that Gadd45b mRNA was rapidly and significantly increased 8- and 11-fold by 30 minutes and 1 hour, respectively, after treatment with TGF-β1, before decreasing (Figure 3A and B). Expression of transcripts for Gadd45a or Gadd45g was detected in C10 cells by RT-PCR only after extended amplification at much lower levels (data not shown). These results suggest that GADD45b may play a role in TGF-β1-mediated apoptosis in C10 cells.

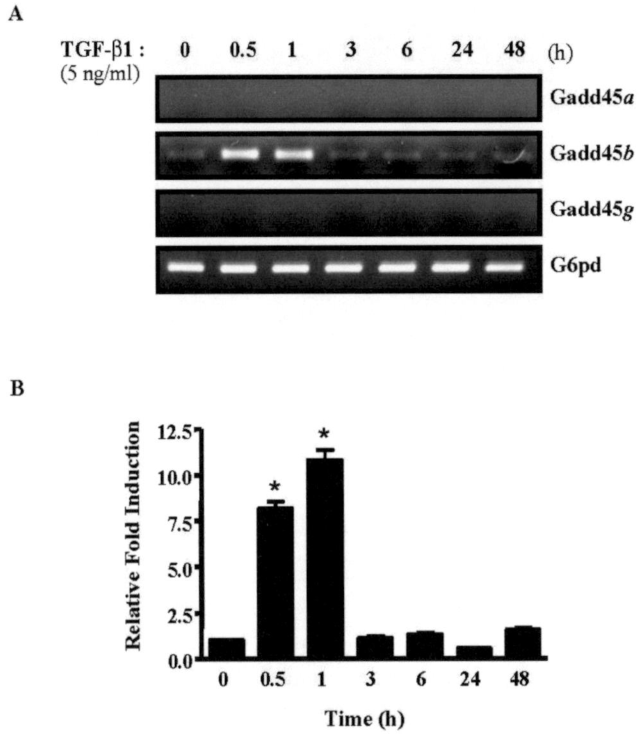

Fig. 3. TGF-β1 increases expression of Gadd45b mRNA in C10 cells.
Time course of expression of Gadd45 mRNA transcripts after stimulation by TGF-β1 using A, semi-quantitative and B, quantitative real-time RT-PCR amplification. Total RNA was prepared, reverse-transcribed and equal amounts of first-strand cDNA were amplified by PCR with Gadd45a-, Gadd45b- and Gadd45g -specific primers. G6pd, glucose-6-phosphate dehydrogenase. B, Relative expression of the Gadd45b gene in C10 cells treated with TGF-β1. The results shown are the means S.E. of two independent experiments performed in duplicate. *, $p < 0.001$ versus control.

3.4 GADD45b enhances the timing and sensitivity of TGF-β1-mediated apoptosis

Having demonstrated that p38 MAPK is activated and expression of Gadd45b mRNA is increased coordinately with the induction of apoptosis by TGF-β1 in C10 cells, we next investigated whether overexpression of GADD45b could affect activation of p38 MAPK and lead to apoptosis. To test this, C10 cells were stably transfected with a hemagglutinin (HA)-tagged Gadd45b expression plasmid or empty vector used as control. In GADD45b-expressing cells (G-45b), p38 MAPK was activated in the absence of TGF-β1 treatment, while TGF-β-induced activation of p38 MAPK occurred in control cells (Figure 4A).

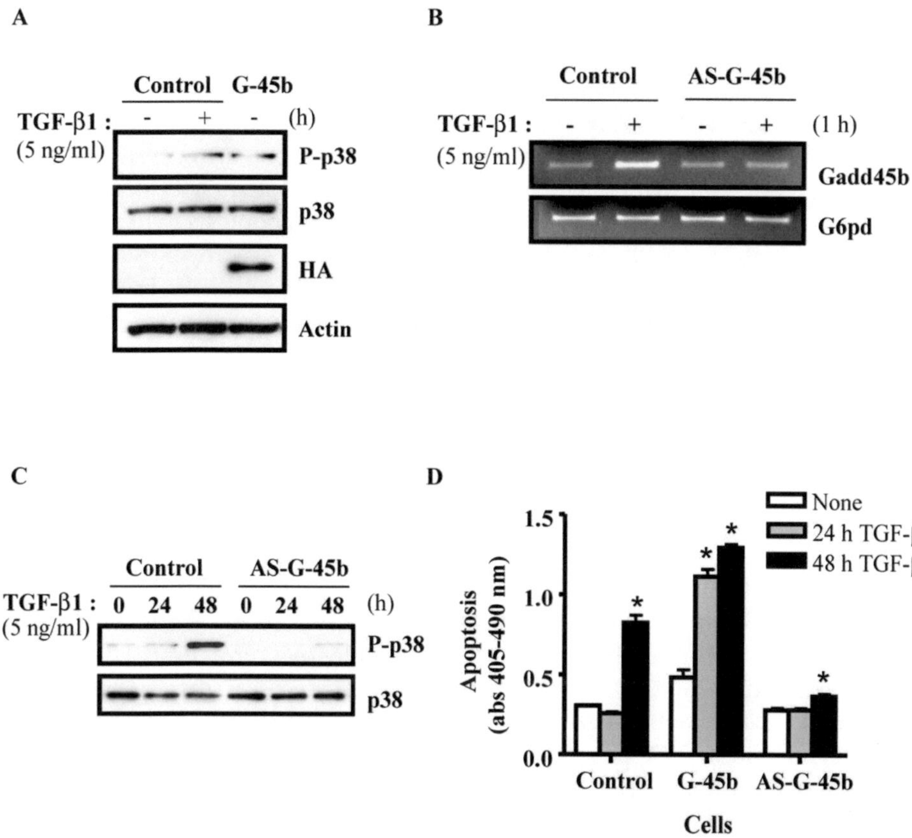

Fig. 4. Overexpression of GADD45b activates p38 MAPK and increases the sensitivity of C10 cells to TGF-β1-mediated apoptosis.
A, C10 cells were stably transfected with either an empty vector (Control) or a hemaggluttinin (HA)-tagged Gadd45b expression vector (G-45b). Total cell lysates prepared from the cells untreated or treated with TGF-β1 for 48 hours were analyzed by immunoblotting. Phosphorylated (P) and non-phosphorylated forms of p38 MAPK are shown in the upper and middle panels, respectively. Expression of HA-tagged GADD45b and actin is shown in the middle and lower panels, respectively. B, Sense Gadd45b transcripts in C10 cells stably transfected with either an empty vector (Control) or an antisense Gadd45b expression vector (AS-G-45b) were subjected to RT-PCR analysis. Following a 1 hour incubation of the cells in the presence or absence of TGF-β1, total RNA was prepared and subjected to RT-PCR amplification using primers specific to the sense Gadd45b transcript. G6pd, glucose-6-phosphate dehydrogenase. C, Phosphorylation of endogenous p38 MAPK in total cell lysates prepared from C10 cells stably transfected with either an empty vector (Control) or an antisense Gadd45b expression vector (AS-G-45b) and untreated or treated with TGF-β1 for 24- and 48 hours, was analyzed by immunoblotting. Phosphorylated (P) and non-phosphorylated forms of p38 MAPK are shown in the upper and lower panels, respectively. D, C10 cells stably transfected with either an empty vector (Control), a Gadd45b expression vector (G-45b) or an antisense Gadd45b expression vector (AS-G-45b) were treated with vehicle (open bars) or TGF-β1 for 24- (gray bars) and 48 hours (dark bars). DNA fragmentation was detected by ELISA assay. *, $p < 0.01$ versus control.

To confirm the effect of GADD45b on activation of p38 MAPK, C10 cells were stably transfected with antisense Gadd45b cDNA (AS-G-45b) to block expression of the endogenous Gadd45b gene. Antisense Gadd45b suppressed endogenous Gadd45b mRNA expression induced by TGF-β1 (Fig 4B), and p38 MAPK activity was substantially reduced 48 hours after treatment with TGF-β1 in AS-G-45b cells compared to control cells (Figure 4C). These results suggest that endogenous GADD45b has a role in p38 MAPK activation. Next, to test whether GADD45b plays a role as a mediator of apoptosis induced by TGF-β1, we examined the ability of these cells to undergo apoptosis with or without TGF-β1. Apoptosis increased by ~50% in G-45b cells compared to control cells in the absence of TGF-β1, and overexpression of GADD45b increased the appearance of apoptosis in C10 cells by 24 hours (Figure 4D). However, apoptosis induced by TGF-β1 decreased in AS-G-45b cells compared to control cells 48 hours after TGF-β1 addition (Figure 4D). This result suggests that expression of endogenous GADD45b is necessary for TGF-β-mediated p38 MAPK activation and apoptosis

3.5 TGF-β1 increases GADD153 mRNA

Because TGF-β1-mediated apoptosis in C10 cells involves increased expression of Gadd45b mRNA only after 0.5- and 1 hour, it is possible that additional proteins may be involved in TGF-β1-mediated apoptosis in these cells. Besides GADD45b, GADD153/CAATT enhancer binding protein homologous protein (CHOP), another member of the GADD family, has been implicated in processes that initiate apoptosis (Corazzari et al., 2003; Maytin et al., 2001; Murphy et al., 2001). We investigated whether GADD153 has a role in TGF-β-mediated apoptosis in C10 cells. Semi-quantitative and real-time RT-PCR amplification showed that Gadd153 mRNA had a gradual, but sustained, increase after TGF-β1 addition (Figure 5A), and by 3 hours, there was a 1.5-fold increase in expression of Gadd153 mRNA that increased significantly to 11- and 9-fold by 24- and 48 hours, respectively (Figure 5B).

We next used actinomycin D and cyclohexamide to investigate whether TGF-β1-induced Gadd153 mRNA expression is transcriptionally regulated and requires prior de novo protein synthesis or not. The addition of actinomycin D, an inhibitor of transcription, inhibited TGF-β1-induced Gadd153 mRNA expression (Figure 5C), indicating that up-regulation of Gadd153 expression is transcriptionally dependent. To address whether the induction of Gadd153 mRNA expression by TGF-β1 requires de novo protein synthesis, the effect of the protein synthesis inhibitor cyclohexamide was examined. Addition of cyclohexamide by itself caused an increase in Gadd153 mRNA levels (Figure 5C). The level of Gadd153 mRNA expression was not significantly changed by addition of cyclohexamide and TGF-β1 together compared to cyclohexamide alone. This suggests that although Gadd153 mRNA is regulated by TGF-β1 in C10 cells, the induction of GADD153 by TGF-β1 depends on prior de novo protein synthesis events. The increase in Gadd153 mRNA level in the presence of cyclohexamide could be explained by an increase in mRNA stability or loss of transcriptional repressors by cyclohexamide.

3.6 GADD153 expression increases with overexpression of GADD45b

Since expression of Gadd45b mRNA is induced early by TGF-β1 in C10 cells, while induction of Gadd153 mRNA occurs more gradually and maximizes at a later time compared to Gadd45b mRNA, we examined whether GADD45b could affect the expression of GADD153.

To test this, we used C10 cells that we had previously stably transfected with a (HA)-tagged sense or antisense Gadd45b expression plasmid. The basal level of GADD153 protein in GADD45b-expressing cells (G-45b) increased in the absence of TGF-β1, and treatment of these cells with TGF-β1 showed further increased expression of GADD153 protein after 24 hours (Figure 6A). However, antisense Gadd45b (AS-G-45b) significantly suppressed endogenous GADD153 protein expression in the absence of TGF-β1 in AS-G-45b cells.

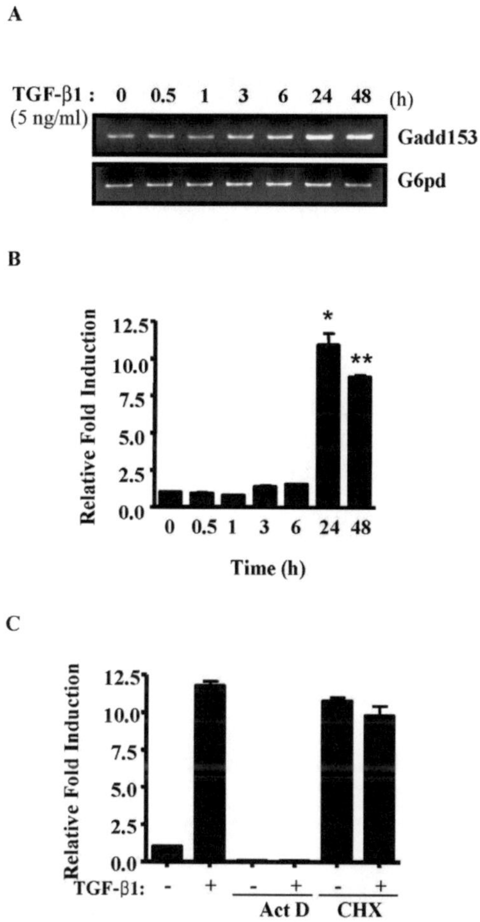

Fig. 5. TGF-β1 increases expression of Gadd153 mRNA in C10 cells.
Time course of expression of Gadd153 mRNA transcripts after stimulation by TGF-β1 using A, semi-quantitative and B, real-time RT-PCR amplification. Total RNA was prepared, reverse-transcribed and equal amounts of the first-strand cDNA were subjected to PCR amplification with specific primers for Gadd153 or glucose-6-phosphate dehydrogenase (G6pd). The results shown are the means S.E. of two independent experiments performed in duplicate. *, $p<0.005$, **, $p < 0.001$ versus control. C, C10 cells were treated with actinomycin (Act D; 1 µg/ml) or cycloheximide (CHX; 5 µg/ml) 1 hour before TGF-β1 addition, and incubated for 24 hours with or without TGF-β1. Total RNA was prepared and subjected to real-time RT-PCR using a primer specific for the Gadd153 transcript. The results shown are the means S.E. of three independent experiments performed in duplicate.

Expression of GADD153 protein was induced by TGF-β1 in C10 cells stably transfected with antisense Gadd45b cDNA, but at levels that were markedly reduced compared to control C10 cells. These results suggest that GADD45b is capable of inducing Gadd153 expression in response to TGF-β1 in C10 cells through a direct or indirect route. The ability of TGF-β1 to stimulate GADD153 expression in AS-G-45b cells could be explained by a residual level of Gadd45b that may be sufficient to stimulate a level of GADD153 expression, or alternatively, both Gadd45b-dependent and Gadd45b-independent mechanisms may exist for stimulating GADD153 expression in C10 cells.

To confirm that endogenous GADD45b has an effect on TGF-β1-induced expression of GADD153, we used a hamster Gadd153 promoter Luciferase reporter construct. Cotransfection of Gadd45b plasmid showed that increasing amounts of Gadd45b using 0.1-, 0.5- and 1-μg of Gadd45b cDNA, augmented transcriptional activity of Gadd153-Luc, with maximal induction occurring using 0.5-μg (Figure 6B). As a control, cotransfection of Gadd45b plasmid had no effect on the transcriptional activity of the TGF-β1-responsive p3TP-Lux reporter. These results suggest that GADD45b is involved in transactivation of the Gadd153 promoter.

Having shown that GADD45b increases the activity of the Gadd153 promoter, we next set out to determine the minimum region of the Gadd153 promoter that was required for induction of Gadd45b. To accomplish this, we utilized a hamster Gadd153 promoter construct (pGadd153-778-+21-Luc) and a series of deletion constructs (pGadd153-225-+21-Luc, pGadd153-165-+21-Luc, pGadd153-105-+21-Luc and pGadd153-36-+21-Luc). Addition of 0.5-μg of Gadd45b cDNA augmented transcriptional activity of pGadd153-778-+21-Luc 3-fold (Figure 6C). Deletion of the Gadd153 promoter up to position –225 still conferred induction by GADD45b. However, deletion of additional nucleotides from –165 to –36 of the Gadd153 promoter resulted in reduced ability of GADD45b to induce the Gadd153 promoter. In addition, cotransfection of Gadd45b with p3TP-Lux showed a minimal effect similar to that of pGadd153-36-+21-Luc, indicating specificity of the effect of GADD45b on GADD153. This suggests the existence of a sequence that is responsive to the effects of GADD45b in region –778 to -225 of the Gadd153 promoter.

3.7 Overexpression of GADD153 activates p38 MAPK and induces apoptosis in the absence of TGF-β1

To address the role of GADD153 inTGF-β1-mediated apoptosis in lung cells, we next investigated whether overexpression of GADD153 could activate p38 MAPK and lead to apoptosis in the absence of TGF-β1 in C10 cells. To test this, C10 cells were stably transfected with a Gadd153 expression vector or empty vector. Figure 7A shows increased expression of GADD153 protein in C10 cells stably transfected with Gadd153 expression plasmid (G-153-1 and G-153-2), but not in control cells. While TGF-β1 treatment induced p38 MAPK activation in control cells, p38 MAPK in GADD153-expressing cells (G-153-1, G-153-2) was activated even in the absence of TGF-β1 (Figure 7B). In GADD153-expressing cells, apoptosis in the absence of TGF-β1 exceeded that in control cells that had been treated with TGF-β1, and sensitivity to TGF-β1-induced apoptosis was increased (Figure 7C and D). To further explore the involvement of p38 MAPK activation in GADD153-expressing cells, we used the potent inhibitor of p38 MAPK, SB203580. Treatment of GADD153-expressing cells with SB203580 strongly inhibited TGF-β1-induced apoptosis at 48 hours (Figure 7D). Our results suggest that the induction of GADD153 by TGF-β1 is part of the TGF-β1-mediated apoptotic pathway, and is upstream of p38 MAPK in this pathway.

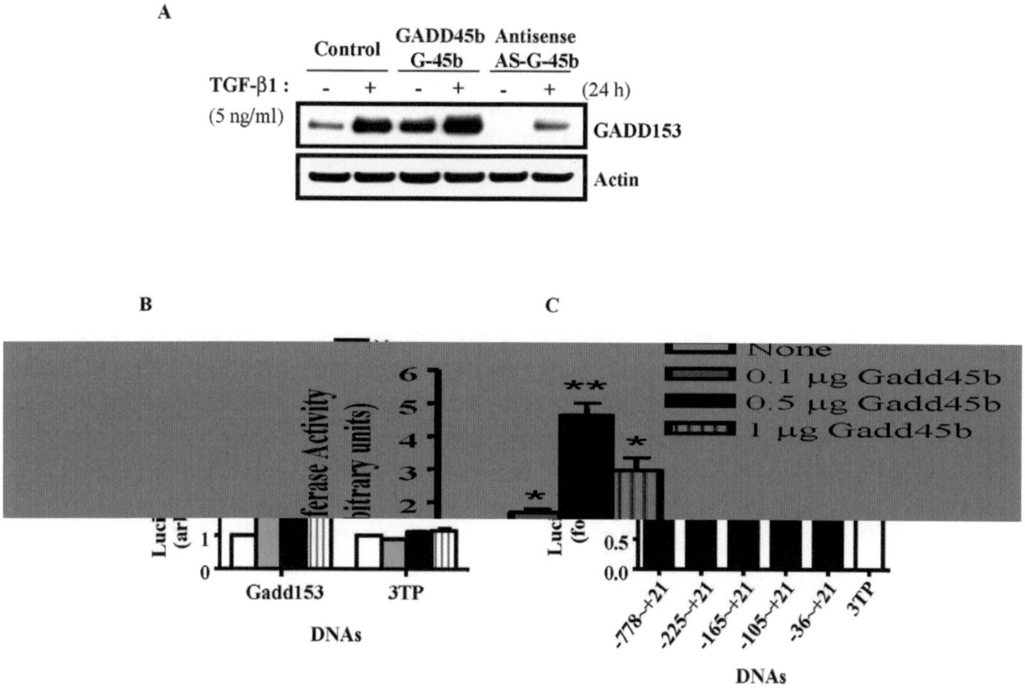

Fig. 6. Effect of GADD45b on transactivation of GADD153.
A, C10 cells stably transfected with either an empty vector (Control), a sense Gadd45b expression vector (G-45b) or an antisense Gadd45b expression vector (AS-G-45b) were treated with TGF-β1 or vehicle for 24 hours, and total cell lysates were analyzed by immunoblotting using GADD153-specific antibodies. Immunoblotting with actin antibodies is shown in the lower panel. B, C10 cells were transiently cotransfected with 0.5-µg Gadd153 (–778-+21)-Luc of the hamster Gadd153 promoter or 3TP-Luc plasmid as a negative control with increasing amounts of the Gadd45b expression plasmid. Cells were harvested 30 hours after transfection and assessed for Luciferase activity. The results shown are the means S.E. of three independent experiments performed. *, $p < 0.05$; **, $p < 0.01$ versus control. C, C10 cells were transiently cotransfected with 0.5-µg of Gadd45b expression plasmid and 0.5-µg of deletion mutants of the hamster Gadd153 promoter, including pGadd153 (-778-+21)-Luc, pGadd153 (-225-+21)-Luc, pGadd153 (-165-+21)-Luc, pGadd153 (-105-+21)-Luc and pGadd153 (-36-+21)-Luc (filled bars) along with p3TP-Lux (open bar). Luciferase activity was measured. The results shown are the means S.E. of two independent experiments performed in triplicate.

3.8 GADD153 expression and TGF-β1-mediated apoptosis is blocked by Smad7

It has previously been reported that GADD45b is activated by TGF-β1 in a Smad-dependent manner (Takekawa et al., 2002; Yoo et al., 2003). Our results showed that GADD153 induction occurs through GADD45b, which in turn, activates p38 MAPK, and leads to apoptosis in the presence of TGF-β1 in C10 cells. These findings evoked the possibility that TGF-β1-mediated apoptosis in C10 cells may be mediated by the Smad pathway. To determine whether the Smad pathway was required for TGF-β-mediated signaling of apoptosis, we asked whether overexpression of Smad7, an inhibitory Smad, would inhibit

this effect in C10 cells. In the Smad7-overexpressing cells detected by Smad7 antibody, expression of GADD153 protein was below the level of detection, and TGF-β1 addition did not result in induction of GADD153 protein as it did in control cells (Figure 8A). The basal level of apoptosis and the sensitivity to TGF-β1-mediated apoptosis was significantly reduced in C10 cells that overexpressed Smad7 (Figure 8B). The morphological changes described earlier did not occur in Smad7-overexpressing C10 cells treated with TGF-β1 (Figure 8C). This indicates that TGF-β1-mediated apoptosis is Smad-dependent and requires induction of GADD153. To confirm that induction of GADD153 is important in determining sensitivity of C10 cells to TGF-β1-mediated apoptosis, we tested the ability of GADD153 to affect apoptosis in C10 cells that overexpressed Smad7. Transient restoration of GADD153 in C10 cells expressing Smad7 significantly augmented apoptosis in the absence of TGF-β1 and the level of apoptosis was not significantly affected by TGF-β1 treatment (Figure 8D). This suggests that the induction of GADD153 expression is a necessary and sufficient step for the induction of apoptosis in C10 cells that overexpress Smad7.
Sensitivity of C10 cells to TGF-β1-mediated apoptosis, we tested the ability of GADD153 to affect apoptosis in C10 cells that overexpressed Smad7. Transient restoration of GADD153 in C10 cells expressing Smad7 significantly augmented apoptosis in the absence of TGF-β1 and the level of apoptosis was not significantly affected by TGF-β1 treatment (Figure 8D). This suggests that the induction of GADD153 expression is a necessary and sufficient step for the induction of apoptosis in C10 cells that overexpress Smad7.

3.9 TGF-β1 regulates IL-6 production through a Smad2-dependent pathway

Since overexpression of Smad7 not only blocked the basal apoptosis, but also resulted in a significant decrease in TGF-β1-mediated apoptosis compared to vector transfected control cells, it may be that TGF-β1 inhibits cell survival signaling pathways as well as activates apoptosis signaling pathways in C10 cells in a Smad-dependent manner. Among the cytokines that have been shown to participate in cellular survival, IL-6 can activate the phosphotidyl inositol-3 kinase (PI3K)/AKT survival pathway (Sierra, 2005). In addition, IL-6 modulates TGF-β1-induced apoptosis via the PI3K/AKT pathway (Chen et al., 1999). To investigate possible crosstalk between TGF-β1 and IL-6, we examined IL-6 production by C10 cells that stably overexpress Smad7. Basal production of IL-6 was found to be 5-fold higher in Smad7-overexpressing C10 cells compared to control cells (Figure 9A), and IL-6 production increased by accumulation in Smad7-overexpressing C10 cells after addition of TGF-β1. In contrast, no significant change in IL-6 production occurred in control C10 cells after treatment with TGF-β1. This result suggests that inhibition of the Smad signaling pathway by Smad7 leads to increased production of IL-6 in C10 cells.

To investigate whether serine/threonine kinase AKT, a downstream target of PI3K, is involved, we also examined activation of AKT in C10 cells overexpressing Smad7. Figure 9B shows phosphorylation, and thus activation, of AKT in Smad7-overexpressing C10 cells. Activation of AKT was maintained at the basal level for up to 24 hours after treatment with TGF-β1 in C10 cells that overexpress Smad7, while activation of AKT was not detected in control C10 cells. To address the effect of IL-6 on TGF-β1-induced apoptosis, C10 cells were treated with either TGF-β1 or increasing amounts of IL-6. TGF-β1 induced apoptosis, while addition of IL-6 increased the ability of C10 cells to survive without TGF-β1 (Figure 9C). The ability of IL-6 to promote cell survival in C10 cells was detected using an IL-6 concentration as low as 1-ng/ml, maximized these effects using 10-ng/ml IL-6 and sustained these effects using 50- and 100-ng/ml IL-6. Next, to investigate whether IL-6 affects apoptosis induced by TGF-β1, C10 cells were treated with TGF-β1 and IL-6 in combination using concentrations of 10-, 50- or 100-ng/ml of IL-6. In the presence of TGF-β1, no treatments with IL-6 protected C10 cells from apoptosis induced by TGF-β1 (Figure 9D). These findings suggest that IL-6 promotes cell survival in the absence of TGF-β1 in C10 cells, but does not inhibit apoptosis induced by TGF-β1, and also suggest that the apoptotic pathway may be predominant over IL-6-mediated survival in these cells.

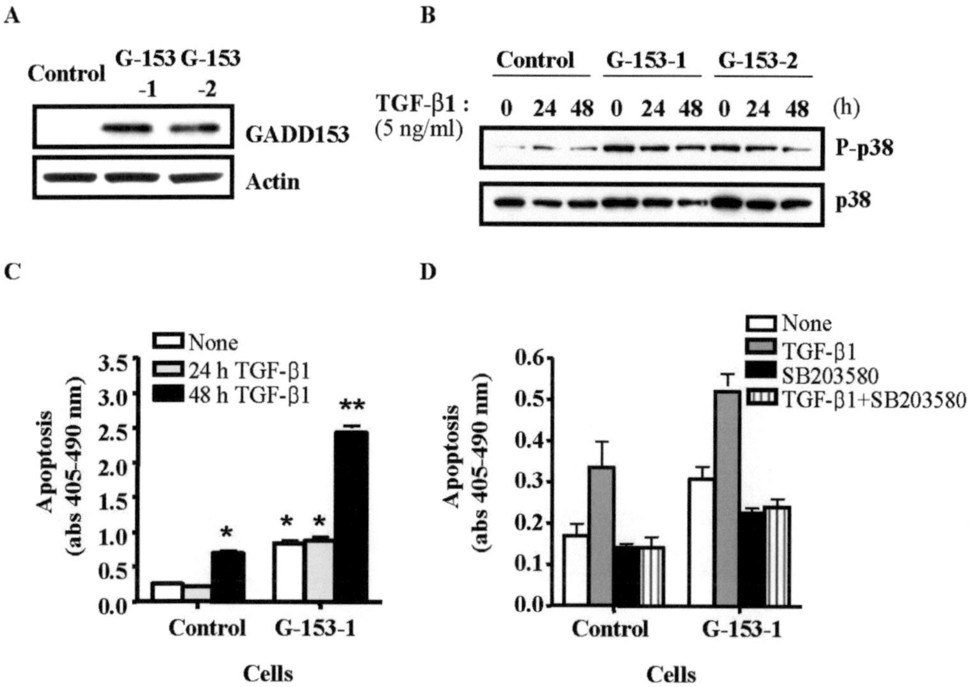

Fig. 7. Overexpression of GADD153 activates p38 MAPK and increases TGF-β1-mediated apoptosis in C10 cells.
A, C10 cells were stably transfected with either an empty vector (Control) or a Gadd153 expression vector (G-153-1 and G-153-2). Total cell lysates were isolated and immunoblotting was performed using GADD153-specific antibodies. Immunoblotting with actin antibodies is shown in the lower panel. B, Phosphorylation of endogenous p38 MAPK in total cell lysates prepared from C10 cells stably transfected with either an empty vector (Control) or a Gadd153 expression vector (G-153-1 and G-153-2) and treated with TGF-β1 or vehicle for 24- and 48 hours was analyzed by immunoblotting. Phosphorylated (P) and non-phosphorylated forms of p38 MAPK are indicated in the upper and lower panels, respectively. C, C10 cells stably transfected with either an empty vector (Control) or a Gadd153 expression vector (G-153-1) were treated with vehicle (open bars) or with TGF-β1 for 24- (gray bars) and 48 hours (dark bars). DNA fragmentation was detected by ELISA assay. *, $p < 0.01$; **, $p < 0.001$ versus control. D, C10 cells stably transfected with either an empty vector (Control) or a Gadd153 expression vector (G-153-1) were treated with vehicle (open bars), TGF-β1 (gray bars), 10 μM SB203580 (dark bars) or TGF-β1 and SB203580 in combination (lined bars) for 48 hours. DNA fragmentation was detected by ELISA assay.

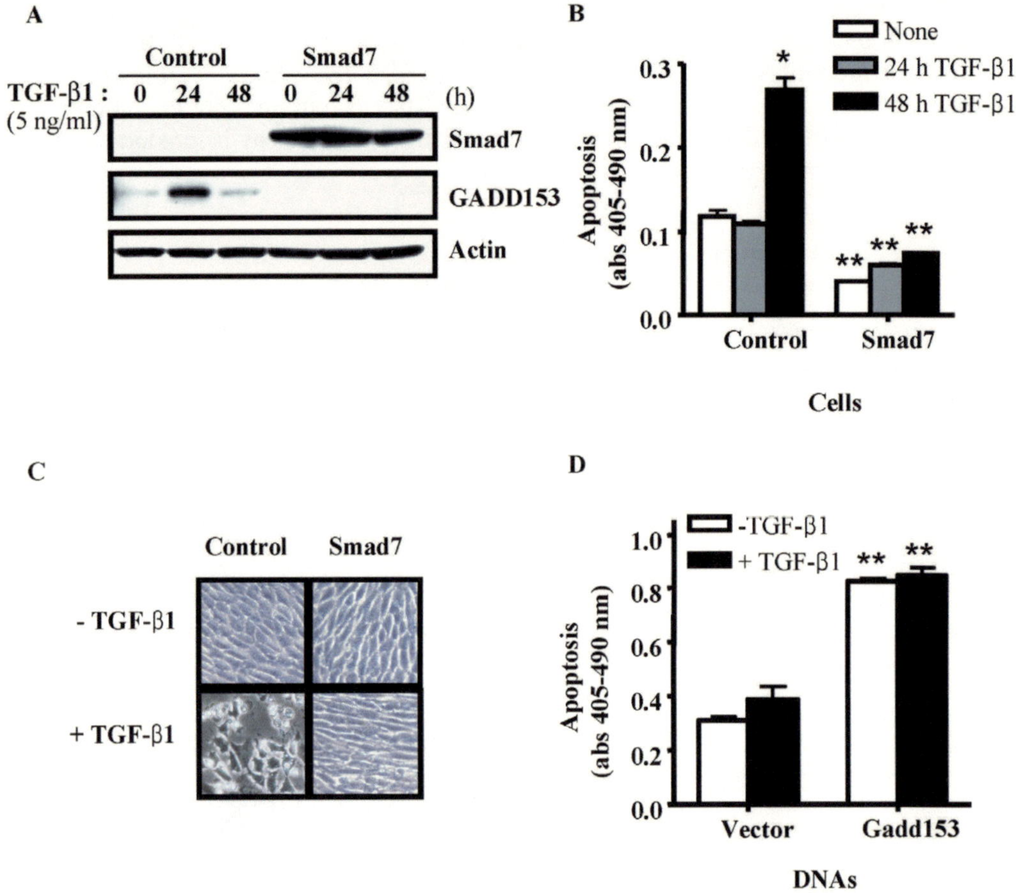

Fig. 8. Overexpression of Smad7 blocks GADD153 expression and TGF-β1-mediated apoptosis.
A, C10 cells were stably transfected with either an empty vector (Control) or a Flag-tagged Smad7 expression vector (Smad7) and treated with TGF-β1 for 24- and 48 hours. Total cell lysates were isolated and immunoblotting was performed using Smad7 and GADD153 antibodies. Immunoblotting with actin antibodies is shown in the lower panel. B, C10 cells stably transfected with either an empty vector (Control) or a Smad7 expression vector (Smad7) were treated with vehicle (open bars) or with TGF-β1 for 24- (gray bars) and 48 hours (dark bars). DNA fragmentation was detected by ELISA assay. *, $p < 0.05$, **, p, < 0.01 versus control. C, Morphology of C10 cells stably transfected with either an empty vector (Control) or a Smad7 expression vector (Smad7) by phase contrast microscopy at 48 hours after treatment with or without TGF-β1. D, C10 cells stably transfected with a Smad7 expression vector were transiently transfected with either an empty vector (Vector) or Gadd153 cDNA expression vector (Gadd153) and cultured with vehicle (open bars) or TGF-β1 (filled bars) for 48 hours. DNA fragmentation was detected by ELISA assay.
** $p < 0.01$ versus control.

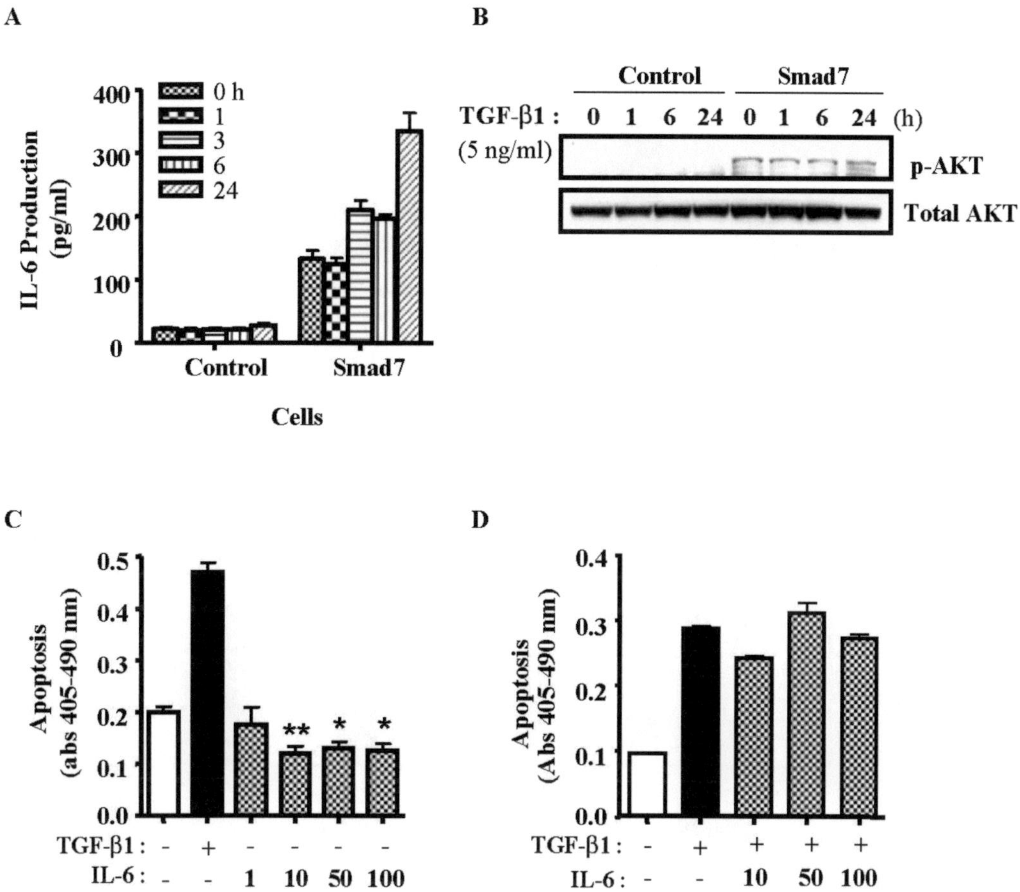

Fig. 9. Overexpression of Smad7 increases IL-6 production in the presence or absence of TGF-β1.

C10 cells were stably transfected with either an empty vector (Control) or a Flag-tagged Smad7 expression vector (Smad7). A, The cells were treated with TGF-β1 for the indicated times. Conditioned media were isolated and the level of IL-6 protein production was detected using a Quantikine assay as described in Materials and Methods. The results shown are the means S.E. of two independent experiments performed in triplicate. B, Time course of phosphorylation of endogenous AKT after stimulation by TGF-β1. Total cell lysates were prepared from untreated or TGF-β1-treated cells and used for immunoblotting. Phosphorylated (P) and non-phosphorylated total forms of AKT are indicated in the upper and lower panels, respectively. C,D, C10 cells were treated with vehicle (open bars) or TGF-β1 (filled bars) or IL-6 (1-, 10-, 50- or 100-ng/ml) (stippled bars) in C, or a combination of TGF-β1 and IL-6 (10-, 50- or 100-ng/ml) (stippled bars) in D, for 48 hours as indicated. DNA fragmentation was detected by ELISA assay at 48 hours after treatments.

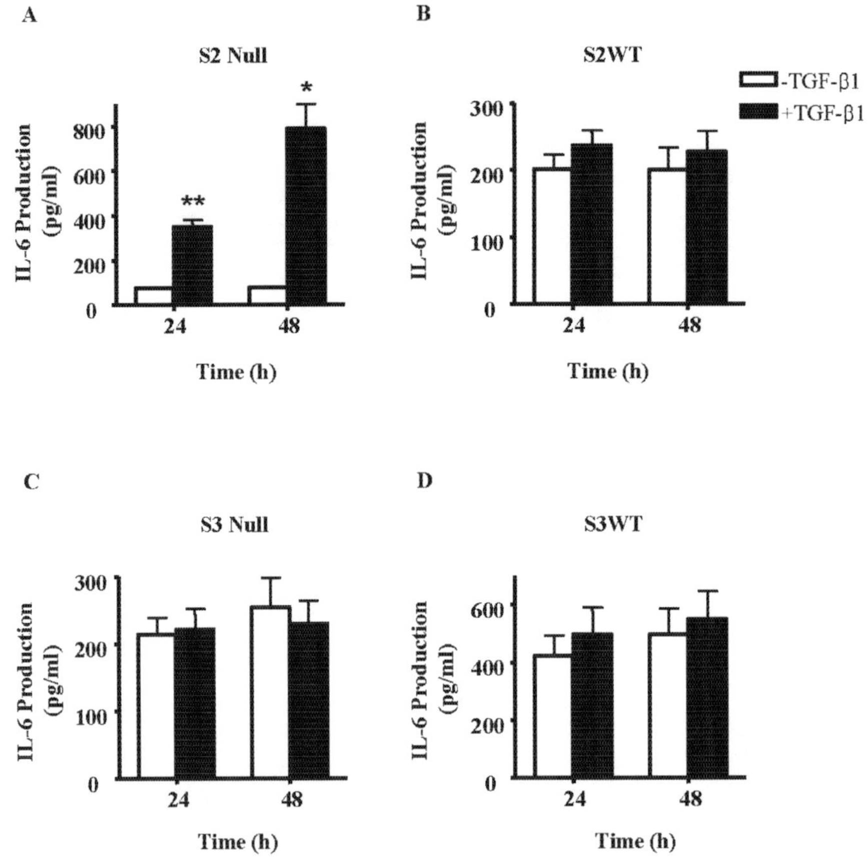

Fig. 10. Production of IL-6 in embryo fibroblasts derived from Smad2- and Smad3-deficient mice and their wildtype littermates.
Embryo fibroblasts from A, Smad2 null, B, Smad2 wildtype, C, Smad3 null and D, Smad3 wildtype mice were cultured with vehicle (open bars) or TGF-β1 (filled bars) for 24- and 48 hours. Conditioned media were isolated and the level of secreted IL-6 protein in pg/ml was detected using a Quantikine assay as described in Materials and Methods. The results shown are the means S.E. of two independent experiments performed in duplicate.
*, $p < 0.01$, **, $p < 0.001$ versus control.

Finally, to determine which Smad affects expression of IL-6, we examined the secretion of IL-6 in embryo fibroblasts from Smad2- and Smad3-deficient mice and their wildtype littermates. Treatment of Smad2 null mouse embryo fibroblasts (MEFs) with TGF-β1 demonstrated that production of IL-6 was enhanced by TGF-β1 7-fold by 24 hours that increased to 15-fold by 48 hours, while no change was detected in the amount of IL-6 that was produced from wildtype MEFs (Figure 10B). In contrast, no change in IL-6 production was detected in Smad3 null and wildtype MEFs after treatment with TGF-β1 for up to 48 hours. This suggests that TGF-β1 regulates IL-6 production via Smad2, but not via Smad3, in C10 cells.

4. Discussion

The present study was undertaken to investigate the potential effect of TGF-β1 on apoptosis in immortalized normal mouse lung C10 cells. We reasoned that it would be easier to understand the mechanism of TGF-β1-mediated apoptosis in normal epithelial cells in which the TGF-β1 signaling pathway was functional than in tumor cells in which the TGF-β1 pathway may not be functional. Addition of TGF-β1 to C10 cells activated the p38 MAPK pathway, and the p38 MAPK inhibitor SB203580 significantly reduced the TGF-β1-mediated apoptotic response. These findings suggest that activation of p38 MAPK is involved in TGF-β1-mediated apoptosis in C10 cells. It has been reported that stress-activated protein kinases like p38 MAPK can mediate pro-apoptotic signals from TGF-β Receptors in multiple cell types, including lung cells (Undevia et al., 2004). Interestingly, although ERK1/ERK2 and JNK activation is associated with TGF-β Receptor-mediated apoptosis in some cell types, addition of TGF-β1 to C10 cells had only a marginal effect on activation of ERK and no effect on JNK. Thus, ERK and JNK do not appear to play essential roles in TGF-β1-mediated apoptosis in these lung cells.

TGF-β1-mediated apoptosis in C10 cells has revealed an unexpected degree of complexity. TGF-β1-mediated apoptosis in C10 cells is dependent on signaling through Smads and p38 MAPK. The delayed kinetics of p38 MAPK activation in TGF-β1-mediated apoptosis in C10 cells suggest that one or more additional components may be involved in this process. Earlier reports have provided strong evidence that GADD45b is a critical upstream component in the apoptotic pathway of TGF-β1 in human pancreatic carcinoma cells and mouse hepatocytes (Takekawa et al., 2004; Yoo et al., 2003). A recent report outlined a role for Smad3 and Smad4 in activating Gadd45b through its third intron to facillitate G2 progression following addition of TGF-β1 (Major & Jones, 2004). We examined the expression of Gadd45b mRNA in response to TGF-β1 in C10 cells. As in earlier reports, TGF-β1 induces expression of GADD45b in C10 cells. Overexpression of GADD45b accelerates the appearance of apoptosis in C10 cells by at least 24 hours, and down-regulation of GADD45b expression with an antisense construct inhibits TGF-β-mediated apoptosis. These results suggest that GADD45b participates in TGF-β1-mediated apoptosis in C10 cells.

The participation of GADD45b in TGF-β1-mediated apoptosis in C10 cells does not rule out the possible involvement of other factors that may cooperate with GADD45b in TGF-β1-mediated apoptosis. The time interval between the initial induction of Gadd45b mRNA expression by TGF-β1 stimulation and the appearance of apoptosis suggest that other factors may be involved. We explored the possible involvement of other GADD family members, including GADD5a and GADD45g. However, transcripts for Gadd45a or Gadd45g in the absence or presence of TGF-β1 were detected only at very low levels in C10 cells. Earlier reports showed that the stress-inducible transcription factor GADD153/CHOP induced apoptosis in mammalian cells through p38 MAPK-dependent and -independent mechanisms (Corazzari et al., 2003; Maytin et al., 2001; Murphy et al., 2001). GADD153 has been implicated in apoptosis, and cells isolated from Gadd153 null mice have been shown to be resistant to apoptosis-inducing regimes (Zinszner et al., 1998). In our study, Gadd153 mRNA had a gradual and sustained increase in Gadd153 mRNA after treatment with TGF-β1 that reached a maximum at 24- to 48 hours. The timing of Gadd153 mRNA induction is consistent with the appearance of TGF-β1-mediated apoptosis in C10 cells. Addition of actinomycin D and cyclohexamide showed that up-regulation of GADD153 expression is dependent on transcription and requires de novo protein synthesis. This suggests that although Gadd153 mRNA is regulated by TGF-β1 in C10 cells, the induction of GADD153 by TGF-β1 depends on prior protein synthesis events.

Our results demonstrate that expression of GADD153 protein is induced in C10 cells stably transfected with Gadd45b cDNA, while it is markedly reduced in antisense Gadd45b-expressing cells compared to control C10 cells untreated or treated with TGF-β1. Cotransfection of Gadd45b plasmid with Gadd153-Luc showed that increasing amounts of Gadd45b cDNA augmented transcriptional activity of Gadd153-Luc. These results suggest that GADD45b has a role in transactivation of GADD153 expression in response to TGF-β1 in C10 cells in a direct or indirect manner. This is the first report of regulation of GADD153 by GADD45b. Our findings also show that the induction of GADD153 is sufficient to activate p38 MAPK and to trigger apoptosis in the absence of TGF-β1 in C10 cells.

In this study, we also demonstrated that GADD153 induction by TGF-β1 and TGF-β1-mediated apoptosis was completely inhibited in C10 cells when Smad signaling was blocked by Smad7. Transient restoration of GADD153 in C10 cells overexpressing Smad7 significantly augmented apoptosis in the absence of TGF-β1, and the level of apoptosis was not affected by TGF-β1 treatment. Our results suggest that GADD153 is a determining factor in TGF-β1-mediated apoptosis in C10 cells and induction of GADD153 may be useful to potentiate apoptosis in cells in which the TGF-β1 signaling pathway is not functional or only minimally functional, which is often the case in tumor cells.

In addition to the p38 MAPK regulated apoptosis pathway, we also identified crosstalk between TGF-β1 and IL-6 in C10 cells. In C10 cells that overexpress Smad7, the basal level of IL-6 production was higher than in control cells and activation of AKT occurred without TGF-β1. Addition of IL-6 alone resulted in increased survival, and IL-6 in combination with TGF-β1 failed to block apoptosis induced by TGF-β1. The slow kinetics of delayed onset of TGF-β1-induced apoptosis may be attributed to the activation of the PI3K/AKT cell survival pathway during the early stage of TGF-β treatment (Yu et al., 2002). Activation of the AKT pathway by TGF-β1 has been shown to be mediated by a p38 MAPK-mediated mechanism (Horowitz et al., 2004). Activation of AKT in response to TGF-β1 addition does not appear to play an important role in normal C10 cells, indicating that this pathway probably does not participate in delaying the onset of apoptosis. However, if events occur which lead to the overexpression of Smad7, and thus decreased Smad-dependent TGF-β1 signaling, the activation of AKT may play a more prominent role. It has been reported that overexpression of Smad7 induced tumorigeniciy in human colon carcinoma cells by blocking TGF-β-induced growth inhibition and apoptosis (Halder et al., 2005). It appears that the TGF-β1/p38 MAPK-mediated apoptosis pathway in which GADD45b and GADD153 participate as intermediates, plays a more prominent role than the IL-6/AKT pathway does in C10 cells as outlined in Figure 11. Although our scenario depicts direct activation of GADD153 by GADD45b, this may or may not occur. Other factors may be involved. In addition, the survival pathway may be a less frequently used pathway in normal C10 cells compared to the apoptosis pathway. The predominance of these pathways may also change in tumor cells. Future studies will be needed to examine he role of these alternative pathways and crosstalk signaling that may be involved or abrogated in tumor cells.

TGF-β1 induces GADD45b expression in a Smad-dependent manner. GADD45b then activates GADD153, which, in turn, activates p38 MAPK. Activated p38 MAPK results in apoptosis. This may be the predominant pathway in C10 cells. Alternatively, TGF-β may down-regulate IL-6 production through Smad2-dependent signaling. Elevated IL-6 may be able to induce activation of AKT to block or reduce apoptosis and increase cell survival. If

Smad signaling is blocked by Smad7 or reduced by another agent or phenomenon, it may be sufficient to confer a pro-survival/apoptosis-resistant phenotype to C10 cells.

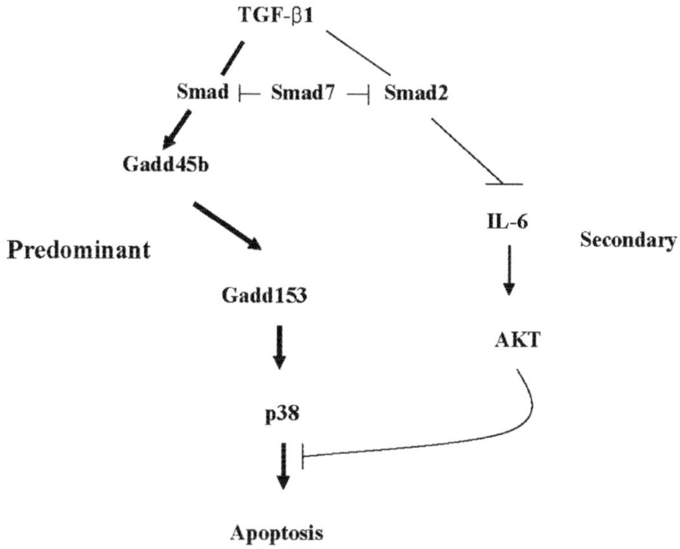

Fig. 11. A possible mechanism of TGF-β1-mediated apoptosis in mouse lung epithelial C10 cells.

5. Conclusion

Resistance to apoptosis has been shown to be one of the characteristics of cancer cells during progressive tumorigenesis (Hanahan & Weinberg, 2000). Thus, it would be promising for the treatment of cancer, to activate TGF-β1-mediated apoptosis by modulating the function of TGF-β1 in specific tumor cell types. Our study has shown that in lung C10 cells that overexpress GADD153, both the basal level and sensitivity to apoptosis are increased, suggesting that the induction of GADD153 is an important step in the sensitivity of these lung cells to apoptosis. Future studies will need to be performed to evaluate whether increased levels of GADD153 can be stimulated effectively to increase TGF-β-mediated apoptosis in lung tumor cells in which this does not occur or occurs less frequently, and thus, bring about their destruction, and an effective therapy that can be used in the treatment of lung cancer.

6. Acknowledgements

We thank the late Dr. A. Roberts (NCI, Bethedsa, MD) for HA-tagged Gadd45b plasmid, antisense Gadd45b plasmids, Smad-dependent reporter plasmids and MEFs from Smad2- and Smad3-deficient mice, Dr. S-J Kim (NCI, Bethesda, MD) for Flag-tagged Smad7 plasmid and Dr. A. Fornace Jr. (Georgetown University Medical Center, Washington, DC) for Gadd153 plasmids. We are grateful for comments given to us by Drs. P. Blumberg, K. Flanders, T. Moody and C. Stuelten (NCI, Bethesda, MD) during the preparation of this chapter article. This research was supported by the Intramural Research Program of the NIH, National Cancer Institute, Center for Cancer Research.

7. References

Albright, C.D., Salganik R.I., Craciunescu, C.N., Mar, M.H., & Zeisel S.H. (2003) Mitochondrial and Microsomal Derived Reactive Oxygen Species Mediate Apoptosis Induced by Transforming Growth Factor β1 in Immortalized Rat Hepatocytes. *Journal of Cellular Biochemistry*, Vol. 89, No. 2, (May 2003), pp. 254-261

Abe, T., Ouyang, H., Migita, T., Kato, Y., Kimura, M., Shiiba, K., Sunamura, M., Matsuno, S., & Horii, A. (1996) The Somatic Mutation Frequency of the Transforming Growth Factor β Receptor Type II Gene Varies Widely Among Different Cancers with Microsatellite Instability. *European Journal of Surgical Oncology*, Vol. 22, No. 5, (October 1996), pp. 474-477

Albright, C.D., Salganik R.I., Craciunescu, C.N., Mar, M.H., & Zeisel S.H. (2003) Mitochondrial and Microsomal Derived Reactive Oxygen Species Mediate Apoptosis Induced by Transforming Growth Factor β1 in Immortalized Rat Hepatocytes. *Journal of Cellular Biochemistry*, Vol. 89, No. 2, (May 2003), pp. 254-261

Amoroso, S.R., Huang, N., Roberts, A.B., Potter, M., & Letterio, J.J. (1998) Consistent Loss of Functional Transforming Growth Factor β Receptor Expression in Murine Plasmacytomas. *Proceedings of the National Academy of Science USA*, Vol. 95, No. 1, (January 1998), pp. 189-194

Annes, J.P., Munger, J.S., & Rifkin, D.B. (2003) Making Sense of Latent TGFβ Activation. *Journal of Cell Science*, Vol. 116, Pt. 2, (June 2003), pp. 217-224

Arandjelovic, S., Freed T.A., & Gonias S.L. (2003) Growth Factor-binding Sequence in Human Alpha2-Macroglobulin Targets the Receptor-binding Site in Transforming Growth Factor-β. *Biochemistry*, Vol. 42, No. 5, (May 2003), pp. 6121-6127

Arteaga, C.L., Coffey, R.J. Jr., Dugger, T.C., McCutchen, C.M., Moses, H.L., Lyons, R.M. (1990) Growth Stimulation of Human Breast Cancer Cells with Anti-Transforming Growth Factor β Antibodies: Evidence for Autocrine Negative Regulation by Transforming Growth Factor β. *Cell Growth & Differentiation*, Vol. 1, No. 18, (August 1990), pp. 367-374

Barcellos-Hoff, M.H. (1996) Latency and Activation in the Control of TGF-β. *Journal of Mammary Gland Biology Neoplasia*, Vol. 1, No. 4, (October 1996), pp. 353-363

Barcellos-Hoff, & M.H., Ewan, KB. (2000) Transforming Growth Factor Type-β and Breast Cancer. Mammary Gland Development. *Breast Cancer Research*, Vol. 2, No. 2, (February 2000), pp. 92-99

Bartram, U., & Speer, C. P. (2004) The Role of Transforming Growth Factor β in Lung Development and Disease. *Chest*, Vol. 125, No. 2, (February 2004), pp. 754-765

Berger, M. (2002) Inflammatory Mediators in Cystic Fibrosis Lung Disease. *Allergy and Asthma Proceedings*, Vol. 23, No. 1, (January-February 2002), pp. 19-25

Bhatia, M., & Moochhala, S. (2004) Role of Inflammatory Mediators in the Pathophysiology of Acute Respiratory Distress. *Journal of Pathology*, Vol. 202, No. 2, (February 2004), pp. 145-156

Böttinger, E.P., Jakubczak, J.L., Haines, D.C., Bagnall, K., & Wakefield, L.M. (1997) Transgenic Mice Overexpressing a Dominant-negative Mutant Type II Transforming Growth Factor β Receptor Show Enhanced Tumorigenesis in the Mammary Gland and Lung in Response to the Carcinogen 7,12-dimethylbenz-[a]-anthracene. *Cancer Research*, Vol. 57, No. 24, (December 1997), pp. 5564-5570

Brown, T.L., Patil, S., Basnett, R.K., & Howe, P.H. (1998) Caspase Inhibitor BD-fmk Distinguishes Transforming Growth Factor-β-induced Apoptosis from Growth Inhibition. *Cell Growth & Differentiation*, Vol. 9, No. 10, (October 1998), pp. 869-875

Chen, R.H., & Chang, T.Y. (1997) Involvement of Caspase Family Proteases in Transforming Growth Factor-β-induced Apoptosis. *Cell Growth & Differentiation*, Vol. 8, No. 7, (July 1997), pp. 821-827

Chen, R. H., Chang, M. C., Su, Y. H., Tsai, Y. T., & Kuo, M. L. (1999) Interleaukin-6 Inhibits Transforming Growth Factor--β-induced Apoptosis through the Phosphotidylinositol 3-Kinase/AKT and Signal Transducers and Activators of Transcription 3 Pathways. *Journal of Biological Chemistry*, Vol. 274, No. 33, (August 1999), pp. 23013-23019

Chen, R.H., Ebner, R., & Derynck, R. (1993) Inactivation of the Type II Receptor Reveals Two Receptor Pathways for the Diverse TGF-β Activities. *Science*, Vol. 260, No. 5112, (May 1993), pp. 1135-1338

Chen, T., Carter, D., Garrigue-Antar, L., & Reiss, M. (1998) Transforming Growth Factor β type I Receptor Kinase Mutant Associated with Metastatic Breast Cancer. *Cancer Research*, Vol. 58, No. 21, (November 1998), pp. 4805-4810

Chen, T., Triplett, T., Dehner, B., Hurst, B., Colligan, B., Pemberton, J., Graff, J.R., & Carter, J.H. (2001) Transforming Growth Factor-β Receptor Type I Gene is Frequently Mutated in Ovarian Carcinomas. *Cancer Research*, Vol. 61, No. 12, (June 2001), pp. 4679-4682

Chin, B.Y., Petrache, I., Choi, A.M., & Choi, M.E. (1999) Transforming Growth Factor β1 Rescues Serum Deprivation-induced Apoptosis via the Mitogen-Activated Protein Kinase (MAPK) Pathway in Macrophages. *Journal of Biological Chemistry*, Vol. 274, No. 16, (April 1999), pp. 11362-11368

Choi, K.S., Lim, I.K., Brady, J.N., & Kim, S.J. (1998) ICE-like Protease (Caspase) is Involved in Transforming Growth Factor β1-mediated Apoptosis in FaO Rat Hepatoma Cell Line. *Hepatology*, Vol. 27, No. 2, (February 1998), pp. 415-421

Chung, Y.J., Song, J.M., Lee, J.Y., Jung, Y.T., Seo, E.J., Choi, S.W., & Rhyu, M.G. (1996) Microsatellite Instability-associated Mutations Associate Preferentially with the Intestinal Type of Primary Gastric Carcinomas in a High-risk Population. *Cancer Research*, Vol. 56, No. 20, (October 1996), pp. 4662-4665

Corazzari, M., Lovat, P. E., Oliverio, S., Pearson, A. D., Piacentini, M., & Redfern, C. P. (2003) Growth and DNA Damage-inducible Transcription Factor 153 Mediates Apoptosis in Response to Fenretinide but not Synergy Between Fenretinide and Chemotherapeutic Drugs in Neuroblastoma. *Molecular Pharmacology*, Vol. 64, No. 6, (December 2003), pp. 1370-1378

Cui, W., Fowlis, D.J., Bryson, S., Duffie, E., Ireland, H., Balmain, A., & Akhurst, R.J. (1996) TGFβ1 Inhibits the Formation of Benign Skin Tumors but Enhances Progression to Invasive Spindle Cell Carcinomas in Transgenic Mice. *Cell*, Vol. 86, No. 4, (August 1996), pp. 531-542

Derynck, R., Akhurst, R.J., & Balmain, A. (2001) TGF-β Signaling in Cancer: A Double-edged Sword. *Trends in Cell Biology, Vol.* 29, No. 2, (October 2001), pp. 117-129

Edlund, S., Bu, S., Schuster, N., Aspenstrom, P., Heuchel, R., Heldin, N.-E., ten Dijke, P., Heldin, C.-H., & Landstrom, M. (2003) Transforming Growth Factor ß1-induced Apoptosis of Prostate Cancer Cells Involves Smad7-dependent Activation of p38 by TGF-β-activated Kinase 1 and Mitogen-Activated Protein Kinase Kinase 3. *Molecular Biology of the Cell*, Vol. 14, No. 2, (February 2003), pp. 529-544

Eisma, R.J., Spiro, J.D., von Bilberstein, S.E., Lindquist, R., & Kreutzer, D.L. (1996) Decreased Expression of Transforming Growth Factor β Receptors on Head and Neck Tumor Cells. *American Journal of Surgery*, Vol. 172, No 6, (December 1996), pp. 641-645

Elliott, R. L., & Blobe, G. C. (2005) Role of Transforming Growth Factor Beta in Human Cancer. *Journal of Clinical Oncology*, Vol. 23, No. 9, (March 2005), pp. 2078-2093

Fafeur, V., O'Hara, B., & Böhlen, P. (1993) A Glycosylation-deficient Endothelial Cell Mutant with Modified Responses to Transforming Growth Factor-β and Other Growth Inhibitory Cytokines: Evidence for Multiple Growth Inhibitory Signal Transduction Pathways. *Molecular Biology of the Cell*, Vol. 4, No. 2, (February 1993), pp. 135-144

Franchi, A., Gallo, O., Sardi, I., & Santucci, M. (2001) Downregulation of Transforming Growth Factor β Type II Receptor in Laryngeal Carcinogenesis. *Journal of Clinical Pathology*, Vol. 54, No. 3, (March 2001), pp. 201-204

Fornace, A. J., Jr., Nebert, D. W., Hollander, M. C., Luethy, J. D., Papathanasiou, M., Fargnoli, J., & Holbrook, N. J. (1989) Mammalian Genes Coordinately Regulated by Growth Arrest Signals and DNA-damaging Agents. *Molecular and Cellular Biology*, Vol. 9, No. 10, (October 1989), pp. 4196-4203

Gentry, LE, Lioubin MN, Purchio AF, Marquardt H. (1988) Molecular Events in the Processing of Recombinant Type I Pre-Pro-Transforming Growth Factor β to the Mature Polypeptide. *Molecular & Cellular Biology, Vol.* 8, No. 10, (October 1988), pp. 4162-4168

Gerber, A., Wille, A., Welte, T., Ansorge, S., & Buhling, F. (2001) Interleukin-6 and Transforming Growth Factor-β1 Control Expression of Cathepsins B and L in Human Lung Epithelial cells. *Journal of Interferon Cytokine Research*, Vol. 21, No. 1, (January 2001), pp. 11-19

Glick, A.B., Flanders, K.C., Danielpour, D., Yuspa, S.H., & Sporn, M.B. (1989) Retinoic Acid Induces Transforming Growth Factor-β2 in Cultured Keratinocytes and Mouse Epidermis. *Cell Regulation*, Vol. 1, No. 1, (November 1989), pp. 617-626

Go, C., Li, P., & Wang, X.-J. (1999) Blocking Transforming Growth Factor β Signaling in Transgenic Epidermis Accelerates Chemical Carcinogenesis: A Mechanism Associated with Increased Angiogenesis. *Cancer Research*, Vol. 59, No. 12, (June 1999), pp. 2861-2868

Gobbi, H., Dupont, W.D., Simpson, J.F., Plummer, W.D., Schuyler, P.A., Olson, S.J., Arteaga, C.L., & Page, D.L. (1999) Transforming Growth Factor β and Breast Cancer Risk in Women with Mammary Epithelial Hyperplasia. *Journal of the National Cancer Institute*, Vol. 91, No. 24, (December 1999), pp. 2096-2101

Goggins, M. (1998) Genetic Alterations of the Transforming Growth Factor β Receptor Genes in Pancreatic and Biliary Adenocarcinomas. *Cancer Research*, Vol. 58, No. 23, (December 1998), pp. 5329-5332

Grady, W.M., Myeroff, L.L., Swinler, S.E., Rajput, A., Thiagalingam, S., Lutterbaugh, J.D., Neumann, A., Brattain, M.G., Chang, J., Kim, S.-J., Kinzler, K.W., Vogelstein, B., Willson, J.K., & Markowitz, S. (1999) Mutational Inactivation of Transforming Growth Factor β Receptor Type II in Microsatellite Stable Colon Cancers. *Cancer Research*, Vol. 59, No. 2, (January 1999), pp. 320-324

Groth, S., Schulze M., Kalthoff, H., Fändrich, F., & Ungefroren, H. (2005) Adhesion and Rac1-dependent Regulation of Biglycan Gene Expression by TGF-β. *Journal of Biological Chemistry*, Vol. 280, No. 39, (September 2005), pp. 33190-33199

Hagimoto, N., Kuwano, K., Inoshima, I., Yoshimi, M., Nakamura, N., Fujita, M., Maeyama, T., & Hara, N. (2002) TGF-β1 as an Enhancer of Fas-mediated Apoptosis of Lung Epithelial cells. *Journal of Immunology*, Vol. 168, No. 12, (June 2002), pp. 6470-6478

Hagimoto, N., Kuwano, K., Miyazaki, H., Kunitake, R., Fujita, M., Kawasaki, M., Kaneko, Y., & Hara, N. (1997) Induction of Apoptosis and Pulmonary Fibrosis in Mice in Response to Ligation of Fas Antigen. *American Journal of Respiratory Cell and Molecular Biology*, Vol. 17, No. 3, (September 1997), pp. 272-278

Hahn, S.A., Hoque, A.T., Moskaluk, C.A., da Costa, L.T., Schulte, M., Rozenblum, E., Seymour, A.B., Weinstein, C.L., Yeo, C.J., Hruban, R.H., & Kern, S.E. (1996) Homozygous Deletion Map at 18q21.1 in Pancreatic Cancer. *Cancer Research*, Vol. 56, No. 3, (February 1996), pp. 490-494

Halder, S. K., Beauchamp, R. D., & Datta, P. K. (2005) Smad7 Induces Tumorigenicity by Blocking TGF-β-induced Growth Inhibition and Apoptosis. *Experimental Cell Research*, Vol. 307, No. 1, (July 2005), pp. 231-246

Han, S.U., Kim, H.T., Seong, Do H., Kim, Y.S., Park, Y.S., Bang, Y.J., Yang, H.K., & Kim, S.-J. (2004) Loss of Smad3 Expression Increases Susceptibility to Tumorigenicity in Human Gastric Cancer. *Oncogene*, Vol. 23, No. 7, (February 2004), pp. 1333-1341

Hanahan, D., & Weinberg, R. A. (2000) The Hallmarks of Cancer. *Cell*, Vol. 100, No. 1, (January 2000), pp. 57-70

Hanson, R. W. (1998) Biological Role of the Isoforms of C/EBP Minireview Series. *Journal of Biological Chemistry*, Vol. 273, No. 44, (October 1998), p.28543

Heldin, C.H., Miyazono, K., & ten Dijke, P. (1997) TGF-β Signaling from Cell Membrane to Nucleus through SMAD Proteins. *Nature*, Vol. 390, No. 6659, (December 1997), pp. 465-471

Herrera, B., Alvarez, A.M., Sanchez, A., Fernandez, M., Roncero, C., Benito, M., & Fabregat, I. (2001) Reactive Oxygen Species (ROS) Mediates the Mitochondrial-dependent Apoptosis Induced by Transforming Growth Factor β in Fetal hepatocytes. *FASEB Journal*, Vol. 15, No. 3, (March 2001), pp. 741-751

Hodge, S., Hodge, G., Flower, R., Reynolds, P.N., Scicchitano, R., & Holmes, M. (2002) Up-regulation of Production of TGF-β and IL-4 and Down-regulation of IL-6 by Apoptotic Human Bronchial Epithelial Cells. *Immunology and Cell Biology*, Vol. 80, No. 6, (December 2002), pp. 537-543

Horowitz, J. C., Lee, D. Y., Waghray, M., Keshamouni, V. G., Thomas, P. E., Zhang, H., Cui, Z., & Thannickal, V. J. (2004) Activation of the Pro-survival Phosphotidylinositol 3-Kinase/AKT Pathway by Transforming Growth Factor-β1 in Mesenchymal Cells is Mediated by p38 MAPK-Dependent Induction of an Autocrine Growth Factor. *Journal of Biological Chemistry*, Vol. 279, No. 2, (January 2004), pp. 1359-1367

Howe, J.R. (1998) Mutations in the Smad4/DPC4 Gene in Juvenile Polyposis. *Science*, Vol. 280, No. 5366, (May 1998), pp. 10986-1088

Hyytiäinen, M., Penttinen, C., & Keski-Oja, J. (2004) Latent TGF-β Binding Proteins: Extracellular Matrix Association and Roles in TGF-β Activation. *Critical Reviews in Clinical Laboratory Science*, Vol. 41, No. 3, (March 2004), pp. 233-264

Iglesias, M., Frontelo, P., Gamallo, C., & Quintanilla, M. (2000) Blockade of Smad4 in Transformed Keratinocytes Containing a Ras Oncogene Leads to Hyperactivation of the Ras-dependent Erk Signaling Pathway Associated with Progression to Undifferentiated Carcinomas. *Oncogene*, Vol. 19, No. 36, (August 2000), pp. 4134-4145

Izumoto, S., Arita, N., Ohnishi, T., Hiraga, S., Taki, T., Tomita, N., Ohue, M., & Havakawa, T. (1997) Microsatellite Instability and Mutated Type II Transforming Growth Factor-β Receptor Gene in Gliomas. Cancer Letters, Vol. 112, No. 2, (January 1997), pp. 251-256

Jakowlew, S.B., Mathias, A., Chung, P., & Moody, T.M. (1995) Expession of Transforming Growth Factor-β Ligand and Receptor Messenger RNAs in Lung Cancer Cell Lines. *Cell Growth & Differentiation*, Vol. 6, No. 4, (April), pp. 465-476

Jakowlew, S.B., Moody, T.M., & Mariano, J.M. (1998) Transforming Growth Factor-β Expression in Mouse Lung Cancinogenesis. *Experimental Lung Research*, Vol. 24, No. 4, (July-August), pp. 579-593

Javelaud, D., & Mauviel, A. (2005) Crosstalk Mechanisms between the Mitogen-activated Protein Kinase Pathways and Smad Signaling Downstream of TGF-β: Implications for Carcinogenesis. *Oncogene*, Vol. 24, No. 37, (August 2005), pp. 5742-5750

Kamaraju, A.K., & Roberts, A.B. (2005) Role of Rho/ROCK and p38 MAP Kinase Pathways in Transforming Growth Factor- β-mediated Smad-dependent Growth Inhibition of Human Breast Cancer cells in vivo. *Journal of Biological Chemistry*, Vol. 280, No. 2, (January 2005), pp. 1024-1036

Kang, S.H., Bang, Y.J., Im, Y.H., Yang, H.K., Lee, D.A., Lee, H.Y., Lee, H.S., Kim, N.K., & Kim, S.-J. (1999) Transcriptional Repression of the Transforming Growth Factor β Type I Receptor Gene by DNA Methylation Results in the Development of TGF-β Resistance in Human Gastric Cancer. *Oncogene*, Vol. 18, No. 51, (December 1999), pp. 7280-7286

Kang, Y., Prentice, M.A., Mariano, J.M., Davarya, S., Linnoila, R.I., Moody, T.W., Wakefield, L.M., & Jakowlew, S.B. (2000) Transforming Growth Factor-β1 and its Receptors in Human Lung Cancer and Mouse Lung Carcinogenesis. *Experimental Lung Research*, Vol. 26, No. 8, (December 2000), pp. 685-707

Kawate, S., Takenoshita, S., Ohwada, S., Mogi, A., Fukusato, T., Makita, F., Kuwano, H., & Morishita, Y. (1999) Mutation Analysis of the Transforming Growth Factor β Type II Receptor, Smad2, and Smad4 in Hepatocellular Carcinoma. *International Journal of Oncology*, Vol. 14, No. 1, (January 1999), pp. 127-131

Kim, K.Y., Kim, B.C., Xu, Z., & Kim, S.-J. (2004) Mixed Lineage Kinase 3 (MLK3)-activated p38 MAP Kinase Mediates Transforming Growth Factor-β-induced Apoptosis in Hepatoma Cells. *Journal of Biological Chemistry*, Vol. 279, No. 28, (July 2004), pp. 29478-29484

Kim, S.-J., Im, Y.-H., Markowitz, S.D., Bang, & Y.J. (2000) Molecular Mechanisms of Inactivation of TGF-β Receptors During Carcinogenesis. *Cytokine & Growth Factor Reviews*, Vol. 11, No. 1-2, (March-June 2000), pp. 159-168

Kishimoto, T., Akira, S., Narazaki, M., & Taga, T. (1995) Interleukin-6 Family of Cytokines and GP130. *Blood*, Vol. 86, No. 4, (August 1995), pp. 1243-1254

Kong, F.M., Washington, M.K., Jirtle, R.L., & Anscher, M.S. (1996) Plasma Transforming Growth Factor-β1 Reflects Disease Status in Patients with Lung Cancer after Radiotherapy: A Possible Tumor Marker. *Lung Cancer*, Vol. 16, No. 1, (December 1996), pp. 47-59

Larisch, S., Yi, Y., Lotan, R., Kerner, H., Eimerl, S., Parks, T.W., Gottfried, Y., Birkey Reffey, S., De Caestecker, M.P., Danielpour, D., Book-Melamed, N., Timberg, R., Duckett, C.S., Lechleider, R.J., Steller, H., Orly, J., Kim, S.-J., & Roberts, A.B. (2000) A Novel Mitochondrial Septin-like Protein, ARTS, Mediates Apoptosis Dependent on its P-Loop Motif. *Nature Cell Biology*, Vol. 2, No. 12, (December 2000), pp. 915-921

Le, H.-V., Minn, A.J., & Massagué, J. (2005) Cyclin-dependent Kinase Inhibitors Uncouple Cell Cycle Progression from Mitochondrial Apoptotic Functions in DNA-damaged Cancer Cells. *Journal of Biological Chemistry*, Vol. 35, No. 36, (September 2005), pp. 32018-32025

Lu, S.L., Zhang, W.C., Akiyama, Y., Nomizu, T., & Yuasa, Y. (1996) Genomic structure of the Transforming Growth Factor β type II Receptor Gene and its Mutations in Hereditary Nonpolyposis Colorectal Cancers. *Cancer Research*, Vol. 56, No. 20, (October 1996), pp. 4595-4598

Luethy, J. D., Fargnoli, J., Park, J. S., Fornace, A. J., Jr., & Holbrook, N. J. (1990) Isolation and Characterization of the Hamster gadd153 Gene. Activation of Promoter Activity by Agents that Damage DNA. *Journal of Biological Chemistry*, Vol. 265, No. 27, (September 1990), pp. 16521-16526

Luttges, J., Galehdari, H., Brocker, V., Schwarte-Waldhoff, I., Henne-Bruns, D., Kloppel, G., Schmiegel, W., Hahn, S.A. (2001) Allelic Loss is Often the First Hit in the Biallelic Inactivation of the p53 and DPC4 Genes During Pancreatic Carcinogenesis. *American Journal of Pathology*, Vol. 158, No. 5, (May 2001), pp. 1677-1683

Maitra, A., Molberg, K., Albores-Saavedra, J., & Lindberg, G. (2000) Loss of Dpc4 Expression in Colonic Adenocarcinomas Correlates with the Presence of Metastatic Disease. *American Journal of Pathology*, Vol. 157, No. 4, (October 2000), pp. 1105-1111

Major, M. B., & Jones, D. A. (2004) Identification of a gadd45b 3' Enhancer that Mediates SMAD3- and SMAD4-dependent Transcriptional Induction by Transforming Growth Factor-β. *Journal of Biological Chemistry*, Vol. 279, No. 7, (February 2004), pp. 5278-5287

Malkinson, A. M., Dwyer-Nield, L. D., Rice, P. L., & Dinsdale, D. (1997) Mouse Lung Epitheliall Cell Lines-Tools for the Study of Differentiation and the Neoplatsic Phenotype. *Toxicology*, Vol. 123, No. 1-2, (November 1997), pp. 53-100

Massagué, J. (1998) TGF-β Signal Transduction. *Annual Review of Biochemistry*, Vol. 67, pp. 753-791

Markowitz, S., Wang, J., Myeroff, L., Parsons, R., Sun, L., Lutterbaugh, J., Fan, R.S., Zborowska, E., Kinzler, K.W., Vogelstein, B., Brattain, M.G., & Willson, J.K.V. (1995) Inactivation of the Type II TGF-β Receptor in Colon Cancer cells with Microsatellite Instability. *Science*, Vol. 268, No. 5215, (June 1995), pp. 1336-1338

Massagué, J. (2000) How Cells Read TGF-β Signals. *Nature Reviews in Molecular and Cell Biology*, Vol. 1, No. 3, (December 2000), pp. 169-178

Massagué, J., Blain, S.W., & Lo, R.S. (2000) TGF-β Signaling in Growth Control, Cancer, and Heritable Disorders. *Cell*, Vol. 103, No. 2, (October 2000), pp. 295-309

Massagué, J., & Wotton, D. (2000) Transcriptional Control by the TGF-β/Smad Signaling System. *EMBO Journal*, Vol. 19, No. 8, (April 2000), pp. 1745-1754

Maytin, E. V., Ubeda, M., Lin, J. C., & Habener, J. F. (2001) Stress-inducible Transcription Factor CHOP/gadd153 Induces Apoptosis in Mammalian Cells via p38 Kinase-Dependent and -Independent Mechanisms. *Experimental Cell Research*, Vol. 267, No. 2, (July 2001), pp. 193-204

Minn, A.J., Kang, Y., Serganova, I., Gupta, G.P., Giri, D.D., Doubrovin, M., Ponomarev, V., Gerald, W.L., Blasberg, R., & Massagué, J. (2005) Distinct Organ-specific Metastatic Potential of Individual Breast Cancer Cells and Primary Tumors. *Journal of Clinical Investigation*, Vol. 115, No. 1, (January 2005), pp. 44-55

Mita, H., Tsutsui, J., Takekawa, M., Witten, E. A., & Saito, H. (2002) Regulation of MTK1/MEKK4 Kinase Activiity by its Autoinhibitory Domain and GADD45 Binding. *Molecular and Cellular Biology*, Vol. 22, No. 13, (July 2002), pp. 4544-4555

Montuenga, L.M., Mariano, J.M., Prentice, M.A., Cuttitta, F., & Jakowlew, S.B. (1998) Coordinate Expression of Transforming Growth Factor-β1 and Adrenomedullin in Rodent Embryogenesis. *Endocrinology*, Vol. 139, No. 9, (September 1998), pp. 3946-3957

Moodley, Y. P., Misso, N. L., Scaffidi, A. K., Fogel-Petrovic, M., McAnulty, R. J., Laurent, G. J., Thompson, P. J., & Knight, D. A. (2003) Inverse Effects of Interleukin-6 on Apoptosis of Fibroblasts from Pulmonary Fibrosis and Normal Lungs. *American Journal of Respiratory, Cell and Molecular Biology*, Vol. 29, No.4, (October 2003), pp. 490-498

Moses, H.L., Tucker, R.F., Leof, E.B., Coffey, R.J. Jr., Halper, J., & Shipley, G.D. (1985) Type β Transforming Growth Factor is a Growth Stimulator and a Growth Inhibitor. In: *Cancer Cells 3*, Feramisco, J., Ozanne, B., & Stiles, C. (Eds.), 67-71, Cold Spring Harbor Laboratory, Cold Spring Harbor, New York

Motyl, T., Grzelkowska, K., Zimowska, W., Skierski, J., Wareski, P., Ploszaj, T., & Trzeciak, L. (1998) Expression of Bcl-2 and Bax in TGF-β1-induced Apoptosis of L1210 Leukemic Cells. *European Journal of Cell Biology*, Vol. 75, No. 4, (April, 1998), pp. 367-374

Moustakas, A., & Heldin, C.-H. (2005) Non-Smad TGF-β Signals. *Journal of Cell Science*, Vol. 118, Pt. 16, (August 2005), pp. 3573-3584

Murphy, T. C., Woods, N. R., & Dickson, A. J. (2001) Expression of the Transcription Factor GADD153 is an Indicator of Apoptosis for Recombinant Chinese Hamster Ovary (CHO) Cells. *Biotechnology and Bioengineering*, Vol. 75, No. 6, (December 2001), pp. 621-629

Öklü, R., & Hesketh, R. (2000) The Latent Transforming Growth Factor-β Binding Protein (LTBP) Family. *Biochemical Journal*, Vol. 352, Pt. 3, (December 2000), pp. 601-610

Pardali, K., Kowanetz, M., Heldin, & C.-H. Moustakas A. (2005) Smad Pathway-specific Transcriptional Regulation of the Cell Cycle Inhibitor p21(WAF1/Cip1). *Journal of Cellular Physiology*, Vol. 204, No. 1, (July 2005), pp. 260-272

Parekh, T.V., Gama, P., Wen, X., Demopoulos, R., Munger, J.S., Carcangiu, M.L., Reiss, M., & Gold, L.I. (2002) Transforming Growth Factor β Signaling is Disabled Early in Human Endometrial Carcinogenesis Concomitant with Loss of Growth Inhibition. *Cancer Research*, Vol. 62, No. 10, (May 2002), pp. 2778-2790

Park, S.H. (2005). Fine Tuning and Cross-talking of TGF-β Signal by Inhibitory Smads. *Journal of Biochemistryand Molecular Biology*, Vol. 38, No. 1, (January 2005), pp. 9-16

Park, J.I., Lee, M. G., Cho, K., Park, B. J., Chae, K. S., Byun, D. S., Ryu, B. K., Park, Y. K., & Chi, S. G. (2003) Transforming Growth Factor-β1 Activates Interleukin-6 Expression in Prostate Cancer Cells through the Synergistic Collaboration of the Smad2, p38-NF-κB, JNK, and Ras Signaling Pathways. *Oncogene*, Vol. 22, No. 28, (July 2003), pp. 4314-4332

Park, J. S., Luethy, J. D., Wang, M. G., Fargnoli, J., Fornace, A. J., Jr., McBride, O. W., & Holbrook, N. J. (1992) Isolation, Characterization and Chromosomal Localization of the Human GADD153 Gene. *Gene*, Vol. 116, No. 2, (July 1992), pp. 259-267

Riggins, G.J., Thiagalingam, S., Rozenblum, E., Weinsten, C.L., Kern, S.E., Hamilton, S.R., Wilson, J.K.V., Markowitz, S.D., Kinzler, K.W., & Vogelstein, B. (1996) Mad-related Genes in the Human. *Nature*, Vol. 13, No. 3, (July 1996), pp. 347-349

Ron, D., & Habener, J. F. (1992) CHOP, a Novel Developmentally Regulated Nuclear Protein that Dimerizes with Transcription Factors C/EBP and LAP and Functions as a Dominant-Negative Inhibitor of Gene Transcription. *Genes & Development*, Vol. 6, No. 3, (March 1992), pp. 439-453

Saltzman, A., Munro, R., Searfoss, G., Franks, C., Jaye, M., & Ivashchenko, Y. (1998) Transforming Growth Factor-β-mediated Apoptosis in the Ramos B-Lymphoma Cell line is Accompanied by Caspase Activation and Bcl-XL Downregulation. *Experimental Cell Research*, Vol. 242, No. 1, (July 1998), pp. 244-254

Sanchez-Capelo, A. (2005) Dual Role for TGF-β1 in Apoptosis. *Cytokine & Growth Factor Reviews*, Vol. 16, No. 1, (February 2005), pp. 15-34

Schiemann, W.P., Pfeifer, W.M., Levi, E., Kadin, M.E., & Lodish, H.F. (1999) A Deletion in the Gene for Transforming Growth Factor β Type I Receptor Abolishes Growth Regulation by Transforming Growth Factor β in a Cutaneous T-Cell Lymphoma. *Blood*, Vol. 94, No. 8, (October 1999), pp.2854-2861

Schiffer, M., Bitzer, M., Roberts, I.S., Kopp, J.B., ten Dijke, P., Mundel, P., & Böttinger, E.P. (2001) Apoptosis in Podocytes induced by TGF-β and Smad7. *Journal of Clinical Investigation*, Vol. 108, No. 6, (September 2001), pp. 807-816

Schlapbach, R., Spanaus, K.S., Malipiero, U., Lens, S., Tasinato, A., Tschopp, J., & Fontana, A. (2000) TGF-β Induces the Expression of the FLICE-inhibitory Protein and Inhibits Fas-mediated Apoptosis of Microglia. *European Journal of Immunology*, Vol. 30, No. 12, (December 2000), pp. 3680-3688

Schmittgen, T. D., Lee, E.J., Jiang, J., Sarkar, A., Yang, L., Elton, T.S., & Chen, C. (2008) Real-time PCR Quantification of Precursor and Mature MicroRNA. *Methods*, Vol. 44, No. 1, (January 2008), pp. 31-38

Schulte-Hermann, R., Bursch, W., Kraupp-Grasl, B., Oberhammer, F., Wagner, A., & Jirtle, R. (1993) Cell Proliferation and Apoptosis in Normal Liver and Preneoplastic Foci. *Environmental Health Perspectives*, Vol. 101 Suppl 5, (December 1993), pp. 87-90

Schuster, N., & Krieglstein, K. (2002) Mechanisms of TGF-β-Mediated Apoptosis. *Cell and Tissue Research*, Vol. 307, No. 1, (January 2002), pp. 1-14

Shahar, I., Fireman, E., Topilsky, M., Grief, J., Kivity, S., Spirer, Z., & Ben Efraim, S. (1996) Effect of IL-6 on Alveolar Fibroblast Proliferation in Interstitial Lung Diseases. *Clinical Immunology and Immunopathology*, Vol. 79, No. 3, (June 1996), pp. 244-251

Sierra, A. (2005) Metastases and their Microenvironments: Linking Pathogenesis and Therapy. *Drug Resistance Update*, Vol. 8, No. 4, (August 2005), pp. 247-257

Smith, G. J., Le Mesurier, S. M., de Montfort, M. L., & Lykke, A. W. (1984) Development and Characterization of Type 2 Pneumocyte-related Cell Lines from Normal Adult Mouse Lung. *Pathology*, Vol. 16, No. 4, (October 1984), pp. 401-405

Stander, M., Naumann, U., Wick, W., & Weller, M. (1999) TGF-β and p21: Multiple Molecular Ttargets of Decorin-mediated Suppression of Neoplastic Growth. *Cell Tissue Research*, Vol. 296, No. 2, (May 1999), pp. 221-227

Sun, L., Wu, G., Willson, J.K., Zborowska, E., Yang, J., Rajkarunanayake, I., Wang, J., Gentry, L.E., Wang, X.-F., & Brattain, M.G. (1994) Expression of Transforming Growth Factor β Type II Receptor Leads to Reduced Malignancy in Human Breast Cancer MCF-7 Cells. *Journal of Biological Chemistry*, Vol. 269, No.42 , (October 1994), pp. 26449-26455

Taga, T. (1997) The Signal Transducer GP130 is Shared by Interleukin-6 Family of Haematopoietic and Neurotrophic Cytokines. *Annals of Medicine*, Vol. 29, No. 1, (February 1997), pp. 63-72

Takanami, I., Tanaka, F., Hashizume, T., Kikuchi, K., Yamamoto, Y., Yamamoto, T., & Kodaira, S. (1997) Transforming Growth Factor-β Isoforms Expressions in Pulmonary Adenocarcinomas as Prognostic Markers: An Immunohistological Study of One Hundred and Twenty Patients. *Oncology*, Vol. 54, No. 2, (March-April 1997), pp. 122-128

Takekawa, M., & Saito, H. (1998) A Family of Stress-inducible GADD45-like Proteins Mediate Activation of the Stress-Responsive MTK1/MEKK4 MAPKKK. *Cell*, Vol. 95, No. 4, (November 1998), pp. 521-530

Takekawa, M., Tatebayashi, K., Itoh, F., Adachi, M., Imai, K., & Saito, H. (2002) Smad-Dependent GADD45b Expression Mediates Delayed Activation of p38 MAP Kinase by TGF-β. *EMBO Journal*, Vol. 21, No. 23, (December 2002), pp. 6473-6482

Tang, B., Böttinger, E. P., Jakowlew, S. B., Bagnall, K. M., Mariano, J., Anver, M. R., Letterio, J. J., & Wakefield, L. M. (1998) Transforming Growth Factor-β1 is a New Form of Tumor Suppressor with True Haploid Insufficiency. *Nature Medicine*, Vol. 4, No. 7, (July 1998), pp. 802-807

ten Dijke, P., Miyazono, K., & Heldin, C.-H. (2000) Signaling Inputs Converge on Nuclear Effectors in TGF-β Signaling. *Trends in Biochemical Science*, Vol. 25, No. 2, (February 2000), pp. 64-70

Teramoto, T., Kiss, A., & Thorgeirsson, S.S. (1998) Induction of p53 and Bax during TGF-β1 Initiated Apoptosis in Rat Liver Epithelial Cells. *Biochemical and Biophysical Research Communications*, Vol. 251, No. 1, (October 1998), pp. 56-60

Tucker, RF, Shipley GD, Moses HL, Holley RW: Growth Inhibitor from BSC-1 Cells Closely Related to Type β Transforming Growth Factor. *Science*, Vol. 226, No. 4675, (November 1984), pp. 705-707

Turco, A., Coppa, A., Aloe, S., Baccheschi, G., Morrone, S., Zupi, G., & Colletta, G. (1999) Overexpression of Transforming Growth Factor β- Type II Receptor Reduces Tumorigenicity and Metastatic Potential of K-ras-transformed Thyroid Cells. *International Journal of Cancer*, Vol. 80, No. 1, (January 1999), pp. 85-91

Uchida, K., Nagatake, M., Osada, H., Yatabe, Y., Kondo, M., Mitsudomi, T., Masuda, A., & Takahashi, T. (1996) Somatic *in vivo* Alterations of the JV18-1 Gene at 18q21 in Human Lung Cancers. *Cancer Research*, Vol. 56, No. 24, (December 1996), pp. 5583-5585

Undevia, N. S., Dorscheid, D. R., Marroquin, B. A., Gugliotta, W. L., Tse, R., & White, S. R. (2004) Smad and p38-MAPK Signaling Mediates Apoptotic Effects of Transforming Growth Factor-β1 in Human Airway Epithelial Cells. *American Journal of Physiology Lung Cellular and Molecular Physiology*, Vol. 287, No. 3, (September 2004), pp. L515-L524

U.S. Cancer Statistics Working Group. United States Cancer Statistics: 1999-2007 Incidence and Mortality Web-based Report. Available at: (http://apps.need.cdc.gov/uscs/)Atlanta (GA), Department of Health and Human Services, Centers for Disease Control and Prevention, and National Cancer Institute; 2010

Vincent, F., Hagiwara, K., Ke, Y., Stoner, G.D., Demetrick, D.J., & Bennett, W.P. (1996) Mutation Analysis of the Transforming Growth Factor β Type II Receptor in Sporadic Human Cancers of the Pancreas, Liver, and Breast. *Biochemical & Biophysical Research Communications*, Vol. 223, No. 3, (June 1996), pp. 561-564

Vujaskovic, Z., & Groen, H.J. (2000) TGF-β, Radiation-induced Pulmonary Injury and Lung Cancer. *International Journal of Radiation Biology*, Vol. 76, No. 4, (April 2000), pp. 511-516

Walia, B., Wang, L., Merlin, D., & Sitaraman, S. V. (2003) TGF-β Down-Regulates IL-6 Signaling in Intestinal Epithelial Cells: Critical Role of SMAD-2. *FASEB Journal*, Vol. 17, No. 14, (November 2003), pp. 2130-2132

Wang, J., Han, W., Zborowska, E., Liang, J., Wang, X., Willson, J.K.V., Sun, L., & Brattain, M.G. (1996) Reduced Expression of Transforming Growth Factor β Type I Receptor Contributes to the Malignancy of Human Colon Carcinoma Cells. *Journal of Biological Chemistry*, Vol. 271, No. 29, (July 1996), pp. 17366-17371

Wang, J., Sun, L., Myeroff, L., Wang, X., Gentry, L.E., Yang, J., Liang, J., Zborowska, E., Markowitz, S.D., Willson, J.K., Brattain, M.G. (1995) Demonstration that Mutation of the type II Transforming Growth Factor β Receptor Inactivates its Tumor Suppressor Activity in Replication Error-positive Colon Carcinoma Cells. *Journal of Biological Chemistry*, Vol. 270, No. 37, (September 1995), pp. 22044-22049

Whitman, M. (1997) Signal Transduction. Feedback from Inhibitory SMADs. *Nature*, Vol. 389, No. 6651, (October 1997), pp. 549-551

Wrana, J.L., & Attisano, L. (2000) The Smad Pathway. *Cytokine & Growth Factor Reviews*, Vol. 11, No. 1-2, (March-June 2000), pp. 5-13

Xie, W., Bharathy, S., Kim, D., Haffty, B.G., Rimm, D.L., & Reiss, M. (2003) Frequent Alterations of Smad Signaling in Human Head and Neck Squamous Cell Carcinomas: A Tissue Microarray Study. *Oncology Research*, Vol. 14, No. 2, (February 2003), pp. 61-73

Xie, W., Mertens, J.C., Reiss, D.J., Rimm, D.L., Camp, R.L., Haffty, B.G., & Reiss, M. (2002) Alterations of Smad Signaling in Human Breast Carcinoma are Associated with Poor Outcome: A Tissue Microarray Study. *Cancer Research*, Vol. 62, No. 2, (January 2002), pp. 497-505

Xie, W., Rimm, D.L., Lin, Y., Shih, W.J., & Reiss, M. (2003) Loss of Smad Signaling in Colorectal Cancer is Associated with Advanced Disease and Poor Prognosis. *Cancer Journal*, Vol. 9, No. 4, (July-August 2003), pp. 302-312

Xu, X., Brodie, S.G., Yang, X., Im, Y.H., Parks, W.T., Chen, L., Zhou, Y.X., Weinstein, M., Kim, S.-J., & Deng, C.X. (2000) Haploid Loss of the Ttumor Suppressor Smad4 (Dpc4) Initiates Gastric Polyposis and Cancer in Mice. *Oncogene*, Vol. 19, No. 15, (April 2000), pp. 1868-1874

Yan, W., Vellucci, V.F., & Reiss, M. (2000) Smad Protein Expression and Activation in Transforming Growth Factor-β Refractory Human Squamous Cell Carcinoma Cells. *Oncology Research*, Vol. 12, No. 3, (March 2000), pp. 157-167

Yanagisawa, K., Osada, H., Masuda, A., Kondo, M., Saito, T., Yatabe, Y., Takagi, K., Takahashi, T., & Takahashi, T. (1998) Induction of Apoptosis by Smad3 and Down-regulation of Smad3 Expression in Response to TGF-β in Human Normal Lung Epithelial Cells. *Oncogene*, Vol. 17, No. 13, (October 1998), pp. 1743-174

Yoo, J., Ghiassi, M., Jirmanova, L., Balliet, A. G., Hoffman, B., Fornace, A. J., Jr., Liebermann, D. A., Böttinger, E. P., & Roberts, A. B. (2003) Transforming Growth Factor-β-induced Apoptosis is Mediated by Smad-dependent Expression of GADD45b through p38 Activation. *Journal of Biological Chemistry*, Vol. 278, No. 44, (October 2003), pp. 43001-43007

Yu, L., Hebert, M. C., & Zhang, Y. E. (2002) TGF-β Receptor-Activated p38 MAP Kinase Mediates Smad-Independent TGF-β Responses, *EMBO Journal*, Vol. 21, No. 14, (July 2002), pp.3749-3759

Zavadil, J., & Böttinger, E. P. (2005) TGF-β and Epithelial-to-Mesenchymal Transitions. *Oncogene*, Vol. 24, No. 37, (August 2005), pp. 5764-5774

Zinszner, H., Kuroda, M., Wang, X., Batchvarova, N., Lightfoot, R. T., Remotti, H., Stevens, J. L., & Ron, D. (1998) CHOP is Implicated in Programmed Cell Death in Response to Impaired Function of the Endoplasmic Reticulum. *Genes & Development*, Vol. 12, No. 7, (April 1998), pp. 982-995

8

Refining the Role of Lgl, Dlg and Scrib in Tumor Suppression and Beyond: Learning from the Old Time Classics

Fani Papagiannouli[1] and Bernard M. Mechler[2,3,4]
[1]*Cell Networks–Cluster of Excellence, Centre for Organismal Studies (COS) and BIOQUANT Center, University of Heidelberg, Heidelberg,*
[2]*Department of Cell Biology, Institute of Physiology, 1st Faculty of Medicine, Charles University, Prague,*
[3]*Deutsches Krebsforschungszentrum, Heidelberg,*
[4]*VIT-University, Vellore, Tamil Nadu,*
[1,3]*Germany*
[2]*Czech Republic*
[4]*India*

1. Introduction

In the course of the 20th century the fruit fly *Drosophila melanogaster* became one of the most studied metazoans and, as all other members of this family, flies can be afflicted by various forms of neoplasia. Pioneering studies in the field of *Drosophila,* mouse somatic cells and human genetics revealed about 40 years ago that cancer development may develop from loss of function in regulatory genes controlling cell growth and differentiation (Gateff and Schneiderman 1969, Gateff 1974, Harris et al. 1969, Knudson 1971). The discovery of mutations causing neoplasia during *Drosophila* development (Gateff 1978) has revealed that cell polarity is significantly affected in the tumor cells. Application of molecular biology for the study of genes controlling *Drosophila* development led to the isolation and characterization of the first tumor suppressor gene (TSG), the *lethal (2) giant larvae (lgl)* (Mechler, McGinnis and Gehring 1985) and consequently placed *Drosophila* at the center of cancer research. *lgl* encodes a cytosolic protein with two WD40 motifs, involved in protein-protein interactions (Wodarz 2000). Lgl can bind to non-muscle myosin II and to the cytoskeleton matrix, along the baso-lateral portion of the plasma membrane in epithelial cells to affect cell polarization (Jakobs et al. 1996, Strand et al. 1994a, Strand, Raska and Mechler 1994b). In addition, Lgl can be a critical factor in the process of steroid-induced cell death during metamorphosis, a process which happens to be independent from the cell polarity function (Farkas and Mechler 2000). Similar to *lgl*, mutations in *discs large-1 (dlg)* and *scribble (scrib)* TSGs can cause tissue overgrowth phenotypes, as homozygous mutations in these genes lead to neoplastic transformation, thereby leading to imaginal disc overgrowth and brain tumors. In these tumors the overproliferating epithelial cells become rounded, rather than polygonal, lose their ability to terminally differentiate and fail to organize an epithelial monolayer (Bilder 2004). *dlg, scrib* and *lgl* mutants fail to pupariate and have a prolonged larval life during which they grow enormously in size and become "giant", bloated and transparent (Papagiannouli 2003). Further analysis revealed defects in apical-basal polarity, followed by loss of epithelial structure; therefore, all three TSGs are classified also as "cell polarity genes" (Wodarz 2000, Woods et al. 1996, Bilder and Perrimon 2000, Li et al. 2001). Dlg is a protein of the MAGUK (membrane - associated guanylate kinases) family, which consists of a class of scaffolding proteins that recruit signaling molecules into localized multimolecular complexes. Dlg localizes at the cytoplasmic side of septate junctions between adjacent epithelial cells, as well as in neuromuscular junctions. It contains 3 PDZ domains involved in protein-protein interactions with membrane or cytoskeletal proteins, an SH3 domain and a GUK domain. The Scrib protein is also a septate junctional protein of the LAP family (Bryant and Huwe 2000), containing four PDZ domains and leucine-rich repeats (LRRs) (Bilder 2001, Wodarz 2000, Mathew et al. 2002) thought to be involved in Ras signaling (Humbert, Russell and Richardson 2003).

The Dlg, Scrib and Lgl proteins are highly conserved in sequence among different species and growing evidence suggests that they are functionally conserved to a large degree since the vertebrate homologues can rescue the polarity defects and tumorous overgrowth of the respective *Drosophila* mutants (Thomas et al. 1997b, Grifoni et al. 2004, Dow et al. 2003). There are four well characterized mammalian Dlg members: Dlg1 (hDlg/SAP97), Dlg2 (PSD-93/Chapsyn-110), Dlg3 (NE-Dlg/SAP102) and Dlg4 (PSD-95/SAP90). All display the characteristic MAGUK structural domains of the *Drosophila* homologue, are involved in polarity establishment and are dysregulated in several cancer lines. There are also two Lgl (Lgl1/Hugl1 and Lgl2/Hugl2) mammalian homologues and only one single Scrib homologue in higher vertebrates. The human Scrib (hScrib) gene shows high homology to the *Drosophila* Scrib and colocalizes with Dlg family members (Humbert et al. 2003). Similarly, loss or alterations in expression of *dlg, scrib* and *lgl* in humans are correlated with more invasive and aggressive tumors (Humbert et al. 2003, Gardiol et al. 2006, Brumby and Richardson 2003, Nakagawa et al. 2004).

2. Tumor suppressors as multitasking proteins

Over the last decades, further work revealed that junction complexes are not just static barriers, limiting the diffusion of proteins along of the cortical cell domains, but have a broader function. As polarity scaffolds are nowadays considered as dynamic organizing centers of site-specific protein targeting or exclusion from adjacent domains that provide guiding cues for signaling molecules and targeted membrane insertion (Lecuit and Wieschaus 2002), studying these classical tumor suppressors in other tissue contexts has gained new interest (Papagiannouli and Mechler 2010). Recent advances in the diverse functions of *dlg, scrib* and *lgl* have defined them as key players in numerous tissues contents and malignancies at different time points throughout development; furthermore, they have revealed their multitasking role in: 1) junction and cytoskeleton establishment, epithelial cell and planar cell polarity, 2) asymmetric neuroblast division, formation of synapses and neuromuscular junctions, nervous system and brain development including memory (Moreau et al. 2010, Chen et al. 2008) and olfaction (Ganguly, Mackay and Anholt 2003, Mao et al. 2008), 3) testis, ovaries and other organ development, 4) cancer initiation, progression and metastasis and 5) mechanism of cooperation with various signaling pathways in different tissue contexts (Ras, SWH, Dpp, JNK, Wg, Egfr etc) (Figure 1). These new and unexpected findings show that Dlg, Scrib and Lgl are dynamic cytoskeletal components which affect epithelial cell structure, polarity and growth behavior by directing the trafficking of proteins to proper plasma membrane surfaces of the cell and by organizing and stabilizing supramolecular adhesion and signaling complexes through their action as scaffolding adaptor molecules (Woods et al. 1996, Bilder, Li and Perrimon 2000, Harris and Lim 2001, Goode and Perrimon 1997, Lee et al. 2003, Gorczyca et al. 2007, Mahoney et al. 2006, Thomas et al. 2000, Chen and Featherstone 2005, Bilder 2001, Humbert et al. 2003).

2.1 Tumor suppressors in polarity establishment and functional cooperation with other polarity and signaling complexes

Epithelial cells are polarized, with apical and baso-lateral domains. These domains are characterized by different components: outer-membrane, trans-membrane and inner-membrane proteins. A belt of adherens junctions (AJs) forming the zonula adherens (ZA) separates the apical domain of the cell membrane from its baso-lateral domain. The ZA complex consists of E-cadherin (E-cad), α-catenin, and Armadillo (the *Drosophila* β-catenin), and serves as a contact interface between neighboring cells and the cytoskeleton. Apically located components include the "Par-complex" consisting of Bazooka/Par3 (multi-PDZ containing protein), *Drosophila* atypical protein kinase C (aPKC), and DmPAR6 (a single-PDZ containing protein) and the "Crumbs-complex" consisting of Crumbs (a trans-membrane protein) and Stardust (a MAGUK protein). The septate junctions are situated in a region underneath the ZA, serve as a barrier, limiting the diffusion of membrane proteins and separate the apical from the basal components. In septate junctions the "Dlg-complex" includes Dlg, Scrib, and Camguk (Cask or Lin2, a MAGUK protein) (Mathew et al. 2002, Humbert et al. 2003), whereas the Lgl protein accumulates at the baso-lateral cortical matrix. In vertebrates the septate junctions are replaced by tight junctions, which are apical rather than basal to the adherens junctions and are composed of two integral membrane proteins, the Occludins and Claudins, and the proteins of the MAGUK family ZO-1, ZO-2 and ZO-3.
In the *Drosophila* embryonic epidermis, mutations in *dlg*, *scrib* or *lgl* cause leakage of the apical protein Crumbs (Bilder et al. 2000, Bilder and Perrimon 2000). *crumbs* overexpression induces expansion of the apical domain and affects the formation of AJs (Wodarz et al. 1995, Grawe et al. 1996), similar to the *scrib* mutant phenotype (Bilder and Perrimon 2000), suggesting that laterally located tumor suppressor proteins regulate apical membrane polarity. Genetic analysis revealed antagonistic interactions between the apical Crumbs- and the lateral Dlg-complex, as *crumbs* and *stardust* mutants are rescued by mutations in *dlg*, *scrib* or *lgl* (Bilder, Schober and Perrimon 2003, Tanentzapf and Tepass 2003). Crumbs has one cytoplasmic motif that links it to the spectrin and actin cytoskeleton and one that interacts with polarity-regulatory factors such as Par6 and Stardust (Bulgakova and Knust 2009). The Par-complex plays a critical role in this antagonistic interaction (Humbert, Dow and Russell 2006), as it restricts the Crumbs-complex apically, and the Par- and Crumbs- complexes act together to exclude the Dlg-complex from the apical membrane (Humbert et al. 2006, Bilder et al. 2003, Tanentzapf and Tepass 2003). This spatial segregation is facilitated by a biochemical interaction between the Scrib and Par complexes through Lgl (Hutterer et al. 2004, Plant et al. 2003, Yamanaka et al. 2003, Betschinger, Mechtler and Knoblich 2003, Langevin et al. 2005). Moreover, in the *Drosophila* ectoderm, phosphorylation of aPKC is required for Lgl to establish the lateral domain and to prevent apical Lgl recruitment (Wirtz-Peitz and Knoblich 2006, Hutterer et al. 2004).

In *Xenopus*, Lgl2 and aPKC act antagonistically to mutually regulate their localization and the establishment of apical-basal polarity in blastomeres (Chalmers et al. 2005). In Mardin-Darby Canine kidney (MDCK) epithelial cells, studies of overexpression and RNAi-induced loss of function revealed that Lgl facilitates the establishment of apical-basal polarity through actively suppressing the formation of the Par-complex formation at the basal domain (Humbert et al. 2006, Yamanaka et al. 2003, Yamanaka et al. 2006). In zebrafish, Lgl2 mutants show an epithelial-to-mesenchymal transition in basal epidermal cells, with loss of hemidesmosome formation and an increase in migratory behavior (Sonawane et al. 2005). At the same time, Lgl2 positively regulates hemidesmosome formation by mediating Integrin alpha 6 (Itga6)-targeting and maintaining its localization, while E-cad negatively regulates Itga6 targeting (Sonawane et al. 2009). Localization of aPKCλ in the basal epidermis is tightly correlated with Itga6 localization and hemidesmosome formation (Sonawane et al. 2009). The role of Lgl and the Par-complex was also analyzed in the polarity establishment of the early *C. elegans* embryo, where they maintain two cortical domains which are sufficient to partition cell fate determinants in the *C. elegans* embryo, by a mechanism of "mutual exclusion" (Hoege et al. 2010). Lgl1 interacts with Par-2 in the posterior of the embryo, but Lgl1 can also compensate the function of Par-2 and restrict the anterior localization of the Par-complex, through a mechanism that involves Lgl phosphorylation (Hoege et al. 2010) and a negative regulation of non-muscle myosin-II at the posterior cortex (Beatty, Morton and Kemphues 2010)

Of particular interest are studies that relate the adenomatous polyposis coli (APC) tumour suppressor to the mammalian Dlg homologues. Dlg1 was isolated in a yeast-two-hybrid screen and was found to directly interact with APC (Humbert et al. 2003, Ishidate et al. 2000). Dlg3 also binds APC, thereby showing that this interaction is probably a common feature of Dlg family members. In the migrating astrocytes, vertebrate Dlg1 binds APC at the leading edge of migrating cells (Etienne-Manneville et al. 2005). In particular, activation of the Par6-PKCζ complex by Cdc42, at the leading edge of migrating cells, promotes the localized association of APC with microtubule plus ends and the assembly of Dlg-containing puncta in the plasma membrane. Scrib also binds APC (Takizawa et al. 2006). As Dlg and Scrib can bind the Wnt signaling component APC, one could hypothesize that loss of Scrib or Dlg could interfere with the normal regulation of the APC-β-catenin complex, thereby leading to pro-migratory effects, if β-catenin is stabilized and allowed to move to the nucleus (Humbert et al. 2006).

In addition, Dlg, Scrib and Lgl play an important role in dorsal closure (DC), during which, the migration of the lateral epidermal leading edge (LE) cells closes the hole of the *Drosophila* dorsal epidermis. Loss of *lgl* results in defective DC (Manfruelli et al. 1996, Arquier et al. 2001) and loss of *scrib* together with one allele of *dlg* also results in incomplete DC (Bilder et al. 2000). Recent studies have shown that during DC the LE cells undergo a mesenchymal-to-epithelial-like transition, during which integrin-mediated localization of the PAK serine/threonine kinase recruits Scrib in septate junction formation, required for epithelial plasticity (Bahri et al. 2010). Wound healing is very similar to the DC in *Drosophila* and Scrib is here again a critical player in the polarization of migrating cells. During wound healing in the astrocytes, Scrib controls Cdc42 through its association with the exchange factor βPIX (Osmani et al. 2006). By regulating Cdc42 activity, Scrib acts upstream of Dlg1 and is involved in the same molecular pathway controlling cell orientation. Cdc42 controls two distinct signaling pathways, promoting: 1) Rac- and PAK-dependent protrusion formation and 2) centrosome and Golgi reorientation through APC clustering and Dlg1 localization at the LE (Osmani et al. 2006).

The role of Dlg, Scrib and Lgl has also been studied in other tissue - specific epithelia. Dlg-1 and Scrib are widely distributed throughout the eye in embryonic and postnatal development and overlap with E-cad and ZO-1 in portions of the cornea and retinal pigment epithelium; in contrast, little, if any, overlap with adhesion proteins is observed in the neural retina (Nguyen, Rivera and Griep 2005). Dlg1 was shown to be required for the development of lens epithelium in a cell autonomous manner as Dlg1 ablation leads to cell structure alterations and disposition of adhesion and cytoskeletal factors such as α-catenin (Rivera et al. 2009). In the intestinal epithelium, Scrib regulates the integrity and plasticity of the epithelial barrier and TJ formation, by binding to the scaffolding protein ZO-1, independently of Lgl1 and Dlg1. The observation that Scrib is downregulated during intestinal inflammation provides the missing link to tumor development during chronic intestinal inflammation (Ivanov et al. 2010). Dlg1 localization at the basolateral side of the intestinal epithelium requires CASK, another MAGUK protein, however *dlg1* mutations there cannot affect epithelial polarity (Lozovatsky et al. 2009). Data from the *C. elegans* intestinal epithelium show that Arp2/3, which promotes nucleation of branched actin, junction initiation and maturation, affects the subcellular distribution of Dlg (Bernadskaya et al. 2011).

Dlg, Scrib and Lgl are also important in follicular epithelium morphogenesis and subsequent polarization of the *Drosophila* oocyte, albeit in a different way as in other epithelia. The work of several groups has shown that Lgl is an essential regulator of posterior follicle cells and that phosphorylation of Lgl together with Par-1 and Par-3 is required for the posterior translocation of oocyte-specific proteins and germline determinants (Fichelson et al. 2010, Doerflinger et al. 2010, Li et al. 2008). Mutation of the aPKC phosphorylation site in Par-1 results in the uniform cortical localization of Par-1 and the loss of cortical microtubules (Doerflinger et al. 2010). Dlg and Scrib are required differentially for patterning in both the anterior and posterior follicular epithelium (Li et al. 2009) and genetically interact with Lgl for posterior follicle cell induction (Li et al. 2011), suggesting a common regulatory pathway in this process. At the same time, Lgl functions in a subdivision of anterior follicle cells into functionally distinct subpopulations and controls collective border cell migration at mid-oogenesis (Li et al. 2011).

The multifunctional role of these TSGs can also be seen in the diverse binding partners and regulators in various cell environments. For example, Scrib1 was found to interact with LPP, a zyxin-related protein, which has been described as a partner in fusion proteins associated with different types of cancers (Petit et al. 2005, Lelievre 2010). Both Scrib and LPP localize at cell-cell contacts whereas LPP is also localized in the focal adhesions and the nucleus. This interaction links Scrib to a communication pathway between cell-cell contacts and the nucleus (Petit et al. 2005). A nuclear shuttling mechanism has also been described for Dlg1 (Carr et al. 2009). Mammalian Scrib regulates also E-cad activity by stabilizing E-cad coupling to catenins (Qin et al. 2005). The stability and function of the mammalian Lgl is regulated by direct binding to the scaffolding RanBPM, a Ran-binding protein (Suresh et al. 2010). Moreover, Dlg1, which is highly expressed in embryonic and adult tissues such as the brain, kidney, ovaries, olfactory bulb and cerebellum, can interact with Dlg3 (Mao et al. 2008). In addition, Dlg1 can interact with the gap junction protein Connexin-32 through its SH3 domain (Duffy et al. 2007). Recent work on caspase target genes has provided evidence that Dlg1 is a direct target of caspase-3 and the unique cleavage site identified separates the C-terminal part of Dlg1 (containing PDZ3, SH3 and GUK domain) from the rest of the protein. Interestingly, this exact C-terminal part is missing from the classical null allele (*dlg*^{m52}) of the *Drosophila* Dlg mutant protein (Gregorc et al. 2005). This cleavage of Dlg1 results in translocation away from sites of cell-cell contacts and is presumably an early step in disassembly of septate and adherens junctions and consequently intercellular detachment (Gregorc et al. 2005).

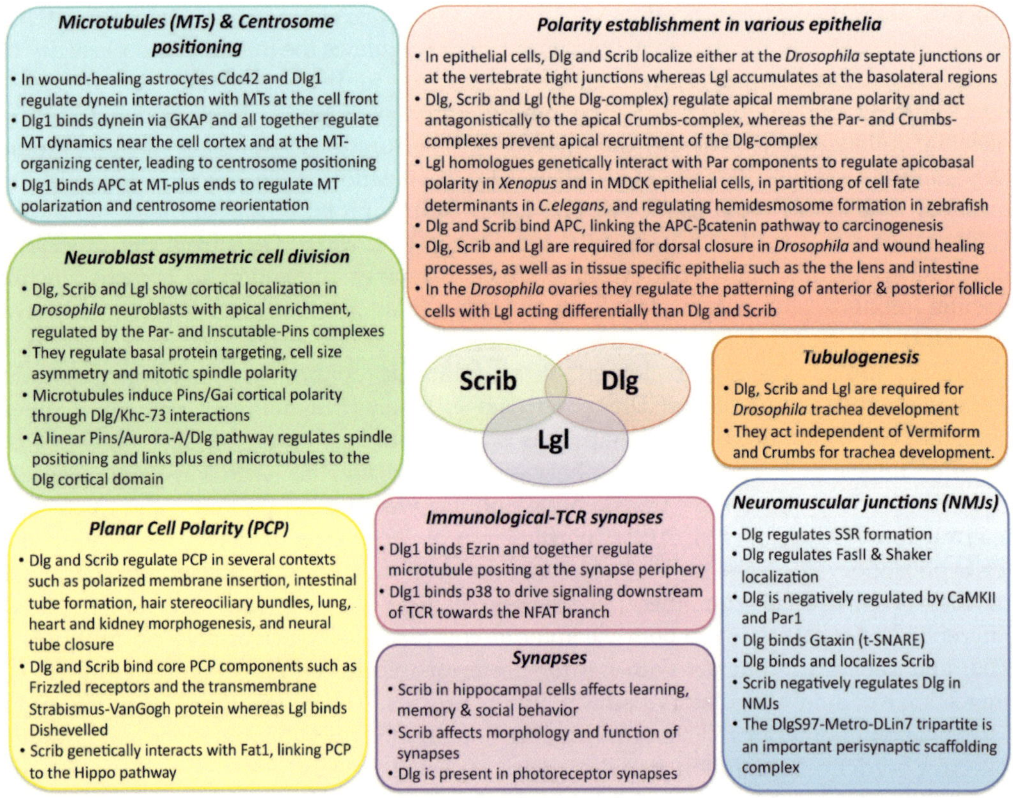

Fig. 1. Overview of the multitasking role of Dlg, Scrib and Lgl in different cellular and tissue contexts.

Dlg is also involved in T-cell receptor (TCR) signaling (Round et al. 2007), as Dlg1 downregulation blocks TCR-induced activation of p38 and the transcription factor NFAT, but not the alternative protein kinase JNK or the NF-κB transcription factor. Dlg1 directly binds p38, to drive signaling downstream of TCR towards the NFAT branch of the cascade and it has been shown to act as an orchestrator of TCR specificity (Round et al. 2007). Rho signaling plays an important role in TJ function and several studies of dominant active and negative mutants of *rhoA*, *Rac* and *cdc42* revealed that they all disrupt the barrier function of TJs, with the most intense effect obtained with dominant active *rhoA* mutants (Gonzalez-Mariscal, Tapia and Chamorro 2008). The RhoA/ROCK signaling pathway participates both in the assembly and disassembly of TJs. Moreover PKN1, a Rho effector protein, participates in the regulation of TJ sealing in the mammary gland by interfering with glycocorticoid signaling, consistent with observations that Rho activation perturbates TJ function in various experimental systems (Fischer et al. 2007). Furthermore, Net1 (neuroepithelioma transforming gene), a RhoGEF specific for the RhoA subfamily of small G proteins, interacts with the PDZ domains of Dlg1 and relocalizes Dlg1 to the nucleus whereas the oncogenic mutant of Net1 sequesters Dlg1 in the cytosol (Garcia-Mata et al. 2007). In particular, Net1 binding to Dlg1 in MCF7 breast cells, which is regulated by E-cad-mediated cell-cell interaction, enhances Net stability and increases Net1 ability to stimulate RhoA activation in these cells (Carr et al. 2009).

2.2 Dlg, Scrib and Lgl in planar cell polarity

The planar cell polarity (PCP) pathway, incorporating the non-canonical Wnt pathway, is best known for directing polarization of cells orthogonal to the apical-basal polarity axis within the plane of an epithelium. Apart from regulating the patterning of external epidermal structures such as wing hair cells in *Drosophila* and ciliary orientation, PCP controls embryonic convergent extension (CE), polarized cell division, cell direction and movement (Yates et al. 2010a). *dlg, scrib* and *lgl* are essential for planar cell polarity (PCP), by establishing a cross-talk between apical-basal and planar cell polarity. Dlg and Scrib have been shown to bind components of the core PCP machinery, including Frizzled receptors and the membrane protein Strabismus/Van Gogh (Stbm/Vang) (Montcouquiol et al. 2006, Kallay et al. 2006, Lee et al. 2003, Hering and Sheng 2002). The direct interaction of Dlg4 with receptors of the Wnt signaling pathway, Frizzled 1-7, link mammalian Dlg to the Frizzled signaling (Humbert et al. 2003, Hering and Sheng 2002). Dlg1 is also required for smooth muscle orientation in the mouse ureter (Mahoney et al. 2006). In addition, Dlg binds through its PDZ1 and PDZ2 domains to Stbm/Vang in order to recruit membrane-associated proteins and lipids from internal membranes to sites of new plasma membrane formation (Lee et al. 2003). In *C. elegans,* the unique PCP protein Vang-1 interacts with the PDZ2 domain of Dlg for its proper localization, which is required for intestinal tube formation, since in *vang-1* mutant embryos the epithelial cells of the intestine are not correctly arranged along the anterior-posterior axis (Hoffmann et al. 2010). Moreover, the Pins/Dlg complex is required to establish PCP during asymmetric cell division in the sensory organ precursor cell of the notum (Bellaiche et al. 2001).

Interestingly, the mouse *scrib* gene genetically interacts with the *vangl2* gene, a mammalian homologue of the *Drosophila stbm/vang* gene, involved in PCP (Montcouquiol et al. 2003). Analysis of PCP in hair cell stereociliary bundles within the cochlea in mammals, showed that Scrib is a prerequisite for the proper localization and function of PCP proteins among which is also Vangl2 (Montcouquiol et al. 2003). Further studies revealed that both mammalian and *Drosophila* Scrib physically interact with Vangl2 (Kallay et al. 2006) and Stbm/Vang (Courbard et al. 2009) respectively, through their PDZ domains to regulate normal development in *Drosophila* wing imaginal discs (Courbard et al. 2009), heart tube and cardiomyocyte organization (Phillips et al. 2007), and neural tube closure (Wen et al. 2010, Wansleeben et al. 2011). Scrib is also implicated in PCP-mediated neural tube closure through binding to Cdx, a homeodomain transcription factor which regulates transcription of the *Ptk7* PCP gene (Savory et al. 2011). A PCP-mediated requirement of Scrib has also been demonstrated for lung development (Wansleeben et al. 2011) and branching morphogenesis (Yates et al. 2010b), for kidney-branching morphogenesis and glomerular maturation (Yates et al. 2010a), and for the tangential migration of facial branchiomotor (FBM) neurons (Walsh et al. 2011). All these later studies provide insights on a very interesting and yet poorly understood role of Scrib on PCP-mediated organogenesis and the interplay of apicobasal and PCP pathways.

Spatial organization of cells and their appendages is controlled through the PCP by a signaling cascade initiated by the protocadherin Fat in *Drosophila*. Fat acts through two distinct branches: the Fat polarity pathway and the Fat tumor suppressor/Hippo pathway. Vertebrates express four Fat molecules, Fat1-4. Indeed, Scrib provided the link between the Fat and the Hippo signaling cascade in vertebrates. Fat1 depletion causes abnormal cyst formation in the zebrafish pronephros, a phenotype underlying a strong genetic and direct interaction between Fat1 and Scrib. The observation that depletion of Yes-associated protein 1, a transcriptional co-activator inhibited by the Hippo pathway, ameliorated the changes caused by *fat1* and *scrib* knockdown, shows that in the absence of Scrib and Fat1, it is the deregulation of the Hippo pathway which contributes to the formation of abnormal pronephric cysts (Skouloudaki et al. 2009).

As already mentioned, the non-canonical Wnt/Wg pathway plays a central role in PCP. A key switch at its branch point appears to be the Dishevelled (Dsh) protein, which is required for both PCP and the canonical Arm/β-Catenin pathway (Wodarz and Gonzalez). Interestingly, a physical and functional interaction has been reported between Lgl and the signaling protein Dishevelled (Dsh) (Dollar et al. 2005). Asymmetric localization of Dsh leads to spatially defined areas of Lgl upregulation, which allows directional tissue morphogenesis and PCP organization of epithelial sheets in *Drosophila* embryos (Kaplan and Tolwinski 2010). In humans, Lgl2 plays a critical role in branching morphogenesis during placental development. Lgl2 regulates cell polarization and polarized-cell invasion guiding trophoblast invasion, yet a connection to the PCP pathway is not established so far (Sripathy, Lee and Vasioukhin 2011).

2.3 Orientation of cell division, spindle, microtubule and centrosome positioning

Orientation of cell division is important in establishing and maintaining normal development and tissue homeostasis from bacteria to mammals. A correct cell division plane is critical during asymmetric cell division, spindle orientation, microtubule and centrosome positioning. Several studies point out the key roles of Dlg, Scrib and Lgl in multiple aspects of cell division orientation.

One of the most well studied systems is the asymmetric division of the *Drosophila* neural stem cells, the so-called embryonic neuroblasts. These studies indicate that *dlg, scrib* and *lgl* have a function in the correct placement of cell-fate determinants, in dividing neuroblasts. Dysregulation of the mechanisms, which control the neuroblast asymmetric division, results in compromised inheritance of cell-fate determinants, triggers neoplastic transformation and promotes brain tumors (Merz et al. 1990, Caussinus and Gonzalez 2005, Betschinger, Mechtler and Knoblich 2006, Lee et al. 2006). Neuroblast division gives rise to a larger daughter cell that remains a neuroblast and a smaller daughter cell that becomes a ganglion mother cell (GMC). This process involves the segregation of the basally localized cell-fate determinants Numb, Prospero (Pros) and Brain tumor (Brat) proteins and their adaptor proteins Partner of Numb (Pon) and Miranda (Mira), into the basal GMC. This segregation is controlled by apically localized components including the Par-complex (Baz/Par3, Par6 and aPKC), as well as the Inscutable (Insc) and Partner of Inscutable (Pins) proteins. Dlg, Scrib and Lgl proteins display a cortical localization, with apical enrichment during early mitosis. Insc and Insc-dependent proteins (Insc/Par pathway) are required for the maintenance and apical enrichment of Dlg and Scrib proteins whereas Dlg controls the cortical recruitment of both Scrib and Lgl. In *dlg, scrib* and *lgl* mutants the localization of the apical proteins is normal but the basal protein targeting is defective, resulting in a reduced apical cortical domain and a smaller size of the apical spindle. Therefore, Dlg, Scrib and Lgl are important in regulating cortical polarity, cell size asymmetry and mitotic spindle asymmetry in *Drosophila* neuroblasts (Albertson and Doe 2003).

The fact that apical Dlg, Scrib and Lgl may promote apical spindle pole growth is consistent with the observation that vertebrate Dlg orthologues physically interact with known microtubule-binding proteins (Albertson and Doe 2003, Brenman et al. 1998, Niethammer et al. 1998, Matsumine et al. 1996, Hanada et al. 2000). In *Drosophila*, kinesin Khc-73 and Dlg induce cortical polarization of Pins/Gai, acting in parallel to the Insc/Par pathway. Interestingly, Khc-73 localizes to astral microtubule plus ends and the Dlg/Khc-73 and Dlg/Pins protein complexes have been found to co-immunoprecipitate, suggesting that microtubules induce Pins/Gai cortical polarity through Dlg/Khc-73 interactions (Siegrist and Doe 2005, Ahringer 2005). The recent identification of an evolutionary conserved $Pins^{LINKER}$ domain uncovered a linear $Pins^{LINKER}$/Aurora-A/Dlg spindle orientation pathway, which links the plus ends of astral microtubules to the Dlg cortical domain (Johnston et al. 2009).

Additionally, Dlg1 is important for centrosome positioning in the astrocytes. During wound-induced cell migration Cdc42 acts through Dlg1, in order to regulate the interaction of dynein with microtubules of the cell front (Manneville, Jehanno and Etienne-Manneville 2010). Dlg1 interacts with dynein via the scaffolding protein GKAP and all three proteins together control microtubule dynamics and organization near the cell cortex and at the microtubule-organizing center (MTOC), ultimately leading to centrosome positioning. Moreover, Dlg1 colocalizes with APC at microtubule plus-ends to promote microtubule polarization and centrosome reorientation (Etienne-Manneville et al. 2005, Etienne-Manneville and Hall 2003). However, the Dlg1-mediated recruitment of dynein is independent of its interaction with APC (Manneville et al. 2010). A crucial function of Dlg1 on microtubules has also been established for immunological synapses (Lasserre et al. 2010, Lasserre and Alcover 2010). Dlg1 and the cell cortex membrane-microfilament linker Ezrin are key players for synapse stability and symmetry. Ezrin silencing alters cell spreading and microtubule network organization at the immune synapse and leads to enhanced T-cell receptor (TCR) signaling (Lasserre et al. 2010). Ezrin-Dlg1 interaction keeps the microtubule architecture at the synapse, which in turn drives signaling microcluster dynamics and downregulation of the TCR receptor signaling. Similar to the role of Dlg1 in MTOC positioning during astrocyte migration (Etienne-Manneville et al. 2005), Ezrin and Dlg1 are necessary for a similar positioning of microtubules at the periphery of the immunological synapse (Lasserre et al. 2010).

Finally, Scrib is required for oriented cell division in the neural keel to promote morphogenesis of the neural tube epithelium (Zigman et al. 2011). Analysis of *scrib* mutants revealed a role of Scrib in controlling clustering of α-catenin foci in dividing progenitors that correspond to the future subapical junctional complexes of the mature epithelium. This function of Scrib, which is independent of the canonical apicobasal polarity and PCP pathways, stresses the importance of single-cell orientation for tissue-level morphogenesis (Zigman et al. 2011).

2.4 Trafficking, exocytosis and polarized membrane insertion

Exocytosis is an important membrane traffic event that mediates the transport of secreted and transmembrane proteins, as well as lipids to the cell surface (Hsu et al. 2004). This transport is highly polarized and tightly regulated, so that the molecular identity of the apical and basolateral membrane domains is maintained. It has already been proposed that the junctions in mammalian epithelial cells promote the correct spatial organization of cellular components by acting as sorting sites for a subset of vesicles (Humbert et al. 2008).

The mechanisms that specify vesicle docking and fusion of intracellular membranes rely on the SNARE proteins, with t-SNAREs localized in a polarized distribution on the target membranes and v-SNAREs on the vesicles. When a v-SNARE encounters its cognate t-SNARE they assemble into a tight complex, which brings together the apposed membranes sufficiently close to each other for fusion to occur. As an example, *Drosophila* embryos with mutated Syntaxin 1 (Syn1), a t-SNARE protein uniformly distributed on target membranes, fail to cellularize (Burgess, Deitcher and Schwarz 1997). The spatial specificity of vesicle trafficking also relies on the tethering of exocytic vesicles, at defined membrane sites, by the eight-subunit exocyst (or Sec6/7) complex. Recent work has shown that the Exo84 component of the exocyst complex is required for membrane trafficking from the recycling endosome to the cell surface and the apical localization of the transmembrane protein Crumbs, whereas the mutant phenotype is suppressed by down-regulation of the Dlg and Lgl proteins (Blankenship, Fuller and Zallen 2007). Interestingly, in yeast the Lgl homologous proteins Sro7p and Sro77p directly interact with Exo84p and the t-SNARE protein Sec9p (Zhang et al. 2005), whereas the mammalian Lgl binds Syntaxin-4, a t-SNARE protein that mediates vesicle fusion, in order to direct protein trafficking (Musch et al. 2002). As the exocyst decides not only what fuses with the plasma membrane but also the site of fusion, we can conclude that Lgl family proteins affect asymmetric protein localization by targeted vesicle fusion (Wirtz-Peitz and Knoblich 2006). Furthermore, type V myosin 2 (Myo2) physically binds Sro7 and negatively regulates Sro7 function in vesicle clustering (Rossi and Brennwald 2011). Myo2 serves in a dual function: to recruit Sro7 to secretory vesicles and to inhibit its Rab-dependent tethering activity until vesicles reach the plasma membrane. Taken together, Sro7 appears to coordinate the spatial and temporal nature of both Rab-dependent tethering and SNARE-dependent membrane fusion of exocytic vesicles with the plasma membrane (Rossi and Brennwald 2011).

Furthermore, Scrib has been shown to have an important role in regulating exocytosis in neuroendocrine cells through its association with the β-Pix-GIT1 complex (Audebert et al. 2004, Humbert et al. 2008). Scrib acts as a membrane anchor for β-Pix, a guanine exchange factor (GEF), which activates Rac1 and recruits it to a functional complex regulating exocytosis of Ca^{++}-regulated hormone release (Momboisse et al. 2009). Since small Rho-GTPases have emerged as key players in membrane trafficking and Rac isoforms have been involved in various processes of exocytosis, this recent work uncovers the actual function of Scrib, β-Pix and Rac1 in exocytosis, in addition to their well-established role in cancer (Momboisse et al. 2009).

While polarized exocytosis of proteins is one of the most studied mechanisms responsible for the maintainance of cell polarity, polarized transport of specific mRNAs represents an alternative pathway (Vasioukhin 2006). It has been demonstrated that Lgl genetically interacts and is present in a complex with the fragile X syndrome protein FMRP, which is responsible for mRNA transport (Zarnescu et al. 2005). This interesting finding suggests that Lgl may be involved in polarity by regulating the localization of specific mRNAs.

Dlg plays an important role in polarized membrane insertion during cellularization. It is known that polarized membrane growth relies on the guiding cues of junctional and peri-junctional proteins (Lecuit and Wieschaus 2002). The *Drosophila* cellularizing blastoderm provides an excellent system for studying the genetic analysis of how polarity is established, reinforced and maintained *in vivo*. During cellularization, an epithelium is formed *de novo* by growth and invagination of plasma membrane between the cortical nuclei, leading to a 20-30 fold increase of membrane surface and formation of the first columnar epithelial cells (~30μm) (Mazumdar and Mazumdar 2002). This process requires the remobilization of the intracellular membrane reservoir from the endoplasmic reticulum (ER) and Golgi. Membrane trafficking is regulated in a way that allows polarized membrane delivery, with the secretory pathway and the membrane-recycling pathway guiding the membrane deposition (Dudu, Pantazis and Gonzalez-Gaitan 2004, Strickland and Burgess 2004). In the secretory pathway, membrane proteins are recruited from post-Golgi vesicles to the lateral domain of growing membranes by the Strabismus/Van Gogh (Stbm/Vang)-Dlg complex. Dlg localizes to the plasma membrane along the newly formed invaginating membrane, whereas Stbm/Vang is localized initially to the Golgi. Both Stbm/Vang and Dlg are required for membrane deposition during cellularization and their simultaneous overexpression induces expansion of the lateral membrane (Lee et al. 2003). In the membrane-recycling pathway, the apical membrane is internalized through a Dynamin-dependent process, travels through the Rab5 early endosome and Rab11 recycling endosome acting together with Nuf, and finally becomes exocytosed at the lateral membrane (Dudu et al. 2004, Strickland and Burgess 2004, Pelissier, Chauvin and Lecuit 2003, Riggs et al. 2003, Lecuit 2004).

2.5 Critical functions in neuromuscular junctions and synapses

One of the most broadly used systems to study Dlg and Scrib function has been the neuromuscular junctions (NMJs). Dlg was shown to be present in glutamatergic larval NMJs. Glutamate receptors (GluR) in *Drosophila* NMJs are of two different types, comprised of either GluIIA (A-type) or GluIIB (B-type) subunits, as well as the common subunits GluIIC, GluIID and GluIIE (Collins and DiAntonio 2007). Dlg controls the subunit composition of the receptor by selectively stabilizing B-type receptors at the synapse, whereas Coracle is required for A-type receptors (Chen and Featherstone 2005, Chen et al. 2005). Dlg is abundantly expressed through the postsynaptic membrane surrounding the presynaptic motor axon terminals. During larval development, the postsynaptic membrane increases enormously leading to a highly convoluted and multilayered postsynaptic membrane structure, the subsynaptic reticulum (SSR). Several years of research in this field have shed light on the role of the different Dlg protein domains (Thomas et al. 2000) and their binding partners (Thomas et al. 2000, Thomas et al. 1997a, Zito et al. 1997), the role of phosphorylation on Dlg regulation (Koh et al. 1999, Beumer et al. 2002, Zhang et al. 2007) and the key role of Dlg on membrane proliferation in the SSR of GluIIB-type receptors (Chen and Featherstone 2005, Roche et al. 2002). The synaptic targeting and localization of Dlg is a stepwise process controlled by different domains of the protein (Thomas et al. 2000). The localization of the postsynaptic Dlg was also investigated during synapse remodeling of larval NMJs, whereby the adult-specific synapses are generated. During synapse dismantling, postsynaptic Dlg becomes diffuse and then undetectable, followed by SSR vacuolization, through a mechanism different than that of GluRs elimination (Liu et al. 2010b).

Dlg is important for proper NMJ establishment as *dlg-* NMJs have defects in synapse structure and function, including an increase in bouton size and number of active zones presynaptically, as well as a poorly developed SSR (Chen and Featherstone 2005). Dlg regulates SSR expansion and is also required for clustering Fasciclin II (FasII) and Shaker proteins (Thomas et al. 1997a, Zito et al. 1997). Dlg-dependent localization of FasII to the *Drosophila* GluRIIB NMJs is negatively regulated by Ca++/calmodulin dependent kinase II (CaMKII) (Koh et al. 1999), with βPS-Integrin (encoded by *myospheroid* in *Drosophila*) acting upstream of CamKII. Upon increased synapse activity, CaMKII phosphorylates Dlg, which dissociates from the synaptic protein complex, releases FasII, and allows for developmental growth in signal response (Beumer et al. 2002). However, *sh* and *fasII* mutations do not affect the SSR, meaning that Dlg plays a role in postsynaptic membrane regulation independent of its interaction to Sh and FasII (Schuster et al. 1996a, Schuster et al. 1996b). Further studies have shown that expression of a constitutively active form of CaMKII abolishes the accumulation of Dlg at synapses, while exerting no significant effect on the presynaptic area and localization of FasII (Morimoto et al. 2010). Postsynaptic targeting of Dlg is negatively regulated by PAR-1, which phosphorylates Dlg at a conserved Ser residue within the GUK domain (Zhang et al. 2007). PAR-1 and Dlg both affect pre- and post-synaptic development and function in a dose-dependent way. PAR-1 overexpression and Dlg inactivation lead both to active zone increase and SSR loss, whereas loss of PAR-1 and Dlg overexpression have the opposite effect and therefore confirm the antagonistic effect of PAR-1 on Dlg (Zhang et al. 2007). Like Dlg, Pumilio (Pum), a known transcriptional regulator of embryonic patterning and germline development, appears to have both pre- and post-synaptic effects in NMJs and is co-localized with Dlg and GluIIB-type boutons (Chen et al. 2008). Notable Pum directly regulates *dlg* by binding to the Dlg-3'UTR, thereby antagonizing the effects of Dlg on neuronal structure and/or function also in the adult mushroom bodies, the anatomical site of memory storage (Chen et al. 2008).

The *Drosophila dlg* gene codes for two isoforms, the DlgA and DlgS97 collectively referred to as Dlg, which have been individually studied in NMJs. Both isoforms are present at the NMJs, but mutations that specifically abolish DlgS97 leave FasII largely unaffected (Albornoz et al. 2008). DlgS97 exerts its function at the NMJs by binding to Metro, a novel MAGUK protein, which stabilizes the complex of DlgS97 and the adaptor protein DLin-7 (Bachmann et al. 2010). In a remarkably interdependent manner, Metro and DLin-7 act downstream of DlgS97 to control NMJ expansion and proper establishment of synaptic boutons, making this tripartite an important perisynaptic scaffolding complex (Bachmann et al. 2010).

Membrane addition by vesicle fusion commonly involves SNARE proteins. Recent work has shown that Dlg binds and controls postsynaptic localization of the t-SNARE GUK-interacting syntaxin (Gtaxin). Gtaxin is required for proper SSR expansion and controls synaptic and muscle development in a dose-dependent manner (Gorczyca et al. 2007). Gtaxin's closest Homologues, Syntaxin 18 and Ufe1p, can mediate homotypic endoplasmic reticulum (ER) membrane fusion in the absence of other known SNAREs (Lewis and Pelham 1996, Patel et al. 1998, Hatsuzawa et al. 2000). The presumptive role of

Gtaxin as part of the ER-specific vesicle fusion machinery, together with its requirement for SSR development, supports the idea that SSR bears at least some ER-like properties (Gorczyca et al. 2007).

Moreover, Dlg interacts at the synapses with Scrib, through simultaneous binding of both the Dlg-GUK domain and the Scrib-PDZ2 domain to the synaptic protein GUK-holder (Gukh) (Mathew et al. 2002). Apart from an increased number of active zones and reduced SSR, *dlg*⁻ NMJs show severe mislocalizaton of synaptic Scrib. Loss of *scrib* in NMJs results in synaptic vesicle increase, decrease in the number of active zones and a thickened basal lamina, however Dlg localization and the SSR remain unaffected (Mathew et al. 2002). Apparently, the synaptic levels of Scrib have an opposite effect than Dlg in active zone number and Scrib negatively regulates Dlg function in NMJs, in contrast to their cooperation in epithelial cells and neuroblasts (Roche et al. 2002). This probably reflects the ability of Dlg and Scrib to exert their function through binding to different protein partners with distinct functions, according to their availability in the various tissues.

Scrib is also capable of influencing the morphology and function of synapses (Moreau et al. 2010). It is expressed in the soma and dendrites of adult hippocampal pyramidal cells, to regulate neuron maturation, with the synaptic strength and plasticity severely affected in *scrib* mutant mice. In the hippocampus of these mutants, the phenotype is associated with Rac1 activation and defects in actin reorganization, which ultimately affect memory consolidation. Scrib effects on brain function and the corresponding effects on enhanced learning, memory abilities and impaired social behavior, provide a step forward in the dissection of Scrib roles in the pathophysiology of behavior (Moreau et al. 2010). Dlg is also found at the lamina of the photoreceptor synapses. Immuno-electron microscopy revealed that Dlg marks the round profiles of R1-R6 ommatidia terminals and the photoreceptor membrane around the invaginating head of capitate projection organelles, which are the organelles from the surrounding glia (Hamanaka and Meinertzhagen 2010).

2.6 Tubulogenesis and trachea development

A less studied role of these tumor suppressor genes involves their function in tubulogenesis, which is the regulation of epithelial tube morphogenesis and size control in organs such as kidney, lungs, vascular system and the *Drosophila* trachea. So far, several studies pointed the significance of septate junctional proteins in trachea tube-size regulation (Paul et al. 2003, Wu and Beitel 2004) but more recent studies reveal a novel mechanistic framework for understanding epithelial tube size regulation in trachea. In the *Drosophila* trachea, tube dimensions are regulated by the luminal extracellular matrix (ECM). ECM organization requires the apical secretion of the protein Vermiform (Verm), which depends on the basolateral septate junctions (SJs) (Wang et al. 2006, Swanson and Beitel 2006). Scrib and Yurt (Yrt), another SJ-associated protein, cause tracheal tube expansion through a Verm-independent pathway (Laprise et al. 2010). Zygotic loss of *scrib, dlg* and *lgl* result in excessively long dorsal trunks, indicating that these genes are critical for tube size control. Zygotic loss of *lgl* expression causes fully penetrant defects in SJ paracellular barrier function, whereas zygotic *scrib* and *dlg* mutants do not have compromised transepithelial barriers. Furthermore, Lgl together with Crumbs have an additional role in apical constriction of tracheal cells, independent of their apicobasal polarity function in trachea epithelial cells (Letizia et al. 2011). Interestingly, Scrib and Crumbs do not display, during trachea elongation, the antagonistic functional interactions they have during apicobasal polarity establishment (Laprise et al. 2010). Therefore, it becomes obvious that the mechanism regulating trachea morphogenesis involves functional interactions between polarity proteins, which are different from those involved in epithelial apicobasal polarity.

2.7 Lgl and salivary gland histolysis in *Drosophila*

Although the architecture of the cells is defective in the neoplastic tissues, the structure of the other tissues is nearly normal, indicating that the loss of cell polarity may not necessarily be the major cause of cell transformation. Therefore, further investigations of *lgl* mutant tissues and organs are important in order to unravel distinct mechanisms with critical roles in tumorigenesis. Along these lines the larval salivary glands constitute a particularly suitable model system for studying developmental cell fate, as the glands are essentially made of one single type of large epithelial cells, containing highly polyploidy nuclei with polytene chromosomes. The salivary glands producc and secrete glue proteins at the onset of metamorphosis and all the cells then degenerate synchronously in a rapid process resulting in a full histolysis of this tissue in about 14 hours. The *lgl* gene critically controls the degenerative process leading to salivary gland histolysis (Farkas and Mechler 2000 and references therein) and recent studies revealed that the *lgl* gene controls this degenerative process, which is induced by the steroid hormone ecdysone during metamorphosis. This process happens to be fully independent from the function of *lgl* in cell polarity (Farkas and Mechler 2000). Previous results have shown that reduced *lgl* expression delays salivary gland histolysis whereas over-expression accelerates this process without affecting larval and pupal development. More recent investigations have shown that the Lgl protein in combination with nonmuscle myosin regulate in the cytoplasm access to chromatin modifiers, remodeling and transcription factors necessary for the implementation of salivary gland degeneration (Farkas et al. 2011). This process is relatively complex and involves the steroid activation of Broad-Complex (BR-C), a BTB/POZ-transcription factor and primary response component in this cascade, which leads to salivary gland histolysis and induction of a set of secondary genes. In wild type salivary glands, chromatin remodeling factors are localized in the nucleus to bind chromatin. In *lgl* salivary glands the BR-C Z1 factor is synthesized, but is unable to bind to chromatin, and accumulates in the cytoplasm and in the cortical nuclear zone devoid of chromatin (Farkas et al. 2011) and additionally the secondary genes remain quiescent (Ashburner 1974; Richards 1976). Through a cascade of gene expression the salivary glands undertake profound morphological changes, characterized by the secretion of cellular components into the lumen of the gland, which ultimately leads to the death of the cells upon activation of death genes and caspases. Although the mechanism by which chromatin access of remodeling and transcription factors is regulated by *lgl* is poorly understood, the occurrence of WD40 motifs in the Lgl protein and the requirement of non-muscle myosin heavy chain suggest that these factors may bind to Lgl in order to be assembled together with other components or alternatively become modified to get access to chromatin.

3. Dlg, Scrib and Lgl in cancer development

3.1 New emerging roles for vertebrate *dlg, scrib* and *lgl*

Neoplastic growth depends on the cooperation of several mutations, ultimately leading to major rearrangements in cellular behavior. Changes in tissue homeostasis, acquisition of invasive cell characteristics and tumor formation are often linked to the loss of epithelial cell polarity. During carcinogenesis, the grade of neoplasia correlates with impaired cell polarity. *dlg, scrib* and *lgl* encode tumor suppressor proteins and orthologs of this evolutionary conserved pathway are lost in human carcinomas with high frequency (Humbert et al. 2003, Humbert et al. 2008, Yamanaka and Ohno 2008, Reischauer et al. 2009). Although the role of these genes in mammals is still not well understood and often controversial, accumulated evidence has shed light on their oncogenic and tumor-suppressing function.

Scrib and Dlg1 are targeted for ubiquitin-mediated proteolysis by the E6 oncoprotein from high-risk strains of human papillomavirus (HPV) (Humbert et al. 2003, Gardiol et al. 1999, Nakagawa and Huibregtse 2000, Tomaic, Pim and Banks 2009), which has a causal role in the development of cervical cancer (Nakagawa et al. 2004). Furthermore, the viral human T-Lymphoma virus type 1 (HTLV1) Tax protein, crucial for viral replication and malignant transformation leading to T-cell leukemia, binds directly to Dlg1 resulting in hyperphosphorylation of Dlg, which promotes abnormal proliferation of cells (Grassmann, Aboud and Jeang 2005, Hall and Fujii 2005). Both Tax and high-risk HPV E6 bind to the PDZ domains of Dlg through their specific PDZ-binding motif (PBM) they contain (Hall and Fujii 2005). In addition, the PBM-containing Tax and APC compete for binding to Dlg (Hall and Fujii 2005), thereby providing insights on how viral proteins interfere with normal cell function. Similarly, the PBM domain of the NSI protein, from the highly pathogenic avian influenza A virus H5N1, contains an ESEV motif, which allows it to bind directly to Dlg, Scrib and other PDZ-containing proteins (Liu et al. 2010a). Notably, NSI proteins, with an ESEA-containing PBM domain, can enhance viral replication up to 4-fold, relocalize Scrib into cytoplasmic puncta concentrated in perinuclear regions and also protect cells from apoptosis. As this latter effect on apoptosis can be reversed by introducing *scrib-siRNAi,* these viruses most likely perform their function by disrupting the Scrib proapoptotic function (Liu et al. 2010a).

Several pieces of evidence show that human Dlg and Scrib are downregulated during malignant progression of colon and lobular breast cancers (Gardiol et al. 2006, Navarro et al. 2005). Both proteins colocalize in colon mucosa and changes in their expression patterns are correlated with loss of tissue architecture during carcinogenesis in the colon (Gardiol et al. 2006). Another study shows that Dlg1, Scrib and Lgl1 are widely distributed in normal ocular tissues, particularly in the retinal neurons, but upon ocular carcinogenesis these proteins are initially mislocalized in retinal layers and subsequently downregulated. The decreased levels of these proteins are related to the late invasive stage of this cancerous process (Vieira et al. 2008). In the mammary epithelia, Scrib depletion disrupts cell polarity, blocks three-dimensional morphogenesis, inhibits apoptosis and induces dysplasia *in vivo* (Zhan et al. 2008). In this tissue type, Scrib cooperates with c-Myc in order to induce epithelial changes and tumors, by blocking activation of the apoptotic pathway. Interestingly, spontaneous mammary tumors in mice and humans exhibit both downregulation and mislocalization of Scrib (Zhan et al. 2008). Decreased expression and changed localization of Scrib is also associated with histopathological differentiation and lymph node metastasis in endometrial cancer (Ouyang, Zhan and Dan 2010) whereas Scrib cytoplasmic mislocalization is also associated with T-cell leukemia (Okajima et al. 2008).

A study performed in colorectal adenomas and adenocarcinomas suggested that Scrib could also be involved in the early steps of colon carcinogenesis (Kamei et al. 2007), as overexpression and cytoplasmic distributions of Scrib were primarily identified as early events of this process. In these colon cells, Scrib accumulation was shown to overlap with the cytoplasmic accumulation of β-Catenin, suggesting that changes in the APC/β-Catenin pathway during colon carcinogenesis could be involved in Scrib mislocalization (Kamei et al. 2007). A very recent study has shown that Scrib is universally overexpressed in cultured tumor cell lines and genetically disparate cancer patient series of tissues such as colon, liver, lung, bladder, breast, ovary, uterus, testis, prostate and CNS (Vaira et al. 2011, Namdarian et al. 2011). Likewise, normal membrane association of Scrib is altered in tumors where Scrib is mislocalized in the cytosol. In a lung adenocarcinoma model, small interfering RNA silencing of Scrib inhibited tumor cell invasion (Vaira et al. 2011). Furthermore, the small non-coding RNA microRNA 296 (miR-296), which is progressively lost during tumor progression in a number of cancers, transcriptionally represses Scrib. In turn, loss of miR-296 causes aberrant increase and mislocalization of Scrib in human tumors, uncovering a new regulation of Scrib in cancer (Vaira et al. 2011). Lgl1 has also been associated with poor clinical prognosis for cancer patients. In colorectal and breast carcinoma lines, ZEB1 (a Zfh-1 family member of transcription factors) regulates the levels of Lgl2 (Reischauer et al. 2009). In zebrafish, the observation that epidermal neoplasia and epidermal-to-mesenchymal transition (EMT) in *lgl2* mutants is promoted by the ErbB signaling, a pathway of high significance in human carcinomas, provides another mechanistic link between neoplasia and TSGs (Reischauer et al. 2009).

3.2 New insights into the mechanisms of cancer initiation and progression

In the last years, a great number of very interesting publications provided us with information on new and unexpected findings on the role of *scrib, lgl* and *dlg* in cancer initiation and the progressive steps leading to tumorigenesis. In particular, these TSGs helped us to understand the role of cell competition and of the tumor microenvironment in tumor survival and progression, as well as the role of JNK-mediated apoptosis in this system. To date, research on *scrib, lgl* and *dlg* has focused on their similar effects and phenotypes, the interdependent localization in various tissues and the cooperation of the three genes in establishing polarity. Nowadays, it becomes obvious that they play a broader role than initially thought, through the cooperation with individual partners and signaling pathways, in a tissue and cell-type specific context. The cellular context and the neighbouring cells of the surrounding tumour environment are recognized as important regulators in cancer progression (Brumby and Richardson 2005, Humbert et al. 2008, Mohamet, Hawkins and Ward 2011, Pagliarini and Xu 2003, Schmeichel 2004, Woodhouse and Liotta 2004). Along these lines, the analysis of cancer-disposing mutations in only a subset of cells or in clones within the context of a wild type surrounding is gaining more interest, compared to the analysis of the multi-step nature of tumor progression in the context of a whole organism, since it offers a reasonable approximation to the clonal nature of human cancers.

Analysis of *scrib*⁻ mutant clones in the *Drosophila* eye imaginal discs has shown that tumor development is suppressed by the JNK-mediated apoptotic pathway activated by the surrounding wild-type cells, whereas the neoplastic and metastatic potential is regained through the synergistic effect of a simultaneous up-regulation of Ras signalling within the same clones (Pagliarini and Xu 2003, Brumby and Richardson 2003, Leong et al. 2009). These results underline the effect of the surrounding normal cells on the transformed *scrib*⁻ clonal cells, which leads to a cell competition similar to the one observed in the mammalian cancers (Etienne-Manneville 2009, Tapon 2003, Kango-Singh and Halder 2004, Vidal et al. 2010, Leong et al. 2009, Wu, Pastor-Pareja and Xu 2010) (Figure 2). In a model for Scrib tumorigenesis, analysis of the downstream pathways in *scrib*⁻ epithelial clones revealed that the polarity defects are mediated by aPKC, independent of Crumbs, whereas an excessive cell proliferation is restrained by JNK-mediated apoptosis. Upon simultaneous activation of either Ras or Notch, JNK-mediated apoptosis is blocked, and Ras/Notch together with JNK cooperatively promote tumor growth and invasion (Leong et al. 2009). In other words, while JNK activation promotes the death of *scrib*⁻ clones, JNK drives tumor progression in the context of *Ras^{v12}scrib*⁻ clones (Vidal 2010). Another report provided a molecular link between loss of polarity and tumorigenesis, since *scrib*⁻, *dlg*⁻ and *lgl*⁻ clonal cells in a wild type surrounding become metastatic only in combination with *Ras^{v12}* activation, resulting in JNK activation and E-cad inactivation (Igaki, Pagliarini and Xu 2006). A study in malpighian tubules proceded a step further, showing that indeed Ras functions downstream of Scrib to regulate the transformation of normal stem cells to cancer stem cells, and that several signal transdunction pathways (including MAPK, RhoA, PKA and TOR) mediate the function of Ras to promote this stem cell transformation (Zeng et al. 2010). Competition between clonal tissues and wild type surrounding can involve several players, since in *Ras^{v12}scrib*⁻ epithelial clones overexpression of *sds22*, a new tumor suppressor gene in *Drosophila,* can prevent tumor formation and metastasis by inhibiting myosin II and JNK activity (Jiang et al. 2011). A genome-wide screen for genes cooperating with *Ras* (Brumby et al. 2011), confirmed the competitive advantage of *Rac1*, *RhoGEF2* and *pbl* together with *Ras* in the clonal system, which leads to JNK upregulation. Remarkably, this JNK activation was sufficient to confer invasive growth in the clonal setting but not in the whole-tissue system. The fact that JNK-mediated tumorigenesis, in cooperation with Ras in the clonal system, resembled the situation in mammalian breast epithelial cells shows that the knowledge gained from clonal analysis in *Drosophila* can help us elucidate tumorigenesis in the mammalian system. Interesting is also that, Rho1 and Rac are critical for the cooperation of Dlg with Ras in the whole-tissue context (Brumby et al. 2011). Along the same line, when *lgl* is mutated in a mosaic tissue, the *lgl*⁻ clonal cells become the "losers" in cell competition. However, simultaneous overexpression of the Ras signalling pathway or of the *yorkie* (yki; a transcription factor, which is suppressed by the Salvator/Warts/Hippo pathway) in *lgl*⁻ clones, causes overgrowths and JNK-mediated apoptosis at the periphery of the transformed clones (Grzeschik et al. 2010a, Grzeschik, Parsons and Richardson 2010b, Tamori et al. 2010, Mair 2010, Alderton 2010, Menendez et al. 2010). Moreover, JNK-mediated elimination of *lgl*⁻ clonal cells was relieved and the overgrowth potential was re-established by upregulation of c-Myc, proving that *lgl*⁻ clonal death is driven mainly by c-Myc-induced cell competition (Froldi et al. 2010). Simultaneous downregulation of the *lgl* and the JNK pathway in the whole-tissue system results in phenotype reversion of tumor growth, absence of the giant larvae and recurrence of pupariation, thereby showing that JNK activity is essential for overgrowth and invasion of *lgl* tumorous discs (Zhu et al. 2010). Among the wide palette of cellular events leading to JNK activation is the dTNF (tumor necrosis factor)/Eiger. Eiger is the sole *Drosophila* member of the TNF superfamily and its dysregulated expression in imaginal disc cells results in JNK-mediated apoptosis (Vidal 2010, Cordero et al. 2010). The role of mammalian TNF in both pro-tumor and anti-tumor function are well documented and recent work suggests that both aspects of TNF function are also conserved in *Drosophila*. On one hand, JNK-dependent cell death in *scrib* and *dlg* clones requires dTNF, consistent with its role as a "tumor death factor" (Igaki 2009). On the other hand, in tumors deficient for *scrib* and *dlg* that also express *Ras*, the TNF signal is converted into a signal which promotes tumor growth and invasion, in accordance with the "tumor promoting" function of mammalian TNF (Cordero et al. 2010). More precisely, upon dTNF downregulation, cell death in *dlg* and *scrib* clones is blocked and *in situ* outgrowths appear, probably by TNF-mediated extra-cellular matrix (ECM) remodelling (Vidal 2010, Cordero et al. 2010). However, a similar effect on clone survival by dTNF knockdown in *lgl* clones was not observed, meaning that there are gene-specificities among the three TSGs (Vidal 2010). When generated in a dTNF mutant background, $Ras^{v12}scrib^{-}$ clones displayed non-invasive *in situ* overgrowth. Similarly, in whole $Ras^{v12}scrib^{-}dTNF^{-}$ animals, development proceeded up to pupal stages, overcoming the "giant larvae" phenotype (Figure 2) (Vidal 2010, Cordero et al. 2010). These recent results suggest that several of the critical overgrowth phenotypes of *scrib, dlg* and *lgl* in the clonal and whole-tissue context are mediated by dTNF and that dTNF pro-tumor function depends partially on JNK activation in tumor cells, which provides a switch from *in situ* to invasive growth. Immunostaining experiments that detected dTNF in a punctuated, intracellular vesicle pattern at the periphery of hemocytes associated with the *dlg*-group clones, indicate that dTNF expression in hemocytes is sufficient for dTNF/JNK pathway activation within *dlg*-group clones, and mark the importance of hemolymph and non-cell autonomous immune response in tumor progression (Vidal 2010, Cordero et al. 2010).

So far, the mechanism by which the surrounding normal tissue exerts antitumor effects against *dlg, scrib* or *lgl* clones remained elucive. New results from clonal analysis in *Drosophila* imaginal discs have shown that JNK activation from the wild type surrounding leads to upregulation of PVR, the *Drosophila* PDGF/VEGF receptor, which subsequently activates the ELMO/Mbc phagocytic pathway, and which in turn eliminates the oncogenic clonal cells by engulfment (Ohsawa et al. 2011). From an evolutionary point of view, the development of such mechanism, which senses and eliminates "neoplastic" tumor-suppressor mutant cells such as those of $scrib^{-}$ and dlg^{-} but not "hyperplastic" ones (in which despite of overproliferation, cells are normally shaped and retain a differentiated epithelial monolayer, such as those of the Hippo pathway and PTEN) (Ohsawa et al. 2011), shows the necessity to specifically eliminate the high-risk malignant neoplastic cells before they confer any harm to the organism. The recent results concerning the function of these TSGs are of great importance as they: (1) promote the basic understanding on cancer development in a tissue and cell-type specific context, (2) recapitulate the situation of cancer development and metastasis in humans, and (3) recognize the advantage of *Drosophila* as a model system of choice in order to elucidate the role of these proteins at a mechanistic level and the molecular wiring that swifts the balance from normal to transformed cells in an otherwise wild type organism.

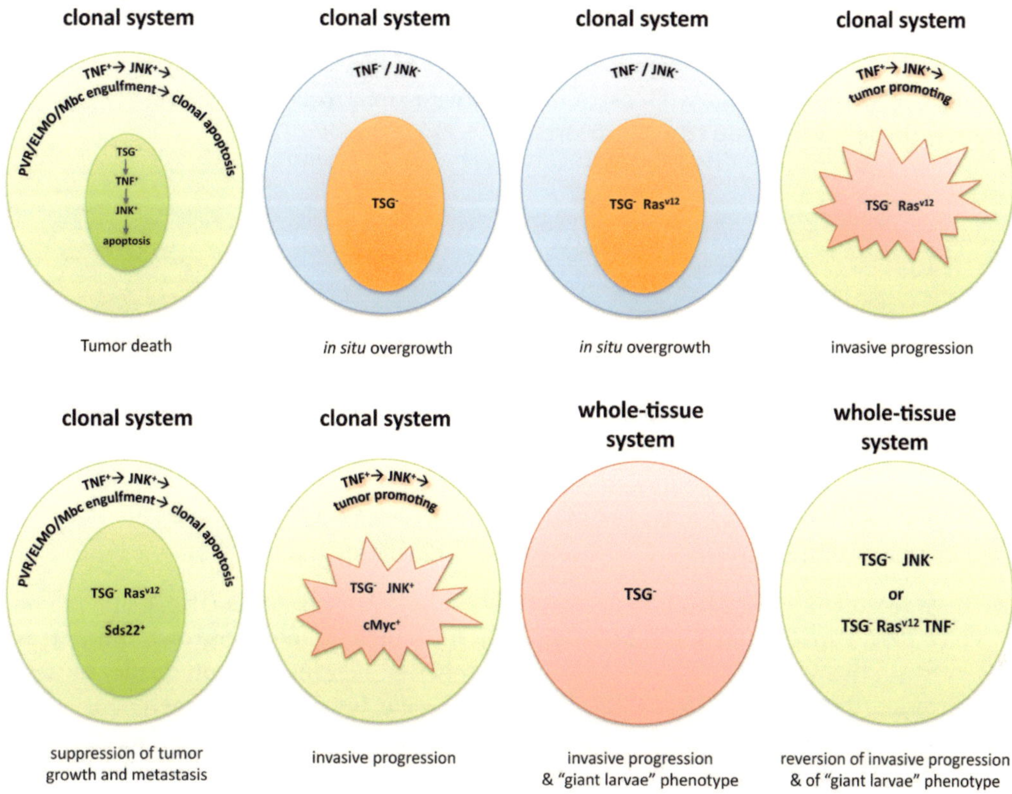

Fig. 2. Simplified model showing the most important genetic interactions of *scrib, dlg* and *lgl* TSGs with the TNF, JNK and Ras signalling pathways at the clonal and the whole-tissue system (for a more detailed analysis and the gene-specific interactions of the individual TSGs refer to the text).

4. Dlg, Scrib and Lgl in the *Drosophila* testis

So far, the role of Dlg, Scrib and Lgl in testis development has been underestimated, as mutations in these genes do not result in tumors. On the other hand, testes do not possess an epithelium similar to the ovarian follicular epithelium, which facilitates the analysis of apicobasal polarity. The more intensive investigation of the *Drosophila* testis in the last 15 years has shed light on basic mechanisms, signaling molecules and cytoskeletal proteins involved in the progressive development of male gonads to adult testis, which provided markers and tools required for subsequent analysis. In the *Drosophila* testis, the somatic cells of the hub form the organizing center that recruits the germline stem cells (GSCs), creating the male stem cell niche (Fuller and Spradling 2007, Lin 2002). Upon asymmetric stem cell division, each GSC produces a new GSC attached to the hub and a distally located gonialblast, whereas each somatic stem cell (SSC) pair divides to generate two SSCs and two somatic cyst cells (SCCs) (Figure 3). The gonialblast divides mitotically four times in 16 interconnected spermatogonial cells surrounded by the two SCCs (Yamashita et al. 2007, Fuller and Spradling 2007, Wong, Jin and Xie 2005). The spermatogonial cells differentiate to primary spermatocytes, which enter the pre-meiotic phase (Fuller 1993). The physical contacts among the testis cell populations are critical as they allow the exchange of signals among GSCs and SSCs as well as SCCs, spermatogonial cells and spermatocytes that promote tissue survival and testis homeostasis.

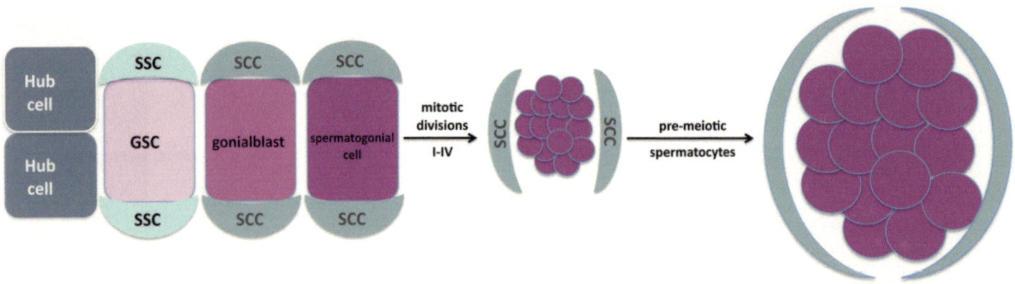

Fig. 3. Diagram depicting early spermatogenesis in *Drosophila*. Abbreviations: GSCs, germline stem cells; SCCs, somatic cyst cells; SSCs, somatic stem cells.

We have recently investigated a new role of *dlg* in the *Drosophila* testis (Papagiannouli and Mechler 2009, Papagiannouli and Mechler 2010). In contrast to the overgrowth phenotypes observed in imaginal discs and brain hemispheres, *dlg* inactivation leads to testis degeneration during early larval development. The *dlg* testes are extremely small, with reduced number of GSCs loosely attached to the hub (Figure 5B, F). The Dlg protein is present in all somatic cells including the hub, SSCs and SCCs (Figure 4A-D) and the specific requirement of *dlg* in these cells is further supported by the finding that the mutant phenotype is rescued by expressing *dlg* in somatic cells but not in germ cells (Papagiannouli and Mechler 2009). In SSCs and early SCCs *dlg* plays a critical role in the establishment of a normal cyst structure, whereas in spermatogonial and spermatocyte stages *dlg* is critical for cyst survival, growth, expansion and maintenance of the integrity of the cysts' microenvironment. Presumably, *dlg* is required for establishing and maintaining a tight connection between GSCs and SSCs around the hub. The connection between gonialblasts and SCC is also maintained during the mitotic divisions. In SSCs and early SCCs, *dlg* acts critically to establish a normal cyst structure, whereas in further spermatogonial and spermatocyte stages *dlg* is significant to the survival, growth and expansion of the cyst (Papagiannouli and Mechler 2010).

A very interesting finding was the formation of wavy and ruffled plasma membrane in *dlg* over-expressing cells capping the spermatocyte cysts. Up to now, there is no mechanism describing how SCCs in *Drosophila* testis grow enormously, elongate and ensheath the germ cells of spermatogonial and spermatocyte cysts or how spermatid differentiation and individualization is guided by the polarized head and tail SCC. One way to interpret this result would be to consider that Dlg regulates the intensity of germ cell encapsulation through the Egfr pathway, which is the major signaling pathway active at the microenvironment of the spermatogonial cysts (Kiger, White-Cooper and Fuller 2000, Tran,

Brenner and DiNardo 2000). Membrane ruffling, detected in somatic cells upon *dlg* over-expression, is highly reminiscent of the formation of lammellipodia-like structures, formed upon up-regulation of Rac1 in SCCs (Sarkar et al. 2007). Rac1 is a downstream component of the Egfr pathway and acts antagonistically to Rho in order to regulate germ cell encapsulation; moreover, Rho activation perturbates TJ function in various experimental systems (Fischer et al. 2007). It has already been shown that Dlg regulates membrane proliferation in a subset of NMJs in a dose-dependent fashion (Budnik et al. 1996) and is an important player in the process of polarized membrane insertion during cellularization (Lecuit and Wieschaus 2000, Dudu et al. 2004, Strickland and Burgess 2004, Lee et al. 2003). The fact that membrane proliferation is also involved in mechanisms such as tissue spreading and cell surface extensions, including membrane ruffles (Lecuit and Pilot 2003, Albertson, Riggs and Sullivan 2005) and combined with our results on SCCs membrane ruffling upon Dlg overexpression, could mean that polarized membrane insertion, mediated by Dlg, might conduct SCCs growth, expansion and spreading over the germ cells of testicular cysts.

Interestingly, our recent results have also shown a requirement of Scrib and Lgl for normal testis development. Scrib and Lgl are localized in the somatic hub, SSCs and SCCs. Scrib is also present in the germline including the spermatocytes and the fusome (Figure 4E-H), with its localization in fusome being dispensable (Lighthouse, Buszczak and Spradling 2008). Lgl has a marked localization at the fusome (Figure 4I-L). The germline localization of Scrib and Lgl is particularly interesting as it distinguishes them from Dlg, which is localized and is exclusively required in the somatic lineage. Examination of 6-7 days-old *scrib* and *lgl* mutant testis from giant larvae, revealed a dramatic reduction in the size of *scrib* and *lgl* testis. *scrib* testes show defects in the male stem cell niche, with less GSCs, gonialblasts and reduction in the transit amplifying spermatogonial cells (Figure 5C, G). The phenotype of the *lgl* testes was more severe, with defects in the male stem cell niche, fewer GSCs loosely attached to the hub and few spermatogonial cysts and with progressive spermatocyte cyst disappearance leading to testis atrophy (Figure 5D, H). The extensive defects in *dlg, scrib and lgl* mutant testes, underline their importance in the establishment and maintenance of the male stem cell niche and proper testis differentiation.

Results obtained in the cancer and testis fields, regarding the role of the microenvironment and of apoptosis, point out the similarities of the basic mechanisms underlying the function of these genes. Our results from the *Drosophila* testis are in agreement with the newly investigated role of these genes in the cancer field. The importance of neighboring cell populations is illustrated in the case of testis where the somatic and germline cells create a microenvironment in the male stem cell niche and in the spermatogonial and spermatocyte cysts, which is required for mutual somatic and germline survival that promotes GSC maintenance and testis differentiation. The effect of Dlg, Scrib and Lgl, when signaling pathways emanating from the somatic and germ cells are affected, and the comparative analysis of apoptosis in the testis and in mosaic clones of the tumor microenvironment are some of the questions we try to investigate. Answering these questions will help us understand how the cell type-specific cellular content (cell intrinsic effects), microenvironment and signaling pathways cooperate with *dlg, scrib* and *lgl* in the various tissues. Although Dlg, Scrib and Lgl act in a slightly variable way in the various tissues and bind to different partners according to the protein availability (Roche et al. 2002), they can still be considered as major players in the pathways they participate in, with a conserved function in the broader sense. Using the knowledge obtained in these systems will allow us to study their function in the testis in a comparative way.

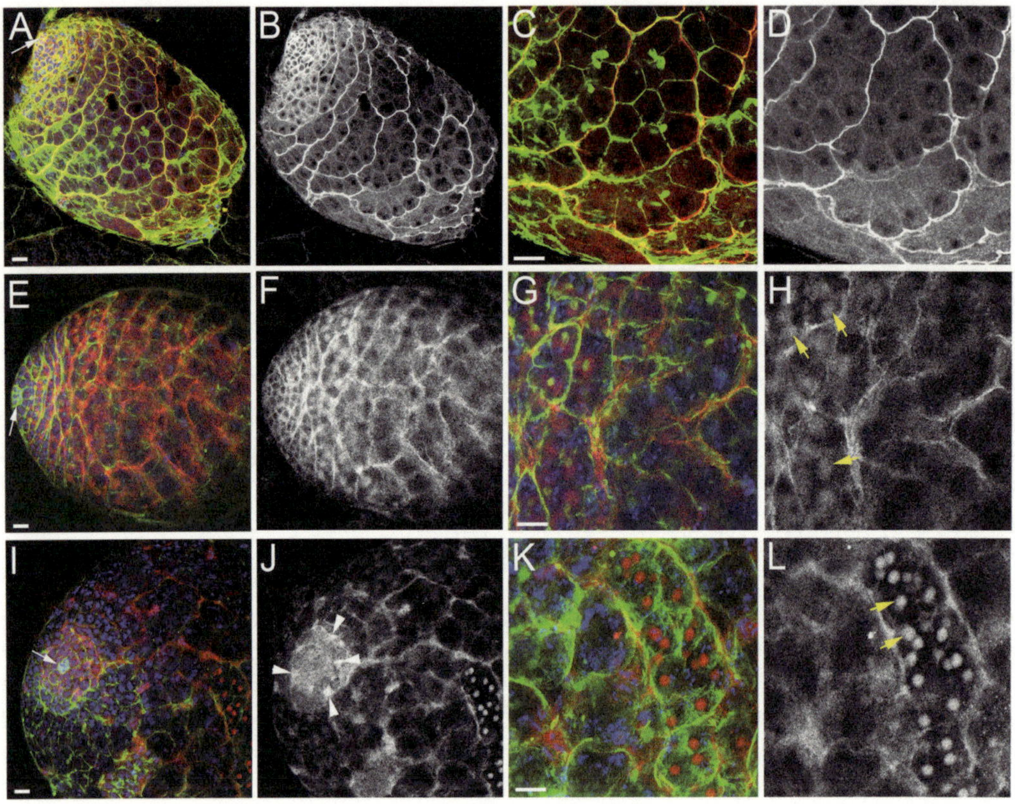

Fig. 4. Pattern of Dlg, Scrib and Lgl distribution in 3rd instar larval testis. (A-D) Wild type testis stained for F-actin with phalloidin (green), DNA with DAPI (blue) and immuno-stained for Dlg (red). (C) and (D) are enlargements of (A) displaying the spermatocyte cysts, (B) and (D) display only the Dlg staining, marking the hub, SSCs and SCCs. (E-H) Scrib-GFP enhancer trap line showing Scrib localization (red) and stained for F-actin with phalloidin (green) and DAPI (blue). (G) and (H) are enlargements of (E) displaying the spermatocyte cysts, (F) and (H) display only the Scrib-GFP, marking the hub, SSCs, SCCs and the spermatocytes with the fusome (yellow arrows). (I-L) Lgl-GFP enhancer trap line showing Lgl localization (red), stained for F-actin with phalloidin (green) and DAPI (blue). (K) and (L) are enlargements of (I) displaying the spermatocyte cysts, (J) and (H) display only the Lgl-GFP, marking the hub, SSCs (arrowheads in J), SCCs and the spermatocytes with the fusome (yellow arrows). Testis hub is oriented towards the left (white arrows). Bar: 15μm.

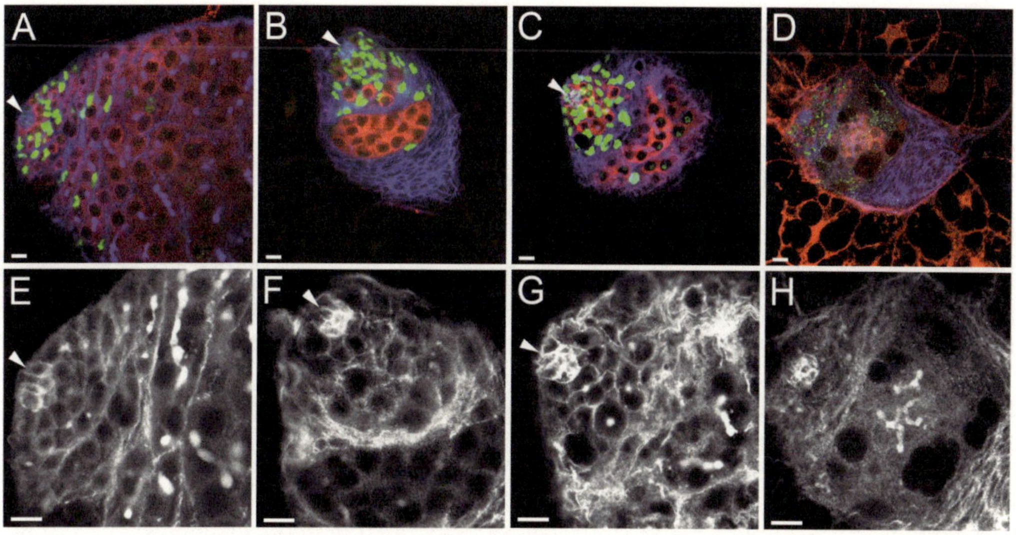

Fig. 5. Testis in wild type, *dlg*, *scrib* and *lgl* 3rd instar larvae. Testes from (A, E) wt, (B, F) *dlg*, (C, G) *scrib* and (D, H) *lgl* larvae stained for Vasa (red), Tj (green), and Arm+α-Spectrin (blue). Low panel pictures (E-H) are enlargements of the hub region shown in (A-D), showing only the co-staining of Arm and α-Spectrin. Testis hub (arrowheads) is oriented towards the left. Bar: 15μm. Staining reveals a dramatic reduction in the size of *scrib* and *lgl* testis. *scrib* testes show defects in the male stem cell niche, with less GSCs, gonialblasts and reduction in the transit amplifying spermatogonial cells. *lgl* testes show defects in the male stem cell niche with fewer GSCs loosely attached to the hub and few spermatogonial cysts, leading to spermatocyte cyst disappearance and testis atrophy, reminiscent of the *dlg* mutant testis (Papagiannouli & Mechler, 2009).

5. Conclusions

Cancer is generally considered as a failure in the normal progression of differentiation. In recent years, developmental biology has contributed a great deal to cancer research. The reason of this success lies mainly in the recognition that cancer is a genetic disease, in which the normal pathway of cell fate and cell differentiation has been altered. The role of the tumor suppressor genes *dlg*, *scrib* and *lgl* as key junctional components in cell-type and tissue specific contexts has been analyzed in this review. It becomes obvious that the cytoskeleton is not seen anymore as a fixed structure but a dynamic and adaptive structure, whose components and regulatory proteins are in constant flux. Furthermore, it organizes the content of the cell, connects the cell with the external environment and coordinates forces that enable the cell to move and change shape. Looking at the cell not as an "inert playground for a few masterminding molecules" (Weiss 1961) but as an integrated whole, "an hierarchical ordered system of mutually interdependent molecular groupings and supramolecular entities" (Weiss 1961, Fletcher and Mullins 2010) can help us understand the role of these TSGs as safeguards of normal development, tissue homeostasis and tumor prevention.

Over the last three decades *Drosophila* has become the organism of choice for molecular and genetic investigations in eukaryotic biology. Its emergence as an animal model system is closely related to the rapid advances in recombinant DNA technology and other methods established in decades of classical genetics and embryology. Given the striking degree of evolutionary conservation of genes and signaling pathways, in particular of disease-causing genes, and the general principles that govern biological processes, sometimes even to the extent that a mouse gene can functionally replace its fly homologue, what we can learn from flies is often relevant to higher organisms, including humans (Gonzalez 2007, Jaekel and Klein 2006). This surprising conservation, together with the recent advances in genetic tools, such as MARCM (Lee and Luo 2001, Wu and Luo 2006), lineage tracing (Potter et al. 2010), multi-color cell labeling (Hadjieconomou et al. 2011, Hampel et al. 2011, Cachero and Jefferis 2011), cell-type specific RNAi (Brand and Perrimon 1993) and genome-wide analysis made *Drosophila* a powerful model organism in elucidating basic cellular and tissue functions and in modeling cancer and other diseases. In the last years, a handful of review articles and conferences focused on the efforts and advances in modeling human diseases in *Drosophila* (Pfleger and Reiter 2008, Crnic and Christofori 2004, Gilbert 2008, Botas 2007, Caldeira et al. 2009, Froldi et al. 2008, Reiter et al. 2001) from cancer, metastasis and neurogenerative diseases to obesity, metabolism and congenital heart disease. All these studies have shown that analysis of human diseases in *Drosophila* can go further than the phenotypic results and the ability to assign a function, in elucidating the mechanisms underlying disease pathology through a straightforward experimental design, thereby providing valuable entry points for later validation in mammalian systems and humans and identify candidate therapeutic agents. The fact that cancer and tumor suppressors underlie almost all basic cellular mechanisms from polarity, cell architecture and adhesion to gene regulation and cell specification, and from trafficking and proper cell compartmentalization to microenvironment signal exchange and neighboring cell competition, prove the necessity of *Drosophila* as a workhorse in unraveling the mechanisms of normal development. Compared with experiments in vertebrates, the large screens facilitated in *Drosophila* due to the low cost, the short generation time, the capacity for experiments with large numbers of animals and the availability of large collections of loss-of-function and overexpression mutant strains together with the power of genetics, that allows researchers to manipulate the fly genome at the level of precision, made the tiny fruit fly the organism of choice in several cases (Botas 2007, Froldi et al. 2008). Finally, the use of innovative technologies such as microarrays and nanotechnology, combined with novel computation and bioinformatics, has allowed genome-wide analysis of *Drosophila*, comprehensive analysis of the chromatin landscape (Kharchenko et al. 2011), cis-regulatory map of the *Drosophila* genome and transcription co-binding relationships (Negre et al. 2011), and high-resolution of transcriptome dynamics throughout development (Graveley et al. 2011). All these studies have laid the carpet for identifying gene networks and complex gene and pathway interactions. Therefore, it becomes clear that we have still a long way to go on the enormous potential to study human genetic conditions and modeling cancer and metastasis in this simple invertebrate.

6. Acknowledgements

We would like to thank the *Drosophila* community for providing us generously with fly stocks and antibodies during the course of this work. This work was supported by DFG/SFB873 to F. Papagiannouli, and by grants GARČR P302/11/1640 to B.M. Mechler and grants MSM 0021620806 and LC535 to the Charles University in Prague.

7. References

Ahringer, J. (2005) Playing ping pong with pins: cortical and microtubule-induced polarity. *Cell,* 123, 1184-6.

Albertson, R. & C. Q. Doe (2003) Dlg, Scrib and Lgl regulate neuroblast cell size and mitotic spindle asymmetry. *Nat Cell Biol,* 5, 166-70.

Albertson, R., B. Riggs & W. Sullivan (2005) Membrane traffic: a driving force in cytokinesis. *Trends Cell Biol,* 15, 92-101.

Albornoz, V., C. Mendoza-Topaz, C. Oliva, J. Tello, P. Olguin & J. Sierralta (2008) Temporal and spatial expression of Drosophila DLGS97 during neural development. *Gene Expr Patterns,* 8, 443-51.

Alderton, G. K. (2010) Tumorigenesis: To the death! *Nat Rev Cancer,* 10, 598.

Arquier, N., L. Perrin, P. Manfruelli & M. Semeriva (2001) The Drosophila tumor suppressor gene lethal(2)giant larvae is required for the emission of the Decapentaplegic signal. *Development,* 128, 2209-20.

Audebert, S., C. Navarro, C. Nourry, S. Chasserot-Golaz, P. Lecine, Y. Bellaiche, J. L. Dupont, R. T. Premont, C. Sempere, J. M. Strub, A. Van Dorsselaer, N. Vitale & J. P. Borg (2004) Mammalian Scribble forms a tight complex with the betaPIX exchange factor. *Curr Biol,* 14, 987-95.

Bachmann, A., O. Kobler, R. J. Kittel, C. Wichmann, J. Sierralta, S. J. Sigrist, E. D. Gundelfinger, E. Knust & U. Thomas (2010) A perisynaptic menage a trois between Dlg, DLin-7, and Metro controls proper organization of Drosophila synaptic junctions. *J Neurosci,* 30, 5811-24.

Bahri, S., S. Wang, R. Conder, J. Choy, S. Vlachos, K. Dong, C. Merino, S. Sigrist, C. Molnar, X. Yang, E. Manser & N. Harden (2010) The leading edge during dorsal closure as a model for epithelial plasticity: Pak is required for recruitment of the Scribble complex and septate junction formation. *Development,* 137, 2023-32.

Beatty, A., D. Morton & K. Kemphues (2010) The C. elegans homolog of Drosophila Lethal giant larvae functions redundantly with PAR-2 to maintain polarity in the early embryo. *Development,* 137, 3995-4004.

Bellaiche, Y., A. Radovic, D. F. Woods, C. D. Hough, M. L. Parmentier, C. J. O'Kane, P. J. Bryant & F. Schweisguth (2001) The Partner of Inscuteable/Discs-large complex is required to establish planar polarity during asymmetric cell division in Drosophila. *Cell,* 106, 355-66.

Bernadskaya, Y. Y., F. B. Patel, H. T. Hsu & M. C. Soto (2011) Arp2/3 promotes junction formation and maintenance in the C. elegans intestine by regulating membrane association of apical proteins. *Mol Biol Cell.*

Betschinger, J., K. Mechtler & J. A. Knoblich (2003) The Par complex directs asymmetric cell division by phosphorylating the cytoskeletal protein Lgl. *Nature,* 422, 326-30.

Betschinger, J., K. Mechtler & J. A. Knoblich (2006) Asymmetric segregation of the tumor suppressor brat regulates self-renewal in Drosophila neural stem cells. *Cell,* 124, 1241-53.

Beumer, K., H. J. Matthies, A. Bradshaw & K. Broadie (2002) Integrins regulate DLG/FAS2 via a CaM kinase II-dependent pathway to mediate synapse elaboration and stabilization during postembryonic development. *Development,* 129, 3381-91.

Bilder, D. (2001) PDZ proteins and polarity: functions from the fly. *Trends Genet,* 17, 511-9.

Bilder, D. (2004) Epithelial polarity and proliferation control: links from the Drosophila neoplastic tumor suppressors. *Genes Dev,* 18, 1909-25.

Bilder, D., M. Li & N. Perrimon (2000) Cooperative regulation of cell polarity and growth by Drosophila tumor suppressors. *Science,* 289, 113-6.

Bilder, D. & N. Perrimon (2000) Localization of apical epithelial determinants by the basolateral PDZ protein Scribble. *Nature,* 403, 676-80.

Bilder, D., M. Schober & N. Perrimon (2003) Integrated activity of PDZ protein complexes regulates epithelial polarity. *Nat Cell Biol,* 5, 53-8.

Blankenship, J. T., M. T. Fuller & J. A. Zallen (2007) The Drosophila homolog of the Exo84 exocyst subunit promotes apical epithelial identity. *J Cell Sci,* 120, 3099-110.

Botas, J. (2007) Drosophila researchers focus on human disease. *Nat Genet,* 39, 589-91.

Brand, A. H. & N. Perrimon (1993) Targeted gene expression as a means of altering cell fates and generating dominant phenotypes. *Development,* 118, 401-15.

Brenman, J. E., J. R. Topinka, E. C. Cooper, A. W. McGee, J. Rosen, T. Milroy, H. J. Ralston & D. S. Bredt (1998) Localization of postsynaptic density-93 to dendritic microtubules and interaction with microtubule-associated protein 1A. *J Neurosci,* 18, 8805-13.

Brumby, A. M., K. R. Goulding, T. Schlosser, S. Loi, R. Galea, P. Khoo, J. E. Bolden, T. Aigaki, P. O. Humbert & H. E. Richardson (2011) Identification of Novel Ras-Cooperating Oncogenes in Drosophila melanogaster: A RhoGEF/Rho-Family/JNK Pathway Is a Central Driver of Tumorigenesis. *Genetics,* 188, 105-25.

Brumby, A. M. & H. E. Richardson (2003) scribble mutants cooperate with oncogenic Ras or Notch to cause neoplastic overgrowth in Drosophila. *EMBO J,* 22, 5769-79.

Brumby, A. M. & H. E. Richardson (2005) Using Drosophila melanogaster to map human cancer pathways. *Nat Rev Cancer,* 5, 626-39.

Bryant, P. J. & A. Huwe (2000) LAP proteins: what's up with epithelia? *Nat Cell Biol,* 2, E141-3.

Budnik, V., Y. H. Koh, B. Guan, B. Hartmann, C. Hough, D. Woods & M. Gorczyca (1996) Regulation of synapse structure and function by the Drosophila tumor suppressor gene dlg. *Neuron,* 17, 627-40.

Bulgakova, N. A. & E. Knust (2009) The Crumbs complex: from epithelial-cell polarity to retinal degeneration. *J Cell Sci,* 122, 2587-96.

Burgess, R. W., D. L. Deitcher & T. L. Schwarz (1997) The synaptic protein syntaxin1 is required for cellularization of Drosophila embryos. *J Cell Biol,* 138, 861-75.

Cachero, S. & G. S. Jefferis (2011) Double brainbow. *Nat Methods,* 8, 217-8.

Caldeira, J., P. S. Pereira, G. Suriano & F. Casares (2009) Using fruitflies to help understand the molecular mechanisms of human hereditary diffuse gastric cancer. *Int J Dev Biol,* 53, 1557-61.

Carr, H. S., C. Cai, K. Keinanen & J. A. Frost (2009) Interaction of the RhoA exchange factor Net1 with discs large homolog 1 protects it from proteasome-mediated degradation and potentiates Net1 activity. *J Biol Chem,* 284, 24269-80.

Caussinus, E. & C. Gonzalez (2005) Induction of tumor growth by altered stem-cell asymmetric division in Drosophila melanogaster. *Nat Genet,* 37, 1125-9.

Chalmers, A. D., M. Pambos, J. Mason, S. Lang, C. Wylie & N. Papalopulu (2005) aPKC, Crumbs3 and Lgl2 control apicobasal polarity in early vertebrate development. *Development,* 132, 977-86.

Chen, G., W. Li, Q. S. Zhang, M. Regulski, N. Sinha, J. Barditch, T. Tully, A. R. Krainer, M. Q. Zhang & J. Dubnau (2008) Identification of synaptic targets of Drosophila pumilio. *PLoS Comput Biol,* 4, e1000026.

Chen, K. & D. E. Featherstone (2005) Discs-large (DLG) is clustered by presynaptic innervation and regulates postsynaptic glutamate receptor subunit composition in Drosophila. *BMC Biol,* 3, 1.

Chen, K., C. Merino, S. J. Sigrist & D. E. Featherstone (2005) The 4.1 protein coracle mediates subunit-selective anchoring of Drosophila glutamate receptors to the postsynaptic actin cytoskeleton. *J Neurosci,* 25, 6667-75.

Collins, C. A. & A. DiAntonio (2007) Synaptic development: insights from Drosophila. *Curr Opin Neurobiol,* 17, 35-42.

Cordero, J. B., J. P. Macagno, R. K. Stefanatos, K. E. Strathdee, R. L. Cagan & M. Vidal (2010) Oncogenic Ras diverts a host TNF tumor suppressor activity into tumor promoter. *Dev Cell,* 18, 999-1011.

Courbard, J. R., A. Djiane, J. Wu & M. Mlodzik (2009) The apical/basal-polarity determinant Scribble cooperates with the PCP core factor Stbm/Vang and functions as one of its effectors. *Dev Biol,* 333, 67-77.

Crnic, I. & G. Christofori (2004) Novel technologies and recent advances in metastasis research. *Int J Dev Biol,* 48, 573-81.

Doerflinger, H., N. Vogt, I. L. Torres, V. Mirouse, I. Koch, C. Nusslein-Volhard & D. St Johnston (2010) Bazooka is required for polarisation of the Drosophila anterior-posterior axis. *Development,* 137, 1765-73.

Dollar, G. L., U. Weber, M. Mlodzik & S. Y. Sokol (2005) Regulation of Lethal giant larvae by Dishevelled. *Nature,* 437, 1376-80.

Dow, L. E., A. M. Brumby, R. Muratore, M. L. Coombe, K. A. Sedelies, J. A. Trapani, S. M. Russell, H. E. Richardson & P. O. Humbert (2003) hScrib is a functional homologue of the Drosophila tumour suppressor Scribble. *Oncogene,* 22, 9225-30.

Dudu, V., P. Pantazis & M. Gonzalez-Gaitan (2004) Membrane traffic during embryonic development: epithelial formation, cell fate decisions and differentiation. *Curr Opin Cell Biol,* 16, 407-14.

Duffy, H. S., I. Iacobas, K. Hotchkiss, B. J. Hirst-Jensen, A. Bosco, N. Dandachi, R. Dermietzel, P. L. Sorgen & D. C. Spray (2007) The gap junction protein connexin32 interacts with the Src homology 3/hook domain of discs large homolog 1. *J Biol Chem,* 282, 9789-96.

Etienne-Manneville, S. (2009) Scribble at the crossroads. *J Biol,* 8, 104.

Etienne-Manneville, S. & A. Hall (2003) Cdc42 regulates GSK-3beta and adenomatous polyposis coli to control cell polarity. *Nature,* 421, 753-6.

Etienne-Manneville, S., J. B. Manneville, S. Nicholls, M. A. Ferenczi & A. Hall (2005) Cdc42 and Par6-PKCzeta regulate the spatially localized association of Dlg1 and APC to control cell polarization. *J Cell Biol,* 170, 895-901.

Farkas, R., S. Kucharova-Mahmood, L. Mentelova, P. Juda, I. Raska & B. Mechler (2011) Cytoskeletal proteins regulate chromatic access of BR-C transcription factor and Rpd3-Sin3A histone deacetylase complex in Drosophila salivary glands. *Nucleus*, (in print).

Farkas, R. & B. M. Mechler (2000) The timing of drosophila salivary gland apoptosis displays an l(2)gl-dose response. *Cell Death Differ*, 7, 89-101.

Fichelson, P., M. Jagut, S. Lepanse, J. A. Lepesant & J. R. Huynh (2010) lethal giant larvae is required with the par genes for the early polarization of the Drosophila oocyte. *Development*, 137, 815-24.

Fischer, A., H. Stuckas, M. Gluth, T. D. Russell, M. C. Rudolph, N. E. Beeman, S. Bachmann, S. Umemura, Y. Ohashi, M. C. Neville & F. Theuring (2007) Impaired tight junction sealing and precocious involution in mammary glands of PKN1 transgenic mice. *J Cell Sci*, 120, 2272-83.

Fletcher, D. A. & R. D. Mullins (2010) Cell mechanics and the cytoskeleton. *Nature*, 463, 485-92.

Froldi, F., M. Ziosi, F. Garoia, A. Pession, N. A. Grzeschik, P. Bellosta, D. Strand, H. E. Richardson & D. Grifoni (2010) The lethal giant larvae tumour suppressor mutation requires dMyc oncoprotein to promote clonal malignancy. *BMC Biol*, 8, 33.

Froldi, F., M. Ziosi, G. Tomba, F. Parisi, F. Garoia, A. Pession & D. Grifoni (2008) Drosophila lethal giant larvae neoplastic mutant as a genetic tool for cancer modeling. *Curr Genomics*, 9, 147-54.

Fuller, M. T. 1993. *Spermatogenesis*. Cold Spring Harbor, New York: Cold Spring Harbor Laboratory Press.

Fuller, M. T. & A. C. Spradling (2007) Male and female Drosophila germline stem cells: two versions of immortality. *Science*, 316, 402-4.

Ganguly, I., T. F. Mackay & R. R. Anholt (2003) Scribble is essential for olfactory behavior in Drosophila melanogaster. *Genetics*, 164, 1447-57.

Garcia-Mata, R., A. D. Dubash, L. Sharek, H. S. Carr, J. A. Frost & K. Burridge (2007) The nuclear RhoA exchange factor Net1 interacts with proteins of the Dlg family, affects their localization, and influences their tumor suppressor activity. *Mol Cell Biol*, 27, 8683-97.

Gardiol, D., C. Kuhne, B. Glaunsinger, S. S. Lee, R. Javier & L. Banks (1999) Oncogenic human papillomavirus E6 proteins target the discs large tumour suppressor for proteasome-mediated degradation. *Oncogene*, 18, 5487-96.

Gardiol, D., A. Zacchi, F. Petrera, G. Stanta & L. Banks (2006) Human discs large and scrib are localized at the same regions in colon mucosa and changes in their expression patterns are correlated with loss of tissue architecture during malignant progression. *Int J Cancer*, 119, 1285-90.

Gateff, E. (1978) Malignant neoplasms of genetic origin in Drosophila melanogaster. *Science*, 200, 1448-59.

Gateff, E. & H. A. Schneiderman (1969) Neoplasms in mutant and cultured wild-tupe tissues of Drosophila. *Natl Cancer Inst Monogr*, 31, 365-97.

Gateff E, S. H. (1974) Developmental capacities of benign and malignant neoplasms of Drosophila. *Wilhelm Roux' Archiv*, 176.

Gilbert, L. I. (2008) Drosophila is an inclusive model for human diseases, growth and development. *Mol Cell Endocrinol*, 293, 25-31.

Gonzalez, C. (2007) Spindle orientation, asymmetric division and tumour suppression in Drosophila stem cells. *Nat Rev Genet,* 8, 462-72.

Gonzalez-Mariscal, L., R. Tapia & D. Chamorro (2008) Crosstalk of tight junction components with signaling pathways. *Biochim Biophys Acta,* 1778, 729-56.

Goode, S. & N. Perrimon (1997) Inhibition of patterned cell shape change and cell invasion by Discs large during Drosophila oogenesis. *Genes Dev,* 11, 2532-44.

Gorczyca, D., J. Ashley, S. Speese, N. Gherbesi, U. Thomas, E. Gundelfinger, L. S. Gramates & V. Budnik (2007) Postsynaptic membrane addition depends on the Discs-Large-interacting t-SNARE Gtaxin. *J Neurosci,* 27, 1033-44.

Grassmann, R., M. Aboud & K. T. Jeang (2005) Molecular mechanisms of cellular transformation by HTLV-1 Tax. *Oncogene,* 24, 5976-85.

Graveley, B. R., A. N. Brooks, J. W. Carlson, M. O. Duff, J. M. Landolin, L. Yang, C. G. Artieri, M. J. van Baren, N. Boley, B. W. Booth, J. B. Brown, L. Cherbas, C. A. Davis, A. Dobin, R. Li, W. Lin, J. H. Malone, N. R. Mattiuzzo, D. Miller, D. Sturgill, B. B. Tuch, C. Zaleski, D. Zhang, M. Blanchette, S. Dudoit, B. Eads, R. E. Green, A. Hammonds, L. Jiang, P. Kapranov, L. Langton, N. Perrimon, J. E. Sandler, K. H. Wan, A. Willingham, Y. Zhang, Y. Zou, J. Andrews, P. J. Bickel, S. E. Brenner, M. R. Brent, P. Cherbas, T. R. Gingeras, R. A. Hoskins, T. C. Kaufman, B. Oliver & S. E. Celniker (2011) The developmental transcriptome of Drosophila melanogaster. *Nature,* 471, 473-9.

Grawe, F., A. Wodarz, B. Lee, E. Knust & H. Skaer (1996) The Drosophila genes crumbs and stardust are involved in the biogenesis of adherens junctions. *Development,* 122, 951-9.

Gregorc, U., S. Ivanova, M. Thomas, V. Turk, L. Banks & B. Turk (2005) hDLG/SAP97, a member of the MAGUK protein family, is a novel caspase target during cell-cell detachment in apoptosis. *Biol Chem,* 386, 705-10.

Grifoni, D., F. Garoia, C. C. Schimanski, G. Schmitz, E. Laurenti, P. R. Galle, A. Pession, S. Cavicchi & D. Strand (2004) The human protein Hugl-1 substitutes for Drosophila lethal giant larvae tumour suppressor function in vivo. *Oncogene,* 23, 8688-94.

Grzeschik, N. A., L. M. Parsons, M. L. Allott, K. F. Harvey & H. E. Richardson (2010a) Lgl, aPKC, and Crumbs regulate the Salvador/Warts/Hippo pathway through two distinct mechanisms. *Curr Biol,* 20, 573-81.

Grzeschik, N. A., L. M. Parsons & H. E. Richardson (2010b) Lgl, the SWH pathway and tumorigenesis: It's a matter of context & competition! *Cell Cycle,* 9, 3202-12.

Hadjieconomou, D., S. Rotkopf, C. Alexandre, D. M. Bell, B. J. Dickson & I. Salecker (2011) Flybow: genetic multicolor cell labeling for neural circuit analysis in Drosophila melanogaster. *Nat Methods,* 8, 260-6.

Hall, W. W. & M. Fujii (2005) Deregulation of cell-signaling pathways in HTLV-1 infection. *Oncogene,* 24, 5965-75.

Hamanaka, Y. & I. A. Meinertzhagen (2010) Immunocytochemical localization of synaptic proteins to photoreceptor synapses of Drosophila melanogaster. *J Comp Neurol,* 518, 1133-55.

Hampel, S., P. Chung, C. E. McKellar, D. Hall, L. L. Looger & J. H. Simpson (2011) Drosophila Brainbow: a recombinase-based fluorescence labeling technique to subdivide neural expression patterns. *Nat Methods,* 8, 253-9.

Hanada, N., K. Makino, H. Koga, T. Morisaki, H. Kuwahara, N. Masuko, Y. Tabira, T. Hiraoka, N. Kitamura, A. Kikuchi & H. Saya (2000) NE-dlg, a mammalian homolog of Drosophila dlg tumor suppressor, induces growth suppression and impairment of cell adhesion: possible involvement of down-regulation of beta-catenin by NE-dlg expression. *Int J Cancer,* 86, 480-8.

Harris, B. Z. & W. A. Lim (2001) Mechanism and role of PDZ domains in signaling complex assembly. *J Cell Sci,* 114, 3219-31.

Harris, H., O. J. Miller, G. Klein, P. Worst & T. Tachibana (1969) Suppression of malignancy by cell fusion. *Nature,* 223, 363-8.

Hatsuzawa, K., H. Hirose, K. Tani, A. Yamamoto, R. H. Scheller & M. Tagaya (2000) Syntaxin 18, a SNAP receptor that functions in the endoplasmic reticulum, intermediate compartment, and cis-Golgi vesicle trafficking. *J Biol Chem,* 275, 13713-20.

Hering, H. & M. Sheng (2002) Direct interaction of Frizzled-1, -2, -4, and -7 with PDZ domains of PSD-95. *FEBS Lett,* 521, 185-9.

Hoege, C., A. T. Constantinescu, A. Schwager, N. W. Goehring, P. Kumar & A. A. Hyman (2010) LGL can partition the cortex of one-cell Caenorhabditis elegans embryos into two domains. *Curr Biol,* 20, 1296-303.

Hoffmann, M., C. Segbert, G. Helbig & O. Bossinger (2010) Intestinal tube formation in Caenorhabditis elegans requires vang-1 and egl-15 signaling. *Dev Biol,* 339, 268-79.

Hsu, S. C., D. TerBush, M. Abraham & W. Guo (2004) The exocyst complex in polarized exocytosis. *Int Rev Cytol,* 233, 243-65.

Humbert, P., S. Russell & H. Richardson (2003) Dlg, Scribble and Lgl in cell polarity, cell proliferation and cancer. *Bioessays,* 25, 542-53.

Humbert, P. O., L. E. Dow & S. M. Russell (2006) The Scribble and Par complexes in polarity and migration: friends or foes? *Trends Cell Biol,* 16, 622-30.

Humbert, P. O., N. A. Grzeschik, A. M. Brumby, R. Galea, I. Elsum & H. E. Richardson (2008) Control of tumourigenesis by the Scribble/Dlg/Lgl polarity module. *Oncogene,* 27, 6888-907.

Hutterer, A., J. Betschinger, M. Petronczki & J. A. Knoblich (2004) Sequential roles of Cdc42, Par-6, aPKC, and Lgl in the establishment of epithelial polarity during Drosophila embryogenesis. *Dev Cell,* 6, 845-54.

Igaki, T. (2009) Correcting developmental errors by apoptosis: lessons from Drosophila JNK signaling. *Apoptosis,* 14, 1021-8.

Igaki, T., R. A. Pagliarini & T. Xu (2006) Loss of cell polarity drives tumor growth and invasion through JNK activation in Drosophila. *Curr Biol,* 16, 1139-46.

Ishidate, T., A. Matsumine, K. Toyoshima & T. Akiyama (2000) The APC-hDLG complex negatively regulates cell cycle progression from the G0/G1 to S phase. *Oncogene,* 19, 365-72.

Ivanov, A. I., C. Young, K. Den Beste, C. T. Capaldo, P. O. Humbert, P. Brennwald, C. A. Parkos & A. Nusrat (2010) Tumor suppressor scribble regulates assembly of tight junctions in the intestinal epithelium. *Am J Pathol,* 176, 134-45.

Jaekel, R. & T. Klein (2006) The Drosophila Notch inhibitor and tumor suppressor gene lethal (2) giant discs encodes a conserved regulator of endosomal trafficking. *Dev Cell,* 11, 655-69.

Jakobs, R., C. de Lorenzo, E. Spiess, D. Strand & B. M. Mechler (1996) Homo-oligomerization domains in the lethal(2)giant larvae tumor suppressor protein, p127 of Drosophila. *J Mol Biol*, 264, 484-96.

Jiang, Y., K. L. Scott, S. J. Kwak, R. Chen & G. Mardon (2011) Sds22/PP1 links epithelial integrity and tumor suppression via regulation of myosin II and JNK signaling. *Oncogene*.

Johnston, C. A., K. Hirono, K. E. Prehoda & C. Q. Doe (2009) Identification of an Aurora-A/PinsLINKER/Dlg spindle orientation pathway using induced cell polarity in S2 cells. *Cell*, 138, 1150-63.

Kallay, L. M., A. McNickle, P. J. Brennwald, A. L. Hubbard & L. T. Braiterman (2006) Scribble associates with two polarity proteins, Lgl2 and Vangl2, via distinct molecular domains. *J Cell Biochem*, 99, 647-64.

Kamei, Y., K. Kito, T. Takeuchi, Y. Imai, R. Murase, N. Ueda, N. Kobayashi & Y. Abe (2007) Human scribble accumulates in colorectal neoplasia in association with an altered distribution of beta-catenin. *Hum Pathol*, 38, 1273-81.

Kango-Singh, M. & G. Halder (2004) Drosophila as an emerging model to study metastasis. *Genome Biol*, 5, 216.

Kaplan, N. A. & N. S. Tolwinski (2010) Spatially defined Dsh-Lgl interaction contributes to directional tissue morphogenesis. *J Cell Sci*, 123, 3157-65.

Kharchenko, P. V., A. A. Alekseyenko, Y. B. Schwartz, A. Minoda, N. C. Riddle, J. Ernst, P. J. Sabo, E. Larschan, A. A. Gorchakov, T. Gu, D. Linder-Basso, A. Plachetka, G. Shanower, M. Y. Tolstorukov, L. J. Luquette, R. Xi, Y. L. Jung, R. W. Park, E. P. Bishop, T. K. Canfield, R. Sandstrom, R. E. Thurman, D. M. MacAlpine, J. A. Stamatoyannopoulos, M. Kellis, S. C. Elgin, M. I. Kuroda, V. Pirrotta, G. H. Karpen & P. J. Park (2011) Comprehensive analysis of the chromatin landscape in Drosophila melanogaster. *Nature*, 471, 480-5.

Kiger, A. A., H. White-Cooper & M. T. Fuller (2000) Somatic support cells restrict germline stem cell self-renewal and promote differentiation. *Nature*, 407, 750-4.

Knudson, A. G., Jr. (1971) Mutation and cancer: statistical study of retinoblastoma. *Proc Natl Acad Sci U S A*, 68, 820-3.

Koh, Y. H., E. Popova, U. Thomas, L. C. Griffith & V. Budnik (1999) Regulation of DLG localization at synapses by CaMKII-dependent phosphorylation. *Cell*, 98, 353-63.

Langevin, J., R. Le Borgne, F. Rosenfeld, M. Gho, F. Schweisguth & Y. Bellaiche (2005) Lethal giant larvae controls the localization of notch-signaling regulators numb, neuralized, and Sanpodo in Drosophila sensory-organ precursor cells. *Curr Biol*, 15, 955-62.

Laprise, P., S. M. Paul, J. Boulanger, R. M. Robbins, G. J. Beitel & U. Tepass (2010) Epithelial polarity proteins regulate Drosophila tracheal tube size in parallel to the luminal matrix pathway. *Curr Biol*, 20, 55-61.

Lasserre, R. & A. Alcover (2010) Cytoskeletal cross-talk in the control of T cell antigen receptor signaling. *FEBS Lett*, 584, 4845-50.

Lasserre, R., S. Charrin, C. Cuche, A. Danckaert, M. I. Thoulouze, F. de Chaumont, T. Duong, N. Perrault, N. Varin-Blank, J. C. Olivo-Marin, S. Etienne-Manneville, M. Arpin, V. Di Bartolo & A. Alcover (2010) Ezrin tunes T-cell activation by controlling Dlg1 and microtubule positioning at the immunological synapse. *EMBO J*, 29, 2301-14.

Lecuit, T. (2004) Junctions and vesicular trafficking during Drosophila cellularization. *J Cell Sci*, 117, 3427-33.

Lecuit, T. & F. Pilot (2003) Developmental control of cell morphogenesis: a focus on membrane growth. *Nat Cell Biol*, 5, 103-8.

Lecuit, T. & E. Wieschaus (2000) Polarized insertion of new membrane from a cytoplasmic reservoir during cleavage of the Drosophila embryo. *J Cell Biol*, 150, 849-60.

Lecuit, T. & E. Wieschaus (2002) Junctions as organizing centers in epithelial cells? A fly perspective. *Traffic*, 3, 92-7.

Lee, C. Y., R. O. Andersen, C. Cabernard, L. Manning, K. D. Tran, M. J. Lanskey, A. Bashirullah & C. Q. Doe (2006) Drosophila Aurora-A kinase inhibits neuroblast self-renewal by regulating aPKC/Numb cortical polarity and spindle orientation. *Genes Dev*, 20, 3464-74.

Lee, O. K., K. K. Frese, J. S. James, D. Chadda, Z. H. Chen, R. T. Javier & K. O. Cho (2003) Discs-Large and Strabismus are functionally linked to plasma membrane formation. *Nat Cell Biol*, 5, 987-93.

Lee, T. & L. Luo (2001) Mosaic analysis with a repressible cell marker (MARCM) for Drosophila neural development. *Trends Neurosci*, 24, 251-4.

Lelievre, S. A. (2010) Tissue polarity-dependent control of mammary epithelial homeostasis and cancer development: an epigenetic perspective. *J Mammary Gland Biol Neoplasia*, 15, 49-63.

Leong, G. R., K. R. Goulding, N. Amin, H. E. Richardson & A. M. Brumby (2009) Scribble mutants promote aPKC and JNK-dependent epithelial neoplasia independently of Crumbs. *BMC Biol*, 7, 62.

Letizia, A., S. Sotillos, S. Campuzano & M. Llimargas (2011) Regulated Crb accumulation controls apical constriction and invagination in Drosophila tracheal cells. *J Cell Sci*, 124, 240-51.

Lewis, M. J. & H. R. Pelham (1996) SNARE-mediated retrograde traffic from the Golgi complex to the endoplasmic reticulum. *Cell*, 85, 205-15.

Li, M., J. Marhold, A. Gatos, I. Torok & B. M. Mechler (2001) Differential expression of two scribble isoforms during Drosophila embryogenesis. *Mech Dev*, 108, 185-90.

Li, Q., S. Feng, L. Yu, G. Zhao & M. Li (2011) Requirements of Lgl in cell differentiation and motility during Drosophila ovarian follicular epithelium morphogenesis. *Fly (Austin)*, 5, 81-7.

Li, Q., L. Shen, T. Xin, W. Xiang, W. Chen, Y. Gao, M. Zhu, L. Yu & M. Li (2009) Role of Scrib and Dlg in anterior-posterior patterning of the follicular epithelium during Drosophila oogenesis. *BMC Dev Biol*, 9, 60.

Li, Q., T. Xin, W. Chen, M. Zhu & M. Li (2008) Lethal(2)giant larvae is required in the follicle cells for formation of the initial AP asymmetry and the oocyte polarity during Drosophila oogenesis. *Cell Res*, 18, 372-84.

Lighthouse, D. V., M. Buszczak & A. C. Spradling (2008) New components of the Drosophila fusome suggest it plays novel roles in signaling and transport. *Dev Biol*, 317, 59-71.

Lin, H. (2002) The stem-cell niche theory: lessons from flies. *Nat Rev Genet*, 3, 931-40.

Liu, H., L. Golebiewski, E. C. Dow, R. M. Krug, R. T. Javier & A. P. Rice (2010a) The ESEV PDZ-binding motif of the avian influenza A virus NS1 protein protects infected cells from apoptosis by directly targeting Scribble. *J Virol*, 84, 11164-74.

Liu, Z., Y. Chen, D. Wang, S. Wang & Y. Q. Zhang (2010b) Distinct presynaptic and postsynaptic dismantling processes of Drosophila neuromuscular junctions during metamorphosis. *J Neurosci,* 30, 11624-34.

Lozovatsky, L., N. Abayasekara, S. Piawah & Z. Walther (2009) CASK deletion in intestinal epithelia causes mislocalization of LIN7C and the DLG1/Scrib polarity complex without affecting cell polarity. *Mol Biol Cell,* 20, 4489-99.

Mahoney, Z. X., B. Sammut, R. J. Xavier, J. Cunningham, G. Go, K. L. Brim, T. S. Stappenbeck, J. H. Miner & W. Swat (2006) Discs-large homolog 1 regulates smooth muscle orientation in the mouse ureter. *Proc Natl Acad Sci U S A,* 103, 19872-7.

Mair, W. (2010) How normal cells can win the battle for survival against cancer cells. *PLoS Biol,* 8, e1000423.

Manfruelli, P., N. Arquier, W. P. Hanratty & M. Semeriva (1996) The tumor suppressor gene, lethal(2)giant larvae (1(2)g1), is required for cell shape change of epithelial cells during Drosophila development. *Development,* 122, 2283-94.

Manneville, J. B., M. Jehanno & S. Etienne-Manneville (2010) Dlg1 binds GKAP to control dynein association with microtubules, centrosome positioning, and cell polarity. *J Cell Biol,* 191, 585-98.

Mao, P., Y. X. Tao, M. Fukaya, F. Tao, D. Li, M. Watanabe & R. A. Johns (2008) Cloning and characterization of E-dlg, a novel splice variant of mouse homologue of the Drosophila discs large tumor suppressor binds preferentially to SAP102. *IUBMB Life,* 60, 684-92.

Mathew, D., L. S. Gramates, M. Packard, U. Thomas, D. Bilder, N. Perrimon, M. Gorczyca & V. Budnik (2002) Recruitment of scribble to the synaptic scaffolding complex requires GUK-holder, a novel DLG binding protein. *Curr Biol,* 12, 531-9.

Matsumine, A., A. Ogai, T. Senda, N. Okumura, K. Satoh, G. H. Baeg, T. Kawahara, S. Kobayashi, M. Okada, K. Toyoshima & T. Akiyama (1996) Binding of APC to the human homolog of the Drosophila discs large tumor suppressor protein. *Science,* 272, 1020-3.

Mazumdar, A. & M. Mazumdar (2002) How one becomes many: blastoderm cellularization in Drosophila melanogaster. *Bioessays,* 24, 1012-22.

Mechler, B. M., W. McGinnis & W. J. Gehring (1985) Molecular cloning of lethal(2)giant larvae, a recessive oncogene of Drosophila melanogaster. *EMBO J,* 4, 1551-7.

Menendez, J., A. Perez-Garijo, M. Calleja & G. Morata (2010) A tumor-suppressing mechanism in Drosophila involving cell competition and the Hippo pathway. *Proc Natl Acad Sci U S A,* 107, 14651-6.

Merz, R., M. Schmidt, I. Torok, U. Protin, G. Schuler, H. P. Walther, F. Krieg, M. Gross, D. Strand & B. M. Mechler (1990) Molecular action of the l(2)gl tumor suppressor gene of Drosophila melanogaster. *Environ Health Perspect,* 88, 163-7.

Mohamet, L., K. Hawkins & C. M. Ward (2011) Loss of function of e-cadherin in embryonic stem cells and the relevance to models of tumorigenesis. *J Oncol,* 2011, 352616.

Momboisse, F., E. Lonchamp, V. Calco, M. Ceridono, N. Vitale, M. F. Bader & S. Gasman (2009) betaPIX-activated Rac1 stimulates the activation of phospholipase D, which is associated with exocytosis in neuroendocrine cells. *J Cell Sci,* 122, 798-806.

Montcouquiol, M., R. A. Rachel, P. J. Lanford, N. G. Copeland, N. A. Jenkins & M. W. Kelley (2003) Identification of Vangl2 and Scrb1 as planar polarity genes in mammals. *Nature,* 423, 173-7.

Montcouquiol, M., N. Sans, D. Huss, J. Kach, J. D. Dickman, A. Forge, R. A. Rachel, N. G. Copeland, N. A. Jenkins, D. Bogani, J. Murdoch, M. E. Warchol, R. J. Wenthold & M. W. Kelley (2006) Asymmetric localization of Vangl2 and Fz3 indicate novel mechanisms for planar cell polarity in mammals. *J Neurosci,* 26, 5265-75.

Moreau, M. M., N. Piguel, T. Papouin, M. Koehl, C. M. Durand, M. E. Rubio, F. Loll, E. M. Richard, C. Mazzocco, C. Racca, S. H. Oliet, D. N. Abrous, M. Montcouquiol & N. Sans (2010) The planar polarity protein Scribble1 is essential for neuronal plasticity and brain function. *J Neurosci,* 30, 9738-52.

Morimoto, T., M. Nobechi, A. Komatsu, H. Miyakawa & A. Nose (2010) Subunit-specific and homeostatic regulation of glutamate receptor localization by CaMKII in Drosophila neuromuscular junctions. *Neuroscience,* 165, 1284-92.

Musch, A., D. Cohen, C. Yeaman, W. J. Nelson, E. Rodriguez-Boulan & P. J. Brennwald (2002) Mammalian homolog of Drosophila tumor suppressor lethal (2) giant larvae interacts with basolateral exocytic machinery in Madin-Darby canine kidney cells. *Mol Biol Cell,* 13, 158-68.

Nakagawa, S. & J. M. Huibregtse (2000) Human scribble (Vartul) is targeted for ubiquitin-mediated degradation by the high-risk papillomavirus E6 proteins and the E6AP ubiquitin-protein ligase. *Mol Cell Biol,* 20, 8244-53.

Nakagawa, S., T. Yano, K. Nakagawa, S. Takizawa, Y. Suzuki, T. Yasugi, J. M. Huibregtse & Y. Taketani (2004) Analysis of the expression and localisation of a LAP protein, human scribble, in the normal and neoplastic epithelium of uterine cervix. *Br J Cancer,* 90, 194-9.

Namdarian, B., E. Wong, R. Galea, J. Pedersen, X. Chin, R. Speirs, P. O. Humbert, A. J. Costello, N. M. Corcoran & C. M. Hovens (2011) Loss of APKC expression independently predicts tumor recurrence in superficial bladder cancers. *Urol Oncol.*

Navarro, C., S. Nola, S. Audebert, M. J. Santoni, J. P. Arsanto, C. Ginestier, S. Marchetto, J. Jacquemier, D. Isnardon, A. Le Bivic, D. Birnbaum & J. P. Borg (2005) Junctional recruitment of mammalian Scribble relies on E-cadherin engagement. *Oncogene,* 24, 4330-9.

Negre, N., C. D. Brown, L. Ma, C. A. Bristow, S. W. Miller, U. Wagner, P. Kheradpour, M. L. Eaton, P. Loriaux, R. Sealfon, Z. Li, H. Ishii, R. F. Spokony, J. Chen, L. Hwang, C. Cheng, R. P. Auburn, M. B. Davis, M. Domanus, P. K. Shah, C. A. Morrison, J. Zieba, S. Suchy, L. Senderowicz, A. Victorsen, N. A. Bild, A. J. Grundstad, D. Hanley, D. M. MacAlpine, M. Mannervik, K. Venken, H. Bellen, R. White, M. Gerstein, S. Russell, R. L. Grossman, B. Ren, J. W. Posakony, M. Kellis & K. P. White (2011) A cis-regulatory map of the Drosophila genome. *Nature,* 471, 527-31.

Nguyen, M. M., C. Rivera & A. E. Griep (2005) Localization of PDZ domain containing proteins Discs Large-1 and Scribble in the mouse eye. *Mol Vis,* 11, 1183-99.

Niethammer, M., J. G. Valtschanoff, T. M. Kapoor, D. W. Allison, R. J. Weinberg, A. M. Craig & M. Sheng (1998) CRIPT, a novel postsynaptic protein that binds to the third PDZ domain of PSD-95/SAP90. *Neuron,* 20, 693-707.

Ohsawa, S., K. Sugimura, K. Takino, T. Xu, A. Miyawaki & T. Igaki (2011) Elimination of oncogenic neighbors by JNK-mediated engulfment in Drosophila. *Dev Cell,* 20, 315-28.

Okajima, M., M. Takahashi, M. Higuchi, T. Ohsawa, S. Yoshida, Y. Yoshida, M. Oie, Y. Tanaka, F. Gejyo & M. Fujii (2008) Human T-cell leukemia virus type 1 Tax induces an aberrant clustering of the tumor suppressor Scribble through the PDZ domain-binding motif dependent and independent interaction. *Virus Genes,* 37, 231-40.

Osmani, N., N. Vitale, J. P. Borg & S. Etienne-Manneville (2006) Scrib controls Cdc42 localization and activity to promote cell polarization during astrocyte migration. *Curr Biol,* 16, 2395-405.

Ouyang, Z., W. Zhan & L. Dan (2010) hScrib, a human homolog of Drosophila neoplastic tumor suppressor, is involved in the progress of endometrial cancer. *Oncol Res,* 18, 593-9.

Pagliarini, R. A. & T. Xu (2003) A genetic screen in Drosophila for metastatic behavior. *Science,* 302, 1227-31.

Papagiannouli, F. 2003. Gonad formation in discs-large and scribble mutant embryos and larvae of Drosophila melanogaster. In *Combined Faculties for the Natural Sciences and Mathematics,* p. 1-120. Heidelberg: Ruperto-Carola, University of Heidelberg.

Papagiannouli, F. & B. M. Mechler (2009) discs large regulates somatic cyst cell survival and expansion in Drosophila testis. *Cell Res,* 19, 1139-49.

Papagiannouli, F. & B. M. Mechler (2010) discs large in the Drosophila testis: An old player on a new task. *Fly (Austin),* 4.

Patel, S. K., F. E. Indig, N. Olivieri, N. D. Levine & M. Latterich (1998) Organelle membrane fusion: a novel function for the syntaxin homolog Ufe1p in ER membrane fusion. *Cell,* 92, 611-20.

Paul, S. M., M. Ternet, P. M. Salvaterra & G. J. Beitel (2003) The Na+/K+ ATPase is required for septate junction function and epithelial tube-size control in the Drosophila tracheal system. *Development,* 130, 4963-74.

Pelissier, A., J. P. Chauvin & T. Lecuit (2003) Trafficking through Rab11 endosomes is required for cellularization during Drosophila embryogenesis. *Curr Biol,* 13, 1848-57.

Petit, M. M., S. M. Meulemans, P. Alen, T. A. Ayoubi, E. Jansen & W. J. Van de Ven (2005) The tumor suppressor Scrib interacts with the zyxin-related protein LPP, which shuttles between cell adhesion sites and the nucleus. *BMC Cell Biol,* 6, 1.

Pfleger, C. M. & L. T. Reiter (2008) Recent efforts to model human diseases in vivo in Drosophila. *Fly (Austin),* 2, 129-32.

Phillips, H. M., H. J. Rhee, J. N. Murdoch, V. Hildreth, J. D. Peat, R. H. Anderson, A. J. Copp, B. Chaudhry & D. J. Henderson (2007) Disruption of planar cell polarity signaling results in congenital heart defects and cardiomyopathy attributable to early cardiomyocyte disorganization. *Circ Res,* 101, 137-45.

Plant, P. J., J. P. Fawcett, D. C. Lin, A. D. Holdorf, K. Binns, S. Kulkarni & T. Pawson (2003) A polarity complex of mPar-6 and atypical PKC binds, phosphorylates and regulates mammalian Lgl. *Nat Cell Biol,* 5, 301-8.

Potter, C. J., B. Tasic, E. V. Russler, L. Liang & L. Luo (2010) The Q system: a repressible binary system for transgene expression, lineage tracing, and mosaic analysis. *Cell,* 141, 536-48.

Qin, Y., C. Capaldo, B. M. Gumbiner & I. G. Macara (2005) The mammalian Scribble polarity protein regulates epithelial cell adhesion and migration through E-cadherin. *J Cell Biol*, 171, 1061-71.

Reischauer, S., M. P. Levesque, C. Nusslein-Volhard & M. Sonawane (2009) Lgl2 executes its function as a tumor suppressor by regulating ErbB signaling in the zebrafish epidermis. *PLoS Genet*, 5, e1000720.

Reiter, L. T., L. Potocki, S. Chien, M. Gribskov & E. Bier (2001) A systematic analysis of human disease-associated gene sequences in Drosophila melanogaster. *Genome Res*, 11, 1114-25.

Riggs, B., W. Rothwell, S. Mische, G. R. Hickson, J. Matheson, T. S. Hays, G. W. Gould & W. Sullivan (2003) Actin cytoskeleton remodeling during early Drosophila furrow formation requires recycling endosomal components Nuclear-fallout and Rab11. *J Cell Biol*, 163, 143-54.

Rivera, C., I. F. Yamben, S. Shatadal, M. Waldof, M. L. Robinson & A. E. Griep (2009) Cell-autonomous requirements for Dlg-1 for lens epithelial cell structure and fiber cell morphogenesis. *Dev Dyn*, 238, 2292-308.

Roche, J. P., M. C. Packard, S. Moeckel-Cole & V. Budnik (2002) Regulation of synaptic plasticity and synaptic vesicle dynamics by the PDZ protein Scribble. *J Neurosci*, 22, 6471-9.

Rossi, G. & P. Brennwald (2011) Yeast homologues of lethal giant larvae and type V myosin cooperate in the regulation of Rab-dependent vesicle clustering and polarized exocytosis. *Mol Biol Cell*, 22, 842-57.

Round, J. L., L. A. Humphries, T. Tomassian, P. Mittelstadt, M. Zhang & M. C. Miceli (2007) Scaffold protein Dlgh1 coordinates alternative p38 kinase activation, directing T cell receptor signals toward NFAT but not NF-kappaB transcription factors. *Nat Immunol*, 8, 154-61.

Sarkar, A., N. Parikh, S. A. Hearn, M. T. Fuller, S. I. Tazuke & C. Schulz (2007) Antagonistic roles of Rac and Rho in organizing the germ cell microenvironment. *Curr Biol*, 17, 1253-8.

Savory, J. G., M. Mansfield, F. M. Rijli & D. Lohnes (2011) Cdx mediates neural tube closure through transcriptional regulation of the planar cell polarity gene Ptk7. *Development*, 138, 1361-70.

Schmeichel, K. L. (2004) A fly's eye view of tumor progression and metastasis. *Breast Cancer Res*, 6, 82-3.

Schuster, C. M., G. W. Davis, R. D. Fetter & C. S. Goodman (1996a) Genetic dissection of structural and functional components of synaptic plasticity. I. Fasciclin II controls synaptic stabilization and growth. *Neuron*, 17, 641-54.

Schuster, C. M., G. W. Davis, R. D. Fetter & C. S. Goodman (1996b) Genetic dissection of structural and functional components of synaptic plasticity. II. Fasciclin II controls presynaptic structural plasticity. *Neuron*, 17, 655-67.

Siegrist, S. E. & C. Q. Doe (2005) Microtubule-induced Pins/Galphai cortical polarity in Drosophila neuroblasts. *Cell*, 123, 1323-35.

Skouloudaki, K., M. Puetz, M. Simons, J. R. Courbard, C. Boehlke, B. Hartleben, C. Engel, M. J. Moeller, C. Englert, F. Bollig, T. Schafer, H. Ramachandran, M. Mlodzik, T. B. Huber, E. W. Kuehn, E. Kim, A. Kramer-Zucker & G. Walz (2009) Scribble participates in Hippo signaling and is required for normal zebrafish pronephros development. *Proc Natl Acad Sci U S A*, 106, 8579-84.

Sonawane, M., Y. Carpio, R. Geisler, H. Schwarz, H. M. Maischein & C. Nuesslein-Volhard (2005) Zebrafish penner/lethal giant larvae 2 functions in hemidesmosome formation, maintenance of cellular morphology and growth regulation in the developing basal epidermis. *Development*, 132, 3255-65.

Sonawane, M., H. Martin-Maischein, H. Schwarz & C. Nusslein-Volhard (2009) Lgl2 and E-cadherin act antagonistically to regulate hemidesmosome formation during epidermal development in zebrafish. *Development*, 136, 1231-40.

Sripathy, S., M. Lee & V. Vasioukhin (2011) Mammalian Llgl2 is necessary for proper branching morphogenesis during placental development. *Mol Cell Biol.*

Strand, D., R. Jakobs, G. Merdes, B. Neumann, A. Kalmes, H. W. Heid, I. Husmann & B. M. Mechler (1994a) The Drosophila lethal(2)giant larvae tumor suppressor protein forms homo-oligomers and is associated with nonmuscle myosin II heavy chain. *J Cell Biol*, 127, 1361-73.

Strand, D., I. Raska & B. M. Mechler (1994b) The Drosophila lethal(2)giant larvae tumor suppressor protein is a component of the cytoskeleton. *J Cell Biol*, 127, 1345-60.

Strickland, L. I. & D. R. Burgess (2004) Pathways for membrane trafficking during cytokinesis. *Trends Cell Biol*, 14, 115-8.

Suresh, B., S. Ramakrishna, Y. S. Kim, S. M. Kim, M. S. Kim & K. H. Baek (2010) Stability and function of mammalian lethal giant larvae-1 oncoprotein are regulated by the scaffolding protein RanBPM. *J Biol Chem*, 285, 35340-9.

Swanson, L. E. & G. J. Beitel (2006) Tubulogenesis: an inside job. *Curr Biol*, 16, R51-3.

Takizawa, S., K. Nagasaka, S. Nakagawa, T. Yano, K. Nakagawa, T. Yasugi, T. Takeuchi, T. Kanda, J. M. Huibregtse, T. Akiyama & Y. Taketani (2006) Human scribble, a novel tumor suppressor identified as a target of high-risk HPV E6 for ubiquitin-mediated degradation, interacts with adenomatous polyposis coli. *Genes Cells*, 11, 453-64.

Tamori, Y., C. U. Bialucha, A. G. Tian, M. Kajita, Y. C. Huang, M. Norman, N. Harrison, J. Poulton, K. Ivanovitch, L. Disch, T. Liu, W. M. Deng & Y. Fujita (2010) Involvement of Lgl and Mahjong/VprBP in cell competition. *PLoS Biol*, 8, e1000422.

Tanentzapf, G. & U. Tepass (2003) Interactions between the crumbs, lethal giant larvae and bazooka pathways in epithelial polarization. *Nat Cell Biol*, 5, 46-52.

Tapon, N. (2003) Modeling transformation and metastasis in Drosophila. *Cancer Cell*, 4, 333-5.

Thomas, U., S. Ebitsch, M. Gorczyca, Y. H. Koh, C. D. Hough, D. Woods, E. D. Gundelfinger & V. Budnik (2000) Synaptic targeting and localization of discs-large is a stepwise process controlled by different domains of the protein. *Curr Biol*, 10, 1108-17.

Thomas, U., E. Kim, S. Kuhlendahl, Y. H. Koh, E. D. Gundelfinger, M. Sheng, C. C. Garner & V. Budnik (1997a) Synaptic clustering of the cell adhesion molecule fasciclin II by discs-large and its role in the regulation of presynaptic structure. *Neuron*, 19, 787-99.

Thomas, U., B. Phannavong, B. Muller, C. C. Garner & E. D. Gundelfinger (1997b) Functional expression of rat synapse-associated proteins SAP97 and SAP102 in Drosophila dlg-1 mutants: effects on tumor suppression and synaptic bouton structure. *Mech Dev*, 62, 161-74.

Tomaic, V., D. Pim & L. Banks (2009) The stability of the human papillomavirus E6 oncoprotein is E6AP dependent. *Virology*, 393, 7-10.

Tran, J., T. J. Brenner & S. DiNardo (2000) Somatic control over the germline stem cell lineage during Drosophila spermatogenesis. *Nature,* 407, 754-7.

Vaira, V., A. Faversani, T. Dohi, M. Maggioni, M. Nosotti, D. Tosi, D. C. Altieri & S. Bosari (2011) Aberrant Overexpression of the Cell Polarity Module Scribble in Human Cancer. *Am J Pathol.*

Vasioukhin, V. (2006) Lethal giant puzzle of Lgl. *Dev Neurosci,* 28, 13-24.

Vidal, M. (2010) The dark side of fly TNF: an ancient developmental proof reading mechanism turned into tumor promoter. *Cell Cycle,* 9, 3851-6.

Vidal, M., L. Salavaggione, L. Ylagan, M. Wilkins, M. Watson, K. Weilbaecher & R. Cagan (2010) A role for the epithelial microenvironment at tumor boundaries: evidence from Drosophila and human squamous cell carcinomas. *Am J Pathol,* 176, 3007-14.

Vieira, V., G. de la Houssaye, E. Lacassagne, J. L. Dufier, J. P. Jais, F. Beermann, M. Menasche & M. Abitbol (2008) Differential regulation of Dlg1, Scrib, and Lgl1 expression in a transgenic mouse model of ocular cancer. *Mol Vis,* 14, 2390-403.

Walsh, G. S., P. K. Grant, J. A. Morgan & C. B. Moens (2011) Planar polarity pathway and Nance-Horan syndrome-like 1b have essential cell-autonomous functions in neuronal migration. *Development,* 138, 3033-42.

Wang, S., S. A. Jayaram, J. Hemphala, K. A. Senti, V. Tsarouhas, H. Jin & C. Samakovlis (2006) Septate-junction-dependent luminal deposition of chitin deacetylases restricts tube elongation in the Drosophila trachea. *Curr Biol,* 16, 180-5.

Wansleeben, C., L. van Gurp, H. Feitsma, C. Kroon, E. Rieter, M. Verberne, V. Guryev, E. Cuppen & F. Meijlink (2011) An ENU-Mutagenesis Screen in the Mouse: Identification of Novel Developmental Gene Functions. *PLoS One,* 6, e19357.

Weiss, P. 1961. In *The Molecular Control of Cellular Activity,* ed. A. JM, pp. 1–72.: McGraw-Hill.

Wen, S., H. Zhu, W. Lu, L. E. Mitchell, G. M. Shaw, E. J. Lammer & R. H. Finnell (2010) Planar cell polarity pathway genes and risk for spina bifida. *Am J Med Genet A,* 152A, 299-304.

Wirtz-Peitz, F. & J. A. Knoblich (2006) Lethal giant larvae take on a life of their own. *Trends Cell Biol,* 16, 234-41.

Wodarz, A. (2000) Tumor suppressors: linking cell polarity and growth control. *Curr Biol,* 10, R624-6.

Wodarz, A. & C. Gonzalez (2006) Connecting cancer to the asymmetric division of stem cells. *Cell,* 124, 1121-3.

Wodarz, A., U. Hinz, M. Engelbert & E. Knust (1995) Expression of crumbs confers apical character on plasma membrane domains of ectodermal epithelia of Drosophila. *Cell,* 82, 67-76.

Wong, M. D., Z. Jin & T. Xie (2005) Molecular mechanisms of germline stem cell regulation. *Annu Rev Genet,* 39, 173-95.

Woodhouse, E. C. & L. A. Liotta (2004) Drosophila invasive tumors: a model for understanding metastasis. *Cell Cycle,* 3, 38-40.

Woods, D. F., C. Hough, D. Peel, G. Callaini & P. J. Bryant (1996) Dlg protein is required for junction structure, cell polarity, and proliferation control in Drosophila epithelia. *J Cell Biol,* 134, 1469-82.

Wu, J. S. & L. Luo (2006) A protocol for mosaic analysis with a repressible cell marker (MARCM) in Drosophila. *Nat Protoc,* 1, 2583-9.

Wu, M., J. C. Pastor-Pareja & T. Xu (2010) Interaction between Ras(V12) and scribbled clones induces tumour growth and invasion. *Nature,* 463, 545-8.

Wu, V. M. & G. J. Beitel (2004) A junctional problem of apical proportions: epithelial tube-size control by septate junctions in the Drosophila tracheal system. *Curr Opin Cell Biol,* 16, 493-9.

Yamanaka, T., Y. Horikoshi, N. Izumi, A. Suzuki, K. Mizuno & S. Ohno (2006) Lgl mediates apical domain disassembly by suppressing the PAR-3-aPKC-PAR-6 complex to orient apical membrane polarity. *J Cell Sci,* 119, 2107-18.

Yamanaka, T., Y. Horikoshi, Y. Sugiyama, C. Ishiyama, A. Suzuki, T. Hirose, A. Iwamatsu, A. Shinohara & S. Ohno (2003) Mammalian Lgl forms a protein complex with PAR-6 and aPKC independently of PAR-3 to regulate epithelial cell polarity. *Curr Biol,* 13, 734-43.

Yamanaka, T. & S. Ohno (2008) Role of Lgl/Dlg/Scribble in the regulation of epithelial junction, polarity and growth. *Front Biosci,* 13, 6693-707.

Yamashita, Y. M., A. P. Mahowald, J. R. Perlin & M. T. Fuller (2007) Asymmetric inheritance of mother versus daughter centrosome in stem cell division. *Science,* 315, 518-21.

Yates, L. L., J. Papakrivopoulou, D. A. Long, P. Goggolidou, J. O. Connolly, A. S. Woolf & C. H. Dean (2010a) The planar cell polarity gene Vangl2 is required for mammalian kidney-branching morphogenesis and glomerular maturation. *Hum Mol Genet,* 19, 4663-76.

Yates, L. L., C. Schnatwinkel, J. N. Murdoch, D. Bogani, C. J. Formstone, S. Townsend, A. Greenfield, L. A. Niswander & C. H. Dean (2010b) The PCP genes Celsr1 and Vangl2 are required for normal lung branching morphogenesis. *Hum Mol Genet,* 19, 2251-67.

Zarnescu, D. C., P. Jin, J. Betschinger, M. Nakamoto, Y. Wang, T. C. Dockendorff, Y. Feng, T. A. Jongens, J. C. Sisson, J. A. Knoblich, S. T. Warren & K. Moses (2005) Fragile X protein functions with lgl and the par complex in flies and mice. *Dev Cell,* 8, 43-52.

Zeng, X., S. R. Singh, D. Hou & S. X. Hou (2010) Tumor suppressors Sav/Scrib and oncogene Ras regulate stem-cell transformation in adult Drosophila malpighian tubules. *J Cell Physiol,* 224, 766-74.

Zhan, L., A. Rosenberg, K. C. Bergami, M. Yu, Z. Xuan, A. B. Jaffe, C. Allred & S. K. Muthuswamy (2008) Deregulation of scribble promotes mammary tumorigenesis and reveals a role for cell polarity in carcinoma. *Cell,* 135, 865-78.

Zhang, X., P. Wang, A. Gangar, J. Zhang, P. Brennwald, D. TerBush & W. Guo (2005) Lethal giant larvae proteins interact with the exocyst complex and are involved in polarized exocytosis. *J Cell Biol,* 170, 273-83.

Zhang, Y., H. Guo, H. Kwan, J. W. Wang, J. Kosek & B. Lu (2007) PAR-1 kinase phosphorylates Dlg and regulates its postsynaptic targeting at the Drosophila neuromuscular junction. *Neuron,* 53, 201-15.

Zhu, M., T. Xin, S. Weng, Y. Gao, Y. Zhang, Q. Li & M. Li (2010) Activation of JNK signaling links lgl mutations to disruption of the cell polarity and epithelial organization in Drosophila imaginal discs. *Cell Res,* 20, 242-5.

Zigman, M., A. Trinh le, S. E. Fraser & C. B. Moens (2011) Zebrafish neural tube morphogenesis requires Scribble-dependent oriented cell divisions. *Curr Biol,* 21, 79-86.

Zito, K., R. D. Fetter, C. S. Goodman & E. Y. Isacoff (1997) Synaptic clustering of Fascilin II and Shaker: essential targeting sequences and role of Dlg. *Neuron,* 19, 1007-16.

9

Epigenetic and Posttranscriptional Alterations of Tumor Suppressor Genes in Sporadic Pituitary Adenomas

Henriett Butz[1], Károly Rácz[1] and Attila Patócs[1,2,3]

[1]2nd Department of Medicine, Faculty of Medicine, Semmelweis University, Budapest,
[2]Molecular Medicine Research Group, Hungarian Academy of Sciences and Semmelweis University,
[3]Department of Laboratory Medicine, Semmelweis University, Budapest, Hungary

1. Introduction

1.1 Epidemiology of pituitary adenomas

Pituitary adenomas are usually benign tumors. Although many of them do not cause clinical symptoms and remain undetected, some leads to hormonal and/or neurological disorders. Because a large proportion of pituitary adenomas are discovered incidentally, the estimation of their prevalence may be difficult. Recently Daly et al. summarized the reported prevalence rate based on *autopsies* and *radiological* series showing a mean prevalence of 14.4 and 22.3% respectively, and a combined analysis yielded a final prevalence rate of 16.7%. Based on three different *population studies* they found that the mean prevalence is 1:1064 (Daly et al., 2009). The most frequent tumors were prolactinomas, followed by non-functioning and growth-hormone (GH) producing tumors (66.2%, 14.7% and 13.2%, respectively). Based on results of an *international, multicentre study* the prevalence of clinically relevant pituitary adenoma is 1:1388 which is 3-5 times higher than that previously reported (Daly et al., 2009).

According to data obtained from 8276 patients the incidence rate of pituitary adenomas is increasing with age, and they occur more frequently in females in early life and in males in later life. Males had larger tumors than females, and a higher incidence was detected in American Blacks compared with other ethnic groups (McDowell et al., 2011).

1.2 Pathogenetic mechanisms leading to pituitary tumorgenesis

Pituitary adenomas usually occur sporadically and most of them have monoclonal origin (Alexander et al., 1990; Herman et al., 1990). Both *hypothalamic and hypophyseal mechanisms* including alterations in hypothalamic control of pituitary hormone secretion and somatic mutations in pituitary cells have been considered as possible pathogenetic factors in pituitary tumor development. In experimental models overproduction of GH-releasing hormone may lead to the development of GH-secreting adenoma, while decreased level of dopamine may be associated with prolactinoma development.

Familial pituitary adenomas represent only 5% of all pituitary tumors. Most of these tumors are associated with known genetic defects predisposing to hereditary endocrine tumor syndromes. The most common is multiple endocrine neoplasia type 1 (MEN1), a disorder transmitted in an autosomal dominant manner due to mutations of the *MEN1* tumor suppressor gene. However, in about 20-30% of clinically MEN1 cases mutation analysis failed to reveal mutations of the *MEN1* gene. Mutations in cyclin-dependent kinase inhibitor 1B (CDKI1B) gene coding for p27 have been demonstrated in a small subset of patients, and the clinical syndrome has been named MEN4 (Dworakowska & Grossman, 2009).

Another familial disease that includes pituitary adenoma is Carney complex (CNC). This syndrome is caused by mutations of the gene encoding the protein kinase A regulatory subunit-1-alpha (PRKAR1A) (Stratakis et al., 2001). PRKAR1A is known to be an important effector molecule in many endocrine signaling pathways and its defect leads to various endocrine and nonendocrine tumor formation.

A separate entity among familial pituitary tumors is the familial isolated pituitary adenoma (FIPA) presenting most frequently as familial somatotropinomas or prolactinomas. Patients with FIPA are significantly younger, and their adenoma size is larger compared to sporadic pituitary adenoma counterparts. About 15% of the FIPA patients have mutations of the gene encoding the aryl hydrocarbon receptor-interacting protein (AIP), which indicates that the FIPA may have a diverse genetic pathophysiology (Daly et al., 2009; Dworakowska & Grossman, 2009).

Although McCune–Albright syndrome (MAS) is not a hereditary disorder, it represents a genetic condition related to mosaicism for a mutation of the guanine nucleotide-activating alpha-subunit (*GNAS*) gene. In addition, somatic mutation of the *GNAS* gene is present in 30–40% of GH-secreting pituitary adenomas (Lania et al., 2003; Spada et al., 1990,). Mutation of this gene leads to the constitutive activation of the GH receptor and thereby contributes to GH-producing adenoma formation.

Genetic changes of classical tumor suppressor genes (TSGs) such as *TP53, PTEN* and *RB1*, or oncogenes (such as Ras) rarely contribute to pituitary tumorigenesis. However, overactivation of the *PI3K/Akt/mTOR signaling pathway* has been demonstrated in pituitary adenomas as frequently as in other solid tumors (Rodriguez-Viciana et al., 1997). Both expression and phopshorylation of the Akt was increased in all types of pituitary adenomas with a highest rate in non-functioining pituitary adenomas (NFPA) (Musat et al., 2005). In addition to PI3K/Akt/mTOR, the *MAPK cascade* was also found to be involved in cell transformation and proliferation (Ewing et al., 2007; Guan, 1994; Joneson & Bar-Sagi, 1997). Recently, microarray studies indicated that the *WNT and Notch signaling pathways* play a role in the pathogenesis of pituitary adenomas, especially in NFPA (Moreno et al., 2005).

Among *growth factors* the N-terminally truncated isoform of fibroblast growth factor receptor type 4 (pdt-FGFR4) and fibroblast growth factor type 2 (FGF2) were found to be overexpressed in some pituitary tumors, especially in aggressive adenomas while overexpression of bone morphogenic protein type 4 (BMP4) was charactheristic for prolactinomas (Ezzat et al., 1995; Ezzat et al., 2002; Morita et al., 2008; Qian et al., 2004).

Cyclin D, a member of cell cycle regulation was shown to be overexpressed in pituitary adenomas, especially in NFPAs, while numerous cyclin-dependent kinase inhibitors (CDKIs) were reportedly underexpressed due to promoter hypermethylation. These alterations will be discussed.

Another relatively common alteration in pituitary tumors is overexpression of the oncogene *pituitary tumor-transforming 1 (PTTG1)*, that is indirectly involved in cell cycle through an interaction with p53 and induction of p21 (Salehi et al., 2008). PTTG1 was found to be overexpressed in most pituitary adenomas, particularly in hormone-secreting and aggressively behaving tumors (X. Zhang et al., 1999).

2. Epigenetic mechanisms

Epigenetic mechanisms denote gene expression variability without coding sequence alteration. These mechanisms have important role in development, X chromosome inactivation, and modulation of gene expression in tissue specific manner. Epigenetic machinery includes *DNA methylation, histone modifications* and regulation of gene expression posttranscriptionally by small, *non-coding RNA molecules.*

The compact DNA structure called chromatin is built from nucleosome units. These nucleosomes consist of approximately 150-200 bp of DNA, which is coiled twice around an octamer protein complex composed of core histones (H2A, H2B, H3 and H4). The adjacent nucleosomes are connected by the "linker" H1 histone. From nucleosomes DNA is assembled into a higher structure by covalent modifications of histone proteins. These modifications include methylation, acetylation, phosphorylation and ubiquitination at the N- and C-terminal domains of core histones. DNA and histone modifications influence DNA compactation thereby affect DNA availability for transcription factors and determine transcriptional activity.

2.1 DNA methylation

DNA methylation occurs as a methyl-group on 5′ position of cytosine in a CpG dinucleotide (5-methylcytosine). Although CpG dinucleotides are relatively infrequent (~1 per 100 bp) throughout the genome, approximately 7% of them are mapped within CpG islands, which in turn are associated with the promoter regions of approximately 40–50% of all transcribed genes (Baylin & Herman, 2000; Gardiner-Garden & Frommer, 1987; Rollins et al., 2006.) and about 45% of all CpGs can be found in repetitive elements (Ehrlich et al., 1982).

Methylation is accomplished by DNA methyltransferases (DNMT). These enzymes create "de novo" (DNMT type 3a and 3b) or maintain (DNMT1) the methylation pattern, which is a replication-dependent process passing off during S-phase of the cell cycle (Klose & Bird, 2006). Methylation of CpG islands cause gene expression silencing by direct inhibition of transcription factors binding and by recruitment of methyl-binding domain proteins (MBDs) occurring in transcription repressor complexes.

CpG island methylation is correlated with condensed heterochromatin. On the contrary, hypomethylation allows an open chromatin structure and it usually occurs in promoter regions of active genes.

In primary human tumors, methylation patterns are frequently disorganized. Promoter regions of genes are often hypermethylated and, therefore, their expressions are silenced. In general, aberrant CpG island methylation tends to be focal, affecting single genes, but not their neighbours (Zardo et al., 2002). Tumor suppressor genes involved in the regulation of cell cycle, apoptosis or genes participating in DNA repair are often silenced by hypermethylation and they do not have other genetic alterations (eg. mutations) (Brena & Costello, 2007). Beside hypermethylation genome-wide hypomethylation was also implicated in tumor development (Feinberg & Vogelstein, 1983; Gaudet et al., 2003).

2.2 Histone modification

Chemical modification of histones (H) frequently targets lysine residues within their N- and C-terminal tails. Core histone modification is frequently called as 'histone code' which determines transcriptional activity by influencing compaction of DNA structure (Jenuwein & Allis, 2001; Turner, 2000). Deacetylated forms of N-tails of H3 and H4 histones have a positive charge that results in a close nucleosome structure because of the negatively charged DNA. Acetylations of lysine residues on histone tails neutralize the positive charge of histones thereby lead to a loose, "opened" chromatin structure (Struhl, 1998) (Fig.1.).

In addition to acetylation, histone modifications may include methylation, phosphorylation, sumoylation, ubiquitination and ADP-ribosylation. Among these mechanisms covalent modifications, such as acetylation of H3 and H4 and methylation pattern on gene expression have been extensively investigated in tumor development. Several enzymes including histone acetyltransferases (HAT), histone deacetylases (HDAC), histone methyltransferases (HMT) and histone demethyltransferases (HDMT) may modify histones. Acetylation of lysine (K) residues associated with H4 and methylation of lysine 9 (K9) in H3 may be present at inactive gene loci. Alternatively, acetylation on K9, K14 and methylation on K4 of H3, or acetylation on K5 of H4 can be found both at active or activating gene loci, reviewed by Tateno et al, 2010 (Tateno et al., 2010; Ezzat, 2008).

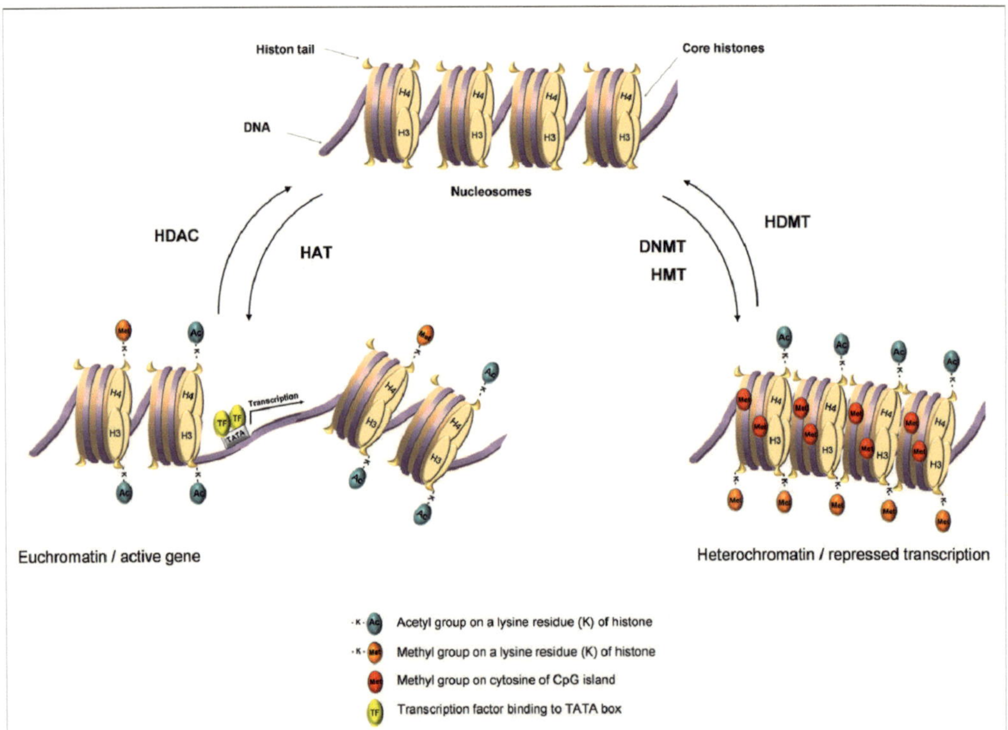

Fig. 1. Histone and DNA modifications.

2.3 Genomic imprinting

Genomic imprinting is related to a special form (or a subgroup) of DNA methylation, which allows monoallelic gene expression in a "parent-of-origin-specific" manner (Wong et al., 2007). Diploid cells have two alleles of each autosomal gene inherited from each parent. Generally both parental alleles are expressed equally, but a subset of genes is expressed by either the maternal or the paternal allele, and this 'genomic imprinting' is regulated by epigenetic mechanisms. This process may be also responsible for tissue specific gene expression.

Imprinted expression is restricted to a few hundred genes in the mammalian genome, most of which are found in small clusters. Imprinted clusters have an imprinting control region (ICR) that is usually 1–5 kb. long, differentially methylated and it regulates the imprinting mechanism across the entire domain. Imprinted genes are regulated also by methylation. Many imprinted genes inside of an imprinted cluster are protein-coding genes, however, recently the role of ncRNAs in imprinting regulation was also raised (Zhou et al., 2010).

The most commonly cited example for imprinting mechanism leading to tumorigenesis is the gene encoding insulin-like growth factor type 2 (IGF2). IGF2 is paternally imprinted in most tissues (Ohlsson et al., 1994). It is an embryonic mitogen and it acts as a paracrine and autocrine regulator of cell proliferation (Yu & Rohan, 2000). In cells that express both parental IGF2 alleles, the increased amount of IGF2 may lead to tumor formation. Loss of imprinting (LOI) of *IGF2* has been reported in many tumors including colorectal carcinomas (Cui et al., 2003), Wilm's tumor (Ogawa et al., 1993), esophageal carcinoma (Zhao et al., 2009), acute lymphoblastic leukemia (Vorwerk et al., 2003) and prostate cancer (Jarrard et al., 1995).

2.4 Regulation by non-coding RNAs (ncRNAs) and microRNAs (miRs)

Thus far small RNAs do not belong tightly to classical epigenetic mechanisms, but based on recent findings we have to classify them into this group as they regulate gene expression without modification of the genetic code. For instance, miRs provide fine tuning of protein expression level, and their role in tumorigenesis has been widely demonstrated.

MicroRNAs belong to non-codingRNAs (ncRNAs) that can regulate gene expression. It was found that about 98% of all transcripts originate from ncRNAs (Mattick, 2001). These arise from exons and introns of protein non-coding genes and from introns of protein-coding genes (Mattick & Makunin, 2005). Non-coding RNAs include transfer-RNAs (tRNAs) involved in mRNA translation, small nucleolar RNAs (snoRNAs) involved in modification of ribosomal RNAs (rRNAs) and small nuclear RNAs (snRNAs) implicated in mRNA splicing (Mattick & Makunin, 2005). Beyond these, several small RNAs (categorized into 13 functional classes) were discovered with diversified biological functions including heterochromatin formation, histone and DNA methylation, mRNA cleavage and transcriptional repression (summarized by Zhou et al., 2010).

MicroRNAs (miRs) are approximately 19-25 nucleotide long, non-coding RNA molecules which posttranscriptionally regulate gene expression via RNA interference by binding 3' untranslated region (3'UTR) of protein coding mRNA (Lagos-Quintana et al., 2001). This pairing is not a perfect match in the case of mammals but it is in plants. By interacting the target mRNAs miRs repress the target protein expression by three major processes: i) mRNA cleavage, ii) mRNA degradation by deadenylation or iii) inhibition of translation initiation. In addition, miRs regulate expression of other types of ncRNAs (Fig.2.).

It has been proposed that 30-50% of all protein coding genes may be controlled by miRs (Chen & Rajewsky, 2006; Lewis et al., 2005). As miRs may influence numerous mRNA they may participate in the regulation of numerous physiological and pathological cellular processes. Their roles were considered in development (Lee & Ambros, 2001), cell proliferation (O'Donnel et al., 2005), differentiation (Chen & Stallings, 2007), apoptosis (Cimmino et al., 2005) and tumorigenesis (reviewed by Deng et al., 2008) including tumors of endocrine system such as the pituitary gland (Bottoni et al., 2005, 2007; Amaral et al., 2009, Butz et al., 2010, 2011).

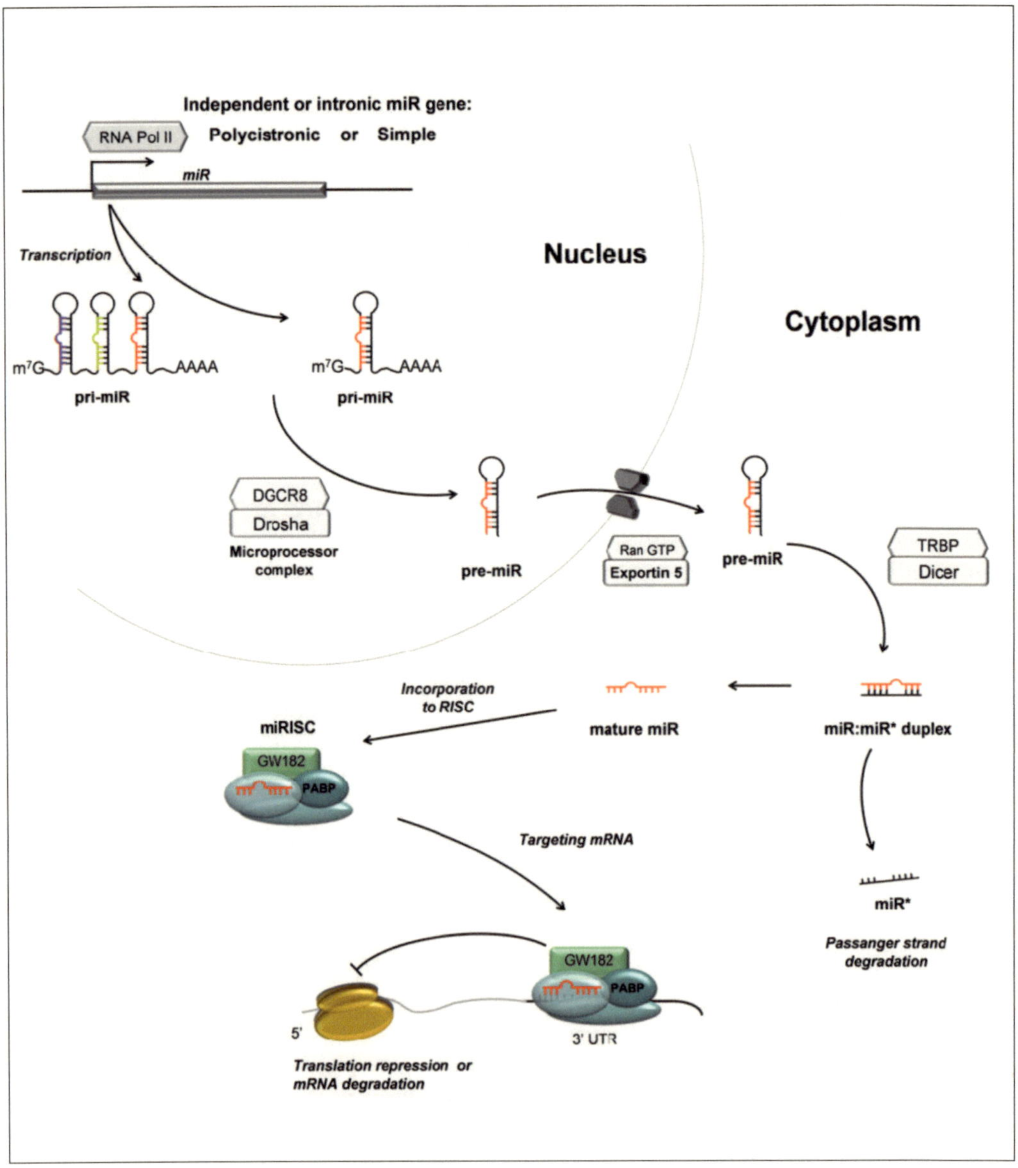

Fig. 2. MicroRNAs' biogenesis and function.

3. Epigenetic alterations involving tumor suppressor genes

3.1 Hypermethylated tumor suppressors

3.1.1 Genes encoding cell cycle regulators

The sensitively balanced cell cycle involves numerous negative and positive regulators. The main proteins involved in this process are the cyclins, cyclin-dependent kinases (CDK) and their inhibitors (CDKI). Alterations of several cell cycle-related genes, especially those involved in the G1/S transition have been associated with pituitary adenomas. Several cell cycle inhibitors (CDKIs) were found to be underexpressed through promoter hypermethylation in pituitary adenomas. CDKIs as members of the INK4 families ($p16^{Ink4a}$, $p15^{Ink4b}$, $p18^{Ink4c}$) and the Cip/Kip ($p21^{Cip1}$, $p27^{Kip1}$, $p57^{Kip2}$) inhibit CDK-cyclin complexes thereby prevent checkpoint transitions (Fig. 3.).

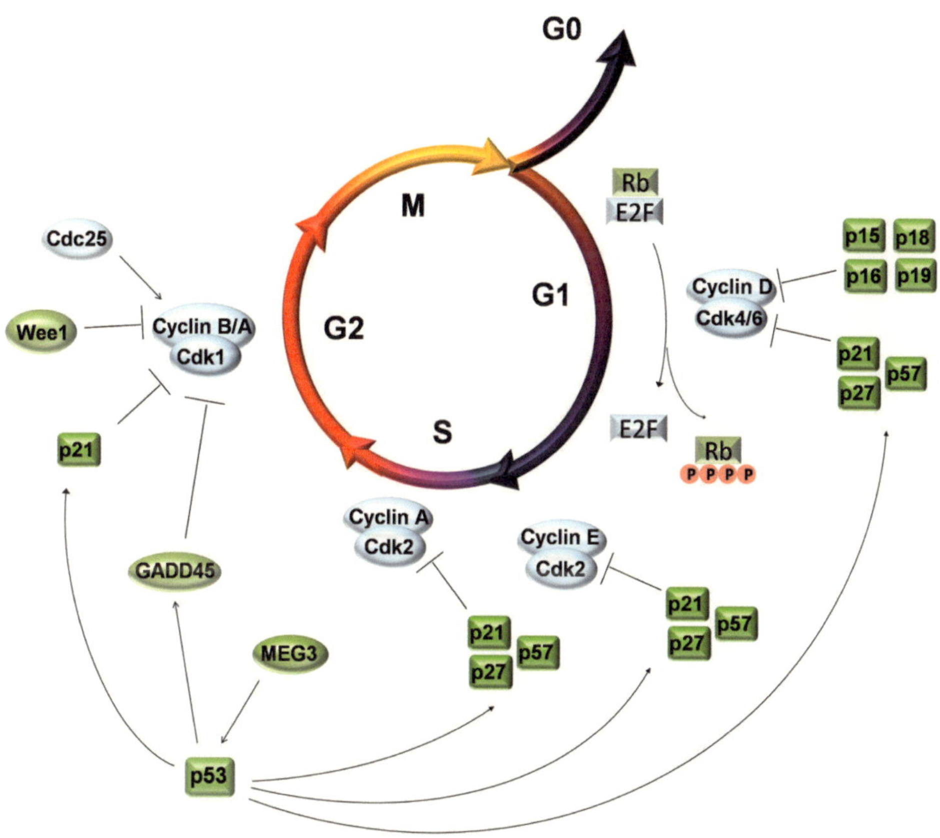

Fig. 3. Regulation of cell cycle.

The restriction point of the G1/S transition requires inactivation of retinoblastoma (Rb) protein via phosphorylation by CDKs. In this process E2F transcription factors are released and transcription of S-phase genes are allowed. The majority of pituitary adenomas express Rb and inactivation of CDKIs (detailed in Table 1) may lead to cell proliferation in pituitary adenomas.

Gene Name	Alterations in pituitary adenomas
pRb (RB1)	• Promoter hypermethylation in 28.6% (12/42) and 35% (12/34) of adenomas (Ogino et al., 2005; Yoshino et al., 2007) • 90% of adenomas expressed Rb (18/20) and in 60% of Rb-non-expressing adenomas promoter methylation was found (Simpson et al., 2000) • LOH of the RB locus in 100% of invasive and malignant tumors (Pei et al., 1995)
p53	• Somatic inactivating mutation and increased expression in 33% (2/6) of pituitary carcinomas (Tanizaki et al., 2007)
p14^ARF^	• Promoter hypermethylation in 6% (2/24) of adenomas (Yoshino et al., 2007)
$p15^{INK4b}$ (CDKN2B)	• Promoter hypermethylation in 32% (11/34) and 35.7% (15/42) of adenomas (Yoshino et al., 2007; Ogino et al., 2005)
$p16^{INK4a}$ (CDKN2A)	• Promoter hypermethylation in 59% (20/34) and 71.4% (30/42) of adenomas (Yoshino et al., 2007; Ogino et al., 2005)
$p18^{INK4c}$ (CDKN2C)	• Promoter hypermethylation in 39.5% (15/38) of adenomas (Kirsch et al., 2009; Morris et al., 2005)
$p21^{Waf1/Cip1}$ (CDKN1A)	• Promoter hypermethylation in 3% (1/34) of adenomas (Yoshino et al., 2007) • Decreased expression in 71% (10/14) of NFPAs (Neto et al., 2005) • Increased expression in 77% (31/40) of hormone producing and 92% (11/12) of GH producing adenomas (Neto et al., 2005)
p27Kip1 (CDKN1B)	• Absence of promoter hypermethylation in 34 pituitary adenomas (Yoshino et al., 2007) • Decreased expression in adenomas especially in corticotrop adenomas (21/21) (Lidhar et al., 1999; Lloyd et al., 1997; Bamberger et al., 1999)
GADD45γ	• Promoter methylation in 58% (19/33) of adenomas (Bahar et al., 2004a; Zhang et al., 2002)
MEG3A	• Promoter methylation (11/11) of adenomas (Gejman et al., 2008; Zhao et al., 2005)
DAPK	• Loss of expression in 59% (10/17) of invasive adenomas caused by hypermethylation (45%) or homozygous deletion (36%) (Simpson et al., 2002)
PTAG	• Loss of expression in 79% (30/38) of adenomas caused by hypermethylation in 20% (Bahar et al., 2004b)
ZAC	• Loss or decreased expression in (34/34) NFPAs (Pagotto et al., 2000)

Table 1. Hypermethylated tumorsuppressors involved in pituitary tumorigenesis.

GADD45γ, also known as *cytokine response 6* (*CR6*) was found to be involved in growth suppression and apoptosis (Zhang et al., 1999). The *GADD45* family genes (*GADD45α: GADD45, GADD45β: MyD118* and *GADD45γ: CR6)* are regulated by p53. They influence the expression of $p21^{WAF1/CIP1}$ and proliferating cell nuclear antigen (PCNA) and have a role in DNA damage repair (Fan et al., 1999; Smith et al., 1994; Xiao et al., 2000). They disrupt interaction between CDK1 kinase and cyclin B1 and, therefore, they suppress cell proliferation not only by inhibiting G1/S transition but they also cause G2/M arrest. (Zhan

et al., 1999). They are also involved in apoptosis regulation by activating MAPK and Jun kinase signaling pathways and they cause DNA fragmentation (Takekawa & Saito, 1998). Further studies demonstrated that they are not expressed in the majority of NFPA and GH- or PRL-secreting tumors. Reexpression of GADD45 in human and rodent pituitary-derived cell lines inhibited cell proliferation suggesting that loss of GADD45 may have a role in pituitary tumorigenesis. Methylation of CpG islands of the GADD45γ gene was identified in 19/33 (58%) of pituitary adenomas including NFPA, GH- and PRL secreting tumors (Bahar et al., 2004a).
Zhao and coworkers showed that a gene named maternally expressed 3 (MEG3) was strongly expressed in normal pituitary gland while its expression was almost undetectable in pituitary tumors and other cancer cell lines (Zhao et al., 2005). In functional studies methylation inhibitor restored *MEG3* expression in human cell lines. MEG3 protein non-coding RNA has multiple splice isoforms and all of them suppress cell growth in vitro by stimulating p53-mediated transactivation (Zhou et al., 2007). All human pituitary cell types express MEG3, while in adenomatous pituitary samples the loss of MEG3 was limited to NFPAs of gonadotroph origin (Gejman et al., 2008). It has been shown that inactivation of the MEG3 gene was exclusively due to methylated CpGs in its promoter. (Zhao et al., 2005; Gejman et al., 2008).

3.1.2 Genes encoding regulators of apoptosis

The gene encoding death-associated protein kinase (DAPK) was found to be frequently altered by epigenetic mechanisms in pituitary tumors. Simpson and his collegues demonstrated that in 34% (11/32) of pituitary tumors expression of the *DAPK* was undetectable and that almost half of the cases had CpG island methylation in the *DAPK* promoter region. In addition, loss of DAPK expression was associated with tumor invasiveness. However, only a minority of non-invasive pituitary adenomas (2/35; 5.7%) showed underexpression of the *DAPK* caused by methylation (Bello et al., 2006). Another protein involved in apoptosis regulation is the pituitary tumor apoptosis gene (PTAG). Its expression was reduced in a significant percent (79%, 30/38) of pituitary adenomas. All corticotropinomas and prolactinomas, 73% of somatotropinomas and 64% of NFPAs showed reduced expression of *PTAG*. Reexpression of *PTAG* alone failed to influence pituitary cell proliferation or cell viability but significantly augmented the apoptotic response to bromocriptin induction. This „apoptosis sensitization" effect was described also in colon cancer (Bahar et al., 2007). It was also suggested that PTAG loss in pituitary adenomas may be an early step in pituitary tumorigenesis leading to a blunted apoptotic response (Bahar et al., 2004b).
Among other methylated genes involved in the regulation of apoptosis in pituitary cells are *ZAC* and *RASSF1*. The *ZAC* (zinc finger protein which regulates apoptosis and cell cycle arrest, or PLAGL1, pleiomorph adenoma gene like-1) encoding a zink finger protein was found to be strongly underexpressed in NFPAs compared to other types of pituitary adenomas or normal pituitary tissue (Pagotto et al., 2000). ZAC inhibited cell proliferation and colony formation in functional *in vitro* experiments and abolished tumor formation in nude mice. It induced apoptosis and cell cycle arrest independently of pRb, $p21^{Waf1/Cip1}$, $p16^{INK4a}$, $p27^{KIP2}$ and $p57^{KIP3}$ (Spengler et al., 1997). Underexpression of ZAC was related either to loss of heterozigosity (LOH) (Pagotto et al., 2000) of the *ZAC* locus or to hypermethylation. *RASSF1A* (Ras association domain family 1) was found to exert a tumor

suppressor function in several neoplasms including pituitary tumors. Qian demonstrated that inactivation of the *RASSF1A* was caused by promoter methylation in 38% of all pituitary adenomas and in 83% of higher grade adenomas (Qian et al., 2005). RASSF1 promoted apoptosis and inhibited cell growth in different cell lines suggesting its general role in apoptosis. This apoptosis promoting effect of RASSF1 was found to be p53-independent (Vos et al., 2000) while its effect on cell proliferation and cell cycle was connected to the prevention of cyclin D1 accumulation (Shivakumar et al., 2002; Song et al., 2004).

3.2 Histone modifications in pituitary adenomas

As mentioned above the key regulators of histone modifications are DNA methyltransferases. Among these enzymes, DNMT3b, a "de novo" DNA methylation enzyme was found to be overexpressed in functioning pituitary adenomas and NFPAs (Zhu et al., 2008a). Using chromatin immunoprecipitation in AtT20 mouse pituitary cells Zhu et al. demonstrated that histone modifications resulted in a change of DNMT3b expression (Zhu et al., 2008a).

Another protein with reduced expression due to histone methylation was fibroblast growth factor receptor type 2 (FGFR2). The FGFR2 gene transcript has two splice variants. Deletion of the FGFR2-IIIb isoform was associated with inaccurate pituitary development (DeMooerloze et al., 2000). FGFR2 was found to be underexpressed in pituitary tumors compared to normal pituitary tissue (Abbass et al., 1997; Zhu et al., 2007a). Underexpression of the FGFR2 gene was also demonstrated in murine adrenocorticotropic hormone secreting pituitary tumor cells (Zhu et al., 2007a). FGFR2 has been previously described as tumor suppressor because in functional experiments its enforced expression impeded cell growth and enhanced apoptosis in thyroid cancer cell lines via attenuation of Ras/BRaf/MAPK phosphorylation (Kondo et al., 2007a). In addition, expression of MAGE-A3 (melanoma antigen family A, 3; cancer/testis antigen family 1, member 3), an FGFR2 signaling target molecule showed an inverse correlation with FGFR2 expression (Kondo et al., 2007b; Zhu et al., 2008b). Activation of FGFR2 signaling resulted in methylation of H3 and deacetylation associated to the MAGE-A3/6 promoter down-regulated its expression (Kondo et al., 2007b). Downregulation of FGFR2 signaling caused hypomethylation of *MAGE-A3* promoter in pituitary tumors originated from female individuals (Ezzat et al., 2008; Zhu et al., 2008b). MAGE-A3 and its protein family are encoded on X chromosome and normally are expressed in placenta, in testicular germ cells and in several tumors such as melanoma, lung cancer and breast cancer (Hussein et al., 2011; Sigalotti et al., 2004; Yanagawa et al., 2011). MAGE-A3 was found to regulate the expression of p53 and p21 and its downregulation resulted in p21 and p53 accumulation that reportedly occurred occasionally in specific cases of pituitary adenomas (see Table 1.) (Ezzat et al., 2008; Zhu et al., 2008a,b).

There may be several links between processes involved in the mechanism of pituitary development and tumorigenesis. An example of this complex crosstalk is the function of Ikaros (Ik), a zinc-finger DNA binding protein implicated in chromatin remodeling, which has a role in the development of GHRH neurons in hypothalamus and plays an important role in pituitary tumorigenesis via its tumor suppressor function (Ezzat et al., 2005a; Winandy et al., 1995). In pituitary corticotroph cells loss of Ik leads to impaired activation of proopiomelanocortin hormone expression and increased mortality (Ezzat et al., 2005a). Ik-deficient mice have reduced GHRH secretion, a shrunk somatotroph population in pituitary and dwarfism (Ezzat et al., 2006). Ik inhibits access of Pit-1 to GH promoter while it facilitates Pit-1 binding to prolactin promoter in mammasomatotroph cells by the histone acetylating-deacetylating system (Ezzat et al., 2005a). Ik is also involved in tumorigenesis and was found to be down-regulated by hypermethylation in human pituitary tumors (Zhu et al., 2007b). One negative isoform of Ik, Ik6 was implicated in pituitary tumorigenesis by promoting pituitary cell survival through enhanced antiapoptotic activity through Bcl-XL induction by chromatin histone acetylation (Ezzat et al., 2005b). In addition to apoptosis regulation Ik6 contributes to dysregulated expression of Ik target genes including growth factor receptors such as FGFR4 which are essential for development. In pituitary tumor cells Ik6 interrupts activation of the FGFR4 promoter through its deacetylation, that results in transcription from a criptic promoter in intron 4 leading to a truncated tumor derived receptor isoform (pituitary derived ptd-FGFR4) with an oncogenic potential (Ezzat et al., 2004; Yu et al., 2003).

3.3 Loss of imprinting

Our knowledge about loss of imptinting (LOI) and its relation to the pituitary tumorigenesis is limited. As imprinting is executed by methylation, altered methylation may lead to LOI. Regarding to the pituitary we already discussed two imprinted tumor suppressor genes, *MEG3A* and *ZAC*, which may be silenced by hypermethylation of both alleles.

In addition, the gene encoding the alpha-subunit of the GTP-binding protein, Gs alpha was found to be expressed only from the maternal allele in normal pituitary tissue. However, some GH-secreting pituitary tumors containing *Gsα* mutation express Gsα from the non-mutated paternal allel too. This biallelic expression was also present in Gsα mutation negative adenomas too (Hayward et al., 2001). In the latter cases relaxation of imprinting occurred.

4. Role of miRs in pituitary adenoma development

Because 30-50% of all protein coding genes may be controlled by miRs (Chen & Rajewsky, 2006; Lewis et al., 2005), it is not surprising that they are implicated in pituitary tumorigenesis. Bottoni et al. described that miR-15a and miR-16-1 may have a pathogenic role in the development GH- and PRL-secreting adenomas (Bottoni et al., 2005). They found that these two miRs were significantly underexpressed in these adenomas. The genes encoding miR-15a and miR-16-1 are located in chromosome 13q14, a region which is frequently deleted in pituitary tumors. These two miRs were found to be negatively correlated with the tumor diameter and miR-16-1 expression showed negative correlation with arginyl-tRNA synthetase (RARS) expression, a putative target in pituitary tumor cells. In addition, RARS associated with the p43 in the aminoacyl-tRNA synthetase complex, and it was suggested that p43 has anti-neoplastic properties in mice. Based on these data it was suggested that in pituitary adenomas miR-16-1 expression may modify RARS level, which associates with p43 in the formation of the ARS complex and that this process may influence tumor growth. Cimmino et al. showed that the antiapoptotic B cell lymphoma 2 (Bcl2) protein is an additional target of miR-16-1. Interaction between miR-16-1 and Bcl-2 may be persent in the majority of B-cell lymphoma cases (Calin et al., 2002; Cimmino et al., 2005). The Bcl2 was found to be overexpressed in approximately one-third of pituitary adenomas, while its expression was not detected in normal pituitary tissues (Wang et al., 1996), suggesting that Bcl2 may be implicated in pituitary tumorigenesis through regulation of apoptosis (Bottoni et al., 2007).

The connection between pituitary development and tumorigenesis is further supported by the dual role of a protein, named high-mobility group A2 (HMGA2). HMGA2 is a small nuclear non-histone chromatic protein involved in the regulation of chromatin structure (Fashena et al., 1992) and gene transcription (Grosschedl et al., 1994). In transgenic mice overexpression of HMGA2 leads to initiation of mixed GH/prolactin secreting pituitary adenomas (Fedele et al., 2002). Although the HMGA2 gene was not expressed in normal pituitary, its expression was present in human prolactinomas and NFPA. In prolactinomas its expression was related to amplification and/or rearrangement of its chromosomal loci (Finelli et al., 2002), but in the case of NFPA genetic alteration was absent (Pierantoni et al., 2005). In 2007 two studies using reporter gene experiments showed that expression of HMGA2 was repressed by miR let-7 (Lee & Dutta, 2007; Mayr et al., 2007). In addition, Qian et al. confirmed an inverse correlation between let-7 and HMGA2 expressions in NFPA (Qian et al., 2009).

Our group using whole genome miR expression profiling combined with bioinformatical tools and luciferase reporter systems showed that Wee1 kinase, a kinase involved in the regulation of G2/M transition, was targeted and downregulated by miRs in pituitary tumor samples compared to normal pituitary tissues (Butz et al., 2010). We showed that both the total and phosphorylated forms of Wee1 protein was decreased in NFPA and GH producing adenomas compared to normal pituitary tissues (Fig. 4A.).

After cloning Wee1 3'UTR into a luciferase reporter plasmid we demonstrated that Wee1 downregulation was, at least in part, due to overexpression of miR-128a, miR-516a-3p and miR-155 in NFPA and overexpression of miR-155 in GH producing adenomas. In addition using site directed mutagenesis we validated binding sites (Fig. 4C.) predicted by three different target prediction algorithms in Wee1 3'UTR for miRs: miR-128a, miR-155 and miR-516a-3p, further confirming that downregulation of Wee1 may be related to the overexpression of these miRs in pituitary adenomas. In another study Qi et al exprerimentally validated two other miRs, miR-195 and miR-372 targeting Wee1 in human embryonic stem cells (hESCs) (Qi et al., 2009). Our group found that miR-195 was moderately overexpressed (1.5 fold) in NFPA and down-regulated in GH-producing adenomas. In pituitary adenomas impairment of cell cycle regulation by Wee1 downregulation may lead to the loss of the G2/M checkpoint, which in turn may allow DNA damage accumulation leading to tumor development (Butz et al., 2010). In addition, multivariate analysis suggested that in non-small-cell lung cancer expression of Wee1 was a prognostic factor: its decreased expression negatively correlated with a higher rate of recurrence and higher Ki-67 proliferation index (Yoshida et al., 2004). Backert et al. reported that Wee1 was underexpressed in colon cancer tissues and cell lines further supporting its tumor suppressor function (Backert et al., 1999).

In addition to cell cycle alterations through Wee1, the TGFβ signaling pathway may also play a role in the pathogenesis of pituitary adenomas. This pathway was shown to exert a prominent role in the regulation of pituitary tumor growth and prolactin secretion from pituitary lactotrope cells, and microarray studies indicated that FSH, LH and TSH β-subunit, which are under TGFβ regulation, are underexpressed in NFPA (Kulig et al., 1999; Wang et al., 2008). In addition, TGFβ administration decreased proliferation and increased apoptosis of HP75 cell line derived from a clinically non-functioning pituitary tumor [Kulig et al., 1999; Danila et al., 2002]. In our study after performing microRNA expression profiling with TaqMan microfluidic card on pituitary adenomas we executed complex bioinformatical procedures including target prediction following pathway analysis using DIANA miR-PathTool software for differentially expressed miRs. Our results suggested involvement of several altered pathways. Of these we selected TGFβ signaling and found that members of TGFβ signaling, Smad3, Smad6 and Smad9 were significantly underexpressed in NFPA compared to normal pituitary tissues using quantitative RT-PCR. In addition, in silico target prediction analysis for Smad3 identified five overexpressed miRs in NFPA compared to normal tissues (miR-135a, miR-140-5p, miR-582-3p, miR-582-5p and miR-938). Our results suggest that these overexpressed miRs may produce downregulation of the TGFβ signaling through Smad3, and these miRs may have a possible role in the complex regulation of the TGFβ signaling pathways involved in the tumorigenesis process of NFPA. (Butz et al., 2011) Also, our miR expression profile analysis suggested that a decrease of TGFβ signaling via Smad3 may result in a shift toward alternative, non-Smad pathways including Ras-MAPK, p38, c-Jun, and PI3K-Akt, which have been already considered as contributing factors in pituitary tumorigenesis (Fig. 5.) (Butz et al., 2011).

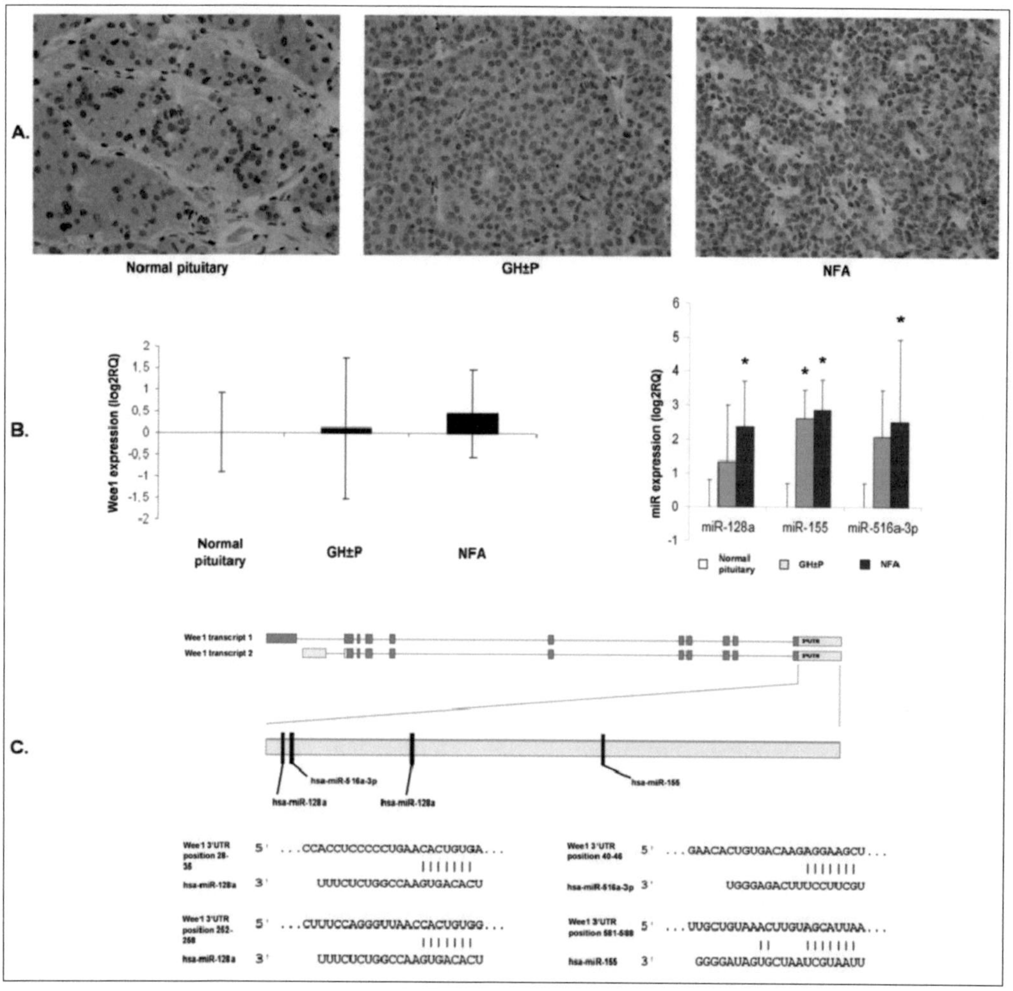

Fig. 4. A: Wee1 immunhistochemistry in normal and adenomatous pituitary. B: Wee1 and its targeting miRs' expression. C: miRs' binding sites at Wee1 3'UTR. (partly presented in paper Journal of Clinical Endocrinology & Metabolism. Vol.95, No.10, (October, 2010), pp. E181-191, ISSN 0021-972X)

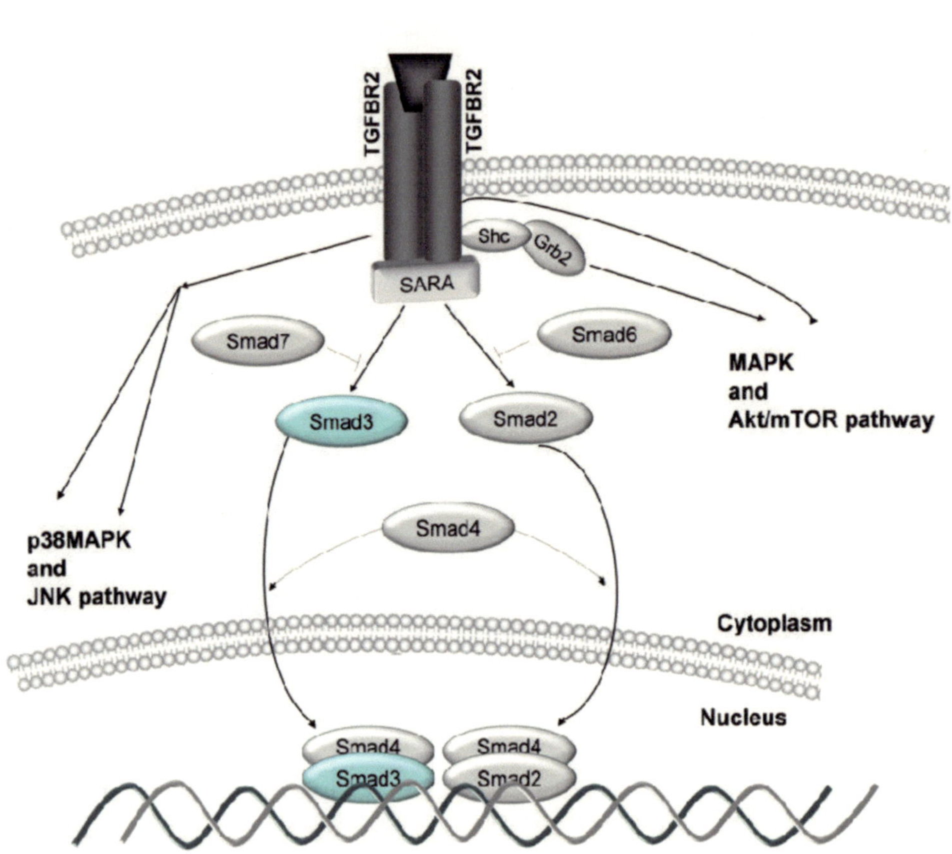

Fig. 5. TGFβ signaling. Smad3 indicated with blue is targeted by several miRs in pituitary.

Another interesting connection between Smad3 and pituitary tumorigenesis arises from a direct interaction of Smad3 with the tumor suppressor menin. Inactivation of menin blocked TGFβ and activin signaling and antagonized their growth-inhibitory properties in anterior pituitary cells (Hendy et al., 2005). It is known that MEN1 gene mutations play a role in MEN1-related pituitary tumorigenesis, but MEN1 gene mutations seem to be very rare in sporadic pituitary adenomas (Prezant et al., 1998; Wenbin et al., 1999). Some reports showed increased menin expression in sporadic pituitary adenomas (Wrocklage et al., 2002). However, there are some conflicting data about menin expression because other reports indicated a significant reduction of menin protein in a high percentage of pituitary adenomas (Theodoropoulou et al., 2004), and studies by several groups using RT-PCR (Asa et al., 1998; Farrel et al, 1999; Satta et al., 1999) showed no differences in MEN1 mRNA levels between pituitary tumors and normal pituitary tissues. All these data may raise the possibility of posttranscriptional mechanisms regulating menin expression via altered expression of miRs. Indeed, in our study we identified 4 miRs (miR-149, miR-570, miR-592, miR-769-5p) potentially targeting MEN1 3'UTR showed a significant overexpression, but further studies are needed to confirm regulation of menin expression by these miRs (Butz et al., 2011).

5. Conclusions and future perspectives

As already shown in several tumor types, the pathogenesis of pituitary adenomas involves epigenetic mechanisms which play a prominent role in the regulation of gene expression. The question is that whether epigenetic alterations, such as DNA and histone modifications are a cause or a consequence in pituitary tumorigenesis. New discoveries and new methodologies in the fields of cell biology, genetics, and genomics open new paths in understanding the complexity of regulatory networks of tumor development. The small RNA systems and their regulatory roles are still uncovered fields in pituitary tumor pathology. To date only miRs of small RNAs have been investigated in pituitary tumorigenesis. It is expected that using novel tools new players and/or new roles for old players will be identified, which may help to develop novel diagnostic and therapeutic approaches.

6. References

Abbass, SA; Asa, SL. & Ezzat, S. (1997). Altered expression of fibroblast growth factor receptors in human pituitary adenomas. *Journal of Clinical Endocrinology & Metabolism*. Vol.82, No.4, (April, 1997), pp. 1160-1166, ISSN 0021-972X

Alexander, JM; Biller, BM; Bikkal, H; Zervas, NT; Arnold, A. & Klibanski, A. (1990). Clinically nonfunctioning pituitary tumors are monoclonal in origin. *Journal of Clinical Investigation*. Vol.86, No.1, (July, 1990), pp. 336-340. ISSN 0021-9738

Amaral, FC; Torres, N; Saggioro, F; Neder, L; Machado, HR; Silva, WA Jr; Moreira, AC. & Castro, M. (2009). MicroRNAs differentially expressed in ACTH-secreting pituitary tumors. *Journal of Clinical Endocrinology & Metabolism*. Vol.94, No.1, (October, 2008), pp.320-323. ISSN 0021-972X

Asa, SL; Somers, K. & Ezzat, S. (1998). The MEN-1 gene is rarely down-regulated in pituitary adenomas. *Journal of Clinical Endocrinology & Metabolism*. Vol.83, No.9, (September, 1998), pp. 3210–3212, ISSN 0021-972X

Backert, S; Gelos, M; Kobalz, U; Hanski, ML; Böhm, C; Mann, B; Lövin, N; Gratchev, A; Mansmann, U; Moyer, MP; Riecken, EO. & Hanski, C. (1999). Differential gene expression in colon carcinoma cells and tissues detected with a cDNA array. *International Journal of Cancer*. Vol.82, No.6, (September, 1999), pp.868-874, ISSN 0020-7136

Bahar, A; Bicknell, JE; Simpson, DJ; Clayton, RN. & Farrell, WE. (2004). Loss of expression of the growth inhibitory gene GADD45gamma, in human pituitary adenomas, is associated with CpG island methylation. *Oncogene*. Vol.23, No.4, (December, 2003), pp. 936-944, ISSN 0950-9232

Bahar, A; Simpson, DJ; Cutty, SJ; Bicknell, JE; Hoban, PR; Holley, S; Mourtada-Maarabouni, M; Williams, GT; Clayton, RN. & Farrell, WE. (2004). Isolation and characterization of a novel pituitary tumor apoptosis gene. *Molecular Endocrinology*. Vol.18, No.7, (July, 2004), pp. 1827-1839, ISSN 0888-8809

Bahar, A; Whitby, P; Holley, S; Hoban, PR; Elder, JB; Deakin, M; Hall, C; Clayton, RN; Williams, GT. & Farrell, WE. (2007). Primary colorectal tumors fail to express the proapoptotic mediator PTAG and its reexpression augments drug-induced apoptosis. *Genes Chromosomes Cancer*. Vol.46, No.2, (February, 2007), pp. 202-212, ISSN 1045-2257

Bamberger, CM; Fehn, M; Bamberger, AM; Lüdecke, DK; Beil, FU; Saeger, W. & Schulte, HM. (1999). Reduced expression levels of the cell-cycle inhibitor p27Kip1 in human pituitary adenomas. *European Journal of Endocrinology*. Vol.140, No.3, (March, 1999), pp. 250-255, ISSN 0804-4643

Baylin, SB. & Herman, JG. (2000). DNA hypermethylation in tumorigenesis. *Trends in Genetics*. Vol.16, No.4, (April, 2000), pp. 168–173, ISSN 0168-9525

Bello, MJ; De Campos, JM; Isla, A; Casartelli, C. & Rey, JA. (2006). Promoter CpG methylation of multiple genes in pituitary adenomas: frequent involvement of caspase-8. *Oncology Reports*. Vol. 15, No.2, (February, 2006), pp. 443-448, ISSN 1021-335X

Bottoni, A; Piccin, D; Tagliati, F; Luchin, A; Zatelli, MC. & Uberti, ECD. (2005). miR-15a and miR-16-1 down-regulation in pituitary adenomas. *Journal of Cell Physiology*. Vol.204, No.1, (July, 2005), pp. 280-285. ISSN 0021-9541

Bottoni, A; Zatelli, MC; Ferracin, M; Tagliati, F; Piccin, D; Vignali, C; Calin, GA; Negrini, M; Croce, CM. & Uberti, ECD. (2007). Identification of differentially expressed microRNAs by microarray: a possible role for microRNA genes in pituitary adenomas. *Journal of Cell Physiology*. Vol.210, No.2, (February, 2007), pp. 370-373, ISSN 0021-9541

Brena, RM & Costello, JF. (2007). Genome-epigenome interactions in cancer. *Human Molecular Genetics*. Vol.16, No.Sp.1, (April, 2007), pp. R96-105, ISSN 0964-6906

Burgers, WA; Fuks, F. & Kouzarides, T. (2002). DNA methyltransferases get connected to chromatin. *Trends in Genetics*. Vol.18, No.6, (June, 2002), pp. 275-277, ISSN 0168-9525

Butz, H; Likó, I; Czirják, S; Igaz, P; Khan, MM; Zivkovic, V; Bálint, K; Korbonits, M; Rácz, K. & Patócs, A. (2010). Down-regulation of Wee1 kinase by a specific subset of microRNA in human sporadic pituitary adenomas. *Journal of Clinical Endocrinology & Metabolism*. Vol.95, No.10, (October, 2010), pp. E181-191, ISSN 0021-972X

Butz, H; Likó, I; Czirják, S; Igaz, P; Korbonits, M; Rácz, K. & Patócs, A. (2011). MicroRNA profile indicates downregulation of the TGFβ pathway in sporadic non-functioning pituitary adenomas. *Pituitary*. Vol.14, No.2, (June, 2011), pp. 112-124, ISSN 1386-341X

Calin, GA; Dumitru, CD; Shimizu, M; Bichi, R; Zupo, S; Noch, E; Aldler, H; Rattan, S; Keating, M; Rai, K; Rassenti, L; Kipps, T; Negrini, M; Bullrich, F. & Croce, CM. (2002). Frequent deletions and downregulation of micro-RNA genes miR15 and miR16 at 13q14 in chronic lymphocytic leukemia. *Proceedings of the National Academy of Sciences of the United States of America*. Vol.99, No.12, (November, 2002), pp. 15524– 15529, ISSN 0027-8424

Chen, K. & Rajewsky, N. (2006). Natural selection on human miRNA binding sites inferred from SNP data. *Nature Genetics*. Vol 38, No.12, (December, 2006), pp. 1452-1456, ISSN 10614036

Chen, Y. & Stallings, RL. (2007). Differential patterns of miRNA expression in neuroblastoma are correlated with prognosis, differentiation, and apoptosis. *Cancer Research*. Vol.67, No.3, (February, 2007), pp. 976-983, ISSN 00085472

Cimmino, A; Calin, GA; Fabbri, M; Iorio, MV; Ferracin, M; Shimizu, M; Wojcik, SE; Aqeilan, RI; Zupo, S; Dono, M; Rassenti, L; Alder, H; Volinia, S; Liu, CG; Kipps, TJ; Negrini, M. & Croce, CM. (2005). miR-15 and miR-16 induce apoptosis by targeting BCL2. *Proceedings of the National Academy of Sciences of the United States of America*. Vol.102, No.39, (September, 2005), pp. 13944–13949. ISSN 00278424

Cui, H; Cruz-Correa, M; Giardiello, FM; Hutcheon, DF; Kafonek, DR; Brandenburg, S; Wu, Y; He, X; Powe, NR. & Feinberg, AP. (2003). Loss of IGF2 imprinting: a potential marker of colorectal cancer risk. *Science.* Vol.299, No.5613, (March, 2003), pp. 1753–1755, ISSN 00368075

Daly, AF; Tichomirowa, MA, & Beckers, A. (2009). The epidemiology and genetics of pituitary adenomas. *Best Practice and Research: Clinical Endocrinology and Metabolism.* Vol.23, No.5, (October, 2009), pp. 543-554, ISSN 1521690X

Danila, DC; Zhang, X; Zhou, Y; Haidar, JN. & Klibanski, A. (2002). Overexpression of wild-type activin receptor alk4-1 restores activin antiproliferative effects in human pituitary tumor cells. *Journal of Clinical Endocrinology & Metabolism.* Vol.87, No.10, (October, 2002), pp.4741–4746, ISSN 0021972X

DeMoerlooze, L; Spencer-Dene, B; Revest, JM; Hajihosseini, M; Rosewell, I. & Dickson, C. (2000). An important role for the IIIb isoform of fibroblast growth factor receptor 2 (FGFR2) in mesenchymal-epithelial signalling during mouse organogenesis. *Development.* Vol.127, No.3, (February, 2000), pp. 483-492, ISSN 09501991

Deng, S; Calin, GA; Croce, CM; Coukos, G. & Zhang, L. (2008).Mechanisms of microRNA deregulation in human cancer. *Cell Cycle.* Vol. 7, No.17, (September, 2008), pp. 2643-2646, ISSN 15384101

Dworakowska, D. & Grossman, AB. (2009). The pathophysiology of pituitary adenomas. *Best Practice and Research: Clinical Endocrinology and Metabolism.* Vol.23, No.5, (October, 2009), pp. 525-541, ISSN 1521690X

Ehrlich, M; Gama-Sosa, M.A; Huang, LH; Midgett, RM; Kuo, KC; McCune, RA. & Gehrke, C. (1982). Amount and distribution of 5-methylcytosine in human DNA from different types of tissues and cells. *Nucleic Acids Research.* Vol.10, No.8, (April, 1982), pp. 2709–2721. ISSN 03051048

Ewing, I; Pedder-Smith, S; Franchi, G; Ruscica, M; Emery, M; Vax, V; Garcia, E; Czirják, S; Hanzély, Z; Kola, B; Korbonits, M. & Grossman, AB. (2007). A mutation and expression analysis of the oncogene BRAF in pituitary adenomas. *Clinical Endocrinology.* Vol.66, No.3, (March, 2007), pp. 348–352, ISSN 03000664

Ezzat, S; Zheng, L; Zhu, XF; Wu, GE. & Asa, SL. (2002). Targeted expression of a human pituitary tumor-derived isoform of FGF receptor-4 recapitulates pituitary tumorigenesis. *Journal of Clinical Investigation.* Vol.109, No.1, (January, 2002), pp. 69-78, ISSN 00219738

Ezzat, S; Mader, R; Yu, S; Ning, T; Poussier, P. & Asa, SL. (2005). Ikaros integrates endocrine and immune system development. *Journal of Clinical Investigation.* Vol.115, No.4, (April, 2005), pp. 1021–1029, ISSN 00219738

Ezzat, S; Smyth, HS; Ramyar, L. & Asa, SL. (1995). Heterogenous in vivo and in vitro expression of basic fibroblast growth factor by human pituitary adenomas. *Journal of Clinical Endocrinology & Metabolism.* Vol.80, No.3, (March, 1995), pp. 878-884, ISSN 0021972X

Ezzat, S; Yu, S. & Asa, SL. (2005). The zinc finger Ikaros transcription factor regulates pituitary growth hormone and prolactin gene expression through distinct effects on chromatin accessibility. *Molecular Endocrinology.* Vol.19, No.4, (April, 2005), pp. 1004–1011, ISSN 08888809

Ezzat, S; Zheng, L. & Asa, SL. (2004). Pituitary tumor-derived fibroblast growth factor receptor 4 isoform disrupts neural cell-adhesion molecule/N-cadherin signaling to diminish cell adhesiveness: a mechanism underlying pituitary neoplasia. *Molecular Endocrinology.* Vol.18, No.10, (October, 2004), pp. 2543–2552, ISSN 08888809

Ezzat, S; Zhu, X; Loeper, S; Fischer, S. & Asa, SL. (2006). Tumor-derived Ikaros 6 acetylates the Bcl-XL promoter to up-regulate a survival signal in pituitary cells. *Molecular Endocrinology.* Vol.20, No.11, (November, 2006), pp. 2976-86, ISSN 08888809

Ezzat, S. (2008). Epigenetic control in pituitary tumors. *Endocr Journal.* Vol.55, No.6, December, 2008), pp. 951-957, ISSN 09188959

Fan, W; Richter, G; Cereseto, A; Beadling, C. & Smith, KA. (1999). Cytokine response gene 6 induces p21 and regulates both cell growth and arrest. *Oncogene.* Vol.18, No.47, (November, 1999), pp. 6573–6582, ISSN 09509232

Farrell, WE; Simpson, DJ; Bicknell, J; Magnay, JL; Kyrodimou, E; Thakker, RV. & Clayton, RN. (1999). Sequence analysis and transcript expression of the MEN1 gene in sporadic pituitary tumours. *British Journal of Cancer.* Vol.80, No.1-2, (April, 1999), pp. 44–50, ISSN 00070920

Fashena, ST; Reeves, R. & Ruddle, NH. (1992). A poly(dA-dT) upstream activating sequence binds high-mobility group I protein and contributes to lymphotoxin (tumor necrosis factor-b) gene regulation. *Molecular and Cellular Biology.* Vol.12, No.2, (February, 1992), pp. 894–903, ISSN 02707306

Fedele, M; Battista, S; Kenyon, L; Baldassarre, G; Fidanza, V; Klein-Szanto, AJ; Parlow, AF; Visone, R; Pierantoni, GM; Outwater, E; Santoro, M; Croce, CM. & Fusco, A. (2002). Overexpression of the HMGA2 gene in transgenic mice leads to the onset of pituitary adenomas. *Oncogene.* Vol.21, No.20, (May, 2002), pp. 3190-3198, ISSN 09509232

Feinberg, AP. & Vogelstein, B. (1983). Hypomethylation distinguishes genes of some human cancers from their normal counterparts. *Nature.* Vol.301, No.5895, (January, 1983), pp. 89–92, ISSN 00280836

Finelli, P; Giardino, D; Rizzi, N; Buiatiotis, S; Virduci, T; Franzin, A; Losa, M. & Larizza, L. (2000). Non random trisomies of chromosomes 5, 8 and 12 in the prolactinoma subtype of pituitary adenomas: conventional cytogenetics and interphase FISH study. *International Journal of Cancer.* Vol.86, No.2, (May, 2000), pp. 344–350 ISSN 00207136

Gardiner-Garden, M. & Frommer, M. (1987). CpG islands in vertebrate genomes. *Journal of Molecular Biology.* Vol.196, No.2, (July, 1987), pp. 261–282, ISSN 00222836

Gaudet, F; Hodgson, JG; Eden, A; Jackson-Grusby, L; Dausman, J; Gray, JW; Leonhardt, H. & Jaenisch, R. (2003). Induction of tumors in mice by genomic hypomethylation. *Science.* Vol.300, No.5618, (April, 2003), pp. 489–492, ISSN 00368075

Gejman, R; Batista, DL; Zhong, Y; Zhou, Y; Zhang, X; Swearingen, B; Stratakis, CA; Hedley-Whyte, ET. & Klibanski, A. (2008). Selective loss of MEG3 expression and intergenic differentially methylated region hypermethylation in the MEG3/DLK1 locus in human clinically nonfunctioning pituitary adenomas. *Journal of Clinical Endocrinology & Metabolism.* Vol.93, No.10, (October, 2008), pp. 4119-4125, ISSN 0021972X

Giacomini, D; Páez-Pereda, M; Theodoropoulou, M; Gerez, J; Nagashima, AC; Chervin, A; Berner, S; Labeur, M; Refojo, D; Renner, U; Stalla, GK. & Arzt, E. (2006). Bone morphogenetic protein-4 control of pituitary pathophysiology. *Frontiers of Hormone Research.* Vol. 35, pp. 22-31, ISSN 03013073

Grosschedl, R; Giese, K. & Pagel, J. (1994). HMG domain proteins: architectural elements in the assembly of nucleoprotein structure. *Trends in Genetics.* Vol.10, No.3, (March, 1994), pp. 94–100, ISSN 01689525

Guan, KL. (1994). The mitogen activated protein kinase signal transduction pathway: from the cell surface to the nucleus. *Cellular Signalling.* Vol, 6., No.6, (August, 1994), pp. 581–589, ISSN 08986568

Hayward, BE; Barlier, A; Korbonits, M; Grossman, AB; Jacquet, P; Enjalbert, A. & Bonthron, DT. (2001). Imprinting of the G(s)alpha gene GNAS1 in the pathogenesis of acromegaly. *Journal of Clinical Investigation.* Vol.107, No.6, (March, 2001), pp. R31-36, ISSN 00219738

Hendy, GN; Kaji, H; Sowa, H; Lebrun, JJ. & Canaff, L. (2005). Menin and TGF-beta superfamily member signaling via the Smad pathway in pituitary, parathyroid and osteoblast. *Hormone and Metabolic Research.* Vol.37, No.6, (June, 2005), pp. 375–379, ISSN 00185043

Herman, V; Fagin, J; Gonsky, R; Kovacs, K. & Melmed, S. (1990). Clonal origin of pituitary adenomas. *Journal of Clinical Endocrinology & Metabolism.* Vol.71, No.6, (December, 1990), pp. 1427-1433, ISSN 0021972X

Hussein, YM; Gharib, AF; Etewa, RL; El-Shal, AS; Abdel-Ghany, ME. & Elsawy, WH. (2011). The melanoma-associated antigen-A3, -A4 genes: relation to the risk and clinicopathological parameters in breast cancer patients. *Molecular Cellular Biochemistry.* Vol.351, No.1-2, (May, 2011), pp. 261-268, ISSN 03008177

Jarrard, DF; Bussemakers, MJ; Bova, GS. & Isaacs, WB. (1995). Regional loss of imprinting of the insulin-like growth factor II gene occurs in human prostate tissues. *Clinical Cancer Research.* Vol.1, No.12, (December, 1995), pp. 1471– 1478, ISSN 10780432

Jenuwein, T. & Allis, CD. (2001). Translating the histone code. *Science.* Vol.293, No.5532, (August, 2001), pp. 1074-1080, ISSN 00368075

Joneson, T. & Bar-Sagi, D. (1997). Ras effectors and their role in mitogenesis and oncogenesis. *Journal of Molecular Medicine.* Vol.75, No.8, (August, 1997), pp. 587–593, ISSN 09462716

Kirsch, M; Mörz, M; Pinzer, T; Schackert, HK. & Schackert, G. (2009). Frequent loss of the CDKN2C (p18INK4c) gene product in pituitary adenomas. *Genes Chromosomes Cancer.* Vol.48, No.2, (February, 2009), pp. 143-154, ISSN 10452257

Klose, RJ. & Bird, AP. (2006). Genomic DNA methylation: the mark and its mediators. *Trends in Biochemical Sciences.* Vol.31, No.2, (February, 2006), pp. 89-97, ISSN 09680004

Kondo, T; Zheng, L; Liu, W; Kurebayashi, J; Asa, SL. & Ezzat, S. (2007). Epigenetically controlled fibroblast growth factor receptor 2 signaling imposes on the RAS/BRAF/mitogen-activated protein kinase pathway to modulate thyroid cancer progression. *Cancer Research.* Vol.67, No.11, (June, 2007), pp. 5461-5470, ISSN 00085472

Kondo, T; Zhu, X; Asa, SL. & Ezzat, S. (2007). The cancer/testis antigen melanoma-associated antigen-A3/A6 is a novel target of fibroblast growth factor receptor 2-IIIb through histone H3 modifications in thyroid cancer. *Clinical Cancer Research.* Vol.13, No.16, (August, 2007), pp. 4713-4720, ISSN 10780432

Kulig, E; Jin, L; Qian, X; Horvath, E; Kovacs, K; Stefaneanu, L; Scheithauer, BW. & Lloyd, RV. (1999). Apoptosis in nontumorous and neoplastic human pituitaries: expression of the Bcl-2 family of proteins. *American Journal of Pathology.* Vol.154, No.3, (March, 1999), pp. 767–774, ISSN 00029440

Lania, A; Mantovani, G. & Spada, A. (2003). Genetics of pituitary tumors: Focus on G-protein mutations. *Experimental Biology and Medicine.* Vol.228, No.9, (October, 2003), pp. 1004-1017, ISSN 15353702

Lagos-Quintana, M; Rauhut, R; Lendeckel, W. & Tuschl, T. (2001). Identification of novel genes coding for small expressed RNAs. *Science.* Vol.294, No.5543, (October, 2001), pp. 853-858, ISSN 00368075

Lee; RC. & Ambros, V. (2001). An exetnsive class of small RNA s in Caenorhabditis elegans. *Science.* Vol.294, No.5543, (October, 2001), pp. 862-864, ISSN 00368075

Lee, YS. & Dutta, A. (2007). The tumor suppressor microRNA let-7 represses the HMGA2 oncogene. *Genes and Development.* Vol.21, No.9, (May, 2007), pp. 1025-30, ISSN 08909369

Lewis, BP; Burge, CB. & Bartel, DP. (2005). Conserved seed pairing, often flanked by adenosines, indicates that thousands of human genes are microRNA targets. *Cell.* Vol.120, No.1, (January, 2005), pp. 15-20, ISSN 00928674

Lidhar, K; Korbonits, M; Jordan, S; Khalimova, Z; Kaltsas, G; Lu, X; Clayton, RN; Jenkins, PJ; Monson, JP; Besser, GM; Lowe, DG. & Grossman, AB. (1999). Low expression of the cell cycle inhibitor p27 Kip1 in normal corticotroph cells, corticotroph tumors, and malignant pituitary tumors. *Journal of Clinical Endocrinology & Metabolism.* Vol.84, No.10, (October, 1999), pp. 3823–3830, ISSN 0021972X

Lloyd, RV; Jin, L; Qian, X. & Kulig, E. (1997). Aberrant p27 kip1 expression in endocrine and other tumors. *American Journal of Pathology.* Vol.150, No.2, (February, 1997), pp. 401–407, ISSN 00029440

Mattick, JS. (2001). Non-coding RNAs: the architects of eukaryotic complexity. *EMBO Reports.* Vol.2, No.11, (November, 2001), pp. 986-991, ISSN 1469221X

Mayr, C; Hemann, MT. & Bartel, DP. (2007). Disrupting the pairing between let-7 and Hmga2 enhances oncogenic transformation. *Science.* Vol.315, No.5818, (March, 2007), pp. 1576-1579, ISSN 00368075

McDowell, BD; Wallace, RB; Carnahan, RM; Chrischilles, EA; Lynch, CF. & Schlechte, JA. Demographic differences in incidence for pituitary adenoma. *Pituitary.* Vol.14, No.1, (March, 2011), pp. 23-30, ISSN 1386341X

Moreno, CS; Evans, CO; Zhan, X; Okor, M; Desiderio, DM. & Oyesiku, NM. (2005). Novel molecular signaling and classification of human clinically nonfunctional pituitary adenomas identified by gene expression profiling and proteomic analyses. *Cancer Research.* Vol.65, No.22, (November, 2005), pp. 10214-10222, ISSN 00085472

Morita, K; Takano, K; Yasufuku-Takano, J; Yamada, S; Teramoto, A; Takei, M; Osamura, RY; Sano, T. & Fujita, T. (2008). Expression of pituitary tumour-derived, N-terminally truncated isoform of fibroblast growth factor receptor 4 (ptd-FGFR4) correlates with tumour invasiveness but not with G-protein alpha subunit (gsp) mutation in human GH-secreting pituitary adenomas. *Clinical Endocrinology.* Vol.68, No.3, (March, 2008), pp. 435-441, ISSN 03000664

Morris, DG; Musat, M; Czirják, S; Hanzély, Z; Lillington, DM; Korbonits, M. & Grossman, AB. (2005). Differential gene expression in pituitary adenomas by oligonucleotide array analysis. *European Journal of Endocrinology.* Vol.153, No.1, (July, 2005), pp. 143-151, ISSN 08044643

Musat, M; Korbonits, M; Kola, B; Borboli, N; Hanson, MR; Nanzer, AM; Grigson, J; Jordan, S; Morris, DG; Gueorguiev, M; Coculescu, M; Basu, S, & Grossman, AB. (2005). Enhanced protein kinase B/Akt signalling in pituitary tumours. *Endocrine-Related Cancer.* Vol.12, No.2, (June, 2005), pp. 423–433, ISSN 13510088

Neto, AG; McCutcheon, IE; Vang, R; Spencer, ML, Zhang, W. & Fuller, GN. (2005). Elevated expression of p21 (WAF1/Cip1) in hormonally active pituitary adenomas. *Annals of Diagnostic Pathology.* Vol.9, No.1, (February, 2005), pp. 6-10, ISSN 10929134

O'Donnell, KA; Wentzel, EA; Zeller, KI; Dang, CV. & Mendell, JT. (2005). c-Myc-regulated microRNAs modulate E2F1 expression. *Nature.* Vol.435, No.7043, (June, 2005), pp. 839–843, ISSN 00280836

Ogawa, O; Becroft, DM; Morison, IM; Eccles, MR; Skeen, JE; Mauger, DC. & Reeve, AE. (1993). Constitutional relaxation of insulin- like growth factor II gene imprinting associated with Wilms' tumour and gigantism. *Natute Genetics.* Vol.5, No.4, (December, 1993), pp. 408–412, ISSN 10614036

Ogino, A; Yoshino, A; Katayama, Y; Watanabe, T; Ota, T; Komine, C; Yokoyama, T. & Fukushima, T. (2005). The p15(INK4b)/p16(INK4a)/RB1 pathway is frequently deregulated in human pituitary adenomas. *Journal of Neuropathology and Experimental Neurology.* Vol.64, No.5, (May, 2005), pp. 398-403, ISSN 00223069

Ohlsson, R; Hedborg, F; Holmgren, L; Walsh, C. & Ekstrom, TJ. (1994) Overlapping patterns of IGF2 and H19 expression during human development: biallelic IGF2 expression correlates with a lack of H19 expression. *Development.* Vol.120, No.2, (Fenruary, 1994), pp. 361- 368, ISSN 09501991

Pagotto, U; Arzberger, T; Theodoropoulou, M; Grübler, Y; Pantaloni, C; Saeger, W; Losa, M; Journot, L; Stalla, GK. & Spengler, D. (2000). The expression of the antiproliferative gene ZAC is lost or highly reduced in nonfunctioning pituitary adenomas. *Cancer Research.* Vol.60, No.24, (December, 2000), pp. 6794-6799, ISSN 00085472

Pei, L; Melmed, S; Scheithauer, B; Kovacs, K; Benedict, WF. & Prager, D. (1995). Frequent loss of heterozygosity at the retinoblastoma susceptibility gene (RB) locus in aggressive pituitary tumors: evidence for a chromosome 13 tumor suppressor gene other than RB. *Cancer Research.* Vol.55, No.8, (April, 1995), pp. 1613-1616, ISSN 00085472

Pierantoni, GM; Finelli, P; Valtorta, E; Giardino, D; Rodeschini, O; Esposito, F; Losa, M; Fusco, A. & Larizza, L. (2005). High-mobility group A2 gene expression is frequently induced in non-functioning pituitary adenomas (NFPAs), even in the absence of chromosome 12 polysomy. *Endocrine-Related Cancer.* Vol.12, No.4, (December, 2005), pp. 867-874, ISSN 13510088

Prezant, TR; Levine, J. & Melmed, S. (1998). Molecular characterization of the men1 tumor suppressor gene in sporadic pituitary tumors. *Journal of Clinical Endocrinology & Metabolism.* Vol.83, No.4, (April, 1998), pp. 1388–1391, ISSN 0021972X

Qi, J; Yu, JY; Shcherbata, HR; Mathieu, J; Wang, AJ; Seal, S; Zhou, W; Stadler, BM; Bourgin, D; Wang, L; Nelson, A; Ware, C; Raymond, C; Lim, LP; Magnus, J; Ivanovska, I; Diaz, R; Ball, A; Cleary, MA. & Ruohola-Baker. H. (2009). microRNAs regulate human embryonic stem cell division. *Cell Cycle.* Vol.8, No.22, (November, 2009), pp. 3729-3741, ISSN 15384101

Qian, ZR; Sano, T; Asa, SL; Yamada, S; Horiguchi, H; Tashiro, T; Li, CC; Hirokawa, M; Kovacs, K. & Ezzat, S. (2004). Cytoplasmic expression of fibroblast growth factor receptor-4 in human pituitary adenomas: relation to tumor type, size, proliferation, and invasiveness. *Journal of Clinical Endocrinology & Metabolism.* Vol.89, No.4, (April, 2004), pp. 1904-1911, ISSN 0021972X

Qian, ZR; Asa, SL; Siomi, H; Siomi, MC; Yoshimoto, K; Yamada, S; Wang, EL; Rahman, MM; Inoue, H; Itakura, M; Kudo, E, & Sano, T. (2009). Overexpression of HMGA2 relates to reduction of the let-7 and its relationship to clinicopathological features in pituitary adenomas. *Modern Pathology.* Vol.22, No.3, (March, 2009), pp. 431-441, ISSN 08933952

Qian, ZR; Sano, T; Yoshimoto, K; Yamada, S; Ishizuka, A; Mizusawa, N; Horiguchi, H; Hirokawa, M. & Asa, SL. (2005). Inactivation of RASSF1A tumor suppressor gene by aberrant promoter hypermethylation in human pituitary adenomas. *Laboratory Investigation.* Vol.85, No.4, (April, 2005), pp. 464-473, ISSN 00236837

Rodriguez-Viciana, P; Warne, PH; Khwaja, A; Marte, BM; Pappin, D; Das, P; Waterfield, MD; Ridley, A. & Downward, J. (1997). Role of phosphoinositide 3-OH kinase in cell transformation and control of the actin cytoskeleton by Ras. *Cell.* Vol.89, No.3, (May, 1997), pp. 457–467, ISSN 00928674

Rollins, RA; Haghighi, F; Edwards, JR; Das, R; Zhang, MQ; Ju, J. & Bestor, TH. (2006). Large-scale structure of genomic methylation patterns. *Genome Research.* Vol.16, No.2, (February, 2006), pp. 157–163, ISSN 10889051

Salehi, F; Kovacs, K; Scheithauer, BW; Lloyd, RV. & Cusimano, M. (2008). Pituitary tumor-transforming gene in endocrine and other neoplasms: a review and update. *Endocrine-Related Cancer.* Vol.15, No.3, (September, 2008), pp. 721-743, ISSN 13510088

Satta, MA; Korbonits, M; Jacobs, RA; Bolden-Dwinfour, DA; Kaltsas, GA; Vangeli, V; Adams, E; Fahlbusch, R. & Grossman, AB. (1999). Expression of menin gene mRNA in pituitary tumours. *European Journal of Endocrinology.* Vol.140, No.4, (April, 1999), pp. 358–361, ISSN 08044643

Shivakumar L, Minna J, Sakamaki T, Pestell R, White MA. (2002). The RASSF1A tumor suppressor blocks cell cycle progression and inhibits cyclin D1 accumulation. *Molecular Cell Biology.* Vol.22, No.12, (June, 2002), pp. 4309–4318, ISSN 02707306

Sigalotti, L, Fratta, E; Coral, S; Tanzarella, S; Danielli, R; Colizzi, F; Fonsatti, E; Traversari, C; Altomonte, M. & Maio, M. (2004). Intratumor heterogeneity of cancer/testis antigens expression in human cutaneous melanoma is methylation-regulated and functionally reverted by 5-aza-2'-deoxycytidine. *Cancer Research.* Vol64, No.24, (December, 2004), pp. 9167-9171, ISSN 00085472

Simpson, DJ; Clayton, RN. & Farrell, WE. (2002). Preferential loss of Death Associated Protein kinase expression in invasive pituitary tumours is associated with either CpG island methylation or homozygous deletion. *Oncogene.* Vol.21, No.8, (February, 2002), pp. 1217-1224, ISSN 09509232

Simpson, DJ; Hibberts, NA; McNicol, AM; Clayton, RN. & Farrell, WE. (2000). Loss of pRb expression in pituitary adenomas is associated with methylation of the RB1 CpG island. *Cancer Research.* Vol.60, No.5, (March, 2000), pp. 1211-1216, ISSN 00085472

Smith, ML; Chen, IT; Zhan, Q; Bae, I; Chen, CY; Gilmer, TM; Kastan, MB; O'Connor, PM. & Fornace, Jr AJ. (1994). Interaction of the p53-regulated protein Gadd45 with proliferating cell nuclear antigen. *Science.* Vol.266, No.5189, (November, 1994), pp. 1376–1380, ISSN 00368075

Song, MS; Song, SJ; Ayad, NG; Chang, JS; Lee, JH; Hong, HK; Lee, H; Choi, N; Kim, J; Kim, H; Kim, JW; Choi, EJ; Kirschner, MW. & Lim, DS. (2004). The tumour suppressor RASSF1A regulates mitosis by inhibiting the APC–Cdc20 complex. *Nature Cell Biology.*Vol.6, No.2, (February, 2004), pp. 129–137, ISSN 14657392

Spada, A; Arosio, M; Bochicchio, D; Bazzoni, N; Vallar, L; Bassetti, M. & Faglia, G. (1990). Clinical, biochemical, and morphological correlates in patients bearing growth hormone-secreting pituitary tumors with or without constitutively active adenylyl cyclase. *Journal of Clinical Endocrinology & Metabolism.* Vol.71, No.6, (December, 1990), pp. 1421-1426, ISSN 0021972X

Spengler, D; Villalba, M; Hoffmann, A; Pantaloni, C; Houssami, S; Bockaert, J. & Journot, L. (1997). Regulation of apoptosis and cell cycle arrest by Zac1, a novel zinc finger protein expressed in the pituitary gland and the brain. *EMBO Journal.* Vol. 16, No.10, (May, 1997), pp. 2814-2825, ISSN 02614189

Stratakis, CA; Kirschner, LS. & Carney, JA. (2001). Clinical and molecular features of the Carney complex: diagnostic criteria and recommendations for patient evaluation. *Journal of Clinical Endocrinology & Metabolism.* Vol.86, No.9, (September, 2001), pp. 4041-4046, ISSN 0021972X

Struhl, K. (1998). Histone acetylation and transcriptional regulatory mechanisms. *Genes and Development.* Vol.12, No.5, (March, 1998), pp. 599-606, ISSN 08909369

Takekawa, M. & Saito, H. (1998). A family of stress-inducible GADD45-like proteins mediate activation of the stress-responsive MTK1/MEKK4/MAPKKK. *Cell.* Vol.95, No.4, (November, 1998), pp. 521–530, ISSN 00928674

Tanizaki, Y; Jin, L; Scheithauer, BW; Kovacs, K; Roncaroli, F & Lloyd, RV. (2007). P53 gene mutations in pituitary carcinomas. *Endocrine Pathology.* Vol. 18, No.4, (December, 2007), pp. 217-222, ISSN 10463976

Tateno, T; Zhu, X; Asa, SL. & Ezzat, S. (2010). Chromatin remodeling and histone modifications in pituitary tumors. *Molecular and Cellular Endocrinology.* Vol.326, No.1-2, (September, 2010), pp. 66-70, ISSN 03037207

Theodoropoulou, M; Cavallari, I; Barzon, L; D'Agostino, DM; Ferro, T; Arzberger, T; Grübler, Y; Schaaf, L; Losa, M; Fallo, F; Ciminale, V; Stalla, GK. & Pagotto, U. (2004). Differential expression of menin in sporadic pituitary adenomas. *Endocrine-Related Cancer.* Vol.11, No.2, (June, 2004), pp. 333–344, ISSN 13510088

Turner, BM. (2000). Histone acetylation and an epigenetic code. *BioEssays.* Vol.22, No.9, (September, 2000), pp. 836–845, ISSN 02659247

Vorwerk, P; Wex, H; Bessert, C; Hohmann, B; Schmidt, U. & Mittler, U. (2003). Loss of imprinting of IGF-II gene in children with acute lymphoblastic leukemia. *Leukemia Research.* Vol.27, No.9, (September, 2003), pp. 807-812, ISSN 01452126

Vos, MD; Ellis, CA; Bell, A; Birrer, MJ. & Clark, GJ. (2000). Ras uses the novel tumor suppressor RASSF1 as an effector to mediate apoptosis. *Journal of Biological Chemistry.* Vol.275, No.46, (November, 2000), pp. 35669-35672, ISSN 00219258

Wang, DG; Johnston, CF; Atkinson, AB; Heaney, AP; Mirakhur, M. & Buchanan, KD. (1996). Expression of bcl-2 oncoprotein in pituitary tumours: Comparison with c-myc. *Journal of Clinical Pathology.* Vol.49, No.10, (October, 1996), pp. 795–797, ISSN 00219746

Wang, Y; Fortin, J; Lamba, P; Bonomi, M; Persani, L; Roberson, MS. & Bernard, DJ. (2008). Activator protein-1 and smad proteins synergistically regulate human follicle-stimulating hormone betapromoter activity. *Endocrinology.* Vol.149, No.11, (November, 2008), pp. 5577–5591, ISSN 00137227

Wenbin, C; Asai, A; Teramoto, A; Sanno, N. & Kirino, T. (1999). Mutations of the MEN1 tumor suppressor gene in sporadic pituitary tumors. *Cancer Letter.* Vol.142, No.1, (July, 1999), pp. 43–47, ISSN 03043835

Winandy, S; Wu, P. & Georgopoulos, K. (1995). A dominant mutation in the Ikaros gene leads to rapid development of leukemia and lymphoma. *Cell.* Vol.83, No.2, (October, 1995), pp. 289–299, ISSN 00928674

Wong, JJ; Hawkins, NJ. & Ward, RL. (2007). Colorectal cancer: a model for epigenetic tumorigenesis. *Gut.* Vol.56, No.1, (January, 2007), pp. 140-148, ISSN 00175749

Wrocklage, C; Gold, H; Hackl, W; Buchfelder, M; Fahlbusch, R. & Paulus, W. (2002). Increased menin expression in sporadic pituitary adenomas. *Clinical Endocrinology.* Vol.56, No.5, (May, 2002), pp. 589-594, ISSN 03000664

Xiao, G; Chicas, A; Olivier, M; Taya, Y; Tyagi, S; Kramer, FR. & Bargonetti, J. (2000). A DNA damage signal is required for p53 to activate gadd45. *Cancer Research.* Vol.60, No.6, (March, 2000), pp. 1711–1719, ISSN 00085472

Yanagawa, N; Tamura, G; Oizumi, H; Endoh, M. & Motoyama, T. (2011). MAGE expressions mediated by demethylation of MAGE promoters induce progression of non-small cell lung cancer.*Anticancer Research.* Vol.31., No.1, (January, 2011), pp. 171-175, ISSN 02507005

Yoshida, T; Tanaka, S; Mogi, A; Shitara, Y. & Kuwano, H. (2004). The clinical significance of Cyclin B1 and Wee1 expression in non-small-cell lung cancer. *Annals of Oncology.* Vol.15, No.2, (February, 2004), pp. 252-256, ISSN 09237534

Yoshino, A; Katayama, Y; Ogino, A; Watanabe, T; Yachi, K; Ohta, T; Komine, C; Yokoyama, T. & Fukushima, T. (2007). Promoter hypermethylation profile of cell cycle regulator genes in pituitary adenomas. *Journal of Neuro-Oncology.* Vol.83, No.2, (June, 2007), pp. 153-162, ISSN 0167594X

Yu, H. & Rohan, T. (2000). Role of the insulin-like growth factor family in cancer development and progression. *Journal of National Cancer Institute.* Vol.92, No.18, (September, 2000), pp. 1472–1489, ISSN 00278874

Yu, S; Asa, SL; Weigel, RJ. & Ezzat, S. (2003). Pituitary tumor AP-2alpha recognizes a cryptic promoter in intron 4 of fibroblast growth factor receptor 4. *Journal of Biological Chemistry.* Vol.278, No.22, (May, 2003), pp. 19597–19602, ISSN 00219258

Zardo, G; Tiirikainen, MIA; Hong, C; Misra, A; Feuerstein, BG; Volik, S; Collins, CC; Lamborn, KR; Bollen, A; Pinkel, D; Albertson, DG. & Costello, JF. (2002). Integrated genomic and epigenomic analyses pinpoint biallelic gene inactivation in tumors. *Nature Genetics.* Vol.32, No.3, (November, 2002), pp. 453–458, ISSN 10614036

Zhan, Q; Antinore, MJ; Wang, XW; Carrier, F; Smith, ML; Harris, CC. & Fornace, Jr AJ. (1999). Association with Cdc2 and inhibition of Cdc2/Cyclin B1 kinase activity by the p53-regulated protein Gadd45. *Oncogene.* Vol.18, No.18, (May, 1999), pp. 2892–2900, ISSN 09509232

Zhang, W; Bae, I; Krishnaraju, K; Azam, N; Fan, W; Smith, K; Hoffman, B. & Lieberman, DA. (1999). CR6: a third member in the MyD118 and GADD45 gene family which functions in negative growth control. *Oncogene.* Vol.18, No.35, (September, 1999), pp. 4899–4907, ISSN 09509232

Zhang, X; Horwitz, GA; Heaney, AP; Nakashima, M; Prezant, TR; Bronstein, MD. & Melmed, S. (1999). Pituitary tumor transforming gene (PTTG) expression in pituitary adenomas. *Journal of Clinical Endocrinology & Metabolism.* Vol.84, No.2, (February, 1999), pp. 761-767, ISSN 0021972X

Zhang, X; Sun, H; Danila, DC; Johnson, SR; Zhou, Y; Swearingen, B. & Klibanski, A. (2002). Loss of expression of GADD45 gamma, a growth inhibitory gene, in human pituitary adenomas: implications for tumorigenesis. *Journal of Clinical Endocrinology & Metabolism.* Vol.87, No.3, (March, 2002), pp. 1262-1267, ISSN 0021972X

Zhao, J; Dahle, D; Zhou, Y; Zhang, X. & Klibanski, A. (2005). Hypermethylation of the promoter region is associated with the loss of MEG3 gene expression in human pituitary tumors. *Journal of Clinical Endocrinology & Metabolism.* Vol.90, No.4, (April, 2005), pp. 2179-2186, ISSN 0021972X

Zhao, R; DeCoteau, JF; Geyer, CR; Gao, M; Cui, H. & Casson, AG. (2009). Loss of imprinting of the insulin-like growth factor II (IGF2) gene in esophageal normal and adenocarcinoma tissues. *Carcinogenesis.* Vol.30, No.12, (October, 2009), pp. 2117–2122, ISSN 01433334

Zhou, H; Hu, H. & Lai, M. (2010). Non-coding RNAs and their epigenetic regulatory mechanisms. *Biology of the Cell.* Vol.102, No.12, (December, 2010), pp. 645-655, ISSN 02484900

Zhou, Y; Zhong, Y; Wang, Y; Zhang, X; Batista, DL; Gejman, R; Ansell, PJ; Zhao, J; Weng, C. & Klibanski, A. (2007). Activation of p53 by MEG3 non-coding RNA. *Journal of Biological Chemistry.* Vol.282, No.34, (August, 2007), pp. 24731-24742, ISSN 00219258

Zhu, X; Asa, SL, & Ezzat, S. (2008). Fibroblast growth factor 2 and estrogen control the balance of histone 3 modifications targeting MAGE-A3 in pituitary neoplasia. *Clinical Cancer Research.* Vol.14, No.7, (April, 2008), pp. 1984-1996, ISSN 10780432

Zhu, X; Asa, SL. & Ezzat, S. (2007). Ikaros is regulated through multiple histone modifications and deoxyribonucleic acid methylation in the pituitary. *Molecular Endocrinology*. Vol.21, No.5, (May, 2007), pp. 1205-1215, ISSN 08888809

Zhu, X; Lee, K; Asa, SL. & Ezzat, S. (2007).Epigenetic silencing through DNA and histone methylation of fibroblast growth factor receptor 2 in neoplastic pituitary cells. *American Journal of Pathology*. Vol.170, No.5, (May, 2007), pp. 1618-1628, ISSN 00029440

Zhu, X; Mao, X; Hurren, R; Schimmer, AD; Ezzat, S. & Asa, SL. (2008). Deoxyribonucleic acid methyltransferase 3B promotes epigenetic silencing through histone 3 chromatin modifications in pituitary cells. *Journal of Clinical Endocrinology & Metabolism*. Vol.93, No.9, (September, 2008), pp. 3610-3617. ISSN 0021972X

10

Genomic and Expression Alterations of Tumor Suppressor Genes in Meningioma Development, Progression and Recurrence

E. Pérez-Magán[1], J. S. Castresana[3], J.A. Rey[2] and B. Meléndez[1]
[1]Virgen de la Salud Hospital, Toledo,
[2]La Paz Hospital, Madrid,
[3]Unidad de Biologia de Tumores Cerebrales-CIFA,
Universidad de Navarra, Pamplona,
Spain

1. Introduction

Meningiomas are solid tumors of the Central Nervous System arising from arachnoid layer cells, which cover the brain and spinal cord. Meningiomas account for about 34% of primary intracranial tumors, with an annual incidence rate of 6.17 per 100,000 person-year, as reported in a recent population-based study (Yee G. 2009). Many small meningiomas go unnoticed during life and are found incidentally in up to 1.4% of people in autopsy series (Rohringer, Sutherland et al. 1989).

In general, meningiomas display a broad range of histological patterns. The current World Health Organization (WHO) classification lists 16 different variants or subtypes, falling into 3 grade designations. The WHO classification of tumors of the nervous system distinguishes between grade I (benign), grade II (atypical) and grade III (anaplastic or malignant) meningiomas (Table 1, Fig. 1) (Perry, Louis et al. 2007). About 90% of all meningiomas are slowly growing benign tumors of WHO grade I. Atypical meningiomas constitute about 6-8% of cases, although using more current definitions, it has been reported in up to 20%. These WHO grade II meningiomas are histologically defined by increased mitotic activity (four or more mitoses per 10 high-power microscopic fields) and/or at least three of the following criteria: increased cellularity, high nucleus/cytoplasm ratio, prominent nucleoli, uninterrupted patternless or sheet-like growth and necrosis. Approximately 2-3% of all meningiomas show histological features of frank malignancy, including a high level of mitotic activity (20 or more mitosis per 10 high-power microscopic fields) and/or a histological appearance similar to sarcoma, carcinoma or melanoma (Perry, Louis et al. 2007).

Tumor recurrence is the major clinical complication in meningiomas, occurring in 10-15% and 25-37% of patients undergoing curative surgery after 5- and 10-year follow-up periods, respectively (Mirimanoff, Dosoretz et al. 1985; Maillo, Orfao et al. 2007). The most important factors that determine the recurrence of meningiomas are the extension of the tumor resection and the histologic grade (Riemenschneider, Perry et al. 2006; Louis, Ohgaki et al. 2007). Therefore, prediction of relapse occurrence in meningiomas during the first few years following diagnostic surgery still remains a major challenge.

Up to date, none of the common genetic alterations of meningiomas have acquired clinical relevance. However, the analysis of these alterations in relation to histological grade has led to a model in which genetic aberrations are presumably involved in the formation of meningiomas, with subsequent alterations associated with tumor progression (Lomas, Bello et al. 2005; Martinez-Glez, Franco-Hernandez et al. 2008).
Meningiomas were among the first solid tumors recognized as being characterized by a specific cytogenetic alteration, which is monosomy 22. Since then, loss of genetic material from chromosome 22 has been the most consistent aberration, observed in up to 70% of tumors (Perry, Louis et al. 2007; Martinez-Glez, Franco-Hernandez et al. 2009).
Familial occurrence of meningiomas is found in patients with neurofibromatosis type 2 (NF2), usually with multiple meningiomas, as also occurs in other non-NF2 families with predisposition to meningioma. Approximately 50% of NF2 patients suffer from meningiomas, making them the second most frequent neoplasm associated with this tumor syndrome. Sporadic meningiomas were then screened for mutations in the NF2 gene, which was found to be frequently inactivated in up to 60-70% of meningiomas. Therefore, the NF2 gene, located at 22q12.2, is considered the main candidate for the genesis of meningiomas, having a role as a tumor suppressor gene (TSG) (Louis DN and JJ 2000; Martínez-Glez V. 2007).

Meningiomas with low risk of recurrence and aggressive growth	
WHO grade I	Meningothelial meningioma Fibrous (fibroblastic) meningioma Transitional (mixed) meningioma Psammomatous meningioma Angiomatous meningioma Microcystic meningioma Secretory meningioma Lymphoplasmacyte-rich meningioma Metaplasic meningioma
Meningiomas with greater risk of recurrence and aggressive growth	
WHO grade II	Chordoid meningioma Clear cell meningioma Atypical meningioma
WHO grade III	Papillary meningioma Rhabdoid meningioma Anaplastic (malignant) meningioma

Table 1. Meningioma grouped by likelihood of recurrence and grade (Perry, Louis et al. 2007).

Other cytogenetic changes secondary to the 22q anomaly, and which are involved in tumor progression to atypical and anaplastic meningiomas, are losses of 1p, 6q, 14q, chr.10, 18q, and gains of 1q, 9q, 12q, 15q, 17q, and 20q (Bello, de Campos et al. 1994; Perry, Gutmann et al. 2004; Perry, Louis et al. 2007; Martinez-Glez, Franco-Hernandez et al. 2009).
Epigenetic alterations seem also to play an important role in the tumorigenesis of meningiomas, as occurs in many other tumor types. These alterations indicate that the silencing by aberrant hypermethylation of gene promoter regions contributes to the genesis and tumor progression of meningiomas (Martinez-Glez, Franco-Hernandez et al. 2008). In

these tumors, aberrant promoter hypermethylation of CpG dinucleotides of several TSG has been described, including *NF2* (26%), *THBS1* (15-30%), *TIMP-3* (24%), *CDKN2A* (10-17%), *MGMT* (6-16%), *p73* (15%), *ER* (15%), *GSTP1* (27%), *RB1* (10%), *DAPK1* (4%), *VHL* (4%) and *CDKN2B* (4-13%) (Bello, Amiñoso et al. 2004; Liu, Pang et al. 2005).

2. Molecular alterations involved in the pathogenesis of meningiomas

2.1 The *NF2* gene

The tumor suppressor gene NF2, located at 22q12.2, is considered the main candidate for the genesis of meningiomas (Martinez-Glez, Franco-Hernandez et al. 2009). Allelic losses of the 22q12.2 chromosomal region encompassing the NF2 gene are found in 40–70% of the sporadic and the vast majority of NF2 associated meningiomas. Additionally, NF2 mutations are found in up to 60-70% of tumors, consistent with a classic two-hit mechanism of tumor suppressor gene inactivation (Ruttledge, Sarrazin et al. 1994). Most of these NF2 mutations are small insertions, deletions, or nonsense mutations affecting splicing sites, with a frequency of NF2 mutations roughly equal among different WHO grades, suggesting that it represents an important initiation rather than progression-associated alteration (Wellenreuther, Kraus et al. 1995).

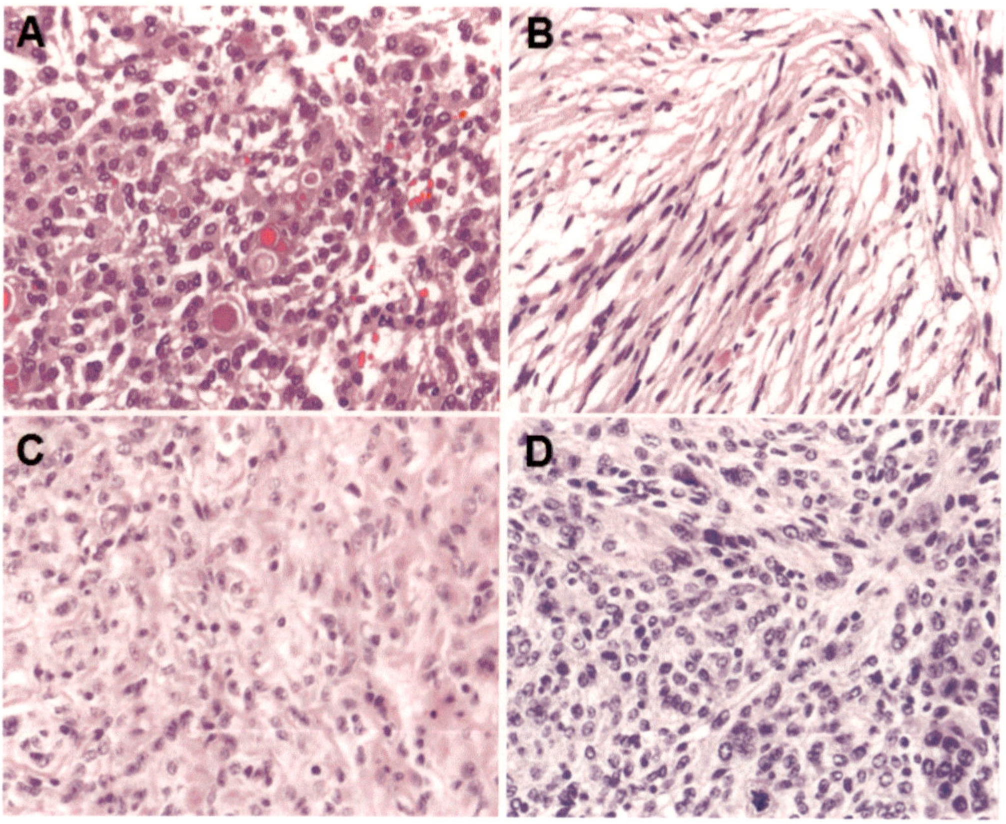

Fig. 1. Histopathological images of a WHO grade I secretory meningioma (A), a WHO grade I fibrous meningioma (B), a WHO grade II atypical meningioma (C), and a WHO grade III anaplastic meningioma (D).

In contrast, differences in the frequency of NF2 alterations have been noted based on variant histology, with higher rates in fibroblastic, transitional and psammomatous than in meningothelial or secretory grade I meningiomas (Wellenreuther, Kraus et al. 1995; Hansson, Buckley et al. 2007; Mawrin and Perry 2010). Thus, NF2 alterations appear to play a preferential role in the mesenchymal like phenotype of meningiomas. Support for this comes from the observation that non-NF2 meningioma families are more likely to develop meningothelial tumors.

Transcriptional silencing by hypermethylation of CpG islands in the promoter region has been accepted as an alternative mechanism to genetic inactivation of tumor-suppressor genes. In fact, site directed mutagenesis demonstrated that a 70-bp region on the *NF2* promoter (-591 to -522 bp from the transcription start site) was essential for the basic expression of the NF2 gene (Kino, Takeshima et al. 2001). At least three CpG sites within this region (at positions -591, -586 and -581) appeared to be of particular importance for silencing of the NF2 gene upon methylation in schwannomas, with the methylation status consistent with the expression/silencing of NF2 mRNA.

In this sense, aberrant methylation of the NF2 gene was detected as the sole alteration in samples of sporadic meningiomas, most of which from grade I tumors (Lomas, Bello et al. 2005). Methylation analysis in two other studies, however, concluded that methylation of the *NF2* promoter is unlikely to play a major role in the silencing of the NF2 gene in meningiomas (van Tilborg, Morolli et al. 2006; Hansson, Buckley et al. 2007).

Alternatively, the NF2 gene may also be inactivated in meningiomas by increased calpain-mediated proteolysis of merlin. Kimura *et al.* demonstrated cleavage of merlin by the ubiquitous protease calpain in meningioma tumors, together with considerable activation of the calpain system resulting in the loss of merlin expression (Kimura, Koga et al. 1998).

The protein product of the *NF2* gene is termed merlin or schwannomin, and meningiomas with associated *NF2* alterations commonly result in a truncated, non-functional merlin protein. Merlin is a member of the 4.1 family of membrane-associated proteins, which also includes proteins ezrin, radixin and moesin. These proteins contribute to the interaction between glycoproteins of the cellular surface and the actin cytoeskeleton, functioning to link cell surface signaling to intracellular pathways (Curto and McClatchey 2008). Thus, alterations in merlin may subtantially affect cell shape and might favor the appearance of a more mesenchymal-like phenotype rather than the epithelioid one, seen more commonly in *NF2* intact meningiomas.

2.2 DAL1/4.1B, a member of the 4.1 protein family

In addition to *NF2,* another gene coding for a member of the 4.1 family of proteins is *DAL1.* This gene encodes for the Protein 4.1B, located on chromosome 18p11.3. *DAL1* gene is generally expressed at high levels in the brain and low levels in the kidney, intestine and testicles (Martinez-Glez, Franco-Hernandez et al. 2008).

DAL1 loss, together with reduced protein expression of its gene product was detected in sporadic meningiomas, affecting more than 70% of tumors regardless of histological grade (Gutmann, Donahoe et al. 2000; Perry, Cai et al. 2000).

This frequency is similar to that of *NF2* absence of protein expression, suggesting that *DAL1,* similarly to *NF2,* could play an important role as an early event in the tumorigenesis of meningiomas.

The similarity between the *DAL1* protein and merlin, with their high levels of expression in the brain and their recurrent loss in meningiomas, led to a mutational study of *DAL1* in a series of sporadic meningiomas (Martinez-Glez, Bello et al. 2005). The low mutational frequency of this gene discounts sequence variations in *DAL1* as the main mechanism underlying participation of this gene in the neoplastic transformation of meningiomas, and suggests that other inactivating mechanism, such as epigenetic changes, may participate in *DAL1* silencing (Martinez-Glez, Bello et al. 2005).

Additional analyses have shown that *DAL1* suppresses the growth and cellular proliferation in meningiomas by activating, among others, the Rac1-dependent c-Jun-NH(2)-kinase signaling pathway (Martinez-Glez, Franco-Hernandez et al. 2008). However, the fact that transgenic mice lacking *DAL1* do not develop tumors (Yi, McCarty et al. 2005), suggests that DAL1 alterations may represent an early progression associated rather than an initiation event for the development of meningiomas. This suggestion is also supported by the observation of losses of chromosome 18 not preferentially of the 18p11.3 region, but instead associated with clinically aggressive tumors.

The absence of expression of two proteins of the Protein 4.1 family in most of sporadic meningiomas suggests that membrane-associated alterations are important events for the development and/or progression of meningiomas. Future experiments however would be necessary to address the functional role of these proteins in leptomeningeal and meningioma cells which may lead to define membrane- or cytoskeletal-associated pathways in tumorigenesis of meningiomas.

2.3 TSCL1 and 14-3-3 are DAL1/4.1B interacting proteins

A potential interaction with protein 4.1B has been reported for the *Tumor Suppressor in Lung Cancer-1* (*TSLC1*) gene, prompting the study of *TSCL1* in meningiomas. *TSCL1* was originally identified as a transmembrane protein involved in specifying cell adhesion. TSLC1 interacts with the actin filament through DAL-1 at the cell-cell attached site where the complex formation of TSLC1 and DAL-1 is dependent on the integrity of actin cytoskeleton (Yageta, Kuramochi et al. 2002).

Surace *et al.* demonstrated that *TSCL1* is expressed in human leptomeningeal tissues, but is absent in 30% to 50% of benign meningiomas, 70% of atypical, and 85% of anaplastic meningiomas. Atypical meningiomas with high proliferative indices and most of WHO grade III meningiomas showed loss of *TSCL1* expression, while atypical meningiomas with brain invasion but low mitotic index had a similar frequency of loss to that of the benign meningiomas (Surace, Lusis et al. 2004).

Moreover, these authors reported a strong correlation between loss of *TSCL1* expression and decreased patient survival. When WHO grade II were stratified by their *TSCL1* expression status, *TSCL1* loss was correlated with reduced patient survival, irrespective of mitotic index. These findings raise the possibility that *TSCL1* may be an independent predictor of survival for patients with atypical meningioma (Surace, Lusis et al. 2004).

Similarly, other study identified 14-3-3 as a 4.1B–specific interacting protein (Yu, Robb et al. 2002). The 14-3-3 family of proteins are adaptor proteins involved in signal transduction regulation, with a role in cell growth, survival or apoptosis. However, impaired 14-3-3 seems not to affect 4.1B function, suggesting additional proteins involved in 4.1B signaling. The potential importance of 14-3-3 proteins for meningioma growth control is underlined by a recent report showing reduced immunoexpression of certain 14-3-3 protein isoforms in aggressive meningiomas (Mawrin and Perry 2010). Thus, the precise roles of protein 14-3-3 interactions with 4.1B have yet to be determined.

2.4 Other 22q tumor suppresor genes

The close association of *NF2* mutations in meningiomas with allelic loss on chromosome 22 suggests that *NF2* is the major meningioma tumor suppressor gene on that chromosome (Xiao, Gallagher et al. 2005; van Tilborg, Morolli et al. 2006; Simon, Boström et al. 2007; James, Lelke et al. 2008; Striedinger, VandenBerg et al. 2008; Martinez-Glez, Franco-Hernandez et al. 2009; Shen, Nunes et al. 2009). Nonetheless, deletion studies of chromosome 22 have detected losses and translocations of genetic material outside the *NF2* region, thus raising the possibility of other meningioma genes residing on chromosome 22. Candidate genes, among others, include *BAM22, BCR* and *TIMP3* (Fig 2).

BAM22 gene belongs to the human β-adaptin gene family. Adaptins are essential for the formation of clathrin coated vesicles in the course of intracellular transport of receptor-ligand complexes.

The *BAM22* gene has been proposed as a second chromosome 22 locus important in meningioma development, after the neurofibromatosis type 2 gene (Peyrard, Fransson et al. 1994; Guilbaud, Peyrard et al. 1997).

Recently, reduced expression of breakpoint cluster region (BCR) mRNA was found. It has appeared to be downregulated in meningiomas with loss of heterozygosity of 22q. The *BCR* gene is an extremely interesting tumor suppressor candidate, since NF2 and BCR proteins perform similar functions (Wozniak, Piaskowski et al. 2008). BCR contains a serine/threonine kinase that functions as a GTPase-activating protein for p21. The inactivation of *BCR* as well as *NF2* might lead to hyperactivation of RAC pathway, and together with the downregulation of the gene, suggest that *BCR* can be considered as a tumor suppressor candidate (Wozniak, Piaskowski et al. 2008).

Matrix metalloproteinases (MMPs) are proteases capable of degrading extracellular matrix proteins. They are involved in the cleavage of cell surface receptors, the release of apoptotic ligands, and chemokine/cytokine inactivation, playing an important role on cell proliferation, migration (adhesion/dispersion), differentiation, angiogenesis, apoptosis and host defense. The *TIMP3* (tissue inhibitor of metalloproteinase 3) gene on 22q12.3 codes for a protein that can specifically inhibit MMPs by covalent binding to the active site of the enzymes and thus reduces the invasion and the metastatic potential of tumor cells. In addition, overexpression of TIMP3 *in vitro* induces apoptosis and suppresses tumor growth and angiogenesis in different cell line models (Barski, Wolter et al. 2010).

Numerous reports have demonstrated the loss of expression of TIMP3 in meningiomas using diverse approaches, such as microarray expression profiling, real-time reverse transcription PCR analyses or immunohistochemical protein expression studies (Carvalho, Smirnov et al. 2007; Fèvre-Montange, Champier et al. 2009; Barski, Wolter et al. 2010; Pérez-Magán, Rodríguez de Lope et al. 2010). In addition, hypermethylation of the promoter region of *TIMP3* gene has been analyzed showing controversial results (Bello, Amiñoso et al. 2004; Liu, Pang et al. 2005). Recently, *TIMP3* hypermethylation has been associated with meningioma progression, due to 67% of anaplastic meningiomas showed hypermethylation of the *TIMP3* promoter, while this was true for only 22% of atypical and 17% of benign meningiomas. In addition, *TIMP3* hypermethylation and transcriptional downregulation were found exclusively in meningioma with allelic losses on 22q12, in contrast to *NF2* mutation (Barski, Wolter et al. 2010; Pérez-Magán, Rodríguez de Lope et al. 2010). Taken togheter, all these results point out *TIMP3* as an important candidate tumor suppressor gene located in 22q, besides *NF2*.

Other genes located on chromosome 22q have also been proposed as possible TSG candidates: *MN1, SMARCB1, LARGE, RRP22* and *GAR22*. The *MN1* gene (22q12.1) was found to be disrupted by a balanced translocation in meningioma, although more recent studies suggest a role as a co-activator of the oncogenic transcription than as a TSG (Martínez-Glez V. 2007; Perry, Louis et al. 2007). The protein encoded by the *SMARCB1* gene (22q12.3) is part of a complex that relieves repressive chromatin structures, allowing the transcriptional machinery to access its targets more effectively.

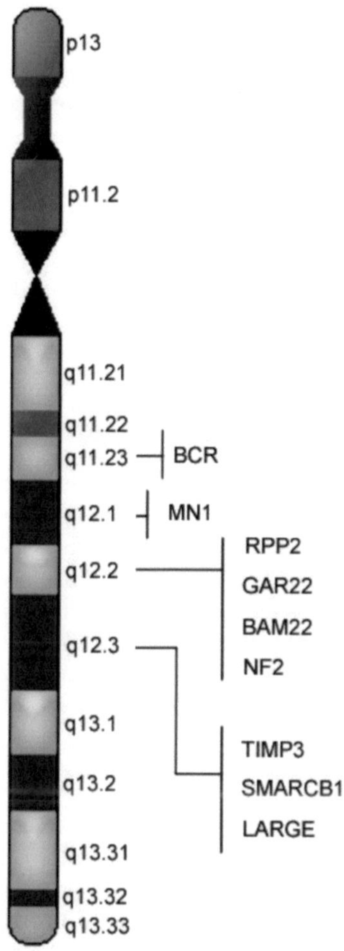

Fig. 2. View of chromosome 22 including candidate TSG involved in meningiomas.

This gene has been found to be a tumor suppressor, and mutations in it have been associated with malignant rhabdoid tumors (Oruetxebarria, Venturini et al. 2004; Martinez-Glez, Franco-Hernandez et al. 2008). In addition, the *LARGE* gene (22q12.3) might be involved in genomic rearrangements associated with tumors (Martinez-Glez, Franco-Hernandez et al. 2008). This gene, which is one of the largest in the human genome, encodes a member of the N-acetylglucosaminyltransferase gene family. Other genes identified in the long arm of chromosome 22 are tumor suppressor genes and are located on 22q12.2, near to NF2: *RRP22* and *GAR22*. The *RRP22* have been identified as a novel, farnesylated member of the Ras superfamily that exhibits the properties of a potential neural-specific tumor suppressor and is implicated in the regulation of nucleolar transport processes (Elam, Hesson et al. 2005). The protein encoded by the gene *GAR22*, a member of the GAS2 family, is an actin-associated protein expressed at high levels in growth-arrested cells (Goriounov, Leung et al. 2003)

3. Molecular alterations involved in meningioma progression

Meningiomas are generally thought to progress from low-grade to high-grade tumors, although this is not always easy to demonstrate clinically. Indeed, none of the typical genetic aberrations found in meningiomas have acquired clinical relevance. Nevertheless, the analysis of the genetic aberrations in relation to the histologic grade pointed out that malignant progression in meningiomas is associated with the acquisition of additional genetic changes, in a stepwise model for acquisition of chromosomal gains and losses during meningioma progression (Weber, Boström et al. 1997).

As mentioned before, chromosome 22 monosomy or 22q deletions are the most frequent genetic alteration found in meningiomas, and thus are considered as an early event involved in the pathogenesis of meningiomas. Secondary to 22q alterations, genetic changes most frequently associated with meningiomas include 1p and 14q deletions. Moreover, these alterations have been related to tumoral progression in meningiomas (Leone, Bello et al. 1999; Buckley, Jarbo et al. 2005; Espinosa, Tabernero et al. 2006; Maillo, Orfao et al. 2007; Martinez-Glez, Franco-Hernandez et al. 2008).

Genetic alterations in atypical meningiomas include allelic losses of 1p, 6q, 10, 14q and 18q and gains of 1q, 9q, 12q, 15q, 17q and 20q. Anaplastic meningiomas frequently show losses of 6q, 10q and 14q as well as gains and/or amplifications on 17q23 (Weber, Boström et al. 1997; Louis DN and JJ 2000; Martínez-Glez V. 2007; Martinez-Glez, Franco-Hernandez et al. 2008).

Genetic alterations in atypical meningiomas include allelic losses of 1p, 6q, 10, 14q and 18q and gains of 1q, 9q, 12q, 15q, 17q and 20q. Anaplastic meningiomas frequently show losses of 6q, 10q and 14q as well as gains and/or amplifications on 17q23 (Weber, Boström et al. 1997; Louis DN and JJ 2000; Martínez-Glez V. 2007; Martinez-Glez, Franco-Hernandez et al. 2008).

4. Altered regions in meningioma progression

4.1 Loss of 1p

Loss of 1p represent the most frequent genetic alteration secondary to chromosome 22 tumor suppressor gene inactivation (*NF2*/others), which seems to participate in the genesis of the aggressive meningiomas, as this anomaly is found predominantly in atypical (40-76%) and anaplastic forms (70-100%), as opposed to benign meningiomas (13-26%) (Bello, de Campos et al. 1994; Bello, de Campos et al. 2000; Maillo, Orfao et al. 2007; Pérez-Magán, Rodríguez de Lope et al. 2010).

Loss of heterozygosity assays revealed two regions mainly involved in meningioma progression, including 1p36 and 1p32-34, although other regions less frequently lost were also detected at 1p22 and 1p21.1-p13 (Bello, de Campos et al. 2000). Furthermore, a comprehensive study of DNA copy number profiling analysis in meningiomas revealed three 1p and one 1q candidate sites of genomic imbalance on chromosome 1, which may be relevant for meningioma development and progression (Buckley, Jarbo et al. 2005). Therefore, these regions may contain one or more tumor suppressor genes important for meningioma progression. Candidate genes have been pointed out, among others: *ALPL*, *TAp73*, *EPB41*, *RAD54L*, *GADD45A*, *CDKN2C*, and *LMO4*.

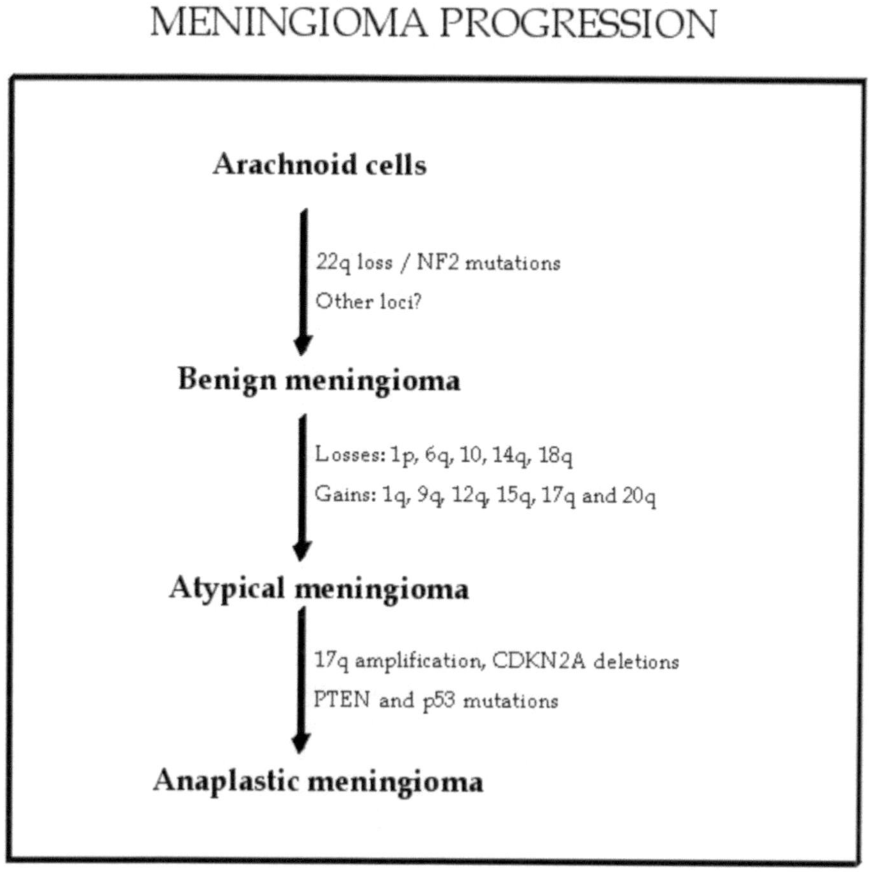

Fig. 3. Molecular alterations associated with tumor progression in meningiomas.

4.1.1 Candidate genes located at 1p36: *ALPL* and *TAp73*

The *ALPL* gene maps to chromosome 1p36.12, and codes for the tissue non-specific form of alkaline phosphatases (APL). In contrast to the brain tissue, the meninges constitutionally exhibit a strong cellular activity of this enzyme, being present in both cytoplasmic membrane and cytosol. Alterations of 1p together with loss of enzyme activity were found in meningiomas, revealing this gene as a good candidate TSG (Müller, Henn et al. 1999). Additionally, the functional expression of the alkaline phosphatase has been related to the mineralization capacity observed in meningiomas, and its loss of expression was associated with increased tumor aggressiveness (Müller, Henn et al. 1999; Sayagués, Tabernero et al. 2007). Further studies of this gene, however, are required.

TAp73 encodes for a protein with significant homology to the p53 tumor suppressor gene throughout its DNA-binding, transactivation, and oligomerization domains. Despite this similarity, animal models showed that p73 is an important player in neurogenesis, sensory pathways and homeostatic control, but its function in tumorigenesis is controversial (Moll and Slade 2004). Mutational analyses of *p73* have been performed in a wide variety of tumor types and, up to date, *p73* is not the target of inactivating mutations in human cancers, including meningiomas (Lomas, Bello et al. 2001). Aberrant *p73* hypermethylation was also analyzed in meningiomas, showing that although it was more frequent in those tumors with 1p deletion, an independent association of *p73* promoter methylation with the grade of malignancy could not be established (Lomas, Amiñoso et al. 2004). Nevertheless, another study detected 1p LOH and *p73* promoter hypermethylation in the malignantly transformed tumors but not in the lower-grade primary ones (Nakane, Natsume et al. 2007).

4.1.2 Candidate genes located at 1p33-32: *EPB41*, *RAD54L* and *CDKN2C*

The *4.1R* gene (1p33-32), or *EPB41*, belongs to the Protein 4.1 family, which also includes the products of the *NF2* and *DAL1* genes, merlin and Protein 4.1B, respectively. *EPB41* was described to function as a tumor suppressor gene in meningiomas, through the demonstration of both, allelic loss of the *4.1R* gene by FISH, and loss of Protein 4.1R expression in sporadic meningiomas and cell lines by using immunohistochemical assays and western blotting. Moreover, *in vitro* functional experiments in meningioma cell lines supported a tumor suppressor function in these tumors (Robb, Li et al. 2003). Opposite results were obtained by Piaskowski *et al.* (2005) who find no change of mRNA expression between meningionmas with 1p LOH and those without it (Piaskowski, Rieske et al. 2005).

The human homologue of the *Saccharomyces cerevisiae RAD54* DNA repair gene (*hRAD54*) is located at 1p32 (Rasio, Murakumo et al. 1997). The protein encoded by this gene plays a role in homologous recombination related repair of DNA double-strand breaks. The *RAD54L* gene was proposed as a candidate for a tumor-associated gene in neoplasms that display 1p allelic imbalance, such as in meningiomas. However, mutational analysis of this gene in a series of 25 oligodendrogliomas and 18 meningiomas failed to identify any deletions or inactivating mutations of the gene (Mendiola, Bello et al. 1999; Bello, de Campos et al. 2000; Bello, de Campos et al. 2000).

The $p18^{INKC}$ gene (*CDKN2C*, 1p32) is a member of the INK4 family of cycline-dependent kinase (CDK) inhibitors, together with $p16^{INK4a}$, $p15^{INK4b}$, and $p19^{INK4d}$. These inhibitors participate in cell cycle regulation by inhibiting the activity of CDK–cyclin complexes. *CDKN2C* was considered a potential tumor suppressor gene in meningiomas due to its similarities with other members of the INK4 family.

However, absence of genetic and epigenetic alterations of *CDKN2C*, together with no altered protein expression in meningiomas ruled out this gene as the major target of the frequent 1p32 losses in meningiomas (Santarius, Kirsch et al. 2000; Boström, Meyer-Puttlitz et al. 2001).

4.2 Loss of 14q

Another frequent cytogenetic anomaly in meningiomas is the loss of 14q, which shows increasing frequencies paralleling the increase in tumor grade. Therefore, about a third of benign meningiomas show the 14q loss, while 40-57% and 55-100% of atypical and anaplastic tumors, respectively, present this loss (Weber, Boström et al. 1997; Ozaki, Nishizaki et al. 1999; Cai, Banerjee et al. 2001; Simon, Boström et al. 2007; Tabernero, Maillo et al. 2008). Various studies have described different regions ranging from 14q21 to 14q32 (Weber, Boström et al. 1997; Martinez-Glez, Franco-Hernandez et al. 2008). To date, however, the actual targets of this chromosomal lost have been remained large elusive and thus, no 14q tumor suppressor genes have been confirmed in meningiomas. Nevertheless, several 14q tumor suppressor candidate genes have been evaluated, namely *NDRG2* and *MEG3*.

4.2.1 *NDRG2* (14q11.2)

This gene is a member of the N-myc downstream-regulated gene family. The protein encoded by this gene is a cytoplasmic protein that has been found involved in a variety of cancers. It is expressed in low-grade gliomas, but present at low levels or absent in primary glioblastoma. In meningioma tumors, Lusis *et al.* used a differential gene expression approach leading to the identification of *NDRG2* as a potential meningioma associated tumor suppressor gene that is inactivated during meningioma progression. Furthermore, these authors showed that the loss of NDRG2 expression was significantly associated with hypermethylation of the NDRG2 promoter (Liu, Pang et al. 2005; Lusis, Watson et al. 2005).

4.2.2 *MEG3* (14q32)

Recently, it has been reported that the maternally expressed gene 3 (*MEG3*), which encodes a noncoding RNA, could be a tumor suppressor gene at chromosome 14q32 involved in meningioma progression (Zhang, Gejman et al. 2010). Zhang *et al.* showed that *MEG3* is expressed in normal human meningothelial cells, but is low or absent in the majority of meningioma tumors and meningioma cell lines. Moreover, loss of *MEG3* RNA expression as well as loss of MEG3 gene copy number is more common in higher grade meningiomas, and there is an overall increase in CpG methylation in tumors associated with tumor grade. Finally, *MEG3* RNA expression in human meningioma cell lines strongly suppresses tumor cell growth *in vitro,* which is independent of merlin, and activates p53-mediated transactivation. As an imprinted gene encoding a noncoding RNA, *MEG3* seems to suppress tumor development in meningioma via entirely novel mechanisms (Zhang, Gejman et al. 2010).

4.3 Alterations of 9p: *CDKN2A*, *p14^ARF^*, and *CDKN2B* genes

Losses of chromosome 9p, particularly at the 9p21 region, were frequently found in anaplastic meningiomas but only rarely in atypical and benign meningiomas (Weber, Boström et al. 1997; Boström, Meyer-Puttlitz et al. 2001). Alterations of 9p21 have been found to represent losses of the well-known tumor suppressor genes *CDKN2A* ($p16^{INK4a}$), $p14^{ARF}$, and *CDKN2B* ($p15^{INK4b}$), involved in control of cell-cycle, and inactivated at high frequency in a large variety of human tumors.

Analysis of the alterations (deletions, mutations and promoter hypermethylation) of these tumor suppressor genes in meningiomas revealed that most of anaplastic meningiomas either show homozygous deletions, mutations (mainly in *CDKN2A* and $p14^{ARF}$), or lack of expression of one or more of these genes. Therefore, inactivation of the G1/S-phase cell-cycle checkpoint is an important feature of meningiomas of advanced stage (anaplastic) that likely contributes to the rapid growth and malignant behavior of these tumors, and point it out as a progression associated alteration in meningiomas (Boström, Meyer-Puttlitz et al. 2001). Moreover, by using FISH, other authors reported higher frequencies of 9p or *CDKN2A* alterations in meningiomas, mostly in anaplastic tumors (74% of anaplastic meningiomas, 52% of atypical, and 17% of benign meningiomas). Interestingly, in this study *CDKN2A* deletion was strongly associated with outcome, with 9p deleted anaplastic tumors showing a high risk ratio for death. On the other hand, absence of deletion identified a subset of anaplastic meningioma patients (26%) with prolonged survival (Perry, Banerjee et al. 2002). Therefore, these studies support that chromosome 9p21 deletions are associated with malignant progression of meningiomas, and that it is a poor prognostic factor in anaplastic meningiomas.

4.4 Amplification of 17q region

Amplification of the 17q21-qter region was associated with the mechanism of progression from atypical to anaplastic tumors, due to high-level amplification on 17q was identified in 48-60% of anaplastic meningiomas and in few or none of atypical and benign tumors (Weber, Boström et al. 1997).

The S6 kinase (*S6K*) gene (17q23) was evaluated as the target of the 17q amplification in anaplastic meningiomas, based on its location (Cai, James et al. 2001) and on the observation of increased *S6K* mRNA expression in these tumors compared with benign meningiomas (Surace, Lusis et al. 2004). Experiments performed in meningioma cell lines revealed no effect of S6K overexpression on meningioma cell growth, motility, or adhesion *in vitro*, although S6K overexpression resulted in increased tumor size *in vivo* (Surace, Lusis et al. 2004). Therefore, although previous studies revealed no high-level amplification of the *S6K* candidate gene (Büschges, Ichimura et al. 2002), the study of Surace and coworkers suggests that S6K may be functionally important for meningioma progression (Surace, Lusis et al. 2004). Further studies are needed to map the 17q23 amplicon to determine whether additional genes in this region are amplified in high-grade meningiomas.

5. Molecular pathology of meningioma recurrence

As mentioned before, histological grade and extent of surgical resection are the two most important variables in meningiomas. However, 5% and 40% of benign and atypical tumors, respectively, recur within 5 years even after total gross resection (Riemenschneider, Perry et al. 2006).

The loss of 1p and 14q was suggested as one of the alterations observed in meningioma recurrence (Maillo, Orfao et al. 2007; Tabernero, Espinosa et al. 2007; Pfisterer, Coons et al. 2008). Recently, a higher recurrence rate of meningiomas with 1p36 loss (33%) than that of meningiomas with normal chromosome 1p36 (18%) has been reported (Ruiz, Martínez et al. 2010). In addition, a differential gene expression pattern that distinguishes between original and recurrent meningiomas identified a subset of meningioma recurrence associated genes, and reported novel candidate genes of recurrence. Most of these candidate genes are located at chromosomal regions previously associated with a higher risk of recurrence or malignant progression of meningiomas: 1p, 6q and 14q (Fig 4) (Pérez-Magán, Rodríguez de Lope et al. 2010). Furthermore, an additional comprehensive copy number and gene expression study also identified 6q and 14q loss significantly more common in recurrent tumors and associated with anaplastic histology (Lee, Liu et al. 2010). Finally, an abnormal cDNA gene expression pattern was identified associated with meningiomas displaying genomic deletions at 1p and 14q (Martínez-Glez, Alvarez et al. 2010).

In general, these recurrence-associated genes are underexpressed relative to non-tumoral meningothelial tissue, denoting an overall underexpression of genes in recurrent meningiomas (Lee, Liu et al. 2010; Pérez-Magán, Rodríguez de Lope et al. 2010). Conversely, overexpression of few genes were identified in recurrent meningiomas, remarkably genes of the histone cluster 1 (6p) (Pérez-Magán, Rodríguez de Lope et al. 2010).

Among the 1p candidate genes, the *LMO4* (LIM-only protein 4) gene is one of the candidates consistently reported on several gene expression studies on meningioma recurrence (Carvalho, Smirnov et al. 2007; Fèvre-Montange, Champier et al. 2009; Pérez-Magán,

Rodríguez de Lope et al. 2010) and progression (Carvalho, Smirnov et al. 2007; Fèvre-Montange, Champier et al. 2009). This gene maps to 1p22.3 and belongs to a family of four mammalian LMO proteins which are short transcriptional regulators that play roles in mammalian development; LMO4 is required for the proper closure of the neural tube (Lee, Jurata et al. 2005). Two members of the family, LMO1 and LMO2 act as oncogenes in acute lymphoblastic leukemia and previous studies have defined LMO3 as an oncogene in neuroblastoma (Lu, Lam et al. 2006). Furthermore, overexpression of LMO4 has been reported to induce cell invasion and to be associated with outcome in breast cancer, especially in estrogen receptor negative tumors (Sum, Segara et al. 2005). In pancreatic tumors it was also found overexpressed (Sum, Segara et al. 2005; Yu, Ohuchida et al. 2008), but high LMO4 expression was associated with survival advantage (Murphy, Scarlett et al. 2008).

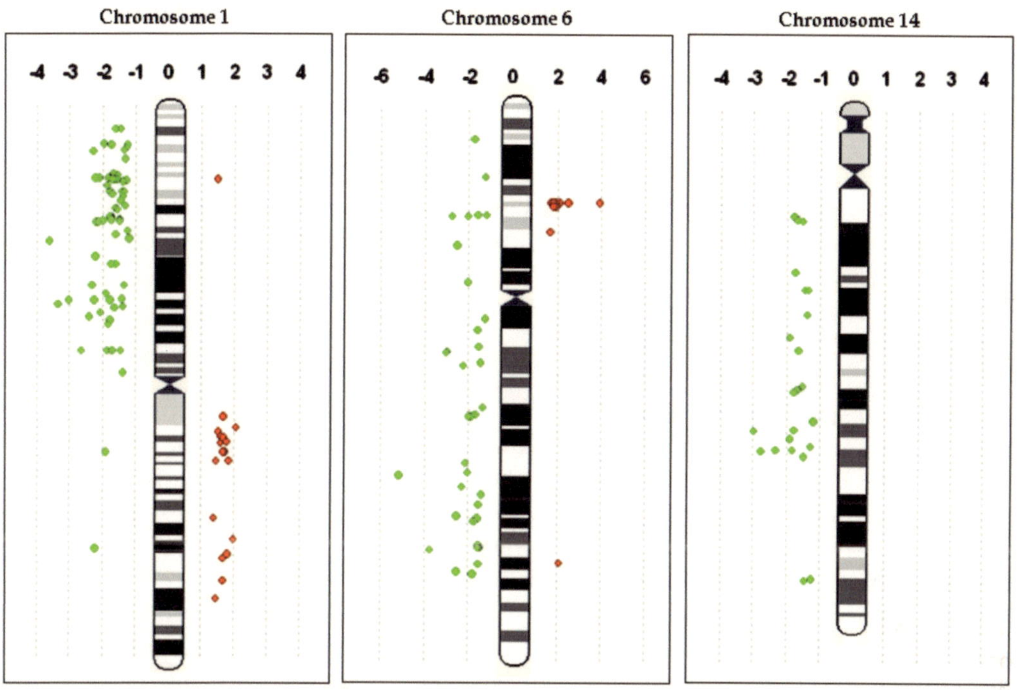

Fig. 4. Location of the genes differentially expressed in original and recurrent meningiomas on chromosomes 1, 6 and 14, plotted according to their map position. Genes with lower (green) and higher (red) levels of expression in recurrences than in original tumors are shown on the left and right, respectively, of the chromosome ideogram.

Surprisingly, underexpression of LMO4 was detected associated with progression and recurrence of meningiomas, as reported on gene expression profiling studies (Carvalho, Smirnov et al. 2007; Fèvre-Montange, Champier et al. 2009); (Pérez-Magán, Rodríguez de Lope et al. 2010). A recent report suggested that LMO4 modulates TGF-β signaling through its interaction with receptor-activated SMADs (Lu, Lam et al. 2006), however its role in meningiomas should be further studied.

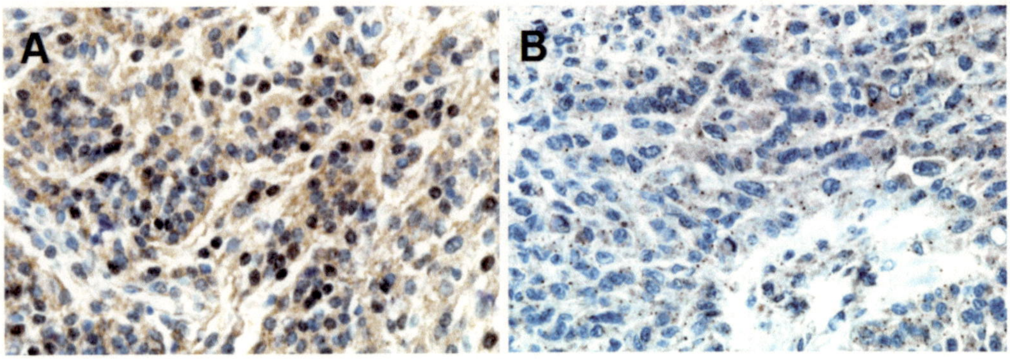

Fig. 5. Immunohistochemistry of meningioma samples with (**A**) positive and (**B**) negative expression of LMO4 (original magnification, ×400).

6. Signal transduction pathways altered in meningiomas

The hallmarks of cancer proposed by Hanahan and Weimberg in a multistep process in which cancer cells acquire the subsequent features that enable them to become tumorigenic and ultimately malignant include: sustaining proliferative signaling, evading growth suppressors, resisting cell death, enabling replicative immortality, inducing angiogenesis, and activating invasion and metastasis (Hanahan and Weinberg 2011). Abnormalities of these processes involve alteratinos of multiple cell signaling pathways affected in meningioma tumorigenesis, such as the beta-catenin/WNT, NOTCH, TGF-beta or p53 pathways (Ragel and Jensen 2010).

6.1 The beta-catenin/WNT pathway

The Wnt (wingless) signaling pathway involves proteins that regulate the production of Wnt signaling molecules, their interaction with receptors, and the physiological responses that result from the exposure of cells to the extracellular Wnt ligands. The series of events that occur when Wnt proteins bind to cell-surface receptors of the Frizzled family ultimately results in a change of the amount of β-catenin that reaches the nucleus.

Studies using microarray-based gene expression profiling identified altered expression of genes associated with the beta-catenin/WNT signaling pathway in meningiomas with losses of 14q, such as the genes for beta-catenin (*CTNNB1*), the regulatory subunit of cyclin-dependent kinase 5 (*CDK5R1*), ectodermal-neural cortex 1 (*ECN1*) and cyclin D1 (*CCND1*), which were upregulated in atypical and anaplastic meningiomas (Wrobel, Roerig et al. 2005). Increased *CTNNB1* and *CDK5R1* mRNA levels may result in aberrant WNT pathway activity due to increased levels of cytoplasmic β-catenin, which may translocate to the nucleus, where it functions as a transcriptional activator of a number of genes.

The beta-catenin/WNT pathway has also been recently implicated as important in meningioma recurrence, showing loss of expression of *SFRP1* (Wrobel, Roerig et al. 2005; Pérez-Magán, Rodríguez de Lope et al. 2010). This gene belongs to the family of the secreted frizzled-related proteins (SFRP), which are able to downregulate Wnt signaling by forming an inhibitory complex with the Frizzled receptors. The role of *SFRP1* as a tumor suppressor has been proposed in many other cancers (Caldwell, Jones et al. 2004; Chung, Lai et al.

2009). In gliomas, lower expression of *SFPR1* and promoter hypermethylation has recently been reported (Götze, Wolter et al. 2009).

6.2 The Notch signaling pathway

The Notch signaling pathway consists of a family of four cell-spanning proteins that enable extracellular-to-intracellular signaling. Ligand proteins bind to the extracellular portion of the Notch protein, resulting in the proteolytic cleavage and release of the intracellular portion. This cleaved portion translocates to the cell nucleus to alter gene expression. This signaling pathway is important for cell-cell communication and has multiple functions during development as well as adult cellular functions. This signaling pathway is dysregulated in many cancers.

Cuevas *et al.* have identified three components of the Notch signaling pathway: the transcription factor, hairy and enhancer of Split1 (HES1), which is induced in meningiomas of all grades; and two members of the Groucho/transducin-like enhancer of Split family of corepressors, TLE2 and TLE3, altered in high grade meningiomas (Cuevas, Slocum et al. 2005).

Furthermore, it has been reported that activated Notch1 and Notch2 receptors induced endogenous HES1 expression and were associated with tetraploidy in meningiomas. Therefore, a novel function for the Notch signaling pathway in generating tetraploidy and contributing to chromosomal instability in meningiomas was reported. This abnormal Notch signaling pathway may be an initiating genetic mechanism for meningioma tumorigenesis and potentially may promote tumor development (Baia, Stifani et al. 2008).

6.3 p53 signaling pathway

Cell-cycle proteins in human tumors comprise both positive and negative regulators. Negative cell cycle regulators include tumor-suppressor genes, of which p53 has been widely studied in different kinds of human tumors. The *p53* gene is located on chromosome 17p13.1 and composed of 11 exons.

p53 protein is a key player in the cellular response to stress. It is a nuclear phosphoprotein that by binding to DNA in a sequence-specific manner functions as a transcription factor regulating a wide diversity of cellular processes such as cell proliferation, differentiation, apoptosis, senescence, DNA repair, or changes in metabolism.

p53 responds to various forms of cellular stresses by activating the expression of downstream genes that inhibit growth, invasion and/or apoptosis, thus functioning as a tumor suppressor (Vousden and Prives 2009).

The expression of p53 protein is mainly regulated at the post-transcription stage and maintained at a very low level in normal cells. MDM2 is an important regulator of p53; it binds to p53 and inhibits its function by concealing the p53 activation domain and by promoting its degradation. In response to DNA damage, the MDM2 binding site of p53 is phosphorylated and the p53–MDM2 interaction is attenuated inducing the rapid accumulation of p53, relieved from MDM2-mediated suppression. The p14ARF protein, another component of the p53 pathway, binds to the p53/MDM2 complex and inhibits MDM2-mediated degradation of p53, which indicates that $p14^{ARF}$ is an upstream regulator of p53 via MDM2. In addition, p53 downregulates the expression of $p14^{ARF}$ and MDM2, in an autoregulatory feedback loop between p53, MDM2, and $p14^{ARF}$ (Zhang, Xiong et al. 1998).

Analysis of this pathway in meningiomas has shown that deregulations of p14-MDM2-p53 pathway may contribute to the malignant progression of meningioma. Amatya *et al.* found that methylation of *p14ARF* gene is more common to atypical and anaplastic meningioma than in benign meningiomas (Amatya, Takeshima et al. 2004). In addition, high expression of p53 was found in atypical and anaplastic meningiomas (Amatya, Takeshima et al. 2001), although low frequency or absence of mutation of *p53* gene was reported by these and other authors (Weber, Boström et al. 1997). Moreover, frequencies of *p14ARF* hypermethylation of the promoter region increases with the tumoral grade in meningiomas, with higher expression of MDM2 protein the cases with methylation of *p14ARF* gene (Amatya, Takeshima et al. 2004).

6.4 TGF-β signaling pathway

The TGF beta signaling pathway is involved in a wide range of cellular process such as cell growth, differentiation and apoptosis among other cellular functions. Therefore, it is a very heavily regulated pathway. The ligands of the TGF-beta superfamily bind to a type II receptor, recruiting and phosphorylating a type I receptor. As a consequence, the type I receptor activates receptor-regulated SMADs (e.g. SMAD2, SMAD3) which can now bind coSMADs (SMAD4). These complexes accumulate in the nucleus where they act as transcription factors and participate in the regulation of target gene expression.

In vitro studies of this pathway in meningioma cell lines suggest that TGF-β has an inhibitory effect on meningioma proliferation, possibly through Smad 2/3 apoptotic pathways (Johnson, Okediji et al. 2004). However, a recent study of the most relevant molecules of the TGF-beta pathway on meningioma tumors concluded that only attenuated TGF-βRIII expression and TGFB growth inhibition may occur in select higher grade meningiomas (Johnson, Shaw et al. 2011).

7. Conclusions

Meningiomas show a broad range of histopathological patterns that in most of the tumors are featured by similar biological and clinical behaviors. Nevertheless, some difficulties still remain, particularly for designation of atypical WHO grade II meningiomas. In addition, different clinical outcomes and recurrence rates even within the same histopathological grade have been observed. Therefore, it is of relevance the identification of prognostic biomarkers for a proper individualized management of the patients. In these sense, useful genetic models for the mechanisms of tumorigenesis and progression in meningiomas have been described, proposing a number of candidate target genes. However, a big amount of genetic and epigenetic research still has to be done in order to identify patients at risk and to translate this information into effective forms of targeted therapies.

8. Acknowledgments

This work was partially supported by grants G-2009_E/04 and PI-2010/045 from Fundación Sociosanitaria de Castilla-La Mancha and the Consejería de Salud y Bienestar Social, Junta de Comunidades de Castilla-La Mancha; and FIS PI08/1662 from the Fondo de Investigaciones Sanitarias (FIS) of the Instituto de Salud Carlos III (Spain).

9. References

Amatya, V. J., Y. Takeshima, et al. (2004). "Methylation of p14(ARF) gene in meningiomas and its correlation to the p53 expression and mutation." Mod Pathol 17(6): 705-710.

Amatya, V. J., Y. Takeshima, et al. (2001). "Immunohistochemical study of Ki-67 (MIB-1), p53 protein, p21WAF1, and p27KIP1 expression in benign, atypical, and anaplastic meningiomas." Hum Pathol 32(9): 970-975.

Baia, G., S. Stifani, et al. (2008). "Notch activation is associated with tetraploidy and enhanced chromosomal instability in meningiomas." Neoplasia 10(6): 604-612.

Barski, D., M. Wolter, et al. (2010). "Hypermethylation and transcriptional downregulation of the TIMP3 gene is associated with allelic loss on 22q12.3 and malignancy in meningiomas." Brain Pathol 20(3): 623-631.

Bello, M., J. de Campos, et al. (1994). "Allelic loss at 1p is associated with tumor progression of meningiomas." Genes Chromosomes Cancer 9(4): 296-298.

Bello, M., J. de Campos, et al. (2000). "High-resolution analysis of chromosome arm 1p alterations in meningioma." Cancer Genet Cytogenet 120(1): 30-36.

Bello, M. J., C. Amiñoso, et al. (2004). "DNA methylation of multiple promoter-associated CpG islands in meningiomas: relationship with the allelic status at 1p and 22q." Acta Neuropathol 108(5): 413-421.

Bello, M. J., J. M. de Campos, et al. (2000). "hRAD54 gene and 1p high-resolution deletion-mapping analyses in oligodendrogliomas." Cancer Genet Cytogenet 116(2): 142-147.

Boström, J., B. Meyer-Puttlitz, et al. (2001). "Alterations of the tumor suppressor genes CDKN2A (p16(INK4a)), p14(ARF), CDKN2B (p15(INK4b)), and CDKN2C (p18(INK4c)) in atypical and anaplastic meningiomas." Am J Pathol 159(2): 661-669.

Buckley, P., C. Jarbo, et al. (2005). "Comprehensive DNA copy number profiling of meningioma using a chromosome 1 tiling path microarray identifies novel candidate tumor suppressor loci." Cancer Res 65(7): 2653-2661.

Büschges, R., K. Ichimura, et al. (2002). "Allelic gain and amplification on the long arm of chromosome 17 in anaplastic meningiomas." Brain Pathol 12(2): 145-153.

Cai, D., R. Banerjee, et al. (2001). "Chromosome 1p and 14q FISH analysis in clinicopathologic subsets of meningioma: diagnostic and prognostic implications." J Neuropathol Exp Neurol 60(6): 628-636.

Cai, D., C. James, et al. (2001). "PS6K amplification characterizes a small subset of anaplastic meningiomas." Am J Clin Pathol 115(2): 213-218.

Caldwell, G., C. Jones, et al. (2004). "The Wnt antagonist sFRP1 in colorectal tumorigenesis." Cancer Res 64(3): 883-888.

Carvalho, L., I. Smirnov, et al. (2007). "Molecular signatures define two main classes of meningiomas." Mol Cancer 6: 64.

Chung, M., H. Lai, et al. (2009). "SFRP1 and SFRP2 suppress the transformation and invasion abilities of cervical cancer cells through Wnt signal pathway." Gynecol Oncol 112(3): 646-653.

Cuevas, I., A. Slocum, et al. (2005). "Meningioma transcript profiles reveal deregulated Notch signaling pathway." Cancer Res 65(12): 5070-5075.

Curto, M. and A. I. McClatchey (2008). "Nf2/Merlin: a coordinator of receptor signalling and intercellular contact." Br J Cancer 98(2): 256-262.

Elam, C., L. Hesson, et al. (2005). "RRP22 is a farnesylated, nucleolar, Ras-related protein with tumor suppressor potential." Cancer Res 65(8): 3117-3125.

Espinosa, A., M. Tabernero, et al. (2006). "The cytogenetic relationship between primary and recurrent meningiomas points to the need for new treatment strategies in cases at high risk of relapse." Clin Cancer Res 12(3 Pt 1): 772-780.

Fèvre-Montange, M., J. Champier, et al. (2009). "Microarray gene expression profiling in meningiomas: differential expression according to grade or histopathological subtype." Int J Oncol 35(6): 1395-1407.

Goriounov, D., C. L. Leung, et al. (2003). "Protein products of human Gas2-related genes on chromosomes 17 and 22 (hGAR17 and hGAR22) associate with both microfilaments and microtubules." J Cell Sci 116(Pt 6): 1045-1058.

Guilbaud, C., M. Peyrard, et al. (1997). "Characterization of the mouse beta-prime adaptin gene; cDNA sequence, genomic structure, and chromosomal localization." Mamm Genome 8(9): 651-656.

Gutmann, D., J. Donahoe, et al. (2000). "Loss of DAL-1, a protein 4.1-related tumor suppressor, is an important early event in the pathogenesis of meningiomas." Hum Mol Genet 9(10): 1495-1500.

Götze, S., M. Wolter, et al. (2009). "Frequent promoter hypermethylation of Wnt pathway inhibitor genes in malignant astrocytic gliomas." Int J Cancer.

Hanahan, D. and R. A. Weinberg (2011). "Hallmarks of cancer: the next generation." Cell 144(5): 646-674.

Hansson, C. M., P. G. Buckley, et al. (2007). "Comprehensive genetic and epigenetic analysis of sporadic meningioma for macro-mutations on 22q and micro-mutations within the NF2 locus." BMC Genomics 8: 16.

James, M., J. Lelke, et al. (2008). "Modeling NF2 with human arachnoidal and meningioma cell culture systems: NF2 silencing reflects the benign character of tumor growth." Neurobiol Dis 29(2): 278-292.

Johnson, M., E. Okediji, et al. (2004). "Transforming growth factor-beta effects on meningioma cell proliferation and signal transduction pathways." J Neurooncol 66(1-2): 9-16.

Johnson, M. D., A. K. Shaw, et al. (2011). "Analysis of transforming growth factor β receptor expression and signaling in higher grade meningiomas." J Neurooncol 103(2): 277-285.

Kimura, Y., H. Koga, et al. (1998). "The involvement of calpain-dependent proteolysis of the tumor suppressor NF2 (merlin) in schwannomas and meningiomas." Nat Med 4(8): 915-922.

Kino, T., H. Takeshima, et al. (2001). "Identification of the cis-acting region in the NF2 gene promoter as a potential target for mutation and methylation-dependent silencing in schwannoma." Genes Cells 6(5): 441-454.

Lee, S. K., L. W. Jurata, et al. (2005). "The LIM domain-only protein LMO4 is required for neural tube closure." Mol Cell Neurosci 28(2): 205-214.

Lee, Y., J. Liu, et al. (2010). "Genomic landscape of meningiomas." Brain Pathol 20(4): 751-762.

Leone, P. E., M. J. Bello, et al. (1999). "NF2 gene mutations and allelic status of 1p, 14q and 22q in sporadic meningiomas." Oncogene 18(13): 2231-2239.

Liu, Y., J. Pang, et al. (2005). "Aberrant CpG island hypermethylation profile is associated with atypical and anaplastic meningiomas." Hum Pathol 36(4): 416-425.

Lomas, J., C. Amiñoso, et al. (2004). "Methylation status of TP73 in meningiomas." Cancer Genet Cytogenet 148(2): 148-151.

Lomas, J., M. J. Bello, et al. (2005). "Genetic and epigenetic alteration of the NF2 gene in sporadic meningiomas." Genes Chromosomes Cancer 42(3): 314-319.

Lomas, J., M. J. Bello, et al. (2001). "Analysis of p73 gene in meningiomas with deletion at 1p." Cancer Genet Cytogenet 129(1): 88-91.

Louis, D. N., H. Ohgaki, et al. (2007). "The 2007 WHO classification of tumours of the central nervous system." Acta Neuropathol 114(2): 97-109.

Louis DN, S. B., Budka H, von Deimling A and and K. JJ (2000). Meningiomas. In: World Health Classification of Tumors: Pathology and Geentics of Tumors of the Nervous System. Lyon.

Lu, Z., K. Lam, et al. (2006). "LMO4 can interact with Smad proteins and modulate transforming growth factor-beta signaling in epithelial cells." Oncogene 25(20): 2920-2930.

Lusis, E., M. Watson, et al. (2005). "Integrative genomic analysis identifies NDRG2 as a candidate tumor suppressor gene frequently inactivated in clinically aggressive meningioma." Cancer Res 65(16): 7121-7126.

Maillo, A., A. Orfao, et al. (2007). "Early recurrences in histologically benign/grade I meningiomas are associated with large tumors and coexistence of monosomy 14 and del(1p36) in the ancestral tumor cell clone." Neuro Oncol 9(4): 438-446.

Martinez-Glez, V., M. Bello, et al. (2005). "Mutational analysis of the DAL-1/4.1B tumour-suppressor gene locus in meningiomas." Int J Mol Med 16(4): 771-774.

Martinez-Glez, V., C. Franco-Hernandez, et al. (2009). "Meningiomas and schwannomas: molecular subgroup classification found by expression arrays." Int J Oncol 34(2): 493-504.

Martinez-Glez, V., C. Franco-Hernandez, et al. (2008). "Microarray gene expression profiling in meningiomas and schwannomas." Curr Med Chem 15(8): 826-833.

Martínez-Glez, V., L. Alvarez, et al. (2010). "Genomic deletions at 1p and 14q are associated with an abnormal cDNA microarray gene expression pattern in meningiomas but not in schwannomas." Cancer Genet Cytogenet 196(1): 1-6.

Martínez-Glez V., F.-H. C., Peña-Granero C., Rey J.A. (2007). Oncogenes and Tumor Suppresor Genes Expression in Meningiomas. MAPFRE MEDICINA.

Mawrin, C. and A. Perry (2010). "Pathological classification and molecular genetics of meningiomas." J Neurooncol 99(3): 379-391.

Mendiola, M., M. J. Bello, et al. (1999). "Search for mutations of the hRAD54 gene in sporadic meningiomas with deletion at 1p32." Mol Carcinog 24(4): 300-304.

Mirimanoff, R. O., D. E. Dosoretz, et al. (1985). "Meningioma: analysis of recurrence and progression following neurosurgical resection." J Neurosurg 62(1): 18-24.

Moll, U. M. and N. Slade (2004). "p63 and p73: roles in development and tumor formation." Mol Cancer Res 2(7): 371-386.

Murphy, N. C., C. J. Scarlett, et al. (2008). "Expression of LMO4 and outcome in pancreatic ductal adenocarcinoma." Br J Cancer 98(3): 537-541.

Müller, P., W. Henn, et al. (1999). "Deletion of chromosome 1p and loss of expression of alkaline phosphatase indicate progression of meningiomas." Clin Cancer Res 5(11): 3569-3577.

Nakane, Y., A. Natsume, et al. (2007). "Malignant transformation-related genes in meningiomas: allelic loss on 1p36 and methylation status of p73 and RASSF1A." J Neurosurg 107(2): 398-404.

Oruetxebarria, I., F. Venturini, et al. (2004). "P16INK4a is required for hSNF5 chromatin remodeler-induced cellular senescence in malignant rhabdoid tumor cells." J Biol Chem 279(5): 3807-3816.

Ozaki, S., T. Nishizaki, et al. (1999). "Comparative genomic hybridization analysis of genetic alterations associated with malignant progression of meningioma." J Neurooncol 41(2): 167-174.

Perry, A., R. Banerjee, et al. (2002). "A role for chromosome 9p21 deletions in the malignant progression of meningiomas and the prognosis of anaplastic meningiomas." Brain Pathol 12(2): 183-190.

Perry, A., D. X. Cai, et al. (2000). "Merlin, DAL-1, and progesterone receptor expression in clinicopathologic subsets of meningioma: a correlative immunohistochemical study of 175 cases." J Neuropathol Exp Neurol 59(10): 872-879.

Perry, A., D. Gutmann, et al. (2004). "Molecular pathogenesis of meningiomas." J Neurooncol 70(2): 183-202.

Perry, A., D. Louis, et al., Eds. (2007). World Health Organization Classification of Tumours. Lyon, IARC Press.

Peyrard, M., I. Fransson, et al. (1994). "Characterization of a new member of the human beta-adaptin gene family from chromosome 22q12, a candidate meningioma gene." Hum Mol Genet 3(8): 1393-1399.

Pfisterer, W. K., S. W. Coons, et al. (2008). "Implicating chromosomal aberrations with meningioma growth and recurrence: results from FISH and MIB-I analysis of grades I and II meningioma tissue." J Neurooncol 87(1): 43-50.

Piaskowski, S., P. Rieske, et al. (2005). "GADD45A and EPB41 as tumor suppressor genes in meningioma pathogenesis." Cancer Genet Cytogenet 162(1): 63-67.

Pérez-Magán, E., A. Rodríguez de Lope, et al. (2010). "Differential expression profiling analyses identifies downregulation of 1p, 6q, and 14q genes and overexpression of 6p histone cluster 1 genes as markers of recurrence in meningiomas." Neuro Oncol 12(12): 1278-1290.

Ragel, B. T. and R. L. Jensen (2010). "Aberrant signaling pathways in meningiomas." J Neurooncol 99(3): 315-324.

Rasio, D., Y. Murakumo, et al. (1997). "Characterization of the human homologue of RAD54: a gene located on chromosome 1p32 at a region of high loss of heterozygosity in breast tumors." Cancer Res 57(12): 2378-2383.

Riemenschneider, M., A. Perry, et al. (2006). "Histological classification and molecular genetics of meningiomas." Lancet Neurol 5(12): 1045-1054.

Robb, V., W. Li, et al. (2003). "Identification of a third Protein 4.1 tumor suppressor, Protein 4.1R, in meningioma pathogenesis." Neurobiol Dis 13(3): 191-202.

Rohringer, M., G. R. Sutherland, et al. (1989). "Incidence and clinicopathological features of meningioma." J Neurosurg 71(5 Pt 1): 665-672.

Ruiz, J., A. Martínez, et al. (2010). "Clinicopathological variables, immunophenotype, chromosome 1p36 loss and tumour recurrence of 247 meningiomas grade I and II." Histol Histopathol 25(3): 341-349.

Ruttledge, M. H., J. Sarrazin, et al. (1994). "Evidence for the complete inactivation of the NF2 gene in the majority of sporadic meningiomas." Nat Genet 6(2): 180-184.

Santarius, T., M. Kirsch, et al. (2000). "Molecular analysis of alterations of the p18INK4c gene in human meningiomas." Neuropathol Appl Neurobiol 26(1): 67-75.

Sayagués, J., M. Tabernero, et al. (2007). "[Cytogenetic alterations in meningioma tumors and their impact on disease outcome]." Med Clin (Barc) 128(6): 226-232.

Shen, Y., F. Nunes, et al. (2009). "Genomic profiling distinguishes familial multiple and sporadic multiple meningiomas." BMC Med Genomics 2: 42.

Simon, M., J. Boström, et al. (2007). "Molecular genetics of meningiomas: from basic research to potential clinical applications." Neurosurgery 60(5): 787-798; discussion 787-798.

Striedinger, K., S. VandenBerg, et al. (2008). "The neurofibromatosis 2 tumor suppressor gene product, merlin, regulates human meningioma cell growth by signaling through YAP." Neoplasia 10(11): 1204-1212.

Sum, E., D. Segara, et al. (2005). "Overexpression of LMO4 induces mammary hyperplasia, promotes cell invasion, and is a predictor of poor outcome in breast cancer." Proc Natl Acad Sci U S A 102(21): 7659-7664.

Surace, E., E. Lusis, et al. (2004). "Functional significance of S6K overexpression in meningioma progression." Ann Neurol 56(2): 295-298.

Surace, E., E. Lusis, et al. (2004). "Loss of tumor suppressor in lung cancer-1 (TSLC1) expression in meningioma correlates with increased malignancy grade and reduced patient survival." J Neuropathol Exp Neurol 63(10): 1015-1027.

Tabernero, M., A. Maillo, et al. (2008). "Gene Expression Profiles of Meningiomas are Associated with Tumor Cytogenetics and Patient Outcome." Brain Pathol.

Tabernero, M. D., A. B. Espinosa, et al. (2007). "Patient gender is associated with distinct patterns of chromosomal abnormalities and sex chromosome linked gene-expression profiles in meningiomas." Oncologist 12(10): 1225-1236.

van Tilborg, A. A., B. Morolli, et al. (2006). "Lack of genetic and epigenetic changes in meningiomas without NF2 loss." J Pathol 208(4): 564-573.

Vousden, K. H. and C. Prives (2009). "Blinded by the Light: The Growing Complexity of p53." Cell 137(3): 413-431.

Weber, R., J. Boström, et al. (1997). "Analysis of genomic alterations in benign, atypical, and anaplastic meningiomas: toward a genetic model of meningioma progression." Proc Natl Acad Sci U S A 94(26): 14719-14724.

Wellenreuther, R., J. A. Kraus, et al. (1995). "Analysis of the neurofibromatosis 2 gene reveals molecular variants of meningioma." Am J Pathol 146(4): 827-832.

Wozniak, K., S. Piaskowski, et al. (2008). "BCR expression is decreased in meningiomas showing loss of heterozygosity of 22q within a new minimal deletion region." Cancer Genet Cytogenet 183(1): 14-20.

Wrobel, G., P. Roerig, et al. (2005). "Microarray-based gene expression profiling of benign, atypical and anaplastic meningiomas identifies novel genes associated with meningioma progression." Int J Cancer 114(2): 249-256.

Xiao, G., R. Gallagher, et al. (2005). "The NF2 tumor suppressor gene product, merlin, inhibits cell proliferation and cell cycle progression by repressing cyclin D1 expression." Mol Cell Biol 25(6): 2384-2394.

Yageta, M., M. Kuramochi, et al. (2002). "Direct association of TSLC1 and DAL-1, two distinct tumor suppressor proteins in lung cancer." Cancer Res 62(18): 5129-5133.

Yee G., R. R., Philips C et al. (2009). CBTRUS Statistical Report:Primary Brain and Central Nervous System Tumors Diagnosed in Eighteen States in 2002-2006. Hinsdale, IL.

Yi, C., J. H. McCarty, et al. (2005). "Loss of the putative tumor suppressor band 4.1B/Dal1 gene is dispensable for normal development and does not predispose to cancer." Mol Cell Biol 25(22): 10052-10059.

Yu, J., K. Ohuchida, et al. (2008). "LIM only 4 is overexpressed in late stage pancreas cancer." Mol Cancer 7: 93.

Yu, T., V. A. Robb, et al. (2002). "The 4.1/ezrin/radixin/moesin domain of the DAL-1/Protein 4.1B tumour suppressor interacts with 14-3-3 proteins." Biochem J 365(Pt 3): 783-789.

Zhang, X., R. Gejman, et al. (2010). "Maternally expressed gene 3, an imprinted noncoding RNA gene, is associated with meningioma pathogenesis and progression." Cancer Res 70(6): 2350-2358.

Zhang, Y., Y. Xiong, et al. (1998). "ARF promotes MDM2 degradation and stabilizes p53: ARF-INK4a locus deletion impairs both the Rb and p53 tumor suppression pathways." Cell 92(6): 725-734.

11

Control of Retinal Development by Tumor Suppressor Genes

Robert Cantrup, Gaurav Kaushik and Carol Schuurmans
Department of Biochemistry & Molecular Biology,
Hotchkiss Brain Institute,
Alberta Children's Hospital Research Institute,
University of Calgary
Canada

1. Introduction

Tumor suppressor genes are so named because of their actions in preventing cancer - but it is often overlooked that they also have normal functions in non-pathological cellular contexts. Here we review the evidence that tumor suppressor genes are key regulators of developmental events, focusing on the neural retina as a model system. At no other time during an organism's lifespan are the biological processes that tumor suppressor genes control - including cell division, differentiation, migration and programmed cell death, more pronounced than during the embryonic and early postnatal period. The developing retina serves as an excellent model of tissue development based on its experimental accessibility, well-characterized cell types, and sophisticated laminar organization. The retina also has an important physiological function - processing light signals so that vision is possible. Visual processing requires functional neural circuits, the formation of which requires that appropriate numbers of the correct types of neuronal and glial cells differentiate during development. Here we introduce our current knowledge of how the retina develops and then review the evidence that tumor suppressor genes control several aspects of this process, including: 1) cell division/proliferation, 2) appropriate cell fate specification/differentiation, 3) cell migration, and 4) cellular apoptosis. By better understanding the normal functions that tumor suppressor genes play in the developing embryo, we are better positioned to understand why their deregulated expression leads to tumor growth and cancer.

1.1 Retinal structure and morphogenesis

The retina is the neural layer of the eye and is responsible for converting light photons into electrical impulses that are transmitted to the brain. It is comprised of one glial and six neuronal cell types that are organized into three nuclear layers: 1) an outer nuclear layer (ONL) of rod and cone photoreceptors, which receive light signals; 2) an inner nuclear layer (INL) of supporting Müller glial cells and bipolar, horizontal and amacrine cell interneurons, which refine and transmit signals from photoreceptors; and 3) a ganglion cell layer (GCL) of retinal ganglion cells (RGCs) - the output neurons of the retina (Figure 1).

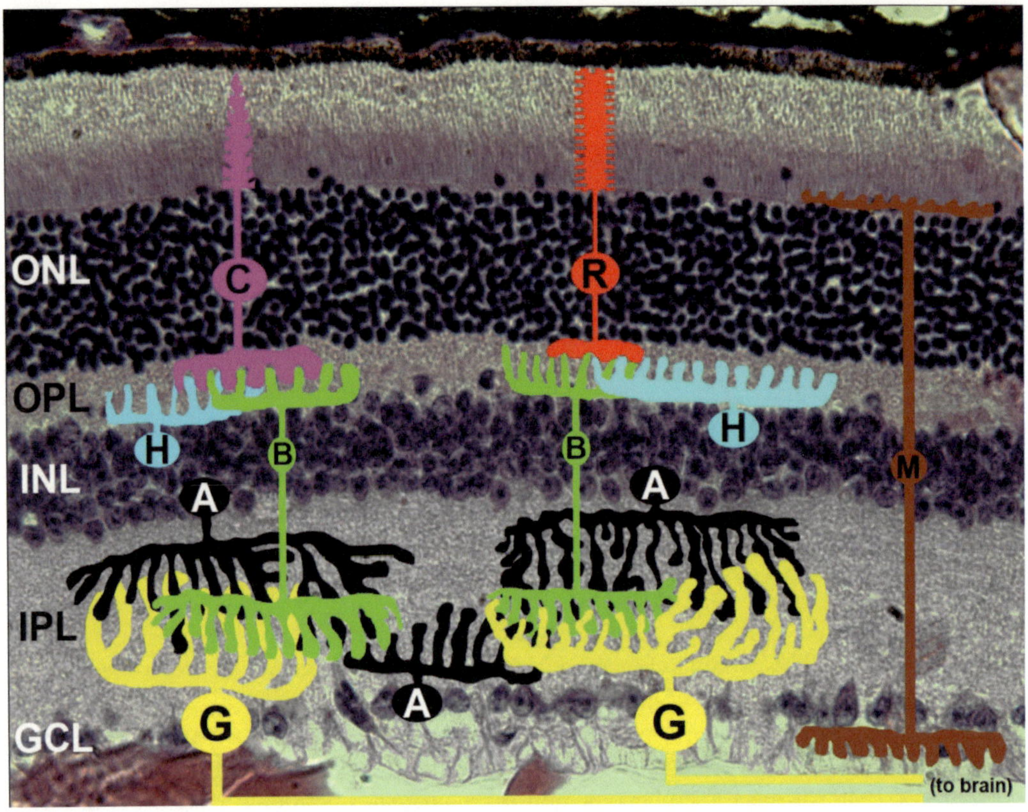

Fig. 1. Structure and connectivity of the mature retina. Animated neurons are drawn on top of a photomicrograph of a hematoxylin & eosin stained adult retina. Rod and cone photoreceptors are located in the ONL, horizontal, amacrine and bipolar cell interneurons and Müller glia are located in the INL, and RGCs and displaced amacrine cells are in the GCL. Light enters the eye and is first processed by the outer segments of rod and cone photoreceptors in the ONL. This information is then passed to the OPL, where connections between photoreceptors and bipolar cells are made, and signals are modulated by horizontal cells. Finally, bipolar cell axons pass visual information to RGC dendrites in the IPL - signaling that is refined by amacrine cells. Information is finally transmitted by RGC axons to the brain for further processing. (A,amacrine cell, B,bipolar cell; C,cone photoreceptor; G, retinal ganglion cell; GCL, ganglion cell layer; H, horizontal cell; INL, inner nuclear layer; IPL, inner plexiform layer; M, Müller glia; ONL, outer nuclear layer; OPL, outer plexiform layer; R, rod photoreceptor).

The GCL also contains some displaced amacrine cells. The three nuclear layers are separated by two synaptic layers; the inner plexiform layer (IPL), which separates the GCL/INL and the outer plexiform layer (OPL), which separates the INL/ONL.

In the embryo, the retina begins as a small bilateral outpocketing of the rostral diencephalon, first emerging at around embryonic day (E) 8.5 in mice (Svoboda and O'Shea 1987; Wawersik and Maas 2000; Fuhrmann 2010). As the evaginated diencephalon comes into contact with the surface ectoderm, it induces formation of the lens placode in the overlying epithelium. At E9.5, the lens vesicle signals to the adjacent diencephalic neuroepithelial cells to invaginate and form an optic cup (Svoboda and O'Shea 1987; Fuhrmann 2010). The inner and outer layers of the optic cup form the neural retina and retinal pigmented epithelium (RPE), respectively. Thus, by E10.5 the neural retina is morphologically distinct, and is comprised of actively proliferating, progenitor cells (Kagiyama et al. 2005; Hirashima et al. 2008). Based on lineage tracing and clonal analyses, all seven retinal cell types are generated from this common pool of multipotent retinal progenitor cells (Turner and Cepko 1987; Holt et al. 1988; Wetts and Fraser 1988; Fekete et al. 1994; Alexiades and Cepko 1997). There is also, however evidence for the existence of some restricted retinal cell lineages (Alexiades and Cepko 1997; Li et al. 2004; Pearson and Doe 2004; Cayouette et al. 2006). Currently, the proportion of retinal progenitors that are multipotent versus lineage-restricted is not known (Cayouette et al. 2003; Cayouette et al. 2006).

1.2 Retinal cell fate specification and differentiation

Retinal cell differentiation commences at around E10.5 in mouse and is not complete until postnatal day (P) 12, preceding in a medial-to-lateral gradient (Young 1985a; Wallace 2011). The seven retinal cell types are generated in a stereotyped, overlapping sequence and can be grouped into two major, overlapping phases; a prenatal and postnatal phase (Young 1985b; Young 1985a; Stiemke and Hollyfield 1995; Cepko et al. 1996) (Figure 2). In the prenatal phase, RGCs first begin to differentiate, starting at approximately E10.5, followed closely by horizontal cells and cone photoreceptors, and slightly later by amacrine cells. This prenatal phase of retinal histogenesis peaks around E15.5 and continues until approximately P2 in mice. In the postnatal phase of retinal cell differentiation, which peaks around P0, rod photoreceptors, bipolar cells and Müller glia are generated (Cepko et al. 1996; Livesey and Cepko 2001; Wallace 2011). Strikingly, the order of cellular differentiation is grossly conserved across vertebrate species despite a wide variance in the overall length of the differentiation period that ranges from 25 hours in *Xenopus* [i.e. stage 28-stage 40; (Holt et al. 1988)] to approximately 3 weeks in rodents (Young 1985b; Rapaport et al. 2004).

Over the course of cellular differentiation, temporal cues are thought to gradually reduce developmental plasticity such that progenitor cells become biased towards a smaller number of cell fates (Competence Model), resulting in the stereotyped order of cellular differentiation (Cepko et al. 1996; Livesey and Cepko 2001). In both multipotent and lineage biased progenitors, transcription factors act combinatorially to specify distinct retinal cell fates at different developmental times (Inoue et al. 2002). Thus, by changing the repertoire of transcription factors that are expressed and active, unique temporal identities are specified and appropriate differentiation programs are initiated (Cepko et al. 1996). Many transcription factors that participate in retinogenesis act in a combinatorial manner to specify retinal cell fates (Hatakeyama et al. 2001; Inoue et al. 2002). As a consequence, misexpression of any one transcription factor does not necessarily induce the generation of the cell types that would be predicted based on its pattern of expression and loss-of-function phenotype. For example, *Math3* and *Mash1* are expressed in bipolar cells, a cell type that is absent in *Math3;Mash1* double mutants, but misexpression of either of these two basic-helix loop-helix (bHLH) proteins alone promotes rod rather than bipolar genesis (Tomita et al. 2000). In contrast, misexpression of *Math3* or *Mash1* in conjunction with the homeodomain protein *Chx10* leads to bipolar cell genesis (Hatakeyama et al. 2001). Similarly, amacrine cells are specified by the combined activities of the bHLH protein NeuroD in conjunction with the homeodomain proteins Pax6 or Six3 (Inoue et al. 2002), whereas Math3 can specify a horizontal cell fate in combination with Pax6 or Six3, and a bipolar cell fate in combination with Chx10 (Hatakeyama et al. 2001; Inoue et al. 2002).

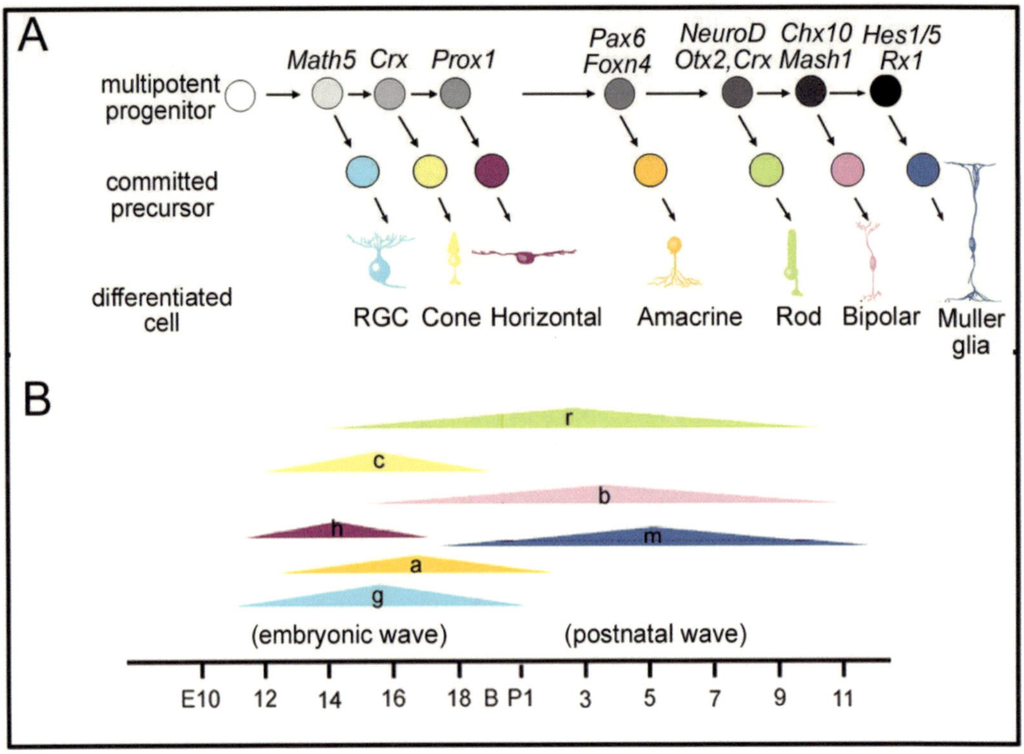

Fig. 2. Sequential generation of retinal cells during development.
(A) The competence model of retinal cell differentiation. Progenitors are gradually restricted in their developmental potential, resulting in the differentiation of different retinal cell types as developmental time proceeds. RGCs are born first, quickly followed in an overlapping manner by cones, horizontal cells, and amacrine cells (embryonic phase), and rod photoreceptors, bipolar cells and Müller glia (postnatal phase). (B) A schematic illustrating that retinal cell neurogenesis occurs in roughly two distinct but overlapping waves.

1.3 Retinal cell migration

The three-layered structure of the retina is reminiscent of the six-layered organization of the neocortex. However, while neocortical neurons are born in non-overlapping waves and migrate radially to sequentially populate the layers in an 'inside-out' manner (i.e., deep-layers formed first, followed by more superficial layers) (Caviness 1982; Caviness et al. 1995; Takahashi et al. 1999), the timing of differentiation and the migratory routes of retinal neurons are more complex. For example, during the early-phase of retinal cell differentiation, RGCs, horizontal cells, amacrine cells and cone photoreceptors have overlapping birthdates, but distinct destinations: RGCs and some amacrine cells migrate to the GCL, horizontal cells and some amacrine cells migrate to the INL and cone photoreceptors migrate to the ONL (Baye and Link 2008; Galli-Resta et al. 2008). How are these distinct migratory routes established? The logic behind radial cell migration begins with an understanding of how retinal progenitor cells divide. Most retinal progenitors have a radial morphology and maintain contact with both the apical and basal surfaces of the retinal neuroepithelium (Figure 3). During the cell cycle, retinal progenitors undergo interkinetic nuclear migration in a cell cycle-dependent fashion, such that mitotic divisions, and hence neuronal birth, occur at the apical surface of the retina (Turner et al. 1990). Horizontal cell precursors are an exception to the rule, as they undergo non-apical mitoses near their final location in the INL (Figure 3, 4) (Godinho et al. 2007), while other cell types are all thought to be born at the apical surface. As RGCs differentiate, they lose their apical attachment, retaining a basal extension that becomes an axon and is thought to help drag RGCs into the GCL (Poggi et al. 2005; Zolessi et al. 2006) (Figure 3). In contrast, amacrine cells lose both apical and basal contacts upon differentiation, and must somehow respond to unknown environmental cues as they migrate into their final positions in the INL and GCL (Galli-Resta et al. 2008) (Figure 3). Finally, cone photoreceptors remain at their apical site of birth - where the future ONL will develop (Figure 3). Similarly, in the second phase of differentiation, rod photoreceptors remain in the apical compartment post-differentiation, whereas bipolar cells and Müller glia must migrate into the INL (Figure 4).

The retina also has a unique three-dimensional architecture in the tangential plane, with the cell bodies of cone photoreceptors, amacrine cells, horizontal cells and RGCs migrating tangentially to position themselves at regular intervals to allow complete sampling of the visual field. These non-random cellular arrays are known as mosaics and evenly tile the retinal field (Galli-Resta et al. 2008). Individual cellular mosaics are characterized by minimal distances between like-cells - a spacing that is achieved by processes that include self-avoidance or isoneuronal repulsion and repulsion of like-neighbours or heteroneuronal repulsion (Grueber and Sagasti 2010). While the molecular cues that establish retinal cell mosaics are poorly understood, individual retinal mosaics are known to develop cell autonomously and are not influenced by the mosaics of other cell types (Rockhill et al. 2000).

1.4 Retinal cell death during development

Apoptosis is also known as programmed cell death, and is a process whereby a cell induces its own death through a well characterized caspase-mediated signalling pathway. During development, neurogenesis and apoptosis are both required to occur in a balanced fashion so that appropriate numbers of each retinal cell type are present in the mature organ. Strikingly, in the CNS, 20-70% of neurons undergo apoptosis (Burek and Oppenheim 1996). While it is still not known why organisms generate extra cells and then have to delete them, the process of apoptosis has been conserved throughout evolution and is essential for proper tissue morphogenesis and to determine the final size of tissues and organs (Burek and Oppenheim 1996; Bahr 2000; Buss and Oppenheim 2004). During embryonic retinal development there are three waves of cell apoptosis. First, during the optic cup stage (E10-E11), apoptosis is primarily observed in the presumptive RPE and optic stalk (Pei and Rhodin 1970; Silver and Hughes 1973). Next, a second wave of apoptosis is observed during the stage of optic fissure closure (E11 to E12), with apoptotic retinal progenitor cells observed at the fissure site (Silver and Robb 1979; Hero 1990). The third wave of apoptosis happens during the optic nerve enlargement stage (E15.5-E17.5). At this stage, neuroepithelial cells close to the optic nerve head undergo degeneration (Silver and Robb 1979). Cell apoptosis is also observed in all three layers in postnatal stage retinae, occurring in a central to peripheral gradient. Studies in rat retinae indicate that around 5%, 50%, and

51% of the ONL, INL, and GCL populations undergoes programmed cell death, respectively (Voyvodic et al. 1995). Cell apoptosis starts in the GCL, and lasts from P2 to P11 with a peak at P2-P5 (Young 1984). Two phases of apoptosis are then observed in the INL, with amacrine cell degeneration peaking at P3-P8, followed by bipolar and Müller glial cell degeneration peaking at P8-P11. Photoreceptor cell apoptosis lasts for two weeks, with a peak from P5 to P9 (Young 1984).

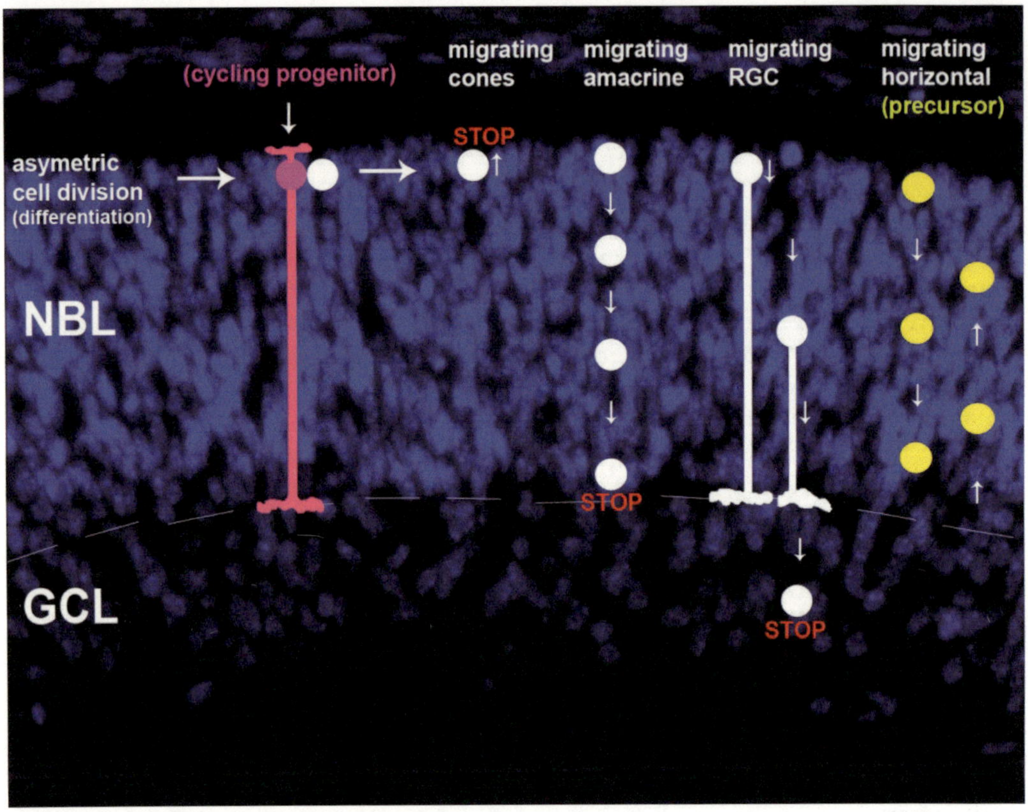

Fig. 3. Site of neuronal birth and migration patterns for retinal neurons born in the early embryonic phase of retinal cell differentiation.

Cells are schematized on top of a photomicrograph of an E15.5, DAPI stained retina. Cycling progenitors (pink) maintain contacts with the apical and basal surface of the retinal neuroepithelium. Retinal progenitors then divide asymmetrically at the apical surface of the neuroblast layer (NBL), giving rise to immature neurons that must migrate to their correct laminar positions within the retina. Cone cells differentiate at the apical surface, where they will remain and form the future ONL (not shown). Amacrine cells differentiate at the apical surface, lose their apical and basal contacts, and then migrate through the NBL to reach the INL (and some go to the GCL). RGCs differentiate at the apical surface and lose their apical contact but maintain their basal contact - an extension that will help RGCs migrate into the forming GCL. During this time, horizontal cell precursors continue to migrate along the apico-basal axis of the NBL, not undergoing terminal differentiation and finding their final position until postnatal stages.

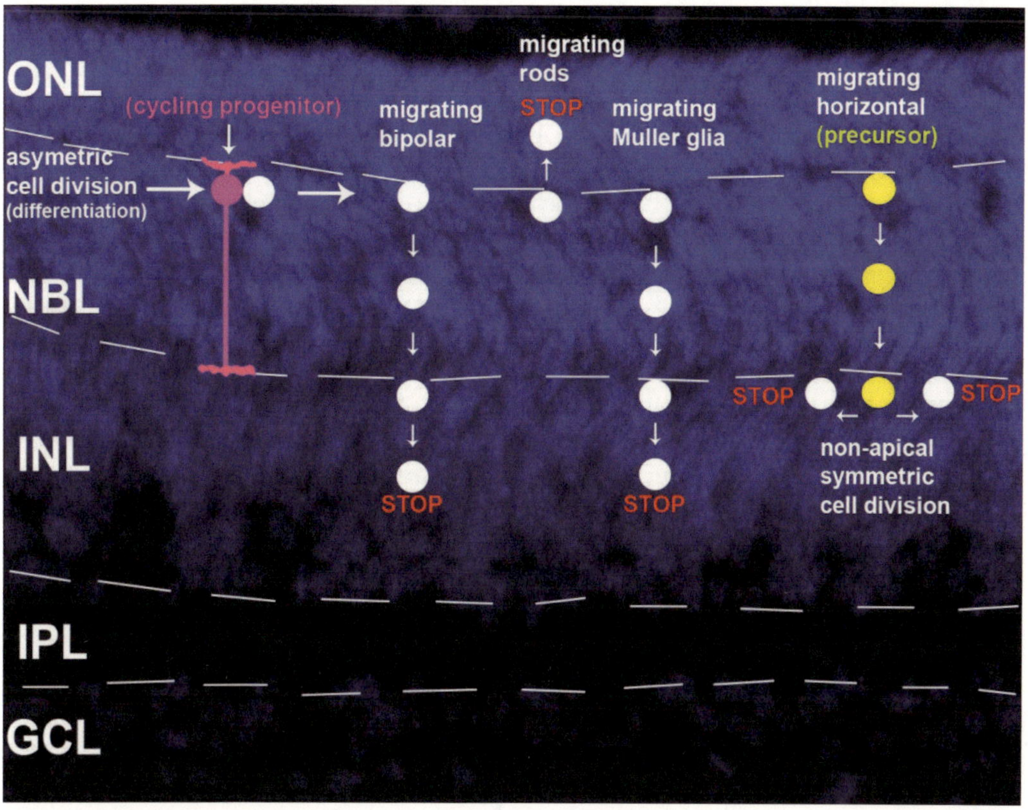

Fig. 4. Site of neuronal birth and migration patterns for retinal neurons born in the late postnatal phase of retinal cell differentiation.
Retinal cells are schematized on top of a photomicrograph of a P3, DAPI stained retina. Cycling progenitors (pink) divide asymmetrically at the apical surface of the NBL to eventually give rise to immature neurons that must migrate to their correct laminar position within the retina. Bipolar cells migrate through the NBL basally and into the middle of the forming INL. Rods remain at the apical surface of the retina, where the ONL is developing. Müller glia migrate in a similar fashion to bipolar cells to reach the INL. Horizontal cell precursors migrate into the apical surface of the forming INL, undergo a terminal symmetric division and migrate in a tangential fashion to find their final position in the INL.

The molecules involved in the apoptotic pathway have been extensively studied in several systems, including the retina (Burek and Oppenheim 1996). While a comprehensive summary is beyond the scope of this review, apoptotic molecules identified in the retina include death receptors, excitotoxic factors, proapoptotic Bcl-2 family proteins, proteases, DNases and transcription factors (for review, see (Isenmann et al. 2003)).
This review will summarize what is currently known and what are some unanswered questions about established tumor suppressor genes and their roles in different stages of retinal histogenesis.

2. Tumor suppressor genes regulate retinal progenitor cell proliferation

2.1 Introduction to the cell cycle

All tissues, including the retina, are genetically programmed to acquire an optimal size, which is determined both by the total number of cells and the sizes of individual cells (Gomer 2001). A major open question is how retinal progenitors know when to switch from making one cell type to the next so that appropriate numbers of each of the seven cell types are generated. In the retina, the choice of cell fate is intimately coupled, albeit not absolutely linked, to the timing of cell cycle exit. Given the central role that tumor suppressor genes play in regulating cell cycle exit, it is therefore not surprising that they are emerging as key regulators of the normal cell cycle in the developing retina. A general introduction to the cell cycle and the tumor suppressor genes that operate in this pathway is highlighted below.

During the cell cycle, dividing cells must replicate their DNA (S-phase) and then segregate a 2N complement of chromosomes into each daughter cell during mitosis (M-phase). S-phase and M-phase of the cell cycle are separated by two Gap phases (G1 before S and G2 before M), in which key checkpoints regulate entry into the next cell cycle phase. An important checkpoint in G1 is the restriction point, where the decision is made to either commit to another round of cell division or to exit the cell cycle and enter G0 (i.e., stop dividing). Two major classes of regulatory molecules control cell cycle progression - the cyclins and cyclin-dependent kinases (CDKs), which together form functional complexes (Nigg 1995). In general, CDKs are constitutively expressed whereas cyclin expression is more tightly regulated and restricted to specific cell cycle stages (Nigg 1995). Progression past the restriction point in G1 is regulated by complex formation between CDK4 or CDK6 with members of the Cyclin D family (D1/D2/D3). Active Cyclin D-CDK4/6 complexes phosphorylate the retinoblastoma protein (Rb), an important tumor suppressor gene that controls G1 progression (Paternot et al. 2010). When Rb is in its hypo-phosphorylated form, it is bound to E2F transcription factors, an interaction that is dissociated by hyperphosphorylation of Rb, releasing the E2F proteins so that they can initiate the transcription of genes required in S-phase of the cell cycle (Figure 5).

The CDK/cyclin complexes that operate in G1 phase of the cell cycle are negatively regulated by cyclin dependent kinase inhibitors (CDKIs), which block cell cycle progression. CDKIs fall into two families: 1) Cip/Kip ($p21^{Cip1}$, $p27^{Kip1}$ and $p57^{Kip2}$) and 2) INK4 ($p16^{INK4a}$, $p15^{INK4b}$, $p18^{INK4c}$, and $p19^{INK4d}$) (Besson et al. 2008). In the Cip/Kip family, $p57^{Kip2}$ and $p27^{Kip1}$ are considered tumor suppressor genes as mutations in these genes are associated with tumor formation in humans (Lee and Kim 2009; Guo et al. 2010). In contrast, $p21^{Cip1}$ is not often mutated in human cancers, but its deletion is associated with tumor formation in mouse models, suggesting that it does have tumor suppressor properties ((Franklin et al. 2000; Poole et al. 2004; Gartel 2009) and references therein). Moreover, $p21^{Cip1}$ mediates cell cycle exit induced in response to DNA damage by *p53*, a well known tumor suppressor that is frequently mutated in human cancers (Gartel 009). Finally, in the INK4 family, $p16^{INK4a}$ and $p19^{INK4d}$ are known tumor suppressor genes that block the assembly of Cdk4/6-cyclin D complexes, thereby inhibiting progression through G1 into S phase of the cell cycle (Besson et al. 2008; Wesierska-Gadek et al. 2010).

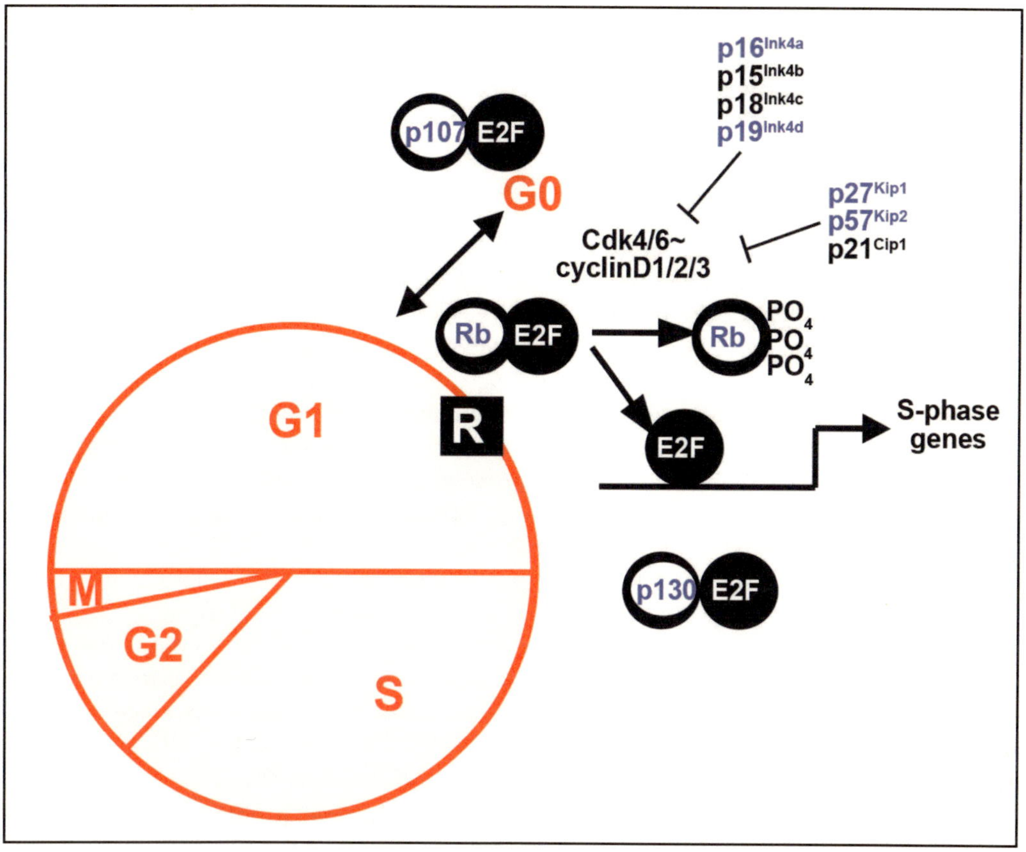

Fig. 5. Tumor suppressor genes and the cell cycle. Schematic illustration of the major phases of the eukaryotic cell cycle.
Progression through the restriction point (R) in G1 is controlled by Cdk4/6~cyclinD1-D3 complexes, which phosphorylate the Rb protein. When Rb is hypophosphorylated, it is bound to E2F transcription factors. When Rb is hyperphosphorylated, it releases E2F transcription factors, which can induce the expression of genes required for progression into S-phase of the cell cycle. The related pocket proteins p107 and p130 also complex with E2F transcription factors. The activities of Cdk4/6~cyclinD1-D3 complexes are negatively regulated by CDKIs of the Cip/Kip and INK4 families. Cell cycle regulators that are known tumor suppressor genes are listed in blue.

2.2 CDKIs regulate retinal progenitor cell proliferation

Of the Cip/Kip family members, only $p27^{Kip1}$ and $p57^{Kip2}$ have been studied extensively in the developing retina. During embryogenesis and in the early postnatal period, $p27^{Kip1}$ and $p57^{Kip2}$ are each expressed in a few scattered progenitor cells in the outer neuroblast layer (ONBL) as well as in a few postmitotic cells that are forming the INL. However, $p27^{Kip1}$ and $p57^{Kip2}$ are not co-expressed in the retina, suggesting that they function in distinct populations of retinal cells (Dyer and Cepko 2000; Dyer and Cepko 2001). The few cells that express CDKIs in the ONBL are thought to be those that are exiting the cell cycle and differentiating. Indeed, withdrawal of the growth factor EGF from cultured retinal progenitor cells induces *p27^Kip1^* expression in association with cell cycle exit and cellular differentiation (Levine et al. 2000). In gain of function experiments in E14.5 retinal progenitors, *p27^Kip1^* promote premature cell cycle exit and differentiation (Dyer and Cepko 2000; Levine et al. 2000; Dyer and Cepko 2001). Conversely, in *p27^Kip1^* mutants, uncommitted retinal progenitor cells, but not committed precursor cells, divide excessively during late retinogenesis (Levine et al. 2000; Dyer and Cepko 2001). Similar results were obtained in *Xenopus* retina. In gain-of-function experiments, *p27^Xic1^* promotes cell cycle exit while loss-of-function conversely promotes retinal progenitor cell proliferation (Ohnuma et al. 1999). *p57^Kip2^* is similarly sufficient and required for cell cycle exit of retinal progenitors, but it functions during an early stage of retinal development, with ectopic cell divisions observed as early as E14.5 in knock-out mice (Dyer and Cepko 2000; Dyer and Cepko 2001).

In the murine retina, the INK4 family member $p19^{INK4d}$ is expressed in retinal progenitors at all embryonic and postnatal stages tested (Cunningham et al. 2002). Mutation of $p19^{INK4d}$ results in increased retinal progenitor cell proliferation during early postnatal stages (Cunningham et al. 2002). Prolonged retinal progenitor cell proliferation is also observed in $p19^{INK4d}$;$p27^{Kip1}$ double null retinae, including at P18, a stage when no BrdU+ proliferating cells are normally detected in the murine retina (Cunningham et al. 2002). The cause of the ectopic cell divisions was shown to be re-entry into the cell cycle by differentiated retinal neurons, including horizontal and amacrine cells (Cunningham et al. 2002).

The activities of $p27^{Kip1}$ and $p19^{INK4d}$ are thus not temporally restricted in the retina - they function both in the embryonic and postnatal stages of retinal development to control cell cycle exit. In contrast, $p57^{Kip2}$ is only required during the embryonic early stage of retinal development to control cell cycle exit (Levine et al. 2000; Dyer and Cepko 2001).

2.3 *Rb* and its family members regulate retinal progenitor cell proliferation

The retinoblastoma protein (Rb) encoded by the *Rb1* gene was the first tumor suppressor gene identified (Chinnam and Goodrich 2011). In humans, mutation of *RB1* results in retinoblastoma, a devastating childhood tumor of the eye that robs children of their vision (DiCiommo et al. 2000). Rb prevents progression from G1 into S phase of the cell cycle by binding E2F transcription factors - an inhibition that is released by CDK4/6-cyclinD-mediated phosphorylation of Rb (Frolov and Dyson 2004; Burkhart and Sage 2008; Paternot et al. 2010). Rb is a pocket-protein that is highly related to two other family members, p107 and p130, which are similar in both sequence and function, also acting as nuclear phosphoproteins (Ewen et al. 1991; Hannon et al. 1993). Like Rb, p107 and p130 also act as negative regulators of cell proliferation through interactions with E2F transcription factors (Zhu et al. 1993; Claudio et al. 1994). It is now known that different Rb family proteins associate with different E2Fs at different times during the cell cycle (Bernards 1997).

In mouse models, animals heterozygous for an *Rb* null allele die at 6-8 months of age due to pituitary gland tumours, but display no evidence of retinal abnormalities, proliferation defects, or retinoblastoma (Clarke et al. 1992; Jacks et al. 1992). This is in keeping with evidence in humans that both *Rb* alleles must be mutated for tumors to arise (DiCiommo et al. 2000). In contrast, animals homozygous for an *Rb* null allele die in the embryonic period - between E12-E15 (Clarke et al. 1992; Jacks et al. 1992). While a detailed analysis of retinal development is not possible at these early stages, it is notable that no gross abnormalities or enhanced proliferation were observed in surviving *Rb* mutant embryos at E13.5 (Zhang et al. 2004). However, more S-phase cells were observed in retinae from homozygous *Rb* null mutants that were explanted at E13.5 and cultured for 6 days *in vitro* (DIV - equivalent to early postnatal retinae *in vivo*) (Zhang et al. 2004). This suggested that *Rb* may only be required to regulate the cell cycle during early postnatal stages of retinal development, a model that was tested further with the advent of the Cre-LoxP system, and the ability to conditionally knock-out (cKO) *Rb* in the retina (Chen et al. 2004; MacPherson et al. 2004; Zhang et al. 2004). Using a Nestin-Cre driver, *Rb* cKO retinae were generated, and ectopic S- and M-phase progenitors were detected in the presumptive IPL/GCL at E18.5, although overall numbers of dividing cells were not significantly increased (MacPherson et al. 2004). Despite the increases in ectopic cycling and mitotic cells, paternal Nestin-Cre *Rb* cKO show no evidence of retinoblastoma but also die at early postnatal stages (MacPherson et al. 2004), likely due to the broad effect of deleting Rb in most of the developing brain.

One reason why *Rb* mutants may not display defects in retinal development may be because of compensation by *p107* and *p130* family members. Analyses of retinal development in *Rb;p107* double mutants was initially precluded by the death of these embryos by E11.5 (Robanus-Maandag et al. 1998). To circumvent this problem, chimeric embryos were generated with *Rb;p107* double mutant embryonic stem cells (Robanus-Maandag et al. 1998). *Rb;p107* double mutant chimeric embryos develop retinoblastoma by E17.5, with tissue hyperplasia originating in retinal cells committed to the amacrine cell lineage (Robanus-Maandag et al. 1998). Subsequently, the floxed *Rb* allele was used to analyze *Rb* mutations in combination with conventional $p107^{-/-}$ (Chen et al. 2004), $p130^{-/-}$ (MacPherson et al. 2004) or $p130^{-/-}$; $p107^{+/-}$ (Ajioka et al. 2007) mutations. Using a Pax6α-Cre driver, *Rb* cKO mice were generated, knocking out *Rb* in peripheral and not central retinal progenitors; this mutant allele was analyzed on a $p107^{-/-}$ background (Chen et al. 2004). At P0, in both *Rb* cKOs and *Rb* cKO; *p107* double knockouts, BrdU+ cells were not increased in number, but were ectopically positioned throughout the differentiated zones of the retina, where dividing cells are not usually detected (Chen et al. 2004). It was not until P8 (and up to P18) that *Rb* cKOs and *Rb* cKO; *p107* double knockouts displayed an overall increase in the number of BrdU+ cells (Chen et al. 2004; MacPherson et al. 2004). *Rb* cKO;*p107* double null mice also developed retinoblastoma as early as P8, with larger tumors apparent in older animals (Chen et al. 2004). Many of the ectopic BrdU+ cells were amacrine cells in *Rb* cKO and *Rb* cKO;*p107* double mutants, while tumors cells rarely expressed markers of photoreceptors, bipolar cells, or RGCs (Chen et al. 2004). Similar results were observed in *Rb* cKO;*p130* double knockout mice generated with a nestin-cre driver, which also developed retinoblastomas in adulthood, with tumors comprised of syntaxin+ and calretinin+ amacrine cells and not other retinal cell types (MacPherson et al. 2004). Thus, the Rb family of pocket proteins have an important role in regulating cell cycle exit in committed amacrine cell precursors, furthermore suggesting that amacrine cells may be the cell of origin for retinoblastoma.

While *Rb* cKO; *p107-/-* and *Rb* cKO; *p130-/-* double knockouts generated with Pax6α-cre and Nestin-cre drivers, respectively, both develop retinoblastomas derived from amacrine cell precursors, it was recently demonstrated that in *Rb* cKO;*p130-/-;p107+/-* animals that were generated with a Chx10-cre driver (commonly referred to as "p107 single" mice as they only express this one pocket protein), metastatic retinoblastoma develops in adults, with tumor cells derived from fully differentiated and synaptically coupled horizontal cells that have de-differentiated and re-entered the cell cycle (Ajioka et al. 2007). In contrast, in human retina, perinatal-derived retinoblastoma (most clinical cases of human familial retinoblastoma are detected during early infancy in children), which requires bi-allelic *Rb1* mutation and/or inactivation, seems to arise from *Rb* mutant cells of the cone photoreceptor precursor lineage (Xu et al. 2009), rather than an amacrine or horizontal cell lineage as in mouse (Chen et al. 2004; Ajioka et al. 2007). The oncogenes *MDM2* and *n-Myc* are highly expressed in cone precursors and are required for the propagation of human retinoblastoma (Xu et al. 2009). It was also found that the cone-specific transcription factors *RXRγ* and *TRβ2* are also required for retinoblastoma proliferation and survival in several human retinoblastoma cell lines (Xu et al. 2009). Moreover, *RXRγ* was found to positively regulate the expression of the oncogene *MDM2* (Xu et al. 2009). Given the evidence found in this human study, it is difficult to say which of the currently generated mouse models of retinoblastoma most closely resemble (or successfully "model") bonafide human retinoblastoma. Further studies will be needed to understand the differences observed in mouse models and in human tumors with respect to the cell of origin for retinoblastoma.

2.4 *Zac1* and *Tgfβ2* regulate retinal progenitor cell proliferation

Zac1 is a tumor suppressor gene encoding a zinc finger transcription factor that promotes cell cycle arrest and apoptosis in cell lines, while germline mutations are associated with numerous carcinomas (Abdollahi et al. 1997; Spengler et al. 1997; Pagotto et al. 2000; Bilanges et al. 2001; Abdollahi et al. 2003; Koy et al. 2004). Similarly, we have shown that *Zac1* is required to elicit apoptosis and cell cycle arrest in the developing murine retina (Ma et al. 2007a). In *Zac1* null mutants, the retina becomes hypercellular in late retinogenesis, an increase in cell number that is associated with ectopic cell divisions in the early postnatal retina (Ma et al. 2007a). Conversely, in gain-of-function experiments, misexpression of *Zac1* blocks retinal cell proliferation (Ma et al. 2007a). Currently, it is not known how *Zac1* promotes cell cycle exit, either in tumor cells or in retinal progenitor cells (Spengler et al. 1997; Ma et al. 2007a). It seems unlikely that *Zac1* regulates retinal cell cycle exit through $p27^{Kip1}$ or $p57^{Kip2}$, as *Zac1* has a distinct requirement in late retinal progenitors, while $p57^{Kip2}$ functions in early progenitors, and $p27^{Kip1}$ functions throughout retinogenesis (Ma et al. 2007a).

We found that *Zac1* is required to induce expression of *transforming growth factor βII* (*TGFβII*) in the retina (Ma et al. 2007a). Notably, *TGFβII* is also a known tumor suppressor gene, and was shown to negatively regulate the proliferation of retinal progenitor cells and Müller glia (Close et al. 2005). Interestingly, previous reports have indicated that *TGFβ* regulates $p27^{Kip1}$ expression (Ravitz and Wenner 1997), whereas *Zac1* does not regulate $p27^{Kip1}$ expression (Ma et al. 2007a). However, Zac1 is known to associate with and modulate the activity of several transcriptional regulators, including p53 (Huang and Stallcup 2000; Huang et al. 2001). *p53* is a well known tumor suppressor that is required for the cellular response to TGFβ signaling in *Xenopus* mesoderm (Cordenonsi et al. 2003; Cordenonsi et al. 2007).

3. Tumor suppressor genes regulate retinal cell death

3.1 CDKIs regulate retinal cell death

Compensatory mechanisms exist in the retina to ensure that the final ratios of individual cell types remain constant, with excess proliferation often balanced by an increase in apoptosis. This is indeed the case in $p27^{Kip1}$ and $p57^{Kip2}$ mutants, where increases in cell death are thought to counterbalance the increased retinal progenitor cell proliferation observed in these mutants (Dyer and Cepko 2000; Levine et al. 2000; Dyer and Cepko 2001). While

19^{INK4d} knockout mouse retinae reported no change in apoptosis at postnatal stages (P10, P14, and P18), *p19^{INK4d};p27^{Kip1}* double knockouts did show increased apoptosis at P10 and P14 (Cunningham et al. 2002). Thus, despite the increase in cell proliferation, cell number is not dramatically changed in *p19^{INK4d};p27^{Kip1}* double null because apoptosis in these retinae is five times higher than in wild-type retinae (Cunningham et al. 2002). This cell death was unable to be rescued upon co-deletion of *p53*, as *p19^{INK4d};p27^{Kip1};p53* triple knockout mouse retinae also showed increased levels of apoptosis at postnatal stages (Cunningham et al. 2002), indicating the underlying mechanism of death signalling is *p53*-independent.

3.2 *Rb* and its family members regulate retinal cell death

In all *Rb* mutant eyes, including in conventional *Rb* knockouts at E13.5 (Zhang et al. 2004), chimeric *Rb* knockouts (from E16 onwards) (Robanus-Maandag et al. 1998), and in *Rb* cKOs generated with Nestin-Cre (at E18.5) (MacPherson et al. 2004) or Pax6α-cre (from P0) (Chen et al. 2004; MacPherson et al. 2004), an increase in cell death was observed. Notably, this increase in cell death was no longer evident in E13.5 retinal explants from conventional *Rb* knockouts that were cultured for 12 DIV (similar to late postnatal stages *in-vivo*), suggesting that *Rb* is required to prevent apoptosis only during embryonic and early postnatal stages (Zhang et al. 2004). It was also reported that amacrine cells seem to be spared from apoptosis since they were not dramatically reduced in number in Rb mutants, unlike other retinal cell types (MacPherson et al. 2004). The mechanism behind the excessive cell death in Rb mutants is independent of *p53*, as *Rb* cKO;*p53* double knockout retinae displayed the same increase in apoptosis observed in *Rb* cKO single mutants (MacPherson et al. 2004). *Rb;p107* double chimeric knockouts (Robanus-Maandag et al. 1998) or *Rb* cKO;*p107* double knockouts generated with Nestin-cre (MacPherson et al. 2004) or Pax6α-cre (Chen et al. 2004) also displayed enhanced apoptosis from E17.5 onwards. The cells that were more prone to apoptosis in double knockout retinae was investigated in more detail, demonstrating that RGCs and other cell types undergo extensive cell death, but amacrine cells were selectively spared from apaoptosis (Chen et al. 2004). The authors of this study argue strongly that because amacrine cells are intrinsically death resistant in double *Rb* cKO;*p107* knockouts, they are capable of forming retinoblastomas, and that resistance to cell death may be a general feature of tumor formation. However, what remains to be determined is why amacrine cells are protected from cell death in Rb mouse mutants, while all other retinal cell types seem to undergo apoptosis when the pocket proteins are mutated.

3.3 *Zac1* regulates retinal cell death

Our analysis of *Zac1* mutant retinae revealed that there are fewer apoptotic cells in E18.5 explants cultured for both 4 and 8 DIV (Ma et al. 2007a). However, misexpression of *Zac1* was not sufficient to induce cell death in the murine retina (Ma et al. 2007a), although it was sufficient to induce apoptosis in the Xenopus retina (Ma et al. 2007b), as well as in mouse or human cell lines (Spengler et al. 1997; Varrault et al. 1998). Interestingly, an isoform of human *Zac1* lacking the first 2 zinc fingers (Zac1Δ2) has a reduced capacity to induce apoptosis and an increased ability to arrest cell cycle progression, suggesting that these two functions are carried out independently of one another (Bilanges et al. 2001). How *Zac1* induces apoptosis in the retina and elsewhere, remains to be determined.

4. Tumor suppressor genes and retinal cell fate specification

In the retina, the choice of cell fate is intimately coupled, albeit not absolutely linked, to the timing of cell cycle exit. This raises the question of how cell fate specification and cell cycle exit decisions are coordinated.

4.1 The CDKIs $p27^{Kip1}$ and $p57^{Kip2}$ influence cell fate decisions in the retina

Misexpression of $p27^{Xic1}$ in *Xenopus* promotes Müller glial cell genesis, while conversely, inactivating $p27^{Xic1}$ decreases Müller glial cell number (Ohnuma et al. 1999). $p27^{Xic1}$ also has the ability to modulate the capacity of transcription factors to specify retinal cell fates in *Xenopus.* For example, *Xath5* has a more potent ability to induce an RGC fate when co-expressed with $p27^{Xic1}$, whereas *Xath5* promotes alternative "later" fates when cell cycle progression is stimulated by cyclin E1 (Ohnuma et al. 2002). In murine systems, $p27^{Kip1}$ appears to function differently than its *Xenopus* homolog. For instance, misexpression of $p27^{Kip1}$ in mouse or rat retinal cells increases the number of rod photoreceptors that differentiate (Levine et al. 2000; Dyer and Cepko 2001), suggesting that $p27^{Kip1}$ may specify a photoreceptor cell fate. Providing further support for this idea, rat embryonic retinal progenitors express high levels of p27^{Kip1} in response to the withdrawal of EGF from the culture media, leading to cell cycle exit and preferential photoreceptor differentiation (Levine et al. 2000). However, if $p27^{Kip1}$ is instead misexpressed together with Notch in mouse retinae, Müller glial cells are increased in number, indicative of a collaborative interaction between Notch and $p27^{Kip1}$ in the specification of a Müller glial cell fate (Levine et al. 2000).

Despite these striking gain-of-function phenotypes, in mammalian loss-of-function experiments, conventional $p27^{Kip1}$ knockout mouse display no overall changes in the final proportions of retinal cells that differentiate (Levine et al. 2000; Dyer and Cepko 2001). This indicates that while $p27^{Kip1}$ is sufficient to alter cell differentiation in mammalian retinae, it seems to not be required to do so. This is in contrast to $p57^{Kip2}$, which does appear to have an essential role in cell fate specification in the mammalian retina (Dyer and Cepko 2000). In the mature mouse retina, p57^{Kip2} expression is restricted to a subset of amacrine cells (Dyer and Cepko 2000). In $p57^{Kip2}$ knockouts, more calbindin+ amacrine cells are generated, while all other cell types are generated in proper numbers (Dyer and Cepko 2000). Currently, it is not known how $p57^{Kip2}$ influences the genesis of calbindin+ amacrine cells, but it may be through collaborative interactions with transcription factors that are involved in specifying the identity of this amacrine cell subpopulation.

4.2 Rb pocket proteins influence cell fate decisions in the retina

The mutation of *Rb* by several genetic means results in a reduction in rod photoreceptor differentiation in the retina, including: 1) in conventional *Rb* knockout mice (E13.5 retinal explants cultured for 12 DIV) (Zhang et al. 2004), 2) following infection of floxed *Rb* retinae with a cre-expressing retrovirus (Zhang et al. 2004), and 3) in *Rb* cKO retinae generated with Nestin-cre (MacPherson et al. 2004) or Pax6α-cre (MacPherson et al. 2004) drivers. RGCs and bipolar cells were also reduced in *Rb* cKO retinae generated with the Pax6α-cre driver (MacPherson et al. 2004), and in *Rb* cKO;*p107* double knockout retinae generated with the Pax6α-cre driver, which also had fewer rod photoreceptors (Chen et al. 2004). The loss of photoreceptors, bipolar cells, and RGCs in *Rb* mutants is likely due to increased apoptosis (Chen et al. 2004; MacPherson et al. 2004). The only evidence that *Rb* is involved in controlling the terminal differentiation of a retinal cell type comes from the analysis of starburst amacrine cells, which require Rb-mediated inhibition of E2f3a, a cycle regulator and oncogene, in order to differentiate (Chen et al. 2007).

4.3 *Zac1* and *TgfβII* regulate retinal cell fate specification through novel pathways

Zac1 mutants develop supernumerary rod photoreceptors and amacrine cells, acting in a cell autonomous fashion to block rod cell differentiation, while acting non cell autonomously to block amacrine cell development (Ma et al. 2007a). Mechanistically, we showed that *Zac1* regulates amacrine cell number via a negative feedback loop that acts as a cell number sensor (Ma et al. 2007a). We found that *Zac1* acts in amacrine cells late in retinogenesis to positively regulate TGFβII expression, which then acts as a negative feedback signal to limit amacrine cell production (Ma et al. 2007a). We found that members of the TGFβ family of ligands (TGFβII) and receptors (TGFβ receptors I and II) are expressed in amacrine cells in wildtype retinae but *Zac1* mutant retinae express significantly less TGFβII and consequently, phosphorylated Smad2/3, a downstream effector, are reduced (Ma et al. 2007a). After showing that retinal explants exposed to exogenous antibodies towards TGFβ receptor II also generate more amacrine cells, we showed that adding exogenous TGFβII to *Zac1* mutant retinal explants rescued the supernumary amacrine cell phenotype (Ma et al. 2007a). Finally, we analyzed the E18.5 retinae of conditional *TGFβ receptor II* knockout mice and also showed qualitatively that there are more amacrine cells present in mutant retinae relative to wildtype (Ma et al. 2007a). A Zac1-TGFβII negative regulatory loop thus controls amacrine cell differentiation in the retina, ensuring that appropriate numbers of these cell differentiate.

5.Tumor suppressor genes and retinal cell migration

5.1 Cell cycle regulators and retinal lamination

The role of CDKIs has been best studied in the cell cycle, but there is growing evidence that CDKIs regulate multiple other processes, including cytoskeletal dynamics and cell migration (Besson et al. 2008). In the developing nervous system, $p27^{Kip1}$ has been implicated in regulating the migration of neocortical neurons, using domains of the protein that are not involved in cell cycle regulation (Nguyen et al. 2006). Consistent with a potential migratory role for $p27^{Kip1}$ in the developing retina, in the mature $p27^{Kip1}$ knockout mouse retinae, bipolar, horizontal and possibly a few amacrine cell bodies are displaced from their regular positions within the INL (Levine et al. 2000). Also, in $p19^{INK4d}$; $p27^{Kip1}$ double knockout mouse retinae, there is apparent displacement of Müller glia and rod photoreceptors from their normal positions in the INL and ONL, respectively (Cunningham et al. 2002). However, the dysplasia of Müller glial cells and rods is reported to be almost completely rescued in $p19^{INK4d}$; $p27^{Kip1}$; *p53* triple knockout retinae (Cunningham et al. 2002), which suggests that p53 contributes to the p19/p27-dependent migration of rods and Müller glia. It was also reported that *Rb* cKO retinae generated with a Chx10-cre driver have ectopic Pax6+ cells in the ONL (Donovan and Dyer 2004), indicating that *Rb* regulates the proper radial migration of amacrine and/or RGCs to their proper layer within the developing retina. Finally, our analysis of *Zac1* mutant retinae revealed that amacrine cells migrate aberrantly, forming an ectopic cellular layer between the GCL and INL (Ma et al. 2007a). This suggests that *Zac1* is required to regulate the proper migration of amacrine cells in the retina. In all cases, it is poorly understood how tumor suppressor genes regulate cellular migration at the molecular level.

5.2 PI3K/PTEN signaling and retinal lamination

Pten (phosphatase and tensin homolog) encodes a lipid and protein phosphatase that is a negative regulator of the PI3K pathway. *Pten* is also a potent tumour suppressor, with loss of 10q23 heterozygosity commonly found in malignant glioblastomas (Li et al. 1997) and somatic *Pten* mutations found in multiple carcinomas (Steck et al. 1997; Ali et al. 1999). In the nervous system, *Pten* mutations are associated with hypertrophy of the cerebellum, neocortex and hippocampus (Backman et al. 2001; Groszer et al. 2001; Kwon et al. 2006; Lehtinen et al. 2011). *Pten* mutants also display defects in cell migration, lamination, dendrite arborization and myelination in different CNS domains (Marino et al. 2002; Yue et al. 2005; Kwon et al. 2006; Fraser et al. 2008). When *Pten* was deleted in the retinal pigment epithelium (RPE), photoreceptor degeneration was observed (Kim et al. 2008). Strikingly, PI3K signalling promotes progenitor cell proliferation and decreased apoptosis in the retina (Pimentel et al. 2002), and influences cell migration in other systems (Rosivatz 2007). Recently, our lab conditionally deleted the tumor suppressor *Pten* from the developing retina using the Pax6α-Cre driver line (Cantrup et al., submitted). We found that amacrine cells and RGCs were disorganized and scattered within the normally cell-sparse IPL, suggesting that PTEN regulates the proper radial migration of both amacrine and RGC's within the developing retina. We also have evidence that PTEN regulates the tangential migration of a subset of amacrine cells. Studies are currently ongoing to determine the molecular and cellular mechanisms by which PTEN regulates cell migration.

6.Tumor suppressor genes not yet characterized in retinal development

6.1 *Runx1*

In other parts of the developing mouse brain, *Runx1* is required for the development of selective spinal cord interneurons (Stifani et al. 2008), hindbrain cholinergic branchiovisceral motor neuron precursors, some sensory neurons in the trigeminal and vestibulocochlear ganglia (Theriault et al. 2004), and olfactory receptor sensory neurons (Theriault et al. 2005). According to GENSAT (gene expression nervous system atlas from NCBI), *Runx1* is expressed in the forming RGC layer at E15.5 in mice. Conventional knockouts for *Runx1* die at E12.5 (Okuda et al. 1996), prohibiting a detailed analysis of mouse retinal development. However, floxed-*Runx1* mice have been made (Kimura et al. 2010) and could be used to generate retinal-specific knock-outs.

6.2 *Tsc1* and *Tsc2*

In cultured rat immature hippocampal neurons, overexpression of *Tsc1* and *Tsc2* together inhibits neurite outgrowth, while conversely, knockdown of either *Tsc1* or *Tsc2* induces neurite growth and increases neurite number (Tavazoie et al. 2005). In the developing mouse neocortex, *Tsc1* conditional knockouts display ectopic axons, an effect also observed in E14.5 organotypic cortical slice cultures in which *Tsc2* is knocked down (Tavazoie et al. 2005). Mouse conventional knockouts for *Tsc1* and *Tsc2* die at E10.5-11.5 (Rennebeck et al. 1998; Kobayashi et al. 2001), prohibiting a detailed analysis of mouse retinal development. Both *Tsc1*- and *Tsc2*-floxed mice have been made (Uhlmann et al. 2002; Hernandez et al. 2007) and could be utilized to study the effect of *Tsc1* or *Tsc2* during retinal development in mice. GENSAT reports a moderate/high mRNA expression of both *Tsc1* and *Tsc2* in the GCL, IPL, INL and RPE at P7 in the mouse retina.

6.3 *Apc*

In the developing mouse cerebral cortex, the conditional loss of *Apc* results in an impaired formation of the radial glial scaffold, which leads to the defective migration of cortical neurons and subsequent layer formation, and the aberrant growth of axonal tracts (Yokota et al. 2009). *Apc* has also shown to be required in the maintenance, differentiation, and migration of neurons derived from adult neural stem cells in the subventricular zone and hippocampus of mice (Imura et al. 2010). GENSAT reports a moderate expression of *Apc* mRNA in the GCL, and a lower relative expression in the rest of retina, and a very high expression in the RPE, all at P7. Mouse conventional knockouts for *Apc* die before gastrulation (around E.5) (Moser et al. 1995), prohibiting any analysis of mouse retinal development. *Apc*-floxed mice have been made (Kuraguchi et al. 2006) and could be utilized to study the effect of *Apc* during retinal development in mice.

6.4 *Nf1* and *Nf2*

The conditional inactivation of *Nf1* results in the selective increase of neural stem cell proliferation and subsequent gliogenesis in the developing brainstem, but not in the developing cerebral cortex (Lee da et al. 2010). Conditional deletion of *Nf2* in GFAP+ cells show increased glial cell proliferation and deletion in adult Schwann cells showed Schwann cell hyperplasia, and other characteristics of neurofibromatosis type 2 (Giovannini et al. 2000). *Nf2* has been deleted in the developing lens as well showing that it is required for proper cell-cycle exit, differentiation and cell polarity of developing mouse lens cells (Wiley et al. 2010). GENSAT reports a moderate ubiquitous expression of *Nf1* mRNA in the neural retina, and a very high expression in the RPE at P7. GENSAT also reports a moderate "salt & pepper" mRNA expression of *Nf2* in retinal progenitors in the neuroblastic layer, and a relative higher expression in the forming GCL at E15.5. Later at P7, there is high *Nf2* expression in both the GCL/INL, and high expression in the RPE. Mouse conventional knockouts for *Nf2* die before gastrulation (around E5) (McClatchey et al. 1997), prohibiting any analysis of mouse retinal development. *Nf2*-floxed mice have been made (Giovannini et al. 2000) and could be utilized to study the effect of *Nf2* during retinal development in mice. Mouse conventional knockouts for *Nf1* die at E12.5-13.5 (Brannan et al. 1994), prohibiting a detailed analysis of mouse retinal development. *Nf1*-floxed mice have been made (Zhu et al. 2001) and could be utilized to study the effect of *Nf1* during retinal development in mice.

6.5 *Cdh1*

In adult mice, it was shown that *Cdh1* regulates the proliferation of neural stem cells in the subventricular zone (Garcia-Higuera et al. 2008). *Cdh1* has also been conditionally knocked out in the developing lens and it generated microphthalmia, iris hyperplasia, and lens epithelial cell deterioration (Pontoriero et al. 2009). GENSAT reports a very high expression of *Cdh1* in the INL and RPE, a moderate expression in the GCL, and a lower expression in rest of the mouse retina, all at P7. To our knowledge, mouse conventional knockouts for *Cdh1* were never made. However, *Cdh1*-floxed mice have been made (Garcia-Higuera et al. 2008) and could be utilized to study the effect of *Cdh1* during retinal development in mice.

7. Summary

Formation of a functional nervous system requires that appropriate numbers of the correct types of neuronal and glial cells are first generated and then migrate to their final destinations. In some regions of the CNS, including the retina, precisely regulated patterns of cell proliferation and migration result in the formation of discrete neuronal layers, each comprised of stereotyped proportions of neuronal subtypes. Defective neuronal layering results in severe functional and visual deficits. In the last few decades, great strides have been made towards understanding how neurons acquire their specific identities during development, revealing a central role for both intrinsic and extrinsic factors. In contrast, the molecular cues that orchestrate tissue morphogenesis are less well understood. Research in the area of tumor suppressor genes has provided key insights into the molecular mechanisms that: 1) control neuronal number by regulating specific patterns of progenitor cell proliferation and differentiation and, 2) guide the complex migratory routes of individual neuronal populations, resulting in the formation of discrete layers in the retina. Such studies may aid in the future design of new stem cell therapies in the clinic, where the current challenge is to direct appropriate numbers of cells to differentiate, migrate and integrate into correct retinal layers, thereby allowing functional recovery.

8. References

Abdollahi, A., Pisarcik, D., Roberts, D., Weinstein, J., Cairns, P., and Hamilton, T.C. 2003. LOT1 (PLAGL1/ZAC1), the candidate tumor suppressor gene at chromosome 6q24-25, is epigenetically regulated in cancer. *J Biol Chem* 278(8): 6041-6049.

Abdollahi, A., Roberts, D., Godwin, A.K., Schultz, D.C., Sonoda, G., Testa, J.R., and Hamilton, T.C. 1997. Identification of a zinc-finger gene at 6q25: a chromosomal region implicated in development of many solid tumors. *Oncogene* 14(16): 1973-1979.

Ajioka, I., Martins, R.A., Bayazitov, I.T., Donovan, S., Johnson, D.A., Frase, S., Cicero, S.A., Boyd, K., Zakharenko, S.S., and Dyer, M.A. 2007. Differentiated horizontal interneurons clonally expand to form metastatic retinoblastoma in mice. *Cell* 131(2): 378-390.

Alexiades, M.R. and Cepko, C.L. 1997. Subsets of retinal progenitors display temporally regulated and distinct biases in the fates of their progeny. *Development* 124(6): 1119-1131.

Ali, I.U., Schriml, L.M., and Dean, M. 1999. Mutational spectra of PTEN/MMAC1 gene: a tumor suppressor with lipid phosphatase activity. *J Natl Cancer Inst* 91(22): 1922-1932.

Backman, S.A., Stambolic, V., Suzuki, A., Haight, J., Elia, A., Pretorius, J., Tsao, M.S., Shannon, P., Bolon, B., Ivy, G.O. et al. 2001. Deletion of Pten in mouse brain causes seizures, ataxia and defects in soma size resembling Lhermitte-Duclos disease. *Nat Genet* 29(4): 396-403.

Bahr, M. 2000. Live or let die - retinal ganglion cell death and survival during development and in the lesioned adult CNS. *Trends Neurosci* 23(10): 483-490.

Baye, L.M. and Link, B.A. 2008. Nuclear migration during retinal development. *Brain Res* 1192: 29-36.

Bernards, R. 1997. E2F: a nodal point in cell cycle regulation. *Biochim Biophys Acta* 1333(3): M33-40.

Besson, A., Dowdy, S.F., and Roberts, J.M. 2008. CDK inhibitors: cell cycle regulators and beyond. *Dev Cell* 14(2): 159-169.

Bilanges, B., Varrault, A., Mazumdar, A., Pantaloni, C., Hoffmann, A., Bockaert, J., Spengler, D., and Journot, L. 2001. Alternative splicing of the imprinted candidate tumor suppressor gene ZAC regulates its antiproliferative and DNA binding activities. *Oncogene* 20(10): 1246-1253.

Brannan, C.I., Perkins, A.S., Vogel, K.S., Ratner, N., Nordlund, M.L., Reid, S.W., Buchberg, A.M., Jenkins, N.A., Parada, L.F., and Copeland, N.G. 1994. Targeted disruption of the neurofibromatosis type-1 gene leads to developmental abnormalities in heart and various neural crest-derived tissues. *Genes Dev* 8(9): 1019-1029.

Burek, M.J. and Oppenheim, R.W. 1996. Programmed cell death in the developing nervous system. *Brain Pathol* 6(4): 427-446.

Burkhart, D.L. and Sage, J. 2008. Cellular mechanisms of tumour suppression by the retinoblastoma gene. *Nat Rev Cancer* 8(9): 671-682.

Buss, R.R. and Oppenheim, R.W. 2004. Role of programmed cell death in normal neuronal development and function. *Anat Sci Int* 79(4): 191-197.

Caviness, V.S., Jr. 1982. Neocortical histogenesis in normal and reeler mice: a developmental study based upon [3H]thymidine autoradiography. *Brain Res* 256(3): 293-302.

Caviness, V.S., Jr., Takahashi, T., and Nowakowski, R.S. 1995. Numbers, time and neocortical neuronogenesis: a general developmental and evolutionary model. *Trends Neurosci* 18(9): 379-383.

Cayouette, M., Barres, B.A., and Raff, M. 2003. Importance of intrinsic mechanisms in cell fate decisions in the developing rat retina. *Neuron* 40(5): 897-904.

Cayouette, M., Poggi, L., and Harris, W.A. 2006. Lineage in the vertebrate retina. *Trends Neurosci* 29(10): 563-570.

Cepko, C.L., Austin, C.P., Yang, X., Alexiades, M., and Ezzeddine, D. 1996. Cell fate determination in the vertebrate retina. *Proc Natl Acad Sci U S A* 93(2): 589-595.

Chen, D., Livne-bar, I., Vanderluit, J.L., Slack, R.S., Agochiya, M., and Bremner, R. 2004. Cell-specific effects of RB or RB/p107 loss on retinal development implicate an intrinsically death-resistant cell-of-origin in retinoblastoma. *Cancer Cell* 5(6): 539-551.

Chen, D., Opavsky, R., Pacal, M., Tanimoto, N., Wenzel, P., Seeliger, M.W., Leone, G., and Bremner, R. 2007. Rb-mediated neuronal differentiation through cell-cycle-independent regulation of E2f3a. *PLoS Biol* 5(7): e179.

Chinnam, M. and Goodrich, D.W. 2011. RB1, development, and cancer. *Curr Top Dev Biol* 94: 129-169.

Clarke, A.R., Maandag, E.R., van Roon, M., van der Lugt, N.M., van der Valk, M., Hooper, M.L., Berns, A., and te Riele, H. 1992. Requirement for a functional Rb-1 gene in murine development. *Nature* 359(6393): 328-330.

Claudio, P.P., Howard, C.M., Baldi, A., De Luca, A., Fu, Y., Condorelli, G., Sun, Y., Colburn, N., Calabretta, B., and Giordano, A. 1994. p130/pRb2 has growth suppressive properties similar to yet distinctive from those of retinoblastoma family members pRb and p107. *Cancer Res* 54(21): 5556-5560.

Close, J.L., Gumuscu, B., and Reh, T.A. 2005. Retinal neurons regulate proliferation of postnatal progenitors and Muller glia in the rat retina via TGF beta signaling. *Development* 132(13): 3015-3026.

Cordenonsi, M., Dupont, S., Maretto, S., Insinga, A., Imbriano, C., and Piccolo, S. 2003. Links between tumor suppressors: p53 is required for TGF-beta gene responses by cooperating with Smads. *Cell* 113(3): 301-314.

Cordenonsi, M., Montagner, M., Adorno, M., Zacchigna, L., Martello, G., Mamidi, A., Soligo, S., Dupont, S., and Piccolo, S. 2007. Integration of TGF-beta and Ras/MAPK signaling through p53 phosphorylation. *Science* 315(5813): 840-843.

Cunningham, J.J., Levine, E.M., Zindy, F., Goloubeva, O., Roussel, M.F., and Smeyne, R.J. 2002. The cyclin-dependent kinase inhibitors p19(Ink4d) and p27(Kip1) are coexpressed in select retinal cells and act cooperatively to control cell cycle exit. *Mol Cell Neurosci* 19(3): 359-374.

DiCiommo, D., Gallie, B.L., and Bremner, R. 2000. Retinoblastoma: the disease, gene and protein provide critical leads to understand cancer. *Semin Cancer Biol* 10(4): 255-269.

Donovan, S.L. and Dyer, M.A. 2004. Developmental defects in Rb-deficient retinae. *Vision Res* 44(28): 3323-3333.

Dyer, M.A. and Cepko, C.L. 2000. p57(Kip2) regulates progenitor cell proliferation and amacrine interneuron development in the mouse retina. *Development* 127(16): 3593-3605.

Dyer, M.A. and Cepko, C.L. 2001. p27Kip1 and p57Kip2 regulate proliferation in distinct retinal progenitor cell populations. *J Neurosci* 21(12): 4259-4271.

Ewen, M.E., Xing, Y.G., Lawrence, J.B., and Livingston, D.M. 1991. Molecular cloning, chromosomal mapping, and expression of the cDNA for p107, a retinoblastoma gene product-related protein. *Cell* 66(6): 1155-1164.

Fekete, D.M., Perez-Miguelsanz, J., Ryder, E.F., and Cepko, C.L. 1994. Clonal analysis in the chicken retina reveals tangential dispersion of clonally related cells. *Dev Biol* 166(2): 666-682.

Franklin, D.S., Godfrey, V.L., O'Brien, D.A., Deng, C., and Xiong, Y. 2000. Functional collaboration between different cyclin-dependent kinase inhibitors suppresses tumor growth with distinct tissue specificity. *Mol Cell Biol* 20(16): 6147-6158.

Fraser, M.M., Bayazitov, I.T., Zakharenko, S.S., and Baker, S.J. 2008. Phosphatase and tensin homolog, deleted on chromosome 10 deficiency in brain causes defects in synaptic structure, transmission and plasticity, and myelination abnormalities. *Neuroscience* 151(2): 476-488.

Frolov, M.V. and Dyson, N.J. 2004. Molecular mechanisms of E2F-dependent activation and pRB-mediated repression. *J Cell Sci* 117(Pt 11): 2173-2181.

Fuhrmann, S. 2010. Eye morphogenesis and patterning of the optic vesicle. *Curr Top Dev Biol* 93: 61-84.

Galli-Resta, L., Leone, P., Bottari, D., Ensini, M., Rigosi, E., and Novelli, E. 2008. The genesis of retinal architecture: an emerging role for mechanical interactions? *Prog Retin Eye Res* 27(3): 260-283.

Garcia-Higuera, I., Manchado, E., Dubus, P., Canamero, M., Mendez, J., Moreno, S., and Malumbres, M. 2008. Genomic stability and tumour suppression by the APC/C cofactor Cdh1. *Nat Cell Biol* 10(7): 802-811.

Gartel, A.L. 2009. p21(WAF1/CIP1) and cancer: a shifting paradigm? *Biofactors* 35(2): 161-164.

Giovannini, M., Robanus-Maandag, E., van der Valk, M., Niwa-Kawakita, M., Abramowski, V., Goutebroze, L., Woodruff, J.M., Berns, A., and Thomas, G. 2000. Conditional biallelic Nf2 mutation in the mouse promotes manifestations of human neurofibromatosis type 2. *Genes Dev* 14(13): 1617-1630.

Godinho, L., Williams, P.R., Claassen, Y., Provost, E., Leach, S.D., Kamermans, M., and Wong, R.O. 2007. Nonapical symmetric divisions underlie horizontal cell layer formation in the developing retina in vivo. *Neuron* 56(4): 597-603.

Gomer, R.H. 2001. Not being the wrong size. *Nat Rev Mol Cell Biol* 2(1): 48-54.

Groszer, M., Erickson, R., Scripture-Adams, D.D., Lesche, R., Trumpp, A., Zack, J.A., Kornblum, H.I., Liu, X., and Wu, H. 2001. Negative regulation of neural stem/progenitor cell proliferation by the Pten tumor suppressor gene in vivo. *Science* 294(5549): 2186-2189.

Grueber, W.B. and Sagasti, A. 2010. Self-avoidance and tiling: Mechanisms of dendrite and axon spacing. *Cold Spring Harb Perspect Biol* 2(9): a001750.

Guo, H., Tian, T., Nan, K., and Wang, W. 2010. p57: A multifunctional protein in cancer (Review). *Int J Oncol* 36(6): 1321-1329.

Hannon, G.J., Demetrick, D., and Beach, D. 1993. Isolation of the Rb-related p130 through its interaction with CDK2 and cyclins. *Genes Dev* 7(12A): 2378-2391.

Hatakeyama, J., Tomita, K., Inoue, T., and Kageyama, R. 2001. Roles of homeobox and bHLH genes in specification of a retinal cell type. *Development* 128(8): 1313-1322.

Hernandez, O., Way, S., McKenna, J., 3rd, and Gambello, M.J. 2007. Generation of a conditional disruption of the Tsc2 gene. *Genesis* 45(2): 101-106.

Hero, I. 1990. Optic fissure closure in the normal cinnamon mouse. An ultrastructural study. *Invest Ophthalmol Vis Sci* 31(1): 197-216.

Hirashima, M., Kobayashi, T., Uchikawa, M., Kondoh, H., and Araki, M. 2008. Anteroventrally localized activity in the optic vesicle plays a crucial role in the optic development. *Dev Biol* 317(2): 620-631.

Holt, C.E., Bertsch, T.W., Ellis, H.M., and Harris, W.A. 1988. Cellular determination in the Xenopus retina is independent of lineage and birth date. *Neuron* 1(1): 15-26.

Huang, S.M., Schonthal, A.H., and Stallcup, M.R. 2001. Enhancement of p53-dependent gene activation by the transcriptional coactivator Zac1. *Oncogene* 20(17): 2134-2143.

Huang, S.M. and Stallcup, M.R. 2000. Mouse Zac1, a transcriptional coactivator and repressor for nuclear receptors. *Mol Cell Biol* 20(5): 1855-1867.

Imura, T., Wang, X., Noda, T., Sofroniew, M.V., and Fushiki, S. 2010. Adenomatous polyposis coli is essential for both neuronal differentiation and maintenance of adult neural stem cells in subventricular zone and hippocampus. *Stem Cells* 28(11): 2053-2064.

Inoue, T., Hojo, M., Bessho, Y., Tano, Y., Lee, J.E., and Kageyama, R. 2002. Math3 and NeuroD regulate amacrine cell fate specification in the retina. *Development* 129(4): 831-842.

Isenmann, S., Kretz, A., and Cellerino, A. 2003. Molecular determinants of retinal ganglion cell development, survival, and regeneration. *Prog Retin Eye Res* 22(4): 483-543.

Jacks, T., Fazeli, A., Schmitt, E.M., Bronson, R.T., Goodell, M.A., and Weinberg, R.A. 1992. Effects of an Rb mutation in the mouse. *Nature* 359(6393): 295-300.

Kagiyama, Y., Gotouda, N., Sakagami, K., Yasuda, K., Mochii, M., and Araki, M. 2005. Extraocular dorsal signal affects the developmental fate of the optic vesicle and patterns the optic neuroepithelium. *Dev Growth Differ* 47(8): 523-536.

Kim, J.W., Kang, K.H., Burrola, P., Mak, T.W., and Lemke, G. 2008. Retinal degeneration triggered by inactivation of PTEN in the retinal pigment epithelium. *Genes Dev* 22(22): 3147-3157.

Kimura, A., Inose, H., Yano, F., Fujita, K., Ikeda, T., Sato, S., Iwasaki, M., Jinno, T., Ae, K., Fukumoto, S. et al. 2010. Runx1 and Runx2 cooperate during sternal morphogenesis. *Development* 137(7): 1159-1167.

Kobayashi, T., Minowa, O., Sugitani, Y., Takai, S., Mitani, H., Kobayashi, E., Noda, T., and Hino, O. 2001. A germ-line Tsc1 mutation causes tumor development and embryonic lethality that are similar, but not identical to, those caused by Tsc2 mutation in mice. *Proc Natl Acad Sci U S A* 98(15): 8762-8767.

Koy, S., Hauses, M., Appelt, H., Friedrich, K., Schackert, H.K., and Eckelt, U. 2004. Loss of expression of ZAC/LOT1 in squamous cell carcinomas of head and neck. *Head Neck* 26(4): 338-344.

Kuraguchi, M., Wang, X.P., Bronson, R.T., Rothenberg, R., Ohene-Baah, N.Y., Lund, J.J., Kucherlapati, M., Maas, R.L., and Kucherlapati, R. 2006. Adenomatous polyposis coli (APC) is required for normal development of skin and thymus. *PLoS Genet* 2(9): e146.

Kwon, C.H., Luikart, B.W., Powell, C.M., Zhou, J., Matheny, S.A., Zhang, W., Li, Y., Baker, S.J., and Parada, L.F. 2006. Pten regulates neuronal arborization and social interaction in mice. *Neuron* 50(3): 377-388.

Lee da, Y., Yeh, T.H., Emnett, R.J., White, C.R., and Gutmann, D.H. 2010. Neurofibromatosis-1 regulates neuroglial progenitor proliferation and glial differentiation in a brain region-specific manner. *Genes Dev* 24(20): 2317-2329.

Lee, J. and Kim, S.S. 2009. The function of p27 KIP1 during tumor development. *Exp Mol Med* 41(11): 765-771.

Lehtinen, M.K., Zappaterra, M.W., Chen, X., Yang, Y.J., Hill, A.D., Lun, M., Maynard, T., Gonzalez, D., Kim, S., Ye, P. et al. 2011. The cerebrospinal fluid provides a proliferative niche for neural progenitor cells. *Neuron* 69(5): 893-905.

Levine, E.M., Close, J., Fero, M., Ostrovsky, A., and Reh, T.A. 2000. p27(Kip1) regulates cell cycle withdrawal of late multipotent progenitor cells in the mammalian retina. *Dev Biol* 219(2): 299-314.

Li, J., Yen, C., Liaw, D., Podsypanina, K., Bose, S., Wang, S.I., Puc, J., Miliaresis, C., Rodgers, L., McCombie, R. et al. 1997. PTEN, a putative protein tyrosine phosphatase gene mutated in human brain, breast, and prostate cancer. *Science* 275(5308): 1943-1947.

Li, S., Mo, Z., Yang, X., Price, S.M., Shen, M.M., and Xiang, M. 2004. Foxn4 controls the genesis of amacrine and horizontal cells by retinal progenitors. *Neuron* 43(6): 795-807.

Livesey, F.J. and Cepko, C.L. 2001. Vertebrate neural cell-fate determination: lessons from the retina. *Nat Rev Neurosci* 2(2): 109-118.

Ma, L., Cantrup, R., Varrault, A., Colak, D., Klenin, N., Gotz, M., McFarlane, S., Journot, L., and Schuurmans, C. 2007a. Zac1 functions through TGFbetaII to negatively regulate cell number in the developing retina. *Neural Dev* 2: 11.

Ma, L., Hocking, J.C., Hehr, C.L., Schuurmans, C., and McFarlane, S. 2007c. Zac1 promotes a Muller glial cell fate and interferes with retinal ganglion cell differentiation in Xenopus retina. *Dev Dyn* 236(1): 192-202.

MacPherson, D., Sage, J., Kim, T., Ho, D., McLaughlin, M.E., and Jacks, T. 2004. Cell type-specific effects of Rb deletion in the murine retina. *Genes Dev* 18(14): 1681-1694.

Marino, S., Krimpenfort, P., Leung, C., van der Korput, H.A., Trapman, J., Camenisch, I., Berns, A., and Brandner, S. 2002. PTEN is essential for cell migration but not for fate determination and tumourigenesis in the cerebellum. *Development* 129(14): 3513-3522.

McClatchey, A.I., Saotome, I., Ramesh, V., Gusella, J.F., and Jacks, T. 1997. The Nf2 tumor suppressor gene product is essential for extraembryonic development immediately prior to gastrulation. *Genes Dev* 11(10): 1253-1265.

Moser, A.R., Shoemaker, A.R., Connelly, C.S., Clipson, L., Gould, K.A., Luongo, C., Dove, W.F., Siggers, P.H., and Gardner, R.L. 1995. Homozygosity for the Min allele of Apc results in disruption of mouse development prior to gastrulation. *Dev Dyn* 203(4): 422-433.

Nguyen, L., Besson, A., Heng, J.I., Schuurmans, C., Teboul, L., Parras, C., Philpott, A., Roberts, J.M., and Guillemot, F. 2006. p27kip1 independently promotes neuronal differentiation and migration in the cerebral cortex. *Genes Dev* 20(11): 1511-1524.

Nigg, E.A. 1995. Cyclin-dependent protein kinases: key regulators of the eukaryotic cell cycle. *Bioessays* 17(6): 471-480.

Ohnuma, S., Hopper, S., Wang, K.C., Philpott, A., and Harris, W.A. 2002. Co-ordinating retinal histogenesis: early cell cycle exit enhances early cell fate determination in the Xenopus retina. *Development* 129(10): 2435-2446.

Ohnuma, S., Philpott, A., Wang, K., Holt, C.E., and Harris, W.A. 1999. p27Xic1, a Cdk inhibitor, promotes the determination of glial cells in Xenopus retina. *Cell* 99(5): 499-510.

Okuda, T., van Deursen, J., Hiebert, S.W., Grosveld, G., and Downing, J.R. 1996. AML1, the target of multiple chromosomal translocations in human leukemia, is essential for normal fetal liver hematopoiesis. *Cell* 84(2): 321-330.

Pagotto, U., Arzberger, T., Theodoropoulou, M., Grubler, Y., Pantaloni, C., Saeger, W., Losa, M., Journot, L., Stalla, G.K., and Spengler, D. 2000. The expression of the antiproliferative gene ZAC is lost or highly reduced in nonfunctioning pituitary adenomas. *Cancer Res* 60(24): 6794-6799.

Paternot, S., Bockstaele, L., Bisteau, X., Kooken, H., Coulonval, K., and Roger, P.P. 2010. Rb inactivation in cell cycle and cancer: the puzzle of highly regulated activating phosphorylation of CDK4 versus constitutively active CDK-activating kinase. *Cell Cycle* 9(4): 689-699.

Pearson, B.J. and Doe, C.Q. 2004. Specification of temporal identity in the developing nervous system. *Annu Rev Cell Dev Biol* 20: 619-647.

Pei, Y.F. and Rhodin, J.A. 1970. The prenatal development of the mouse eye. *Anat Rec* 168(1): 105-125.

Pimentel, B., Rodriguez-Borlado, L., Hernandez, C., and Carrera, A.C. 2002. A Role for phosphoinositide 3-kinase in the control of cell division and survival during retinal development. *Dev Biol* 247(2): 295-306.

Poggi, L., Vitorino, M., Masai, I., and Harris, W.A. 2005. Influences on neural lineage and mode of division in the zebrafish retina in vivo. *J Cell Biol* 171(6): 991-999.

Pontoriero, G.F., Smith, A.N., Miller, L.A., Radice, G.L., West-Mays, J.A., and Lang, R.A. 2009. Co-operative roles for E-cadherin and N-cadherin during lens vesicle separation and lens epithelial cell survival. *Dev Biol* 326(2): 403-417.

Poole, A.J., Heap, D., Carroll, R.E., and Tyner, A.L. 2004. Tumor suppressor functions for the Cdk inhibitor p21 in the mouse colon. *Oncogene* 23(49): 8128-8134.

Rapaport, D.H., Wong, L.L., Wood, E.D., Yasumura, D., and LaVail, M.M. 2004. Timing and topography of cell genesis in the rat retina. *J Comp Neurol* 474(2): 304-324.

Ravitz, M.J. and Wenner, C.E. 1997. Cyclin-dependent kinase regulation during G1 phase and cell cycle regulation by TGF-beta. *Adv Cancer Res* 71: 165-207.

Rennebeck, G., Kleymenova, E.V., Anderson, R., Yeung, R.S., Artzt, K., and Walker, C.L. 1998. Loss of function of the tuberous sclerosis 2 tumor suppressor gene results in embryonic lethality characterized by disrupted neuroepithelial growth and development. *Proc Natl Acad Sci U S A* 95(26): 15629-15634.

Robanus-Maandag, E., Dekker, M., van der Valk, M., Carrozza, M.L., Jeanny, J.C., Dannenberg, J.H., Berns, A., and te Riele, H. 1998. p107 is a suppressor of retinoblastoma development in pRb-deficient mice. *Genes Dev* 12(11): 1599-1609.

Rockhill, R.L., Euler, T., and Masland, R.H. 2000. Spatial order within but not between types of retinal neurons. *Proc Natl Acad Sci U S A* 97(5): 2303-2307.

Rosivatz, E. 2007. Inhibiting PTEN. *Biochem Soc Trans* 35(Pt 2): 257-259.

Silver, J. and Hughes, A.F. 1973. The role of cell death during morphogenesis of the mammalian eye. *J Morphol* 140(2): 159-170.

Silver, J. and Robb, R.M. 1979. Studies on the development of the eye cup and optic nerve in normal mice and in mutants with congenital optic nerve aplasia. *Dev Biol* 68(1): 175-190.

Spengler, D., Villalba, M., Hoffmann, A., Pantaloni, C., Houssami, S., Bockaert, J., and Journot, L. 1997. Regulation of apoptosis and cell cycle arrest by Zac1, a novel zinc finger protein expressed in the pituitary gland and the brain. *Embo J* 16(10): 2814-2825.

Steck, P.A., Pershouse, M.A., Jasser, S.A., Yung, W.K., Lin, H., Ligon, A.H., Langford, L.A., Baumgard, M.L., Hattier, T., Davis, T. et al. 1997. Identification of a candidate tumour suppressor gene, MMAC1, at chromosome 10q23.3 that is mutated in multiple advanced cancers. *Nat Genet* 15(4): 356-362.

Stiemke, M.M. and Hollyfield, J.G. 1995. Cell birthdays in Xenopus laevis retina. *Differentiation* 58(3): 189-193.

Stifani, N., Freitas, A.R., Liakhovitskaia, A., Medvinsky, A., Kania, A., and Stifani, S. 2008. Suppression of interneuron programs and maintenance of selected spinal motor neuron fates by the transcription factor AML1/Runx1. *Proc Natl Acad Sci U S A* 105(17): 6451-6456.

Svoboda, K.K. and O'Shea, K.S. 1987. An analysis of cell shape and the neuroepithelial basal lamina during optic vesicle formation in the mouse embryo. *Development* 100(2): 185-200.

Takahashi, T., Goto, T., Miyama, S., Nowakowski, R.S., and Caviness, V.S., Jr. 1999. Sequence of neuron origin and neocortical laminar fate: relation to cell cycle of origin in the developing murine cerebral wall. *J Neurosci* 19(23): 10357-10371.

Tavazoie, S.F., Alvarez, V.A., Ridenour, D.A., Kwiatkowski, D.J., and Sabatini, B.L. 2005. Regulation of neuronal morphology and function by the tumor suppressors Tsc1 and Tsc2. *Nat Neurosci* 8(12): 1727-1734.

Theriault, F.M., Nuthall, H.N., Dong, Z., Lo, R., Barnabe-Heider, F., Miller, F.D., and Stifani, S. 2005. Role for Runx1 in the proliferation and neuronal differentiation of selected progenitor cells in the mammalian nervous system. *J Neurosci* 25(8): 2050-2061.

Theriault, F.M., Roy, P., and Stifani, S. 2004. AML1/Runx1 is important for the development of hindbrain cholinergic branchiovisceral motor neurons and selected cranial sensory neurons. *Proc Natl Acad Sci U S A* 101(28): 10343-10348.

Tomita, K., Moriyoshi, K., Nakanishi, S., Guillemot, F., and Kageyama, R. 2000. Mammalian achaete-scute and atonal homologs regulate neuronal versus glial fate determination in the central nervous system. *Embo J* 19(20): 5460-5472.

Turner, D.L. and Cepko, C.L. 1987. A common progenitor for neurons and glia persists in rat retina late in development. *Nature* 328(6126): 131-136.

Turner, D.L., Snyder, E.Y., and Cepko, C.L. 1990. Lineage-independent determination of cell type in the embryonic mouse retina. *Neuron* 4(6): 833-845.

Uhlmann, E.J., Wong, M., Baldwin, R.L., Bajenaru, M.L., Onda, H., Kwiatkowski, D.J., Yamada, K., and Gutmann, D.H. 2002. Astrocyte-specific TSC1 conditional knockout mice exhibit abnormal neuronal organization and seizures. *Ann Neurol* 52(3): 285-296.

Varrault, A., Ciani, E., Apiou, F., Bilanges, B., Hoffmann, A., Pantaloni, C., Bockaert, J., Spengler, D., and Journot, L. 1998. hZAC encodes a zinc finger protein with antiproliferative properties and maps to a chromosomal region frequently lost in cancer. *Proc Natl Acad Sci U S A* 95(15): 8835-8840.

Voyvodic, J.T., Burne, J.F., and Raff, M.C. 1995. Quantification of normal cell death in the rat retina: implications for clone composition in cell lineage analysis. *Eur J Neurosci* 7(12): 2469-2478.

Wallace, V.A. 2011. Concise review: making a retina--from the building blocks to clinical applications. *Stem Cells* 29(3): 412-417.

Wawersik, S. and Maas, R.L. 2000. Vertebrate eye development as modeled in Drosophila. *Hum Mol Genet* 9(6): 917-925.

Wesierska-Gadek, J., Maurer, M., Zulehner, N., and Komina, O. 2010. Whether to target single or multiple CDKs for therapy? That is the question. *J Cell Physiol* 226(2): 341-349.

Wetts, R. and Fraser, S.E. 1988. Multipotent precursors can give rise to all major cell types of the frog retina. *Science* 239(4844): 1142-1145.

Wiley, L.A., Dattilo, L.K., Kang, K.B., Giovannini, M., and Beebe, D.C. 2010. The tumor suppressor merlin is required for cell cycle exit, terminal differentiation, and cell polarity in the developing murine lens. *Invest Ophthalmol Vis Sci* 51(7): 3611-3618.

Xu, X.L., Fang, Y., Lee, T.C., Forrest, D., Gregory-Evans, C., Almeida, D., Liu, A., Jhanwar, S.C., Abramson, D.H., and Cobrinik, D. 2009. Retinoblastoma has properties of a cone precursor tumor and depends upon cone-specific MDM2 signaling. *Cell* 137(6): 1018-1031.

Yokota, Y., Kim, W.Y., Chen, Y., Wang, X., Stanco, A., Komuro, Y., Snider, W., and Anton, E.S. 2009. The adenomatous polyposis coli protein is an essential regulator of radial glial polarity and construction of the cerebral cortex. *Neuron* 61(1): 42-56.

Young, R.W. 1984. Cell death during differentiation of the retina in the mouse. *J Comp Neurol* 229(3): 362-373.

Young, R.W. 1985a. Cell differentiation in the retina of the mouse. *Anat Rec* 212(2): 199-205.

Young, R.W. 1985b. Cell proliferation during postnatal development of the retina in the mouse. *Brain Res* 353(2): 229-239.

Yue, Q., Groszer, M., Gil, J.S., Berk, A.J., Messing, A., Wu, H., and Liu, X. 2005. PTEN deletion in Bergmann glia leads to premature differentiation and affects laminar organization. *Development* 132(14): 3281-3291.

Zhang, J., Gray, J., Wu, L., Leone, G., Rowan, S., Cepko, C.L., Zhu, X., Craft, C.M., and Dyer, M.A. 2004. Rb regulates proliferation and rod photoreceptor development in the mouse retina. *Nat Genet* 36(4): 351-360.

Zhu, L., van den Heuvel, S., Helin, K., Fattaey, A., Ewen, M., Livingston, D., Dyson, N., and Harlow, E. 1993. Inhibition of cell proliferation by p107, a relative of the retinoblastoma protein. *Genes Dev* 7(7A): 1111-1125.

Zhu, Y., Romero, M.I., Ghosh, P., Ye, Z., Charnay, P., Rushing, E.J., Marth, J.D., and Parada, L.F. 2001. Ablation of NF1 function in neurons induces abnormal development of cerebral cortex and reactive gliosis in the brain. *Genes Dev* 15(7): 859-876.

Zolessi, F.R., Poggi, L., Wilkinson, C.J., Chien, C.B., and Harris, W.A. 2006. Polarization and orientation of retinal ganglion cells in vivo. *Neural Dev* 1: 2.

12

Properties of Human Tumor Suppressor 101F6 Protein as a Cytochrome b_{561} and Its Preliminary Crystallization Trials

Mariam C. Recuenco[1], Suguru Watanabe[1], Fusako Takeuchi[2], Sam-Yong Park[3] and Motonari Tsubaki[1]
[1]*Department of Chemistry, Kobe University Graduate School of Science,*
[2]*Kobe University Institute for Promotion of Higher Education,*
[3]*Protein Design Laboratory, Yokohama City University, Graduate School of Nanobioscience,*
Japan

1. Introduction

Identification of the physiological roles and elucidation of the molecular mechanisms involving tumor suppressor genes and their gene products are important for a more comprehensive understanding of cancer pathogenesis. Since the Knudson's statistical studies on retinoblastoma, neuroblastoma, and pheochromocytoma, which led to the conclusion that the occurrence of these tumors fits a two-mutation model (Knudson, 1971; Knudson & Strong, 1972), it became recognized that there were some genes that function to inhibit tumor development. The model stated that tumorigenesis results when there are genetic alterations such as deletions and mutations in both alleles of a gene in a cell (Knudson, 1971; Knudson & Strong, 1972). A tumor suppressor gene may have one or more functions related to cell division and differentiation, extracellular communication, tissue formation or senescence (Hollingsworth & Lee, 1991).

Several regions of the human chromosome 3 have been identified as susceptible sites for homozygous deletions and mutations that may lead to inactivation of one or more tumor suppressor genes. A particular tumor suppressor gene candidate *101F6* is located within a narrow 630-kb region on chromosome 3p.21.3, called LUCA (lung cancer region) (Lerman & Minna, 2000; Zabarovsky et al., 2002). Interestingly, the 101F6 protein is expressed in normal lung bronchial epithelial cells and fibroblasts but is lost in most lung cancers (Ohtani et al., 2007). Previous studies have shown that forced expression of the *101F6* gene *via* adenoviral vector-mediated gene transfer (Ji et al., 2002) or *via* nanoparticle injection (Ohtani et al., 2007) caused the inhibition of tumor growth in non-small cell lung cancer cells *in vitro* and *in vivo*. The treated cancer cells were also found to accumulate ascorbate (AsA) when incubated in a medium containing AsA (Ohtani et al., 2007). Apoptosis and autophagy of the cancer cells were reportedly to be enhanced by the treatment and were postulated to be caused by the synergistic action of the *101F6* gene and AsA though the mechanism of the action is still not clear (Ohtani et al., 2007).

The human *101F6* gene was found to encode a protein consisting of 222 amino acids and was predicted to be a member of the cytochrome b_{561} protein family (Tsubaki et al., 2005). Proteins such as adrenal cytochrome b_{561} (Tsubaki et al., 1997), duodenal cytochrome b_{561} (Mckie et al., 2001), and stromal cell-derived receptor 2 (Vargas et al., 2003) that were classified under this family have a common "b561 core domain" consisting of four transmembrane α-helices that have four totally conserved His residues for the binding of two heme *b* groups (Okuyama et al., 1998; Tsubaki et al., 2005). The adrenal cytochrome b_{561}, as a classic representative of this family, is a highly hydrophobic protein, consisting of six transmembrane α-helices with a molecular mass of 28 kDa and is located in the secretory vesicle membranes of adrenal chromaffin cells. This protein is involved in a transmembrane electron transfer reaction from cytosolic AsA to intravesicular monodehydroascorbate (MDA) radical that replenishes reducing equivalents to maintain physiological levels of AsA inside the vesicles (Kobayashi et al., 1998; Seike et al., 2003). AsA is an essential water-soluble vitamin that maintains the activity of copper-containing enzymes such as dopamine β-hydroxylase and peptidylglycine α-amidating monooxygenase by providing electrons to the copper center of the enzyme (Prigge et al., 2000) and to keep the intravesicular side in reduced state to protect otherwise very labile catecholamines. For efficient electron transfer, adrenal cytochrome b_{561} contain a putative AsA-binding motif on the cytosolic side close to the cytosolic heme center and a putative MDA-radical binding motif on the intravesicular side close to the intravesicular heme center, respectively (Okuyama et al., 1998). Such motifs were found to be conserved in other subfamilies of cytochrome b_{561}, including duodenal cytochrome b_{561} and plant cytochrome b_{561} (Tsubaki et al., 2005).

Comparative analysis on the amino acid sequences of seven subfamilies of the cytochrome b_{561} protein family showed that 101F6 protein does not contain the MDA-radical binding motif while the AsA-binding motif was significantly modified ("modified motif 1") (Tsubaki et al., 2005). These results suggested that redox active biofactor(s) other than AsA or MDA radical might be responsible as redox mediators of the 101F6 protein (Tsubaki et al., 2005). It is very intriguing to consider that the 101F6 protein has a role for transmembrane redox signal transduction *via* this unknown redox-linked activity. Therefore, the "modified motif 1" may be a primary candidate for conducting such transmembrane redox reactions (Tsubaki et al., 2005). Thus, clarification of the properties and three-dimensional structure of the 101F6 protein is highly necessary in understanding the role of this transmembrane protein as a tumor suppressor and as a controlling factor in human lung cancer development.

Although the cytochrome b_{561} protein family has a large numbers of its members (human tissues contain 6 members), none of them has ever been successfully crystallized for analysis by X-ray diffraction. Though we have attempted the crystallization for various members of the cytochrome b_{561} family, we have been limited by the amount of samples for more extensive screenings. A major barrier to crystallizing membrane proteins from higher eukaryotes (animals and plants) is the inability to purify sufficient amounts of non-denatured active proteins for conducting the crystallization trials. Indeed, except for the classic cytochrome b_{561} protein from bovine adrenal chromaffin vesicles, purification of cytochrome b_{561} from native tissues has been found to be almost impossible. Further, heterologous expression systems for the membrane protein including the members of the cytochrome b_{561} family, by employing the prokaryote *Escherichia coli*, the yeast *Saccharomyces cerevisiae*, the insect *Sf9* cells, and mammalian cells, showed limited success based on the evaluation of their final qualities and/or quantities. Recently, the methylotrophic yeast, *Pichia pastoris*, has proven to be a very useful system to express and purify milligram quantities of membrane proteins (Abramson et al., 2003; Huang et al., 2003; Jiang et al., 2003). However, instances about its use as a host for the expression of mammalian membrane proteins was limited (Long et al., 2005).

We have previously reported about the functional expression, purification and characterization of recombinant human 101F6 protein, which was expressed as a poly-histidine tagged protein in methylotrophic yeast *Pichia pastoris* (Recuenco et al., 2009). The purified 101F6 protein exhibited characteristic properties as a member of the cytochrome b_{561} protein family, particularly with regards to spectral characteristics and electron transfer activities with AsA and MDA radical. In this paper, we want to present our optimized protocol for the human 101F6 protein expression and purification. Further, we have succeeded in the crystallization of recombinant human 101F6 protein for the first time. We also present preliminary results on the quality of the human 101F6 protein crystals.

2. Materials and methods

2.1 The *Pichia pastoris* expression system

In our present study, we employed the *Pichia pastoris* expression system (*Pichia pastoris* GS115 cells and a pPICZB vector; from Invitrogen Corp., Tokyo, Japan) for the successful expression of human *101F6* gene. As a single-celled microorganism, yeast *Pichia pastoris* is easy to manipulate and is, therefore, very suitable for culture. However, it is a eukaryote and capable of many of post-translation modifications onto the heterologously expressed proteins such as proteolytic processing, folding, disufide bond formation, and glycosylation, which are performed by higher eukaryotic cells. Most importantly, *Pichia pastoris* cell is a very suitable host for the expression of membrane proteins, particularly for integral membrane proteins, because of its eukaryotic nature (*e.g.*, presence of membranes within the cytosolic milieu).

It was proposed that, compared to insect cells (*e.g.*, *Sf9* cell) or other mammalian cultured cells, *Pichia pastoris* cells are much easier to handle, can be grown at lower cost, and can be expressed quicker in a large scale (Asada et al., 2011). Such successful examples for expressing eukaryotic membrane proteins were reported previously (Weiß et al., 1998; Wetterholm et al., 2008; Nakanishi et al., 2009a; Nakanishi et al., 2009b; Alisio & Mueckler, 2010; Ostuni et al., 2010; Mizutani et al., 2011).

2.2 Construction of the expression plasmid pPICZB-101F6-His_8

Procedure for a molecular cloning of the human 101F6 gene was described previously (Recuenco et al., 2009). Construction of the expression plasmid, pPICZB-101F6-His_8, was described previously (Recuenco et al., 2009). Briefly, the thrombin-specific sequence followed by the eight-histidine residue-tag (QPSA<u>LVPRGS</u>SAHHHHHHHH; the underline indicates the thrombin-specific sequence) was introduced at the C-terminus of human 101F6 protein, resulting in a total of 240 aa residue-long with a molecular mass of 25996.9 Da. An eight-histidine residue-tag sequence, instead of a usual six-histidine residue-tag, was added to provide a stronger binding affinity towards Ni-NTA affinity column. Such a poly-histidine-residue tag was employed for the expression of mammalian glucose transporter (eight-histidine residue) (Alisio & Mueckler, 2010) and G-protein coupled receptors (deca-histidine residue) (Yurugi-Kobayashi et al., 2009). Introduction of the tag-sequences at the C-terminus of human 101F6 protein was chosen with considerations about the increase in length of the C-terminal part and its successful protein expression in the ER membranes of *Pichia pastoris* cells.

2.3 Expression and purification of the human wild-type 101F6 protein

The pPICZB-101F6-His$_8$ plasmids obtained from the transformed *E. coli* cells were purified and linearized using *Pme* I and were used for the transformation of *Pichia pastoris* GS115 competent cells according to EasyComp™ transformation protocol (Invitrogen Corp., Tokyo, Japan). Selection was done by plating onto YPDS medium containing 400 µg/mL Zeocin (Invitrogen Corp., Tokyo, Japan), a bleomycin-like compound that kills cells by introducing lethal double-strand breaks in chromosomal DNA. In our screening process, the concentration of Zeocin was increased four times higher than the recommended concentration of 100 µg/mL, to obtain Zeocin hyper-resistant transformants that would have multicopy clones. The Zeocin-resistant protein (the product of the *Sh ble* gene in the pPICZB vector) confers resistance to the transformed cells stoichiometrically, not enzymatically, by binding to and inactivating the drug. Therefore, such transformants may ultimately result in an increase in the level of heterologous 101F6-His$_8$ protein production (Romanos et al., 1998).

Single colonies with a hyper Zeocin-resistant activity from the YPDS-Zeocin plates were inoculated into 1000-mL Erlenmeyer flasks with a baffled bottom containing 250 mL BMGY media (2% glycerol). During the usual induction procedure of such transformants by the addition of methanol (final 2%) as described previously (Recuenco et al., 2009), the color of the medium become reddish, indicating a successful expression of a holo-form of the 101F6 protein in the *Pichia pastoris* cells. After harvesting the induced cells, microsomal fractions were prepared in the presence of protease inhibitor cocktail (Protease Inhibitor Cocktail for General Use (100X); Nacalai Tesque, Kyoto, Japan). Then, the cytochrome b_{561} content based on the absorption at 561 nm was calculated. Typical results showed a total yield of 600~1000 nmoles of cytochrome b_{561} in microsomal fraction obtained from a 250-mL culture after 96 h of incubation (Table 1).

Solubilization of microsomal membrane fraction was conducted with β-octyl glucoside (2%)(Anatrace, Maumee, Ohio, USA). All the following steps were conducted at 4°C or on ice to avoid the formation of aggregates. Further, to obtain a better yield, we skipped the step of DEAE-Sepharose column chromatography, which was included in the original purification procedure (Recuenco et al., 2009). Thus, the solubilized membrane proteins from the microsomal fraction were directly applied to a pre-packed Ni-NTA-Sepharose (GE Healthcare Japan. Tokyo, Japan) column equilibrated with a buffer containing 300 mM NaCl and 10 mM imidazole. Removal of interfering proteins was achieved by washing the column with the buffers containing 20 mM imidazole and 50 mM imidazole. Then, the 101F6-His$_8$ protein was eluted with the buffer containing 300 mM imidazole. The purified sample was promptly desalted with PD-10 column (GE Healthcare Japan, Tokyo, Japan) equilibrated with 50 mM phosphate buffer containing 1 % β-octyl glucoside and 10 % glycerol.

3. Results

3.1 Properties of the purified 101F6-His$_8$ protein

Table 1 shows a typical example for the protein yield and the cytochrome b_{561} content at all the purification steps. From a 250-mL culture, which provides about 16-20 grams of wet cell bodies expressing the 101F6-His$_8$ protein with an approximate cytochrome b_{561} content of 800~900 nmoles, it was possible to purify about 0.60 mg of the recombinant human 101F6-His$_8$ protein with the cytochrome b_{561} content of 180 nmoles, with a purification fold of 56 from the stage of microsomes to the stage of the final desalting. Since the cytochrome b_{561} content at the stage of microsomes would include a considerable amount of other *b*-type cytochromes, such as cytochrome bc_1 complex, the actual yield of the recombinant 101F6-His_8 protein would be much better. Then, the purified 101F6-His_8 protein was evaluated by SDS-PAGE, visible absorption spectroscopy, MALDI-TOF mass spectrometory, redox titration, heme content analysis, in comparison with those of classic chromaffin granule (CG) (*i.e.*, chromaffine vesicle) cytochrome b_{561}.

SDS-PAGE analysis on the purified 101F6-His_8 protein showed a single protein band with its estimated molecular weight around 26 kDa. Achievement of the highly purified sample by a single column chromatography step as in our present study might be possible by the better binding affinity of the 101F6-His_8 protein towards Ni-NTA-Sepharose column, by the introduction of eight-histidine residue-tag at the C-terminus (Alisio & Mueckler, 2010). Occasionally we found a dimer (or trimer) form of the 101F6-His_8 protein monomer upon the SDS-PAGE analysis. We found that such a formation of the dimer (or trimer) form was not due to a disulfide bond formation between the monomers and could be avoided without the heat treatment of the purified sample before the analysis. The great tendency to form aggregates of the 101F6-His_8 protein during the purification steps is likely to be related to a spontaneous formation of the dimer (or trimer) and might be the intrinsic nature of the cytochrome b_{561} protein family more or less (Apps et al., 1984; Duong et al., 1984; Liu et al., 2011).

Visible absorption spectra of the purified 101F6-His_8 protein were analyzed in the region from 700 to 340 nm. The purified 101F6-His_8 protein exhibited typical spectra characteristics as a member of the cytochrome b_{561} family (Tsubaki et al., 1997). A strong Soret band at 414 nm and weak Q bands between 500-600 nm were observed for the oxidized form. Addition of sodium dithionite produced the fully-reduced form with a Soret band at 427 nm and resolved Q bands at 529 (β-band) and at 561 nm (α-band) (Figure 1). For the heme content analysis, the purified 101F6-H_8 protein was converted to a pyridine hemochrome by the addition of pyridine and NaOH according to the method of (Fuhrhop & Smith, 1975) as modified with (Berry & Trumpower, 1987). An extinction coefficient value for heme B pyridine hemochrome of 34.4 $mM^{-1}cm^{-1}$ at 557 nm (in the absolute spectrum) (Fuhrhop & Smith, 1975) was used. Protein concentration was determined by a modified Lowry method (Markwell et al., 1981) and by the Bradford method (Bradford, 1976). Bovine serum albumin was used as a standard in each method. Concentration of the standard solution was assessed spectrophotometrically using an extinction coefficient of 6.60 $\%^{-1}cm^{-1}$ at 280 nm. The heme content of the purified 101F6-His_8 protein was found to be 1.59 (±0.06) mole/mole protein, as calculated from the absolute spectrum at 557 nm of the pyridine hemochrome. This value was slightly less than the calculated value for bovine CG cytochrome b_{561} at 1.70 mole heme/mole protein (Tsubaki et al., 1997). Nevertheless, the value supported the presence of two heme B groups *per* protein in the purified sample, like the classic CG cytochrome b_{561}. This result was also consistent with the result of EPR analysis on the purified form of oxidized 101F6-His_8 (Recuenco et al., unpublished), which showed the presence of two independent heme centers.

Mass spectrometric analyses were conducted with a Voyager DE Pro mass spectrometer (Applied Biosystems, Foster City, California, USA). The estimated molecular mass of the intact 101F6-His_8 was found as 25941.70 Da, very close to the theoretical value corresponding to 1-240 residue (25996.9 Da; average). In total of 240 amino acid residues of the 101F6-His8 protein, we could identify most of the cleaved peptides with coverage of more than 99% and there was no post-translational modification occurred. These results confirmed the successful expression and purification of the intact 101F6-His8 protein.

Purification steps	Total protein (mg)	Total cytochrome b_{561} content (nmol)	Specific content (nmol/mg protein)	Purification Fold	Yield (%)
Microsomes	165.75	861	5.20	1	100
β-octyl glucoside-solubilized	109.20	459	4.20	0.81	53.3
Ni-NTA chromatography/desal/concentrate	0.60	176	293.3	56	20.5

Table 1. Purification of recombinant human 101F6-His8 protein (starting from a culture of 250 mL-scale).

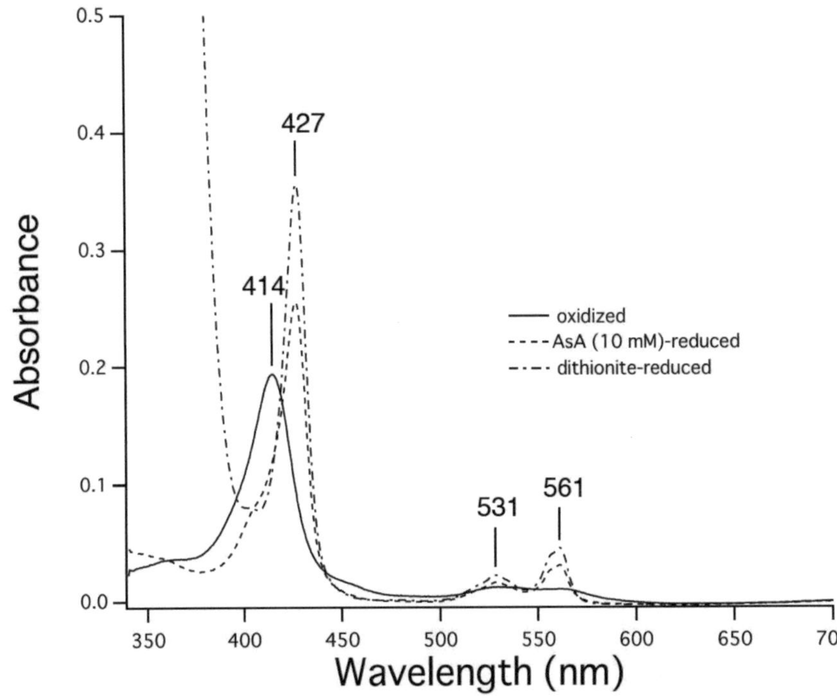

Fig. 1. Visible absorption spectra of purified 101F6-H8 protein. Spectra were measured in oxidized (solid line), AsA (10 mM)–reduced (broken line), and dithionite-reduced (dashed broken line) states with cytochrome b_{561} content of 1.66 μM in 50 mM potassium phosphate buffer (pH 7.0) 1.0% β-octyl glucoside at room temperature.

The 101F6-His_8 protein was found to be reducible by AsA very efficiently. Redox titration analysis showed that its redox behaviour could be simulated satisfactory by assuming the presence of two independent heme *b* prosthetic groups with their midpoint potentials at +89.5 and +13.1 mV, respectively, slightly lower than the corresponding values of bovine CG cytochrome b_{561} (Tsubaki et al., 2000; Takeuchi et al., 2001). Electron accepting activity from AsA to the oxidized 101F6-His_8 protein and electron donating activity from the reduced 101F6-His_8 protein to MDA radical were further analyzed by a stopped-flow and pulse-radiolysis techniques, respectively. The results showed that these two properties are distinct from bovine CG cytochrome b_{561}: (a) very high electron accepting rate constant from ascorbate compared to other cytochrome b_{561} (Kobayashi et al., 1998); (b) absence of initial pH-dependency from AsA to the oxidized heme of 101F6-His_8 protein (Takigami et al., 2003). Details were described elsewhere (Recuenco et al., unpublished results). These properties may be directly related to the tumor suppressor activity of 101F6-His_8 protein in human lung tissues.

3.2 Protein crystallization screening

Purified eight-histidine-tagged human 101F6 protein in 50 mM potassium phosphate buffer (pH 7.0) containing 1% β-octyl glucoside was freed from aggregates by centrifugation at 15,000 rpm for 5 minutes. The supernatant containing the solubilized protein was put in Amicon Ultra-4 centrifugal filter unit (UFC 801096; Nihon Millipore K.K., Tokyo, Japan) and centrifuged at 3,000 rpm to concentrate the protein sample. The concentrated sample was again centrifuged to remove aggregates and then filtered through a 0.22 µm syringe filter. A 0.3 mL sample with a concentration at least 150 µM of cytochrome b_{561} content was enough for screening approximately 1000 different conditions using a crystallization robot, Hydra II Plus One system (Matrix Technologies Corp., Thermo Fischer Scientific Inc., Hudson, New Hampshire, USA). Screening of the crystallization condition was performed by a sitting-drop vapor diffusion method on 96-well Intelli-plates at room temperature. A ratio of 0.3 µL protein and 0.3 µL precipitant over 30 µL well solution was employed. Crystallization screening solutions such as, Classics Neo, Classics Neo II, JCSG+, Mb Class I, MPD, pH clear, pH clear II, $AmSO_4$, PEG I, and PEG II Suite (Qiagen K. K., Tokyo, Japan), were used. After the deposition of the samples, plates were incubated at 20°C for about 14 days.

Crystals with size of 0.020 mm were formed from the following precipitants:

JCSG+ (20 % PEG3350, 0.2 M sodium thiocyanate), Classics Neo (1.0 M imidazole (pH 7.0), and Classics II (25 % PEG3350, 0.2 M ammonium acetate, 0.1 M *bis*-Tris (pH 5.5) (Figure 2). Diffraction data were first measured on an R-axis imaging plate (IP) area detector (Rigaku Corp., Tokyo, Japan) at the Protein Design Laboratory, Yokohama City University. The X-ray diffraction data of the crystals were further collected at the Photon Factory in Tsukuba, Ibaraki, Japan (Beam line; PF-BL5A). The crystals from Classics II (25 % PEG3350 (w/v), 0.2 M ammonium acetate, 0.1 M *bis*-Tris (pH 5.5) were able to produce an X-ray diffraction pattern with a maximum resolution at 8.4 Å (Figure 2B). Further, optimization of the conditions using 20 % PEG3350 (w/v), 0.2M ammonium acetate, 0.1 M *bis*-Tris (pH 5.5) and 15 % PEG3350 (w/v), 0.2 M ammonium acetate, 0.1 M *bis*-Tris (pH 5.5) produced better crystals (Figure 3). The crystals from 15 % PEG3350 (w/v), 0.2M ammonium acetate, 0.1M *bis*-Tris (pH 5.5) produced a diffraction pattern of spots with the highest resolution at 4 Å (Figure not shown).

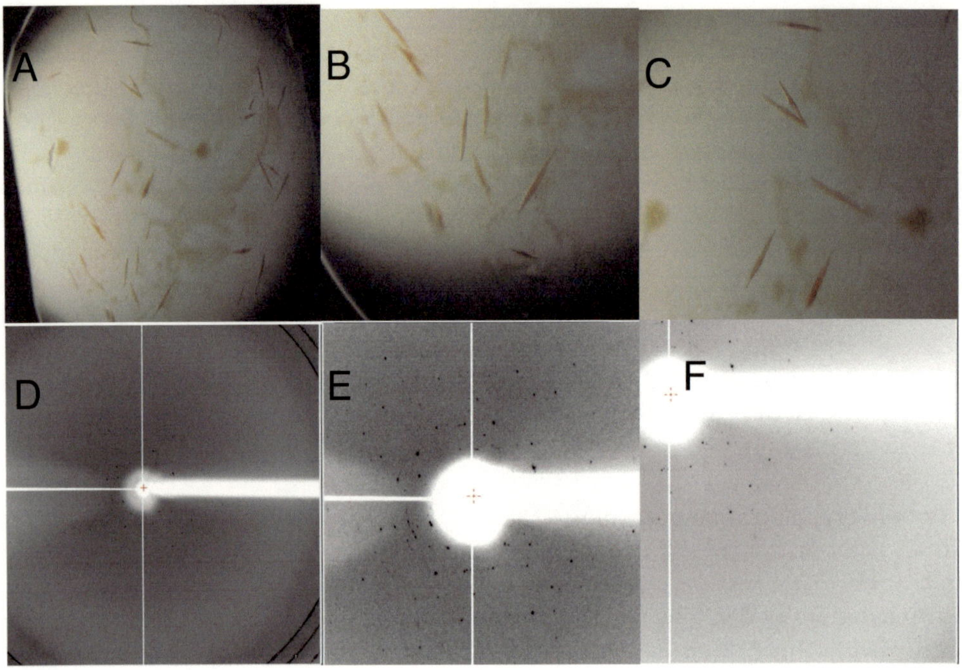

Fig. 2. Screening of crystallization conditions for 101F6-His_8 protein. (A-C) Crystals formed upon crystallization screening with a sitting-drop vapor diffusion method on 96-well plates. Conditions: Precipitant, 25% PEG3350, 0.2M Ammonium acetate, 0.1M *bis*-Tris (pH5.5) solution; Temperature 20 °C; Incubation time 10-14 days; Protein concentration, 150 μM in 50 mM potassium buffer (pH 7.0) containing 1.0 % β-octyl glucoside. (D-F) Diffraction patterns of the 101F6-H_8 crystals obtained from the conditions described above. Highest resolution at 8 Å was obtained at Tsukuba Photon Factory (Beam Line: PF-BL5A, Exposure time=20 sec).

4. Discussion

The candidate tumor suppressor protein 101F6 could be an important factor in cell proliferation and apoptosis. The reported induction of apoptosis in cultured cancer cells and inhibition of tumor growth in mouse models on forced expression of the 101F6 gene (Ji et al., 2002; Ohtani et al., 2007) gave a promising outlook for cancer prevention and treatment. In the present study, the human 101F6 protein was expressed and purified successfully from the yeast *Pichia pastoris* cells. The purified 101F6-His_8 protein was found to be reducible by AsA very efficiently and can donate electrons to MDA radical very rapidly. These new findings provide clues as to the possible role of the 101F6 protein in AsA-recycling that may be linked to processes that ultimately lead to apoptosis (Figure 3). Our view is basically consistent with the proposal by Ohtani et al., in which the exogenously-expressed 101F6 protein in cancer cells enhanced intracellular uptake of AsA, leading to an accumulation of cytotoxic H_2O_2 and synergistic killing of tumor cells through caspase-independent apoptotic and autophagic pathways (Ohtani et al., 2007). Our present view, however, needs further clarification to explain the possible mechanism(s) to enhance the cellular uptake of AsA by the introduction of the 101F6 protein into the ER membranes. Further, the proximate target of the 101F6 protein in the proposed AsA-signaling pathway must be clarified. Importantly, in our scheme in Figure 3, H_2O_2 was not included. Ohtani et al. observed a significant increase in the intracellular accumulation of H_2O_2 in non-small cell lung cancer (NSCLC) cells only in response to exogenous 101F6 and AsA (Ohtani et al., 2007). Therefore, it might be very important to clarify the molecular mechanism concealed in the 101F6 protein in facilitating the formation and accumulation of cytotoxic H_2O_2 by the increased concentration of cytosolic AsA. For these purposes, complete three-dimensional structural information about this hydrophobic membrane protein is highly necessary and it would be very helpful for the understanding of the mechanism of the putative tumor suppression function and, further, in the design of therapeutic agents for cancer.

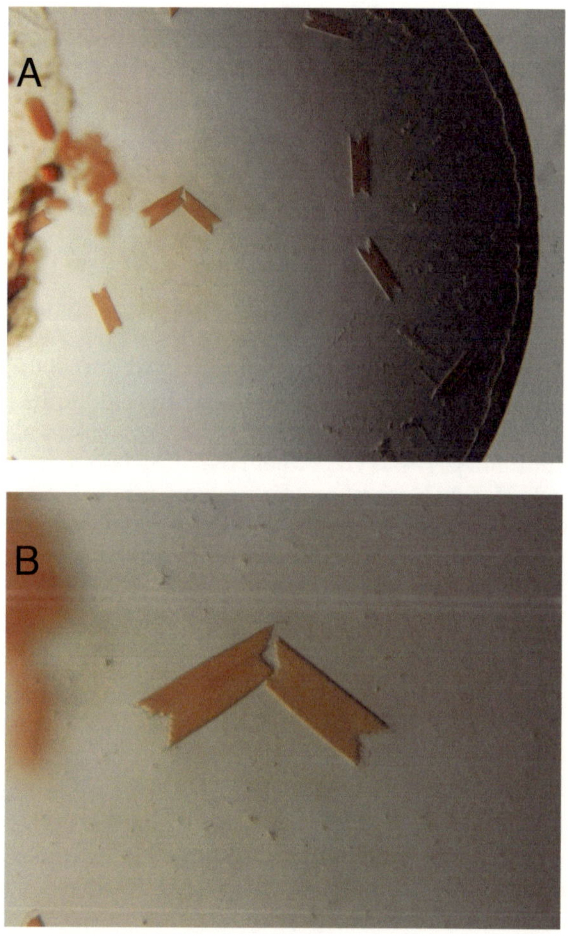

Fig. 3. Crystals formed from crystallization screening with a sitting-drop vapor diffusion method after optimization of precipitant composition. (A and B) 15% PEG3350 (w/v), 0.4M Ammonium acetate, 0.1M *bis*-Tris (pH6.0). Temperature 20°C; Incubation time, 10-14 days; Protein concentration, 150µM of 101F6-His_8 protein in 50 mM potassium phosphate buffer (pH 7.0) containing 1.0 % β-octyl glucoside.

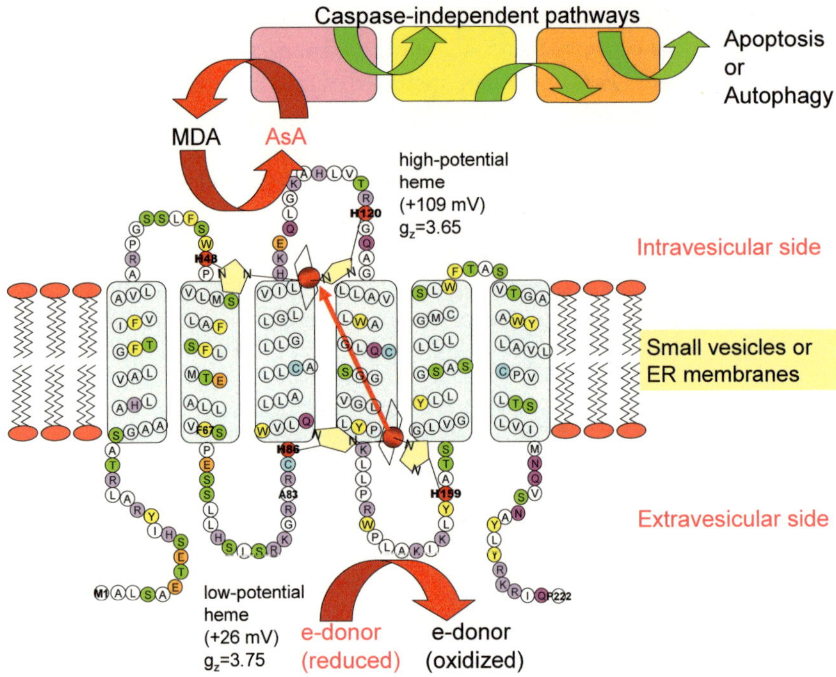

Fig. 4. Proposed topological model and function of the human tumor suppressor 101F6 protein in human cells. The human 101F6 protein contains six transmembrane α-helices and two *b*-type hemes. Alignment with other cytochromes b_{561} identified four histidine residues that might be the axial ligands of two hemes: His48 and His120 for the intravesicular heme; and His86 and His159 for the cytosolic side heme. The 101F6 protein may be located in the small vesicle or ER membranes. The 101F6 protein may function as an electron transfer protein inside the vesicles for AsA recycling. An electron donor donates an electron to the cytosolic heme of the 101F6 protein. The electron is then passed to the intravesicular heme *via* intramolecular electron transfer. MDA radical that might have been generated in some processes in the lumen accepts the electron from the intravesicular heme to re-generate AsA. AsA in the lumen of the vesicles is used as a cofactor to activate a certain target protein that may signal a caspase-independent pathway to induce apoptosis or autophagy.

Purification and crystallization of membrane proteins are considered to be much more difficult than soluble proteins. This difficulty is mostly due to the presence of transmembrane domains, in which hydrophobic α-helical domains were covered with detergent molecules, which was inevitably used for the solubilization of the proteins, forming a micelle structure. Such hydrophobic domains do not have specific interactions with other protein molecules, having a tendency to form non-specific aggregates during the protein purification, therefore, hampered the purification of membrane proteins into a homogenous state. Similar problems occur during the crystallization of a membrane protein. To obtain successful protein crystals of a membrane protein, we may have two strategies; one way is increasing a part of the hydrophilic domain to facilitate the specific interactions among the hydrophilic amino acid residues of the protein. Usually, a monoclonal body specific to such a hydrophilic domain would be used for such purpose. The other way is a choice of detergents. To find the best conditions for crystal growth with a suitable crystal group, one needs large amounts of pure protein sample and suitable detergents (Gutmann, 2007; Wetterholm et al., 2008).

We could obtain enough amounts of nearly homogeneous sample of human 101F6 protein in the form of eight-histidine-tagged fusion protein from the heterologous expression system of yeast *Pichia pastoris* cells. The protein samples were subjected to crystallization trials where initial screening was performed using a crystallization robot and commercially-available protein crystallization precipitants containing varying proportions of different salts, polymers and organic solvents. This allowed the screening of about 1000 different conditions within a very short time and usage of a tiny amount of the protein sample.
The β-octyl glucoside detergent used throughout in this study was a small micelle-forming detergent. Small micelle-forming detergents solubilize membrane proteins efficiently and leave hydrophilic parts of the protein being exposed to the water medium, allowing better interactions with other protein molecule(s) that are required for the formation of protein crystal lattice (Gutmann, 2007). However, if the hydrophobic regions are not well-covered with detergent molecules, aggregation of the membrane protein may occur. Large micelle-forming detergents such as n-dodecyl-β-D-maltoside and polyoxyethylene dodecyl ether can be used to address this problem. But with the use of these detergents, only small portions of the protein may be actually available for the lattice formation with other protein molecules. Thus, the human 101F6 protein should be subjected to a detergent screening to obtain better diffracting crystals and resolve its X-ray structure.

5. Conclusion

Previous studies showed that forced expression of the *101F6* gene in cultured cancer cells and in animal cancer models could significantly inhibit tumor growth. These promising results encouraged our investigation on the properties and function of the 101F6 protein. The human 101F6 protein was successfully expressed as an octahistidine-tagged fusion protein in the methylotropic yeast *Pichia pastoris* and was purified in its functional form. Characterization of the protein revealed that it possesses similar absorption spectra and AsA-reducibility as the prototype bovine CG cytochrome b_{561}. However, the results from kinetic studies on the reduction by AsA and the oxidation by MDA radical indicated different properties in the electron transfer mechanism. Most of the differences may be attributed to the low sequence homology of the 101F6 protein to the bovine CG cytochrome b_{561}. Other previously studied members of the cytochrome b_{561} family are much more similar to each other because of their higher sequence homology. Present study showed that it was possible to produce high quality sample and good diffracting crystals of the octahistidine-tagged 101F6 protein. An extensive screening for the best condition for crystallization should be done with the use of other detergents (such as n-dodecyl-β-D-maltoside), precipitants, and monoclonal antibodies. The detailed protein structure of the 101F6 protein through X-ray crystallography may be attained in the near future.

6. References

Abramson, J., Smirnova, I., Kasho, V., Verner, G., Kaback, H. R. & Iwata, S. (2003). Structure and mechanism of the lactose permease of *Escherichia coli*, *Science*, Vol. 301, No. 5633, pp.610-615, ISSN 0036-8075

Alisio, A. & Mueckler, M. (2010). Purification and characterization of mammalian glucose transporters expressed in *Pichia pastoris*, *Prot. Exp. Purif.*, Vol. 70, No. 1, pp.81-87, ISSN 1046-5928

Apps, D. K., Boisclair, M. D., Gavine, F. S. & Pettigrew, G. W. (1984). Unusual redox behaviour of cytochrome *b*-561 from bovine chromaffin granule membranes, *Biochim. Biophys. Acta,* Vol. 764, No. 1, pp.8-16, ISSN 0005-2728

Asada, H., Uemura, T., Yurugi-Kobayashi, T., Shiroishi, M., Shimamura, T., Tsujimoto, H., Ito, K., Sugawara, T., Nakane, T., Nomura, N., Murata, T., Haga, T., Iwata, S. & Kobayashi, T. (2011). Evaluation of the *Pichia pastoris* expression system for the production of GPCRs for structural analysis, *Microbial Cell Factories,* Vol. 10, No. pp.(in press), ISSN 1475-2859

Berry, E. A. & Trumpower, B. L. (1987). Simultaneous determination of hemes a, b, and c from pyridine hemochrome spectra, *Anal. Biochem.,* Vol. 161, No. 1, pp.1-15, ISSN 0003-2697

Bradford, M. M. (1976). A rapid and sensitive method for the quantitation of microgram quantities of protein utilizing the principle of protein-dye binding, *Anal. Biochem.,* Vol. 72, No. 1-2, pp.248-254, ISSN 0003-2697

Duong, L. T., Fleming, P. J. & Russell, J. T. (1984). An identical cytochrome b561 is present in bovine adrenal chromaffin vesicles and posterior pituitary neurosecretory vesicles, *J. Biol. Chem.,* Vol. 259, No. 8, pp.4885-4889, ISSN 0021-9258

Fuhrhop, J.-H. & Smith, K. M. (1975). Laboratory Methods. *Porphyrins and Metalloporphyrins.* Smith, K. M. (Ed), pp. 755-869, Elsevier Scientific Publishing Co., ISBN 0-444-41375-8, Amsterdam

Gutmann, D. A. P., Mizohata, E., Newstead, S., Ferrandon, S., Henderson, P. J. F., van Veen, H. W. and Byrne, B. (2007). A high-throughput method for membrane protein solubility screening: The ultracentrifugation dispersity sedimentation assay, *Protein Sci.,* Vol. 16, No. 7, pp.1422-1428, ISSN 0961-8368

Hollingsworth, R. E. & Lee, W.-H. (1991). Tumor suppressor genes: new prospects for cancer research, *J. Natl. Cancer Inst.,* Vol. 83, No. 2, pp.91-96, ISSN 0027-8874

Huang, Y., Lemieux, M. J., Song, J., Auer, M. & Wang, D.-N. (2003). Structure and mechanism of the glycerol-3-phospate transportor from *Escherichia coli, Science,* Vol. 301, No. 5633, pp.616-620, ISSN 0036-8075

Ji, L., Nishizaki, M., Gao, B., Burbee, D., Kondo, M., Kamibayashi, C., Xu, K., Yen, N., Atkinson, E. N., Fang, B., Lerman, M. I., Roth, J. A. & Minna, J. D. (2002). Expression of several genes in the human chromosome 3p21.3 homozygous deletion region by an adenovirus vector results in tumor suppressor activities *in vitro* and *in vivo, Cancer Res.,* Vol. 62, No. 9, pp.2715-2720, ISSN 0008-5472

Jiang, Y., Lee, A., Chen, J., Ruta, V., Cadene, M., Chait, B. T. & MacKinnon, R. (2003). X-ray structure of a voltage-dependent K^+ channel, *Nature,* Vol. 423, No. 6935, pp.33-41, ISSN 0028-0836

Knudson, A. G., Jr. (1971). Mutation and cancer: statistical study of retinoblastoma, *Proc. Natl. Acad. Sci. U S A,* Vol. 68, No. 4, pp.820-823, ISSN 0027-8424

Knudson, A. G., Jr. & Strong, L. C. (1972). Mutation and cancer: Neuroblastoma and pheochromocytoma, *Am. J. Hum. Genet.,* Vol. 24, No. 5, pp.514-532, ISSN 0002-9297

Kobayashi, K., Tsubaki, M. & Tagawa, S. (1998). Distinct roles of two heme centers for transmembrane electron transfer in cytochrome b_{561} from bovine adrenal chromaffin vesicles as revealed by pulse radiolysis, *J. Biol. Chem.,* Vol. 273, No. 26, pp.16038-16042, ISSN 0021-9258

Lerman, M. I. & Minna, J. D. (2000). The 630-kb lung cancer homozygous deletion region on human chromosome 3p21.3: Identification and evaluation of the resident candidate tumor suppressor genes, *Cancer Res.,* Vol. 60, No. 21, pp.6116-6133, ISSN 0008-5472

Liu, W., Wu, G., Tsai, A.-L. & Kulmacz, R. J. (2011). High-yield production, purification and characterization of functional human duodenal cytochrome *b* in an *Escherichia coli* system, *Protein Expr. Purif.*, Vol. (in press), No., ISSN 1046-5928

Long, S. B., Campbell, E. B. & MacKinnon, R. (2005). Crystal structure of a mammalian voltage-dependent *Shaker* family K^+ channel, *Science,* Vol. 309, No. 5 August, pp.897-903, ISSN 0036-8075

Markwell, M. A. K., Haas, S. M., Tolbert, N. E. & Bieber, L. L. (1981). Protein determination in membrane and lipoprotein sampled: Manual and automated procedures, *Methods Enzymol.,* Vol. 72, pp.296-303, ISSN 0076-6879

Mckie, A. T., Barrow, D., Latunde-Dada, G. O., Rolfs, A., Sager, G., Mudaly, E., Mudaly, M., Richardson, C., Barlow, D., Bomford, A., Peters, T. J., Raja, K. B., Shirali, S., Hediger, M. A., Farzaneh, F. & Simpson, R. J. (2001). An iron-regulated ferric reductase associated with the absorption of dietary iron, *Science,* Vol. 291, No. 5509, pp.1755-1759, ISSN 0036-8075

Mizutani, K., Yoshioka, S., Mizutani, Y., Iwata, S. & Mikami, B. (2011). High-throughput construction of expression system using yeast Pichia pastoris, and its application to membrane proteins, *Prot. Exp. Purif.,* Vol. 77, No. 1, pp.1-8, ISSN 1046-5928

Nakanishi, N., Rahman, M. M., Sakamoto, Y., Miura, M., Takeuchi, F., Park, S.-Y. & Tsubaki, M. (2009a). Inhibition of electron acceptance from ascorbate by the specific *N*-carbethoxylations of maize cytochrome b_{561}: A common mechanism for the transmembrane electron transfer in cytochrome b_{561} protein family, *J. Biochem.,* Vol. 146, No. 6, pp.857-866, ISSN 0021-924X

Nakanishi, N., Rahman, M. M., Sakamoto, Y., Takigami, T., Kobayashi, K., Hori, H., Hase, T., Park, S.-Y. & Tsubaki, M. (2009b). Importance of conserved Lys83 residue of *Zea mays* cytochrome b_{561} for ascorbate-specific transmembrane electron transfer as revealed by site-directed mutageneis studies, *Biochemistry,* Vol. 48, No. 44, pp.10665-10678, ISSN 0006-2960

Ohtani, S., Iwamura, A., Deng, W., Ueda, K., Wu, G., Jayachandran, G., Kondo, S., Atkinson, E. N., Minna, J. D., Roth, J. A. & Ji, L. (2007). Tumor suppressor 101F6 and ascorbate synergistically and selectively inhibit non-small cell lung cancer growth by caspase-independent apoptosis and autophagy, *Cancer Res.,* Vol. 67, No. 13, pp.6293-6303, ISSN 0008-5472

Okuyama, E., Yamamoto, R., Ichikawa, Y. & Tsubaki, M. (1998). Structural basis for the electron transfer across the chromaffin vesicle membranes catalyzed by cytochrome b_{561}: Analyses of cDNA nucleotide sequences and visible absorption spectra, *Biochim. Biophys. Acta,* Vol. 1383, No. 2, pp.269-278, ISSN 1570-9639

Ostuni, M. A., Lamanuzzi, L. B., Bizouarn, T., Dagher, M.-C. & Baciou, L. (2010). Expression of functional mammal flavocytochrome b_{558} in yeast: Comparison with improved insect cell system, *Biochim. Biophys. Acta,* Vol. 1798, No. 6, pp.1179-1188, ISSN 0005-2736

Prigge, S. T., Mains, R. E., Eipper, B. A. & Amzel, L. M. (2000). New insights into copper monooxygenases and peptide amidation: structure, mechanism and function, *Cell. Mol. Life Sci.,* Vol. 57, No. 8-9, pp.1236-1259, ISSN 1420-682X

Recuenco, M. C., Fujito, M., Rahman, M. M., Sakamoto, Y., Takeuchi, F. & Tsubaki, M. (2009). Functional expression and characterization of human *101F6* protein, a homologue of cytochrome b_{561} and a candidate tumor suppressor gene product, *BioFactors,* Vol. 34, No. 3, pp.219-230, ISSN 0951-6433

Romanos, M., Scorer, C., Sreekrishna, K. & Clare, J. (1998). The generation of multicopy recombinant strains. *Pichia protocols*. Higgins, C. F. & Cregg, J. M. (Ed), pp. 55-72, Humana Press Inc., ISBN 0-89603-421-6, Totowa, NJ

Seike, Y., Takeuchi, F. & Tsubaki, M. (2003). Reversely-oriented cytochrome b_{561} in reconstituted vesicles catalyzes transmembrane electron transfer and supports the extravesicular dopamine b-hydroxylase activity, *J. Biochem.*, Vol. 134, No. 6, pp.859-867, ISSN 0021-924X

Takeuchi, F., Kobayashi, K., Tagawa, S. & Tsubaki, M. (2001). Ascorbate inhibits the carbethoxylation of two histidyl and one tyrosyl residues indispensable for the transmembrane electron transfer reaction of cytochrome b_{561}, *Biochemistry*, Vol. 40, No. 13, pp.4067-4076, ISSN 0006-2960

Takigami, T., Takeuchi, F., Nakagawa, M., Hase, T. & Tsubaki, M. (2003). Stopped-flow analyses on the reaction of ascorbate with cytochrome b561 purified from bovine chromaffin vesicle membanes, *Biochemistry*, Vol. 42, No. 27, pp.8110-8118, ISSN 0006-2960

Tsubaki, M., Kobayashi, K., Ichise, T., Takeuchi, F. & Tagawa, S. (2000). Diethylpyrocarbonate-modification abolishes fast electron accepting ability of cytochrome b_{561} from ascorbate but does not influence on electron donation to monodehydroascorbate radical: Distinct roles of two heme centers for electron transfer across the chromaffin vesicle membranes, *Biochemistry*, Vol. 39, No. 12, pp.3276-3284, ISSN 0006-2960

Tsubaki, M., Nakayama, M., Okuyama, E., Ichikawa, Y. & Hori, H. (1997). Existence of two heme B centers in cytochrome b_{561} from bovine adrenal chromaffin vesicles as revealed by a new purification procedure and EPR spectroscopy, *J. Biol. Chem.*, Vol. 272, No. 37, pp.23206-23210, ISSN 0021-9258

Tsubaki, M., Takeuchi, F. & Nakanishi, N. (2005). Cytochrome b561 protein family: Expanding roles and versatile transmembrane electron transfer abilities as predicted by a new classification system and protein sequence motif analyses, *Biochim. Biophys. Acta*, Vol. 1753, No. 2, pp.174-190, ISSN 1570-9639

Vargas, J. D., Herpers, B., Mckie, A. T., Gledhill, S., McDonnell, J., van der Heuvel, M., Davies, K. E. & Ponting, C. P. (2003). Stromal cell-derived receptor 2 and cytochrome *b*561 are functional ferric reductase, *Biochim. Biophys. Acta*, Vol. 1651, No. 1-2, pp.116-123, ISSN 1570-9639

Weiß, H. M., Haase, W. & Reiländer, H. (1998). Expression of an integral membrane protein, the $5HT_{5A}$ receptor. *Pichia protocols*. Higgins, C. F. & Cregg, J. M. (Ed), pp. 227-239, Humana Press Inc., ISBN 0-89603-421-6, Totowa, NJ

Wetterholm, A., Molina, D. M., Nordlund, P. r., Eshaghi, S. & Haeggström, J. Z. (2008). High-level expression, purification, and crystallization of recombinant rat leukotriene C_4 synthase from the yeast *Pichia pastoris*, *Protein Expr. Purif.*, Vol. 60, No. 1, pp.1-6, ISSN 1046-5928

Yurugi-Kobayashi, T., Asada, H., Shiroishi, M., Shimamura, T., Funamoto, S., Katsuta, N., Ito, K., Sugawara, T., Tokuda, N., Tsujimoto, H., Murata, T., Nomura, N., Haga, K., Haga, T., Iwata, S. & Kobayashi, T. (2009). Comparison of functional non-glycosylated GPCRs expression in *Pichia pastoris*, *Biochem. Biophys. Res. Commun.*, Vol. 380, No. 2, pp.271-276, ISSN 0006-291X

Zabarovsky, E. R., Lerman, M. I. & Minna, J. D. (2002). Tumor suppressor genes on chromosome 3p involved in the pathogenesis of lung and other cancers, *Oncogene*, Vol. 21, No. 45, pp.6915-6935, ISSN 0950-9232

13

Epigenetic Control of Tumor Suppressor Genes in Lung Cancer

Xuan Qiu, Roman Perez-Soler and Yiyu Zou
Albert Einstein College of Medicine,
Department of Medicine/Oncology/Cancer Center, New York,
USA

1. Introduction

Lung cancer is the number one cause of cancer-related deaths worldwide. It claims 1.3 million lives every year (www.who.int/mediacentre) (1). To understand the mechanism of lung carcinogenesis is one of the essential tasks for effective control of lung cancer. Lung cancer and other cancers have long been viewed as "genetic diseases" (2, 3). Particularly, tumor suppressor gene (TSG) deactivation plays a critical role in carcinogenesis.

Historically, majority of the scientific evidence on tumor suppressor gene-related carcinogenesis describes the genetic defects occurring either in the TSGs themselves, such as mutations, or in their environment, such as activation of their inhibitors. Therapeutic applications of such knowledge against cancers have been attempted through reconstituting wild-type TSG products in target cells/tissues by genetic manipulation or biological or chemical molecules, thereby restoring the functions of TSGs and possibly slowing cancer progression.

Ever since the 'two-hit' hypothesis (4) and the first proposal of a potential tumor suppressor gene being involved in the retinoblastomas formation (5), especially after the function of wild-type p53 gene was clearly described (6, 7), the therapeutic research effort has been shifted from optimizing the non-specific radiation and chemotherapy that mainly kill fast-dividing cells to targeting the specific genetic changes. Restoring the function of TSGs has been considered as one of the most promising directions for cancer therapy.

Directly transfecting TSGs into the cancer cells to restore the function of the TSGs and inhibit the tumor growth has become a promising direction to develop novel cancer therapy for the past two decades. Adenoviral and retroviral vectors have been used to deliver TSGs into human tumors by intratumoral or regional administration. The best example is the adenoviral carried wild-type p53 gene used to treat patients with non-small cell lung cancer (NSCLC) by direct intratumoral injection (8). Nonviral gene delivery methods such as cationic liposomes and cationic polymers were also developed for delivering TSGs because of their distinct advantage of lack of immunogenicity (9-11). Our lab has developed a unique cationic liposomal p53 and cationic polymers p53 to treat orthotopic human NSCLC model in mice with intratracheal or aerosol administration, which significantly enhanced the gene delivery efficiency to the airway epithelium and markedly reduced the systemic toxicity, the results showed a great therapeutic potential in the preclinical orthotopic human NSCLC xenografts in mice (12, 13).

However, the overall efficacy of these TSG therapies by direct gene transfection or delivery was limited. One of the important reasons is that most cases of "loss of function" found in tumor tissues are at the mature stage of the carcinogenesis process, at which moment the multiple irreversible genetic defects are established already, therefore, it is very difficult to reverse the carcinogenesis process by restoring or correcting the functions of one or a few TSGs.

More recently, increasing evidence, particularly the "cancer stem cell" model suggests that epigenetic changes, which occur in normal stem or progenitor cells, are the earliest events in cancer initiation (14). Therefore, to catch the early cancer-specific epigenetic changes and reverse them logically becomes a better strategy than those focusing on the irreversible genetic defects.

Multiple research groups have demonstrated that correcting the aberrant methylation in the promoter region of TSGs could inhibit cancer development. Among these studies, we have directly proved the concept in the orthotopic lung cancer models in mice. Briefly, we first proved that azacytidine (Aza), a demethylation agent, could effectively demethylate the hypermethylated promoter of RASSF1a gene (a TSG), at non-cytotoxic concentration range which was a thousand fold lower than its cytotoxic concentration. Then we used intratracheal injection of Aza at a non-cytotoxic dose to treat the airway inoculated NSCLC xenografts in mice, and we found that the demethylation treatment significantly prolonged the life of the tumor-bearing mice, and the locoregional therapy for localized lung cancer in the airway epithelium was significantly superior than the systemic (IV) treatment. Our results demonstrated that the model NSCLC could be inhibited if the TSGs were reactivated by the reversal of the hypermethylation in the promoter regions. In this chapter, we will also discuss the possible application, the advantages and limitation of the current epigenetic methods aimed to enhance cancer therapeutic efficacy by promoting TSGs.

Restoring TSG functions through epigenetic manipulations will be a promising strategy for cancer therapy and prevention, which shifts the focus from treating cells with irreversible genetic lesions to targeting the reversible epigenetic changes. Further work in this field will complement our knowledge of TSG-expression control and enhance our understanding of the carcinogenesis process. This exciting new therapeutic strategy could potentially reduce cancer mortality when applied to populations of individuals at risk.

In this chapter we will briefly summarize the studies describing the aberrant epigenetic alterations in lung cancer and the methods to control carcinogenesis with epigenetic manipulations, particularly, through controlling TSGs. We will also outline advances in the potential use of these epigenetic events for cancer diagnosis, prognosis and targeted epigenetic therapy, and present an experimental study of demethylation therapy at the preclinical level.

2. Epigenetic changes and lung cancer

Epigenetic changes usually are heritable changes in gene expression level without alteration of DNA sequence. Unlike genetic changes, epigenetic changes are reversible. The normal epigenetic process is important for gene expression and genome stability. When this normal process is disrupted, carcinogenesis may start. Therefore, epigenetic changes are considered a key player in the onset and progression of different type of cancers including lung cancer. The most frequently reported epigenetic phenomena are chromatin modifications including post-translational modifications of histones and chromatin modifying complexes, non-coding RNAs mediated regulations, and particularly DNA methylation. Epigenetic processes are finely tuned, undergo many regulations in response to the environment, and involve almost all the signaling pathways described in the literature. Epigenetics plays a crucial role in the control of nuclear architecture and gene activity and constitutes one of the bases of the biological diversity. In the first part of this chapter, we mainly focus on DNA methylation and its links to TSGs and lung cancer.

2.1 DNA methylation and lung cancer

DNA methylation is the most widely studied epigenetic modification restricted to the DNA motif called CpG dinucleotides, i.e. cytosine followed by guanine residues (15). Enriched in genomic regions known as "CpG islands," these CpG dinucleotides are typically at least 200 bp and up to several Kb in length with a high GC percentage, and are mainly found near or at the transcription start site within the promoter of about 40% of mammalian genes. CpG islands play a major role in the process of transcriptional regulation, and the ability of a gene to be or not to be transcribed is correlated with the unmethylated and methylated status of a CpG island, respectively, in the presence of the required co-regulators.

Methylation is the only covalent modification of the DNA in mammalian cells and carries out normal physiological functions during embryonic development (16), genomic imprinting (17), and chromosome-X inactivation (18). However, frequent alterations in DNA methylation are observed in cancers such as hypermethylation of CpG islands at tumor suppressor gene (TSG) loci leading to the loss of their expression, genome-wide hypomethylation in the body of genes and in DNA repetitive sequences leading to genomic instability (16), and altered DNA methyltransferases (DNMTs) expression (17).

DNA hypermethylation in the promoter region of TSGs is frequently found in human lung cancer tissues and cell lines. It was proved to be responsible for silencing the TSG and therefore promoting the initiation and development of the lung carcinogenesis. The best-studied example is the case of p16INK4a (CDKN2A); its promoter hypermethylation prevents the negative control exerted by p16INK4a on RB phosphorylation, thereby promoting cell cycle progression. p16INK4a hypermethylation is considered as one of the earliest event in lung tumorigenesis and increases constantly with disease progression (19, 20). An increasing number of other genes have been investigated for their methlyation status in lung cancer, including h-cadherin (CDH13) (21), 14-3-3σ (22), death associated protein kinase 1 (DAPK1) (23), ras association domain family 1 gene (RASSF1a) (24), caspase-8 (25), retinoic acid receptor β-2 (RAR-β), tissue inhibitor of metalloproteinase 3 (TIMP3), o6-methylguanine DNA methyltransferase (MGMT), E-cadherin (ECAD), gluthatione s-transferase p1 (GSTP1) (26), FHIT (27, 28), ASC/TMS1, HSRBC, TSLC1, DAL-1, and PTEN (29). Since these genes are involved in a broad range of biological processes, such as cancer cell cycle regulation, proliferation, apoptosis, cell adhesion, mobility, and DNA repair, promoter DNA hypermethylation may be a key event in lung carcinogenesis. Furthermore, genome-wide analyses have suggested that the presence of promoter DNA hypermethylation is probably more extensive than previously thought (30-33). For instance, Shames et al. recently identified 132 genes that are methylated with high penetrance in lung cancer cells (32). More strikingly, Brena et al. reported that 4.8% of all CpG island promoters might be aberrantly methylated, suggesting that the expression of about 1,400 genes might be disturbed in lung cancer (30).

Due to the spontaneous hydrolytic deamination under physiological conditions, methylated cytosine can be considered as a potent endogenous mutagen for C to T mutations, therefore

DNA hypermethylation can actually predispose to mutational events (14). Although representing only 1% of the bases in the mammalian genome, methylated cytosine might be responsible for as much as 30% of all transition mutations found in human disease such as cancers (34, 35).

The mechanism of the aberrant hypermethylation in the promoter region of TSGs in human non-small-cell lung cancer especially among smoker patients was described as the overexpression of DNA methyltranferases including DNMT1, DNMT3A and DNMT3B. Interestingly, polymorphisms that influence expression of the DNMT3B gene have been connected with increasing risk of lung cancer (36, 37). An adverse consequence of methylation of CpG sites appears to facilitate the binding for benzo[a]pyrene, a carcinogen, found in cigarette smoke, leading to the formation of major DNA damage hotspots in human lung cancer (38, 39). A well-illustrated example of this phenomenon is the occurrence of some hotspot mutations of the p53 tumor suppressor gene in lung tumors (40, 41).

Clinical evidence also showed that TSG promoter methylation is associated with the smoking history of patients with lung cancer. In lung adenocarcinomas and squamous cell carcinomas, the frequency of p16, MGMT, RASSF1, MTHFR, and FHIT promoter methylation was significantly higher among smokers than never-smokers (42-45); but the promoter methylation of other genes such as RASSF2, TNFRSF10C, BHLHB5, and BOLL was higher in never-smoker lung cancer patients than those of smokers (46, 47), suggesting smoking may target specific genes for methylation.

The roles of methylation in lung cancers for early detection, risk assessment, disease progression, and prognosis have also been studied. DNA methylation may serve as a marker for the early detection of lung cancer when found in the sputum of the patient (19, 48). For example, p16INK4a and MGMT promoter methylation could predict the development of squamous cell carcinoma up to three years before clinical diagnosis (49, 50), and RASSF1A, APC, ESR1, ABCB1, MT1G, and HOXC9 genes were found more frequently methylated in stage I lung adenocarcinomas/squamous cell carcinomas than the non-cancerous lesions (51), whereas the prevalence of hDAB2IP, H-cadherin, DAL-1, and FBN2 methylation was associated significantly with advanced stage of lung cancer (52-54). Altogether, theses studies highlight promoter methylation as a promising epigenetic approach for early detection and prognosis of NSCLC.

Demethylating drugs have great and promising clinical potential based on their ability to restore the expression of epigenetic silenced TSGs and inhibit tumor cell growth, while inducing manageable short-term side effects at the effective doses (55). The 5-aza-2′-deoxycytidine demethylating agent has been reported to increase the survival of chemotherapy-naive NSCLC patients, up to 6 years in some cases (56), although the relatively high dose in the treatment could be suspected to contribute partially cytotoxic effect to the final therapeutic outcome. More therapeutic investigations are underway, aiming at combining the demethylating agents with histone deacetylase inhibitors and attempting to integrate epigenetic therapy with more standard therapy.

2.2 Chromatin modifications and lung cancer

Chromatin is formed by basic units called the nucleosome, which is assembled by wrapping approximately 147 bp of genomic DNA around a histone octamere containing two copies of each of the core histones H2A, H2B, H3 and H4. The core histones possess an amino-terminal tail that protrudes outside of the nucleosome, which are subjected to a wide variety of post-translational covalent modifications such as acetylation, methylation, phosphorylation and ubiquitinylation. Access to the chromatin is thus affected by these modifications and therefore influences almost all DNA-based processes. Consequently, the structure and integrity of the genome and normal patterns of gene expression are potentially affected by the global alterations of histone modification patterns.

The protein complexes that regulate transcription by modifying histones or altering chromatin structure are mainly represented by Histones AcetylTransferases (HATs)/Histones Deacetylases (HDACs) and Histones methyltransferases (HMTs)/Histones Demethylases (DHMTs) complexes that determine the level of acetylation and methylation, respectively, of the amino-terminal domains of nucleosomal histones associated with them, and by ATP-dependent complexes such as SWI/SNF which use the energy of ATP hydrolysis to locally disrupt or alter the association of histones with DNA. Histone deacetylation mediated by HDACs works synergistically to alter the chromatin condensation status and represses transcription with DNMTs and a group of methylated DNA-binding proteins (57). In general, high HDAC activity is associated with condensed, transcriptionally inactive chromatin.

Altered expression pattern of histone and chromatin modifying enzymes have been found in human tumors, and histone modifications may contribute to tumorigenesis (58, 59). A clinical study including 138 lung cancer patients demonstrated that changes in global levels of histone 3 lysine 4 dimethylation (H3K4diMe), histone 3 lysine 9 acetylation (H3K9Ac), and histone 2A lysine 5 acetylation (H2AK5Ac) are predictive of the clinical outcome of lung cancers. Seligson et al (58) discovered that lower cellular levels of H3K4diMe and H3K18Ac predict significantly poorer survival probabilities for lung cancer patients (60). It has been summarized that the status of acetylation and methylation of specific lysine residues contained within the tails of nucleosome core histones is crucial in regulating chromatin structure and gene expression (61, 62).

In addition to this epigenetic function, certain HDACs also exhibit important cytoplasmatic function by controlling the acetylation status and function of numerous cytoplasmic proteins and transcription factors that may be important in carcinogenesis (63). Moreover, Sasaki et al (64) reported that expressions of HDAC1 correlated with the progression of lung carcinomas. Bartling et al (65) found HDAC3 upregulation in squamous lung cancers compared with non-tumor tissues in lung. Osada et al discovered that in a group of 72 lung cancer patients, the reduction of class II HDAC gene expression was clearly associated with poor prognosis (66). These results suggested that HDAC might be involved in lung cancer occurrence, progression, and prognosis and that inhibition of HDAC activity might be a possible target for lung cancer treatment.

Increasing laboratory evidence has illustrated the therapeutic mechanisms of HDACi: e.g., HDAC inhibitor FK228 suppressed the PI3K/Akt (67) and Src/Raf/MEK/ERK1/2 (68) signaling pathways, resulting in the downregulation of the anti-apoptotic proteins Bcl-2 and Bcl-xL, upregulation of the pro-apoptotic protein Bax, and the induction of time-dependent apoptosis in both adenocarcinoma (69) and small cell carcinoma cells (69, 70). Coincident with inhibition of ERK1/2 and PI3K/AKT survival pathways, the HDAC inhibitor FK228 enhanced JNK and p38MAPK signaling (68), whereas an SIRT1 inhibitor, Sirtinol, impaired activation of Ras/MAPK pathways in response to EGF and insulin-like growth factor-I (71). Furthermore, another HDAC inhibitor, trichostatin A, suppressed the levels of COX-2 mRNA and protein expression, which were correlated with an inhibition in prostaglandin E2 synthesis in lung adenocarcinoma cells (69). Clearly, HDACi have a specific antitumor effect and thorough studies analyzing the full potential and mechanism of these drugs with

regards to optimal dose, schedule, patient selection and combination strategies would allow the development of molecules with more effective therapeutic effect.
Recently, targeting HDAC activity using inhibitors of HDAC (HDACi) has become a novel and promising anticancer strategy, in particular in the treatment of advanced NSCLC where phase I and II trials have been completed (72). In addition, several HDACi have been shown to increase the cytotoxic effects of radiation in NSCLC by decreasing DNA repair efficiency and promoting cell death (73). HDACi also showed favorable results when used in combination with standard NSCLC chemotherapeutic agents and are likely to be a novel approach for the treatment of NSCLC because of an anti-growth activity against NSCLC cells (74, 75). Ongoing clinical trials are exploring the use of many new HDACi alone or as part of a combination with existing therapeutic modalities such as chemotherapy or radiotherapy (76).

2.3 Micro-RNAs and lung cancer

Micro-RNAs (miRNAs) are small non-coding RNAs with ~22 nucleotides in length (77, 78). miRNAs control a wide range of biological processes including apoptosis, development, proliferation and differentiation (78). High-throughput analyses have highlighted aberrant miRNA expression profiles in an increasing range of human cancer types (79-81) and all these studies suggested that cancer cells express altered miRNAs patterns consisting of both overexpression and downregulation. Therefore, miRNAs may function either as tumor suppressors or oncogenes and the genomic abnormalities found to influence their activity are the same as those described for protein-coding genes.
To date, both laboratory and clinical studies demonstrate a deregulation of miRNA expression in lung cancer and highlight them as useful diagnostic, pronostic and therapeutic tools. A growing number of miRNAs has been found aberrantly expressed in lung cancer and our understanding of miRNA expression patterns and functions in normal and lung cancer cells is just starting to emerge. Such miRNAs as miR-21, miR-126, miR-31, miR-519c, Let-7a, miR-133B, miR-15a, miR-16, and miR-183 have been found to regulate lung cancer cell proliferation, migration and invasion by targeting specific molecules, including Crk, EGFL7, VEGF, LATS2, PPP2R2A, HIF-1α, NIRF, MCL-1, Bcl-2, cyclins D1, D2 and E1, and Ezrin (82-89).
Growing evidence indicates that miRNA expression profiles confer important clues for clinical diagnosis and prognosis of human lung cancer. MicroRNA microarray analyses have identified profiles which could discriminate lung cancers from noncancerous lung tissues, as well as molecular signatures that differ according to tumor histology (80, 90). Interestingly, recent identification of Has-miR-205 has suggested it to be a highly specific marker for squamous carcinoma (91), therefore a clinical diagnostic assay based on miR-205 expression levels could aid the differential diagnosis of NSCLCs. Since miRNAs are more stable than mRNA and more tissue specific than DNA, their measurement could provide a novel and promising non-invasive approach to discriminate between normal and cancer patient samples. Studies found that aberrant miRNA expression could be used as a marker for the diagnosis of NSCLC in sputum specimen (92) and miRNA expression in peripheral blood or in serum correlated well with its expression in the tumor sample (93).
In terms of prognostic value, several miRNAs are reported to be associated with the clinical outcome of lung cancer. For instance, clinical study indicated that overexpression of mature miR-21 in the tissue and sputum samples could be an independent negative prognostic

factor for overall survival in NSCLC patients (94). Detection of miR-21 expression in sputum as a non-invasive approach for the diagnosis of lung cancer confers better sensitivity than sputum cytology (92). Clinical studies also showed reduced let-7 (81) and miR-34 (95) expression or enhanced miR-146b (96) and miR155 (80) expression with short survival or a high probability of relapse in patients with NSCLC. In patients with NSCLC, a five-miRNA signature including miR-221, let-7a, miR-137, miR-372, and miR-182 was identified and validated as an independent predictor of cancer relapse and survival (97). Remarkably, this signature is valuable even after patient stratification by stage or histology. In addition, expression levels of miR-486, miR-30d, miR-1, and miR-499 in serum could be used to predict survival for patients with NSCLC (98). Overexpression of miR-155 correlates with a poor prognosis when all clinical variables are considered together (80). Since miRNAs are upstream regulators of gene expression, they may be more powerful prognostic markers than their downstream target genes. For example, miR-146b alone was found to have a predictive accuracy for prognosis in ~78% of patients with lung squamous cell carcinoma (96), better than the overall predictive accuracy of 68% for a 50-gene signature (99).

The potential for using miRNAs in lung cancer therapy is now being explored. Let-7 overexpression confers radio-sensitivity to lung cancer cells (100). miR-128b LOH, a direct regulator of EGFR, correlates with clinical response and survival following gefitinib treatment (101). miR-221, miR-222 and miR-17-92 sensitize lung cancer cells to cytotoxic agents (102-104). Such results offer the experimental bases for the use of miRNAs as therapeutic targets. Further experiments are needed to uncover the emerging power of small non-coding RNAs to improve lung cancer therapeutics, and would have significant consequences for cancer patients in clinic.

Accumulative scientific evidence suggests that cancer, particularly lung cancer, is not only a genetic disease (2, 3), but also an epigenetic disease. Laboratory and clinical studies clearly demonstrate that many aberrant epigenetic events occurring before the genetic changes are responsible for the cancer initiation and progression. It has been confirmed that disruption of the normal epigenetic processes promotes lung carcinogenesis and lung tumor growth through complicated mechanisms involving TSGs silencing and oncogene activation. Majority of these disruptions are found to be the consequence of exposure to environmental carcinogens, particularly from cigarette smoking causing heritable epigenetic changes. The management of aberrant epigenetic states as a way to target early lung cancer development or lung tumor progression is therefore a logical therapeutic approach.

In the future, to develop new anti-tumor agents, such as DNMTi or HDACi, and the specific treatment strategies including tumor-targeted drug delivery system and specific administration routes, and to avoid the non-specific toxicity of anti-cancer drugs, will be of particular interest. Indeed, the side effects of these epigenetic compounds may have unscheduled consequences in terms of gene expression, in that they may display growth-promoting effects on tumor cells. As more critical miRNAs are found and the expression of many of them reduced in lung cancer cells, targeting miRNA is becoming a promising strategy in terms of cancer treatment. Administration of synthetic oligonucleotides that mimic endogenous miRNAs might be used to treat specific tumor types if an effective delivery system can be developed. Moreover, targeting oncogenic miRNAs through administration of anti-sense oligonucleotides, called anti-miRNA oligonucleotides (AMO) is coming into focus, given that the use of antagomirs, which are AMOs conjugated with cholesterol, has emerged as an efficient approach to inhibit miRNA activity (105). Further studies to uncover the potential usefulness of chromatin modifying drugs in restoring the loss of expression of tumor suppressor miRNAs are underway. There is no doubt that a more comprehensive dissection of the cellular and molecular pathways controlled by epigenetic processes will provide new insights into cancer related mechanisms and will highlight promising fields for the development of novel therapies to fight lung cancer.

3. A preclinical study to use demethylating agent to treat orthotopic human lung cancer xenografts

Lung cancer has remained as the number one cause of cancer-related deaths worldwide for decades (106). Traditional methods are mainly non-specific cytotoxic radiation therapy and chemotherapy; their non-specificity and therefore, life-threatening toxicity determined their limitation in the application. There is an urgent need to develop more sensitive diagnosis and more effective therapeutic methods to save lung cancer patients. About 90% of lung cancer cases are the end result of cumulative aberrant epigenetic changes and genetic damage to the respiratory epithelium chronically exposed to environmental, particularly tobacco carcinogens (107-109). One of the well accepted mechanisms of carcinogenesis in lung cancer is the aberrant methylation of CpG islands in the promoter regions of tumor suppressor genes (TSGs) leading to underexpression or absence of the proteins of those genes thus propagating tumorigenesis (110).

It has also been proved that the promoter hypermethylation down regulated TSGs can be reversed by DNA-methyltransferase inhibitors (DMTI) like azacytidine (Aza), Aza-2′-deoxycytidine, and Zebularine (11, 111, 112). These agents have been in clinical treatment for NSCLC patients by systemic administration with high doses and limited efficacy.

Inhalation of carcinogens, mainly as a result of tobacco exposure, causes a field cancerization effect thereby placing the entire bronchial epithelium at risk of developing bronchogenic carcinoma. Any strategies that aim at decreasing the incidence of lung cancer or decreasing the incidence of a second primary in a patient with a history of lung cancer would have to have an effect on the entire bronchial epithelium. In the case of a pharmacologic agent, this would be possible and feasible by inhalation of aerosolized solution of the drug. DMTI agents like Aza have the potential to reexpress tumor suppressor genes, which might lead to reversal of premalignant changes, slow the carcinogenesis process, and eventually decrease the incidence of bronchogenic carcinoma (113). Systemic administration of these drugs has been explored in advanced NSCLC patients but not pursued because of significant systemic toxicity (114).

In this part we present a study with two objectives: 1. To prove that whether reversing the hypermethylation in promoter region of the TSGs can make a positive contribution to the therapeutic outcome of lung cancer. 2. To prove whether the airway administration more effective than systemic administration to treat airway localized advanced bronchial premalignancy or endobronchial lung cancer. In this study, we used intratarcheal injection of Aza to treat the orthotopic lung cancer models in mice, the low dose (non-cytotoxic dose) we used mainly brought demethylating effect of Aza and avoided its cytotoxic effect.

3.1 Experimental design and methods

In order to prove whether demethylation on the hypermethylated promoters of TSGs will contribute therapeutic efficacy in the preclinical level, we tested the demethylation function of a typical demethylation agent azacytidine (Aza) in vitro and in vivo. Particularly, we

used intratracheal injection of Aza to treat orthotopic lung cancer xenografts in the efficacy study. The detailed experimental studies are presented below.
We selected three different human non-small cell lung cancer cell lines for the in vitro and in vivo studies: a squamous cell carcinoma cell line H226, a bronchioalveolar carcinoma cell line H358, and a metastatic large cell carcinoma H460 from pleural effusion. All cell lines were purchased from American Type Culture Collection (ATCC, Manassas, VA) and cultured per ATCC's protocols.

3.1.1 In vitro studies

In order to distinguish the cytotoxic effect and demethylation effect of Aza, we used MTT assay to determine the growth inhibition range of Aza and methylation-specific PCR with the samples treated by a set concentrations of Aza to detect the minimal concentration for the effective demethylation at the promoter region of TSGs. MTT assay used was literature method (115), briefly, ~5,000 cells in 0.135 μL RPMI 1640/well were seeded in 96-well plates. After 24 h of culture, Aza at various concentrations was added to the cells. Three days later, the cells were stained with 3-(4,5-dimethylthiazol-2-yl)-2,5-diphenyltetrazolium bromide (MTT) and lysed. The absorbance of each well was measured in a microplate reader at 570 nm. The percent growth inhibition of the cells was calculated as the absorbance of treated cells normalized to no treatment cells.
We selected RASSF1a as the first candidate TSG to prove the concept. Because it was found silenced by promoter hypermethylation in 32.6% of NSCLC patients (116). The human NSCLC cells H226 were treated with Aza at 0.1, 1, and 10 ng/ml. On day 4 after the treatment, the cells were harvested. About 8 x 10^4 cells were used to detect the methylation status of the RASSF1a promoter using EZ DNA Methylation-Direct Kit™ (Zymo Research Corp., Orange, CA, USA), according to the manufacturer's instructions. The bisulfate-converted DNA was then used as a template for methylation-specific PCR reactions using primers specific for either the modified methylated or modified unmethylated promoter sequences of the RASSF1a genes. The primers used have been described previously by others (117). The sequences are: methylated: 5'-GGG TTT TGC GAG AGC GCG-3' (forward) and 5'-GCT AAC AAA CGC GAA CCG-3'(reverse); unmethylated: 5'-GGT TTT GTG AGA GTG TGT TTA G-3'(forward), and 5'-CAC TAA CAA ACA CAA ACC AAA C-3'(reverse). Briefly, PCR reactions contained 1-4 microliters of bisulfate-converted DNA, purified as above, 300 ng each of forward and reverse primers, 45 microliters of Platinum® PCR SuperMix (Invitrogen), and distilled water to a final reaction volume of 50 microliters. PCR amplification conditions were as described in the literature (117), unless otherwise noted. The PCR products were separated on 2% agarose gels containing ethidium bromide and were visualized under UV illumination.

3.1.2 Animal studies

The studies were begun from testing acute toxicity and finding the therapeutic dose. CD-1 mice (Harlan) were used to evaluate and compare the acute toxicities of Aza by the intratracheal or intravenous routes. Two groups of mice (5-8 mice/group) were treated with 90 mg/kg of Aza via intravenous injection (IV) or intratracheal injection (IT), respectively. The dose of 90 mg/kg is the maximum tolerated dose (MTD) of IV Aza in mice. The IV and IT injection methods were described previously (12, 118). Briefly, for the IT the mice were anesthesized with intraperitoneal injection of 30-50 mg/kg of Nembutal or isoflurane inhalation, fixed on the small animal fixing board. The mouth of mouse was open with a forceps; the drug solution or cell suspension was carefully injected into the trachea through mouth via a 22-gage feeding needle attached to a 1 ml syringe. The injection volume did not exceed 100 µl/mouse. If necessary, a "tube" type of light inserting into the mouth can be used to help locate the trachea.

For myelotoxicity assessment, blood (100 µl/mouse, 5 mice/group) was drawn from the tail vein before treatment (at day 0) and on days 4, 7, 14, and 28 after treatment. Red blood cells (RBC) were removed from the blood samples using RBC lysis buffer (eBioscience San Diego, CA) as per the manufacturer's protocol. White blood cells (WBC) were collected and counted with a hematocytometer under a microscope. Blood samples from mice without treatment were used as controls. In the organ toxicity studies, groups of mice given IT of Lactated Ringer's Solution or without treatment were used as vehicle and normal controls, respectively. Creatinine levels, and liver function tests were determined at Antech Diagnosis (Lake Success, NY). Organ pathological examination was performed at different time points. Briefly, 5 mice in each group were euthanized on day 4, 7, 14, and 28 days after administration of the drug. Blood was drawn from the caudal vena cava, and lungs, livers and kidneys were resected and fixed with 10% buffered Formalin. The fixed tissues were processed with standard procedure for H&E staining. The toxicity levels were determined by giving toxicity grade to each tissue sample. The grading based on the general pathology guidelines was 0 to 4, they reflect a percentage of damaged tissue of 0, <10 (mild), 10-30 (moderate), 30-60 (severe), >60 (life threaten), respectively.

To mimic human NSCLC, we developed a mouse model by intratracheal inoculation of human lung cancer cells in nude mice (12). Briefly, the nude mice (in this particular example, male and female NCRNU-M-F nude mice, 6-7 weeks old, purchased from Taconic Farms, Germantown, NY) were given tumor inoculation with 2~5 x 10^6 cells/mouse by IT described above. In this model, we found that the cancer cells initially attached on the airway epithelium of the mice and survived (from day 0 to 10), and then they formed micro nodules in the airway (from day 7 to 21), and finally the tumors invaded lung tissue (from day 14 to 35). The tumors mainly remain in the lung during the rest of lifetime of the mice, and the animal on average die on day 45 to 70 from the lung tumor burden (13). This model mimics the human NSCLCs that develop on the airway epithelium before they invade the lung parenchyma, and it is one of human lung cancer relevant models to evaluate lung cancer therapeutics by different administration routes, particularly by airway administration.

In the antitumor efficacy test, we used a relative low dose of Aza with intratracheal injection to avoid the cytotoxic effect and emphasize the demethylation effect of Aza. Ten days after the intratracheal tumor inoculation, the nude mice were randomly divided into 3 groups of 5 mice each in each test, and were treated with daily intravenous injection (IV) of Aza at 6.25 mg/kg/day x 6 doses or intratracheal injection (IT) of Aza at 2.5 mg/kg/every other day x 3 doses. The IT used the same method of the tumor inoculation described above. These optimal doses for the therapeutic study were determined in prior dose ranging studies. A group of mice without treatment was used as control. Survival was used as the major endpoint to evaluate efficacy.

The same Aza formulation was used for the IT and IV treatment. It was made by dissolving azacytidine powder (Sigma, St Louis, MO) in Lactated Ringer's Injection (Hospira, Inc., Lake Forest, IL) and passing the solution through 0.22 µm filter immediately prior to use.

3.1.3 Statistical analysis

Differences among different groups were analyzed by two-side Log Rank Assay. A difference was considered statistically significant when $p < 0.05$.

3.2 Results

3.2.1 Growth inhibition and demethylation function of Aza in human NSCLC cell lines

Aza has the both functions. In order to know whether Aza's demethylation effect can function at a non-toxic concentration, we measured its cell growth inhibition and demethylation function in the selected human NSCLC cell lines. We found that Aza inhibited the growth of the NSCLC cells in a dose dependent manner as shown in Figure 1. The 50% inhibitory concentrations (IC50) of Aza were 0.6, 3.4, and 4.9 μg/ml in H226, H358, and H460 cells, respectively. In this study, Aza at a concentration below 0.6 μg/ml did not cause significant growth inhibition in all tested cell lines.

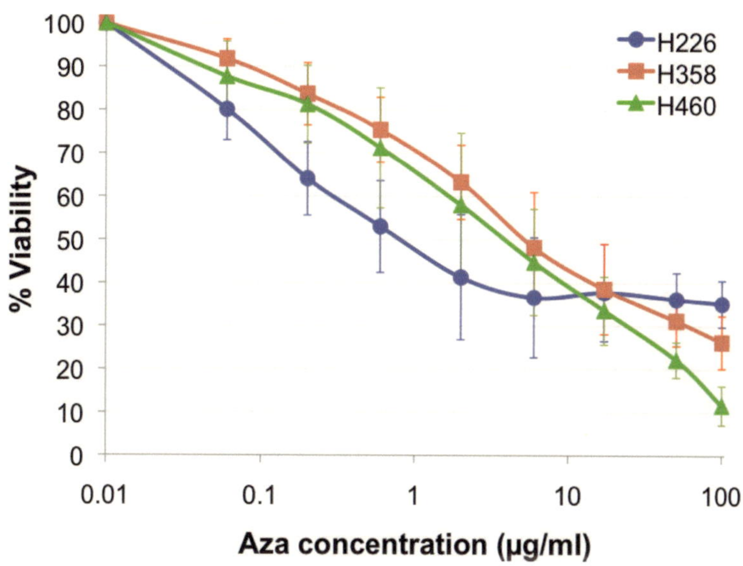

Fig. 1. Growth inhibition of Aza on human NSCLC cell lines. H226, H358, and H460 cells were treated with (5-fold) increasing concentrations of Aza. The percentage of growth inhibition was measured with MTT Assay. The data for each cell line are mean ± standard deviation obtained from 3 independent experiments.

The demethylation function of Aza were detect by a methylation-specific PCR method in the H226 NSCLC cell line at a very low concentration range (0.1 ~ 10 ng/ml). As shown in Figure 2, the unmethylated band (#5) of the promoter of RASSF1a gene was found in the H226 cells at the lowest concentration of 0.1 ng/ml, which is 6000-fold lower than the IC50 of Aza in the same cell line. This indicates that when directly exposing lung cancer cells to Aza, Aza can function as effective demethylation agent at an extremely low concentration without causing any direct cytotoxicity.

3.2.2 Intratracheal administration of Aza results in significantly reduced toxicity

Myelosuppression is the dose-limiting toxicity of intravenously administered Aza when used clinically. In this study, we compared the myelotoxicity of IT and IV Aza at the same dose, 90 mg/kg that is MTD when using IV administration. IT Aza produced significantly less myelotoxicity than IV Aza at the MTD of IV Aza. As shown in Figure 3, IV Aza significantly reduced the total WBC by > 68% on day 4 and 7 ($p < 0.004$) and >38% on day 14 ($p < 0.006$), the WBC count recovered to about 90% of the normal level on day 28. While the only detectable WBC reduction in IT Aza treated mice was about 13% on day 7 ($p < 0.01$). The recovery was faster (on day 14) and complete (>97% of the normal level, $p > 0.5$) compared with IV Aza (Figure 3).

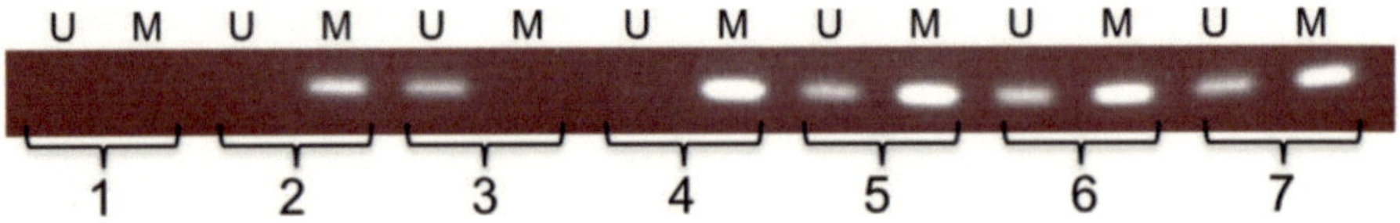

Fig. 2. The demethylation function of Aza in the NSCLC cells. H226 human NSCLC cells (8×10^4 cells) were treated with Aza at 0.1, 1, and 10 ng/ml. The methylation status of the RASSF1a promoter was detected by methylation-specific PCR method using the EZ DNA Methylation-Direct Kit. The pair of bands from 1 to 3 are samples of water, methylated DNA control, and unmethylated DNA control; from 4 to 7 are samples of H226 cells treated with Aza at 0, 0.1, 1, and 10 ng/ml, respectively. The letters "U" and "M" represent unmethylated and methylated detection, respectively.

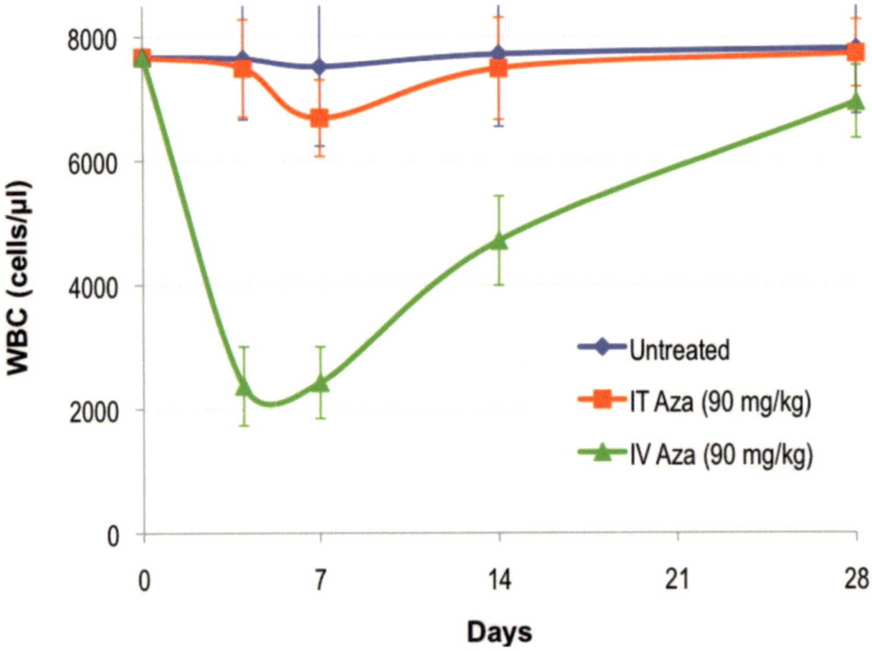

Fig. 3. IT administration of Aza is 5-fold less myelosuppression compared to IV Aza. Aza was administered IT (round dots) or IV (triangle dots) at a dose of 90 mg/kg. Control mice were not given any treatment (square dots). Blood was drawn on day 0, 4, 7, 14, and 28 after treatment. WBC was counted after removal of red blood cells. The data of each group (5-8 mice each) are mean ± standard deviation.

To know whether the IT Aza will cause the locoregional toxicity or systemic toxicity in other organs, an organ toxicity study in a scope of acute toxicity of IT Aza were performed and the IV Aza was used as comparison. At the MTD, the results of serum liver function tests and serum creatinine measurements were normal for all mice and there were no differences among the groups of IT Aza, IV Aza, and no treatment (data not shown). On histopathological evaluation, no liver or kidney toxicities were identified in any treatment group (data not shown). By lung histological evaluation, moderate pulmonary toxicity was observed in all 5 animals in the IT Aza group on day 7 but not at the other time points. Of note is that the IT dose used in these experiments is 12-fold higher dose than the optimized total dose used in the therapeutic experiments. The lung toxicity was described as moderate pneumonitis, characterized by type II pneumocyte hypertrophy, neutrophilic infiltration, and lymphohistiocytic inflammation (Figure 4, photograph 2). As stated, no pulmonary

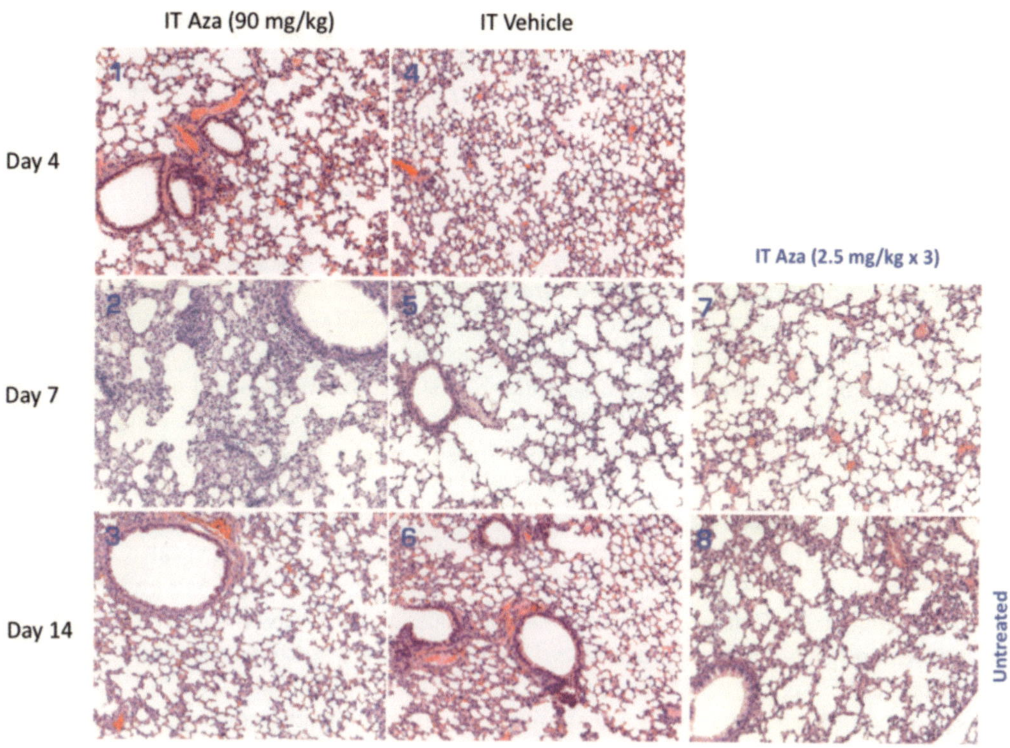

Fig. 4. IT Aza at the therapeutic dose does not produce pulmonary toxicity. ICR mice were intratracheally injected with 90 mg/kg of Aza, 2.5 mg/kg qod x 3 of Aza, or the equal volume of vehicle (Lactated Ringer's Injection). The lungs of mice were resected on day 4, 7, and 14 after injection. Standard H & E staining of lung tissues was used to assess pulmonary toxicity. Photographs 1 to 6 are the lungs from mice receiving 90 mg/kg of IT Aza (1~3) or the same volume of IT vehicle (4~6). Photograph 7 is the lung from mice receiving the therapeutic dose of IT Aza (2.5 mg/kg, qod x 3) on day 7 post the final injection. Photograph 8 is the lung from untreated mice.

toxicity was observed in animals treated with IT Aza on days 4 or 14. At the optimal therapeutic dose (2.5 mg/kg, qod x 3), IT Aza did not cause lung toxicity (Figure 4, photograph 7) and any other toxicity (data not shown). The pulmonary toxicity grades are listed in Table 1. These results indicate that the pulmonary toxicity caused by IT Aza at supratherapeutic doses (the MTD of IV Aza) is moderate (photograph 2) and reversible within 2 weeks (photograph 3). IT Aza at the therapeutic dose, IT vehicle, and IV Aza (data not shown) did not cause detectable pulmonary toxicity.

Day	**4**	**7**	**14**	**28**
IT Aza (90 mg/kg)	0*	2*	0*	0
IT Aza (2.5 mg/kg x 3)	0	0*	0	0
IT Vehicle	0*	0*	0*	0
IV Aza (90 mg/kg)	0	0	0	0
No Treatment	0	0*	0	0

* histopathological photographs are shown in Figure 3.

Table 1. Toxicity grade of lungs of the mice treated with IT Aza

3.2.3 Intratracheal administration of Aza significantly prolonged the survival of mice bearing orthotopic human NSCLC xenografts

To evaluate the efficacy of IT Aza in clinically relevant NSCLC models, we inoculated the human NSCLC cell lines H266, H358, and H460 into the lungs of nude mice via the trachea. These models mimic closely orthotopic human NSCLC. In mice, small mucosal tumor nodules are evident at 1-3 weeks after the inoculation of tumor cells. In the absence of any intervention, the mice succumb to the tumor in 6-10 weeks. The survival curve in these models closely correlates with the tumor burden (13), and can be utilized as an endpoint for the evaluation of treatment efficacy.

Treatments were initiated on day 10 post tumor inoculation. The survival observed in mice treated with IT Aza was compared to that in mice treated with IV Aza and untreated tumor-bearing mice. Animals in each treatment group were given multiple injections; these doses and schedules were optimized in a preliminary study (data not shown). The total dose was 7.5 mg/kg for IT Aza (2.5 mg/kg, qod x 3) and 37.5 mg/kg for IV Aza (6.25 mg/kg, qd x 6). Both dose levels are significantly lower than the corresponding MTD's. Results are shown in Figure 5. IV Aza had limited efficacy against three lung cancer models at the optimal therapeutic dose: the median survival increased by 10% in H226 model (72 vs. 67), , and 22% in the H358 model (73 vs. 60 days, $p > 0.05$) and 60% in the H460 model (80 vs. 50 days, $p < 0.01$), whereas IT Aza demonstrated significantly increased efficacy: the median survival increased by 107% (139 vs. 67), 63%, (98 vs. 60 days, $p < 0.006$), and 142% (121 vs. 50 days, $p < 0.002$) in the H226, H358, and H460 model, respectively. The increased lifespan (%ILS) (119) of IT Aza treated mice bearing H226, H358, or H460 lung tumors was 3.2- to 8.6-fold higher than that of IV Aza treated mice (96.2% vs. 11.2%; 75.8% vs. 21.5%; 131.3% vs. 40.7%). The efficacy of each treatment is summarized in Table 2.

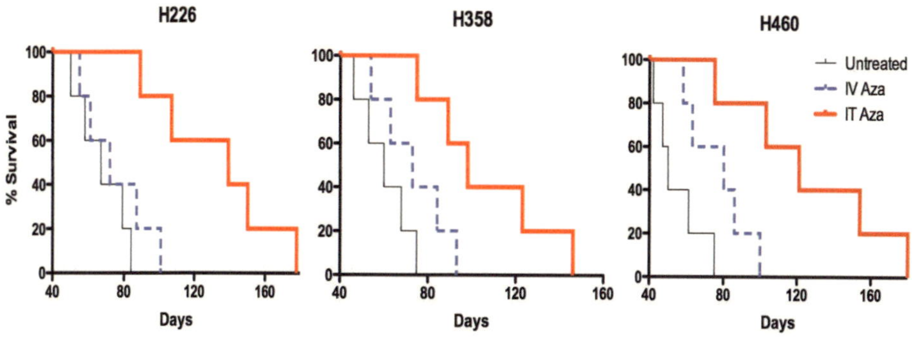

Fig. 5. Intratracheal administration of low dose Aza significantly prolongs survival of mice bearing orthotopic human NSCLC xenografts. Mice intratracheally inoculated with H226 (left), H358 (middle), or H460 (right) human NSCLC cell lines were treated with IT Aza (thick line) or IV Aza (dash line) on day 10 at a dose of 2.5 mg/kg qod x 3 for IT and 6.25 mg/kg daily x 6 for IV. The control was a group of untreated mice (thin line).

		No treatment	IV	IT	IT vs. V	P value
H226	**Median Survival** (Range)	67 (50~84)	72 (55~101)	139 (89~178)	1.93	0.016
	%ILS	0	11.2	96.2	8.59	
H358	**Median Survival** (Range)	60 (46~75)	73 (54~93)	98 (75~146)	1.34	0.018
	%ILS	0	21.5	75.8	3.52	
H460	**Median Survival** (Range)	50 (42~75)	80 (58~100)	121 (75~183)	1.51	0.005
	%ILS	0	40.7	131.3	3.23	

Table 2. Efficacy summary

3.3 Discussion

Azacytidine (Aza) is approved by the Food and Drug Administration for the treatment of myelodysplastic syndromes (11), a preleukemic condition, and has potential for the treatment of other cancers and premalignant conditions as a result of a cytotoxic effect, a DNA demethylating effect, or both. As a cytotoxic agent in proliferating cells, Aza can disrupt RNA metabolism, DNA synthesis, and protein synthesis. Particularly, Aza is incorporated into DNA and inhibits DNA methyltransferases and causes hypomethylation of replicating DNA (120, 121) which can result in re-expression of tumor suppressor genes silenced by hypermethylation. From 1973 to 1977, there were at least 9 clinical studies in solid tumor patients with intravenous Aza, which included 78 lung cancer patients (122). The therapeutic efficacy observed was limited, possibly due to two major reasons: First, the studies were performed in advanced lung cancer patients where reversal of hypermethylation per se may not be sufficient to have a therapeutic impact; second, all the studies were done using systemic administration or a sub-optimal dose schedule, which limits the use of these agents as a result of systemic toxicity. The studies presented here were designed to provide the foundation for the potential use of a regional demethylation strategy for malignant or premalignant conditions of the bronchial epithelium in which DNA hypermethylation plays an important role. We used Aza as a model compound and tested its toxicity and antitumor efficacy by direct delivery in the respiratory airways via the trachea in models of endobronchial human NSCLC. Our studies demonstrate that IT Aza produced a 5-fold reduced myelosuppression (as assessed by WBC nadir) than IV Aza at a dose equivalent to the IV MTD and 3-fold higher antitumor efficacy (as assessed by %ILS) at a dose 5-fold lower than that of IV Aza, the end-result being a 75-fold increased therapeutic index. These results justify continuing exploring regional demethylating therapy for the treatment of malignant or premalignant conditions of the lungs that are easily accessible through the airways, including advanced premalignancy, bronchioalveolar carcinoma, and small parenchymal metastatic disease.

Lung cancers develop in the epithelium in direct contact with the airways because carcinogens reach the lungs through inhalation. Bronchial premalignancy, carcinoma in situ, small primary or metastatic tumors, and some cases of BAC are theoretically more accessible via the endobronchial space than through the bloodstream. Aerosol approaches to the treatment or prevention of these conditions are therefore a more logical therapeutic strategy than systemic treatment. However, in the present studies we used intratracheal administration rather than aerosol administration because the purpose was proof of concept and administration of drugs by aerosolization to mice is inefficient. The major difference between these two types of drug administration (IT vs. aerosol) would be a higher distribution of the drug to the alveolar space with aerosol administration. We are currently conducting studies to validate the results presented here using the clinically available formulation of Aza administered by aerosolization to mice.

Our toxicity studies demonstrate, as expected, that Aza given IT results in a 5-fold reduced myelosuppression, which is the dose-limiting toxicity of IV Aza. Most importantly, IT Aza at 90 mg/kg only caused moderate pulmonary inflammation on day 7 after IT administration. It was encouraging to see that there was no evidence of lung inflammation on day 14 post IT Aza, even when the dose used for IT was as high as the maximum tolerated dose using the IV route. In the efficacy experiments, the optimal total IT dose used was 12 fold lower, a dose did not cause any pulmonary toxicity. To confirm this, we are currently performing more refined lung toxicity studies in the context of our current therapeutic experiments using aerosolized administration.

In the efficacy experiments, the efficacy (%ILS) of IT Aza at a 5-fold lower dose was 3.2- to 8.6-fold superior to that of IV Aza in mice with endobronchial H226, H358, or H460 tumors. These results indicate that the regional administration route into the airways is more efficient than the intravenous route for the treatment of endobronchial tumors. The main therapeutic potential of airway-administered Aza is secondary prevention of NSCLC due to the field cancerization effect of inhaled carcinogens via tobacco smoke. The proposed mechanism would be hypomethylation of CpG islands of the promoter regions of tumor suppressor genes thereby inhibiting development of dysplasia and progression of dysplasia to cancer. In these studies, we used a mouse model of endobronchial tumors but not dysplasia. We are currently developing an animal model of lung premalignancy in mice by exposing them to tobacco carcinogens directly into the upper airways. We plan to test the ability of aerosolized Aza in reversing tumor suppressor gene hypermethylation in this model.

In these studies, the efficacy endpoint was survival secondary to antitumor effect in models of malignancy. In the anticipated clinical scenario, the intermediate efficacy endpoint would be changes in hypermethylation patterns or effective gene reexpression. In this study, the optimal therapeutic dose was 12-fold lower than the maximum tolerated dose (MTD). This finding suggests that this strategy may have a large therapeutic window and that the risk of acute or chronic side effects might be very low if these agents were used at optimal doses rather than MTD. Therefore, determining optimal doses based on pharmacodynamic assessments in patients enrolled in clinical studies with this new therapeutic strategy are essential to minimize the potential side effects. Particularly, the potential carcinogenicity of this approach could become an important limitation if benefit was demonstrated but required chronic administration of unnecessarily high doses of these agents. Therefore, in the context of our initial Phase I clinical study of inhaled Aza we intend to monitor methylation patterns as well as gene reexpression in the target tissue pre and post-therapy to establish an optimal dose based on target effects rather than a maximum tolerated dose.

In vitro, we have proved that Aza can effectively demethylate the hypermethylation in the promoter of tumor suppressor gene at a non-toxic concentration. In vivo, we found that IT Aza are effective against experimental lung cancer by prolonging the life of the mice bearing orthotopic lung tumors without causing any detectable systemic or locoregional toxicity. Here the functions of both the epigenetic effect and the locoregional administration played an important role. We believe that the lung-specific epigenetic treatment with Aza has great potential to reduce the tumor burden by reversing the hypermethylation in the promoters of the tumor suppressor genes and therefore reactivating the silenced genes. This is an important project to be further studied.

4. Acknowledgment

Grant Support: U.S. National Cancer Institute Grants 5R21 CA104297-02 (Yiyu Zou) and 5R01CA154755-02 (Roman Perez-Soler and Yiyu Zou).

5. References

[1] Jemal A, Bray F, Center MM, Ferlay J, Ward E, Forman D. Global cancer statistics. CA Cancer J Clin 2011 Mar-Apr;61(2):69-90.

[2] Sharma S, Kelly TK, Jones PA. Epigenetics in cancer. Carcinogenesis 2010 Jan;31(1):27-36.

[3] Vogelstein B, Kinzler KW. Cancer genes and the pathways they control. Nat Med 2004 Aug;10(8):789-99.

[4] Knudson AG, Jr. Mutation and cancer: statistical study of retinoblastoma. Proc Natl Acad Sci U S A 1971 Apr;68(4):820-3.

[5] Benedict WF, Murphree AL, Banerjee A, Spina CA, Sparkes MC, Sparkes RS. Patient with 13 chromosome deletion: evidence that the retinoblastoma gene is a recessive cancer gene. Science 1983 Feb 25;219(4587):973-5.

[6] Baker SJ, Fearon ER, Nigro JM, *et al.* Chromosome 17 deletions and p53 gene mutations in colorectal carcinomas. Science 1989 Apr 14;244(4901):217-21.

[7] Baker SJ, Markowitz S, Fearon ER, Willson JK, Vogelstein B. Suppression of human colorectal carcinoma cell growth by wild-type p53. Science 1990 Aug 24;249(4971):912-5.

[8] Roth JA, Nguyen D, Lawrence DD, *et al.* Retrovirus-mediated wild-type p53 gene transfer to tumors of patients with lung cancer. Nat Med 1996 Sep;2(9):985-91.
[9] Kim DS, Kim MJ, Lee JY, Kim YZ, Kim EJ, Park JY. Aberrant methylation of E-cadherin and H-cadherin genes in nonsmall cell lung cancer and its relation to clinicopathologic features. Cancer 2007 Dec 15;110(12):2785-92.
[10] Seng TJ, Currey N, Cooper WA, *et al.* DLEC1 and MLH1 promoter methylation are associated with poor prognosis in non-small cell lung carcinoma. British Journal of Cancer 2008 Jul 22;99(2):375-82.
[11] Kaminskas E, Farrell AT, Wang YC, Sridhara R, Pazdur R. FDA drug approval summary: azacitidine (5-azacytidine, Vidaza) for injectable suspension. Oncologist 2005 Mar;10(3):176-82.
[12] Zou Y, Zong G, Ling YH, *et al.* Effective treatment of early endobronchial cancer with regional administration of liposome-p53 complexes. J Natl Cancer Inst 1998 Aug 5;90(15):1130-7.
[13] Zou Y, Zong G, Ling YH, Perez-Soler R. Development of cationic liposome formulations for intratracheal gene therapy of early lung cancer. Cancer Gene Ther 2000 May;7(5):683-96.
[14] Feinberg AP, Ohlsson R, Henikoff S. The epigenetic progenitor origin of human cancer. Nature Reviews Genetics 2006 Jan;7(1):21-33.
[15] Weber M, Hellmann I, Stadler MB, *et al.* Distribution, silencing potential and evolutionary impact of promoter DNA methylation in the human genome. Nat Genet 2007 Apr;39(4):457-66.
[16] Li E, Bestor TH, Jaenisch R. Targeted mutation of the DNA methyltransferase gene results in embryonic lethality. Cell 1992 Jun 12;69(6):915-26.
[17] Li E, Beard C, Jaenisch R. Role for DNA methylation in genomic imprinting. Nature 1993 Nov 25;366(6453):362-5.
[18] Heard E, Clerc P, Avner P. X-chromosome inactivation in mammals. Annu Rev Genet 1997;31:571-610.
[19] Belinsky SA, Palmisano WA, Gilliland FD, *et al.* Aberrant promoter methylation in bronchial epithelium and sputum from current and former smokers. Cancer Res 2002 Apr 15;62(8):2370-7.
[20] Belinsky SA, Nikula KJ, Palmisano WA, *et al.* Aberrant methylation of p16(INK4a) is an early event in lung cancer and a potential biomarker for early diagnosis. Proc Natl Acad Sci U S A 1998 Sep 29;95(20):11891-6.
[21] Sato M, Mori Y, Sakurada A, Fujimura S, Horii A. The H-cadherin (CDH13) gene is inactivated in human lung cancer. Hum Genet 1998 Jul;103(1):96-101.
[22] Osada H, Tatematsu Y, Yatabe Y, *et al.* Frequent and histological type-specific inactivation of 14-3-3sigma in human lung cancers. Oncogene 2002 Apr 4;21(15):2418-24.
[23] Tang X, Khuri FR, Lee JJ, *et al.* Hypermethylation of the death-associated protein (DAP) kinase promoter and aggressiveness in stage I non-small-cell lung cancer. J Natl Cancer Inst 2000 Sep 20;92(18):1511-6.
[24] Dammann R, Li C, Yoon JH, Chin PL, Bates S, Pfeifer GP. Epigenetic inactivation of a RAS association domain family protein from the lung tumour suppressor locus 3p21.3. Nat Genet 2000 Jul;25(3):315-9.

[25] Hopkins-Donaldson S, Ziegler A, Kurtz S, *et al.* Silencing of death receptor and caspase-8 expression in small cell lung carcinoma cell lines and tumors by DNA methylation. Cell Death Differ 2003 Mar;10(3):356-64.

[26] Zochbauer-Muller S, Fong KM, Virmani AK, Geradts J, Gazdar AF, Minna JD. Aberrant promoter methylation of multiple genes in non-small cell lung cancers. Cancer Res 2001 Jan 1;61(1):249-55.

[27] Lin R-K, Hsu H-S, Chang J-W, Chen C-Y, Chen J-T, Wang Y-C. Alteration of DNA methyltransferases contributes to 5'CpG methylation and poor prognosis in lung cancer. Lung Cancer 2007 Feb;55(2):205-13.

[28] Kim H, Kwon YM, Kim JS, *et al.* Elevated mRNA levels of DNA methyltransferase-1 as an independent prognostic factor in primary nonsmall cell lung cancer. Cancer 2006 Sep 1;107(5):1042-9.

[29] Heller G, Zielinski CC, Zochbauer-Muller S. Lung cancer: from single-gene methylation to methylome profiling. Cancer Metastasis Rev 2010 Mar;29(1):95-107.

[30] Brena RM, Morrison C, Liyanarachchi S, *et al.* Aberrant DNA methylation of OLIG1, a novel prognostic factor in non-small cell lung cancer. PLoS Med 2007 Mar 27;4(3):e108.

[31] Rauch TA, Zhong X, Wu X, *et al.* High-resolution mapping of DNA hypermethylation and hypomethylation in lung cancer. Proc Natl Acad Sci U S A 2008 Jan 8;105(1):252-7.

[32] Shames DS, Girard L, Gao B, *et al.* A genome-wide screen for promoter methylation in lung cancer identifies novel methylation markers for multiple malignancies. PLoS Med 2006 Dec;3(12):e486.

[33] Zhong S, Fields CR, Su N, Pan YX, Robertson KD. Pharmacologic inhibition of epigenetic modifications, coupled with gene expression profiling, reveals novel targets of aberrant DNA methylation and histone deacetylation in lung cancer. Oncogene 2007 Apr 19;26(18):2621-34.

[34] Tornaletti S, Pfeifer GP. Complete and tissue-independent methylation of CpG sites in the p53 gene: implications for mutations in human cancers. Oncogene 1995 Apr 20;10(8):1493-9.

[35] Jones PA, Rideout WM, 3rd, Shen JC, Spruck CH, Tsai YC. Methylation, mutation and cancer. Bioessays 1992 Jan;14(1):33-6.

[36] Lee SJ, Jeon HS, Jang JS, *et al.* DNMT3B polymorphisms and risk of primary lung cancer. Carcinogenesis 2005 Feb;26(2):403-9.

[37] Shen H, Wang L, Spitz MR, Hong WK, Mao L, Wei Q. A novel polymorphism in human cytosine DNA-methyltransferase-3B promoter is associated with an increased risk of lung cancer. Cancer Res 2002 Sep 1;62(17):4992-5.

[38] Smith LE, Denissenko MF, Bennett WP, *et al.* Targeting of lung cancer mutational hotspots by polycyclic aromatic hydrocarbons. J Natl Cancer Inst 2000 May 17;92(10):803-11.

[39] Yoon JH, Smith LE, Feng Z, Tang M, Lee CS, Pfeifer GP. Methylated CpG dinucleotides are the preferential targets for G-to-T transversion mutations induced by benzo[a]pyrene diol epoxide in mammalian cells: similarities with the p53 mutation spectrum in smoking-associated lung cancers. Cancer Res 2001 Oct 1;61(19):7110-7.

[40] Denissenko MF, Chen JX, Tang MS, Pfeifer GP. Cytosine methylation determines hot spots of DNA damage in the human P53 gene. Proc Natl Acad Sci U S A 1997 Apr 15;94(8):3893-8.

[41] Magewu AN, Jones PA. Ubiquitous and tenacious methylation of the CpG site in codon 248 of the p53 gene may explain its frequent appearance as a mutational hot spot in human cancer. Mol Cell Biol 1994 Jun;14(6):4225-32.

[42] Kim H, Kwon YM, Kim JS, *et al.* Tumor-specific methylation in bronchial lavage for the early detection of non-small-cell lung cancer. J Clin Oncol 2004 Jun 15;22(12):2363-70.

[43] Liu Y, Lan Q, Siegfried JM, Luketich JD, Keohavong P. Aberrant promoter methylation of p16 and MGMT genes in lung tumors from smoking and never-smoking lung cancer patients. Neoplasia 2006 Jan;8(1):46-51.

[44] Vaissiere T, Hung RJ, Zaridze D, *et al.* Quantitative analysis of DNA methylation profiles in lung cancer identifies aberrant DNA methylation of specific genes and its association with gender and cancer risk factors. Cancer Res 2009 Jan 1;69(1):243-52.

[45] Buckingham L, Penfield Faber L, Kim A, *et al.* PTEN, RASSF1 and DAPK site-specific hypermethylation and outcome in surgically treated stage I and II nonsmall cell lung cancer patients. Int J Cancer 2010 Apr 1;126(7):1630-9.

[46] Kaira K, Sunaga N, Tomizawa Y, *et al.* Epigenetic inactivation of the RAS-effector gene RASSF2 in lung cancers. Int J Oncol 2007 Jul;31(1):169-73.

[47] Tessema M, Yu YY, Stidley CA, *et al.* Concomitant promoter methylation of multiple genes in lung adenocarcinomas from current, former and never smokers. Carcinogenesis 2009 Jul;30(7):1132-8.

[48] de Fraipont F, Moro-Sibilot D, Michelland S, Brambilla E, Brambilla C, Favrot MC. Promoter methylation of genes in bronchial lavages: a marker for early diagnosis of primary and relapsing non-small cell lung cancer? Lung Cancer 2005 Nov;50(2):199-209.

[49] Zochbauer-Muller S, Lam S, Toyooka S, *et al.* Aberrant methylation of multiple genes in the upper aerodigestive tract epithelium of heavy smokers. Int J Cancer 2003 Nov 20;107(4):612-6.

[50] Palmisano WA, Divine KK, Saccomanno G, *et al.* Predicting lung cancer by detecting aberrant promoter methylation in sputum. Cancer Research 2000 Nov 1;60(21):5954-8.

[51] Lin Q, Geng J, Ma K, *et al.* RASSF1A, APC, ESR1, ABCB1 and HOXC9, but not p16INK4A, DAPK1, PTEN and MT1G genes were frequently methylated in the stage I non-small cell lung cancer in China. J Cancer Res Clin Oncol 2009 Dec;135(12):1675-84.

[52] Yano M, Toyooka S, Tsukuda K, *et al.* Aberrant promoter methylation of human DAB2 interactive protein (hDAB2IP) gene in lung cancers. Int J Cancer 2005 Jan 1;113(1):59-66.

[53] Kikuchi S, Yamada D, Fukami T, *et al.* Promoter methylation of DAL-1/4.1B predicts poor prognosis in non-small cell lung cancer. Clin Cancer Res 2005 Apr 15;11(8):2954-61.

[54] Chen H, Suzuki M, Nakamura Y, *et al.* Aberrant methylation of FBN2 in human non-small cell lung cancer. Lung Cancer 2005 Oct;50(1):43-9.

[55] Issa J-PJ. DNA methylation as a therapeutic target in cancer. Clinical Cancer Research 2007 Mar 15;13(6):1634-7.

[56] Momparler RL, Eliopoulos N, Ayoub J. Evaluation of an inhibitor of DNA methylation, 5-aza-2'-deoxycytidine, for the treatment of lung cancer and the future role of gene therapy. Adv Exp Med Biol 2000;465:433-46.
[57] Kopelovich L, Crowell JA, Fay JR. The epigenome as a target for cancer chemoprevention. Journal of the National Cancer Institute 2003 Dec 3;95(23):1747-57.
[58] Seligson DB, Horvath S, McBrian MA, *et al.* Global levels of histone modifications predict prognosis in different cancers. Am J Pathol 2009 May;174(5):1619-28.
[59] Fraga MF, Ballestar E, Villar-Garea A, *et al.* Loss of acetylation at Lys16 and trimethylation at Lys20 of histone H4 is a common hallmark of human cancer. Nat Genet 2005 Apr;37(4):391-400.
[60] Barlesi F, Giaccone G, Gallegos-Ruiz MI, *et al.* Global histone modifications predict prognosis of resected non small-cell lung cancer. J Clin Oncol 2007 Oct 1;25(28):4358-64.
[61] LaVoie HA. Epigenetic control of ovarian function: the emerging role of histone modifications. Mol Cell Endocrinol 2005 Nov 24;243(1-2):12-8.
[62] Esteller M. Cancer epigenomics: DNA methylomes and histone-modification maps. Nat Rev Genet 2007 Apr;8(4):286-98.
[63] Witt O, Deubzer HE, Milde T, Oehme I. HDAC family: What are the cancer relevant targets? Cancer Lett 2009 May 8;277(1):8-21.
[64] Sasaki H, Moriyama S, Nakashima Y, *et al.* Histone deacetylase 1 mRNA expression in lung cancer. Lung Cancer 2004 Nov;46(2):171-8.
[65] Bartling B, Hofmann HS, Boettger T, *et al.* Comparative application of antibody and gene array for expression profiling in human squamous cell lung carcinoma. Lung Cancer 2005 Aug;49(2):145-54.
[66] Osada H, Tatematsu Y, Saito H, Yatabe Y, Mitsudomi T, Takahashi T. Reduced expression of class II histone deacetylase genes is associated with poor prognosis in lung cancer patients. Int J Cancer 2004 Oct 20;112(1):26-32.
[67] Kodani M, Igishi T, Matsumoto S, *et al.* Suppression of phosphatidylinositol 3-kinase/Akt signaling pathway is a determinant of the sensitivity to a novel histone deacetylase inhibitor, FK228, in lung adenocarcinoma cells. Oncol Rep 2005 Mar;13(3):477-83.
[68] Yu XD, Wang SY, Chen GA, *et al.* Apoptosis induced by depsipeptide FK228 coincides with inhibition of survival signaling in lung cancer cells. Cancer J 2007 Mar-Apr;13(2):105-13.
[69] Choi YH. Induction of apoptosis by trichostatin A, a histone deacetylase inhibitor, is associated with inhibition of cyclooxygenase-2 activity in human non-small cell lung cancer cells. Int J Oncol 2005 Aug;27(2):473-9.
[70] Doi S, Soda H, Oka M, *et al.* The histone deacetylase inhibitor FR901228 induces caspase-dependent apoptosis via the mitochondrial pathway in small cell lung cancer cells. Mol Cancer Ther 2004 Nov;3(11):1397-402.
[71] Ota H, Tokunaga E, Chang K, *et al.* Sirt1 inhibitor, Sirtinol, induces senescence-like growth arrest with attenuated Ras-MAPK signaling in human cancer cells. Oncogene 2006 Jan 12;25(2):176-85.
[72] Gridelli C, Rossi A, Maione P. The potential role of histone deacetylase inhibitors in the treatment of non-small-cell lung cancer. Crit Rev Oncol Hematol 2008 Oct;68(1):29-36.

[73] Cuneo KC, Fu A, Osusky K, Huamani J, Hallahan DE, Geng L. Histone deacetylase inhibitor NVP-LAQ824 sensitizes human nonsmall cell lung cancer to the cytotoxic effects of ionizing radiation. Anticancer Drugs 2007 Aug;18(7):793-800.

[74] Komatsu N, Kawamata N, Takeuchi S, *et al.* SAHA, a HDAC inhibitor, has profound anti-growth activity against non-small cell lung cancer cells. Oncol Rep 2006 Jan;15(1):187-91.

[75] Loprevite M, Tiseo M, Grossi F, *et al.* In vitro study of CI-994, a histone deacetylase inhibitor, in non-small cell lung cancer cell lines. Oncol Res 2005;15(1):39-48.

[76] Cang S, Ma Y, Liu D. New clinical developments in histone deacetylase inhibitors for epigenetic therapy of cancer. J Hematol Oncol 2009;2:22.

[77] Esquela-Kerscher A, Slack FJ. Oncomirs - microRNAs with a role in cancer. Nat Rev Cancer 2006 Apr;6(4):259-69.

[78] Calin GA, Croce CM. MicroRNA signatures in human cancers. Nat Rev Cancer 2006 Nov;6(11):857-66.

[79] Volinia S, Calin GA, Liu CG, *et al.* A microRNA expression signature of human solid tumors defines cancer gene targets. Proc Natl Acad Sci U S A 2006 Feb 14;103(7):2257-61.

[80] Yanaihara N, Caplen N, Bowman E, *et al.* Unique microRNA molecular profiles in lung cancer diagnosis and prognosis. Cancer Cell 2006 Mar;9(3):189-98.

[81] Takamizawa J, Konishi H, Yanagisawa K, *et al.* Reduced expression of the let-7 microRNAs in human lung cancers in association with shortened postoperative survival. Cancer Res 2004 Jun 1;64(11):3753-6.

[82] Liu B, Peng XC, Zheng XL, Wang J, Qin YW. MiR-126 restoration down-regulate VEGF and inhibit the growth of lung cancer cell lines in vitro and in vivo. Lung Cancer 2009 Nov;66(2):169-75.

[83] Liu X, Sempere LF, Ouyang H, *et al.* MicroRNA-31 functions as an oncogenic microRNA in mouse and human lung cancer cells by repressing specific tumor suppressors. J Clin Invest 2010 Apr 1;120(4):1298-309.

[84] Cha ST, Chen PS, Johansson G, *et al.* MicroRNA-519c suppresses hypoxia-inducible factor-1alpha expression and tumor angiogenesis. Cancer Res 2010 Apr 1;70(7):2675-85.

[85] He X, Duan C, Chen J, *et al.* Let-7a elevates p21(WAF1) levels by targeting of NIRF and suppresses the growth of A549 lung cancer cells. FEBS Lett 2009 Nov 3;583(21):3501-7.

[86] Crawford M, Batte K, Yu L, *et al.* MicroRNA 133B targets pro-survival molecules MCL-1 and BCL2L2 in lung cancer. Biochem Biophys Res Commun 2009 Oct 23;388(3):483-9.

[87] Bandi N, Zbinden S, Gugger M, *et al.* miR-15a and miR-16 are implicated in cell cycle regulation in a Rb-dependent manner and are frequently deleted or down-regulated in non-small cell lung cancer. Cancer Res 2009 Jul 1;69(13):5553-9.

[88] Wang G, Mao W, Zheng S. MicroRNA-183 regulates Ezrin expression in lung cancer cells. FEBS Lett 2008 Oct 29;582(25-26):3663-8.

[89] Sun Y, Bai Y, Zhang F, Wang Y, Guo Y, Guo L. miR-126 inhibits non-small cell lung cancer cells proliferation by targeting EGFL7. Biochem Biophys Res Commun 2010 Jan 15;391(3):1483-9.

[90] Liang Y. An expression meta-analysis of predicted microRNA targets identifies a diagnostic signature for lung cancer. BMC Med Genomics 2008;1:61.

[91] Lebanony D, Benjamin H, Gilad S, *et al.* Diagnostic assay based on hsa-miR-205 expression distinguishes squamous from nonsquamous non-small-cell lung carcinoma. J Clin Oncol 2009 Apr 20;27(12):2030-7.

[92] Xie Y, Todd NW, Liu Z, *et al.* Altered miRNA expression in sputum for diagnosis of non-small cell lung cancer. Lung Cancer 2010 Feb;67(2):170-6.

[93] Rabinowits G, Gercel-Taylor C, Day JM, Taylor DD, Kloecker GH. Exosomal microRNA: a diagnostic marker for lung cancer. Clin Lung Cancer 2009 Jan;10(1):42-6.

[94] Markou A, Tsaroucha EG, Kaklamanis L, Fotinou M, Georgoulias V, Lianidou ES. Prognostic value of mature microRNA-21 and microRNA-205 overexpression in non-small cell lung cancer by quantitative real-time RT-PCR. Clin Chem 2008 Oct;54(10):1696-704.

[95] Gallardo E, Navarro A, Vinolas N, *et al.* miR-34a as a prognostic marker of relapse in surgically resected non-small-cell lung cancer. Carcinogenesis 2009 Nov;30(11):1903-9.

[96] Raponi M, Dossey L, Jatkoe T, *et al.* MicroRNA classifiers for predicting prognosis of squamous cell lung cancer. Cancer Res 2009 Jul 15;69(14):5776-83.

[97] Yu SL, Chen HY, Chang GC, *et al.* MicroRNA signature predicts survival and relapse in lung cancer. Cancer Cell 2008 Jan;13(1):48-57.

[98] Hu Z, Chen X, Zhao Y, *et al.* Serum microRNA signatures identified in a genome-wide serum microRNA expression profiling predict survival of non-small-cell lung cancer. J Clin Oncol 2010 Apr 1;28(10):1721-6.

[99] Raponi M, Zhang Y, Yu J, *et al.* Gene expression signatures for predicting prognosis of squamous cell and adenocarcinomas of the lung. Cancer Res 2006 Aug 1;66(15):7466-72.

[100] Weidhaas JB, Babar I, Nallur SM, *et al.* MicroRNAs as potential agents to alter resistance to cytotoxic anticancer therapy. Cancer Res 2007 Dec 1;67(23):11111-6.

[101] Weiss GJ, Bemis LT, Nakajima E, *et al.* EGFR regulation by microRNA in lung cancer: correlation with clinical response and survival to gefitinib and EGFR expression in cell lines. Ann Oncol 2008 Jun;19(6):1053-9.

[102] Hayashita Y, Osada H, Tatematsu Y, *et al.* A polycistronic microRNA cluster, miR-17-92, is overexpressed in human lung cancers and enhances cell proliferation. Cancer Res 2005 Nov 1;65(21):9628-32.

[103] Matsubara H, Takeuchi T, Nishikawa E, *et al.* Apoptosis induction by antisense oligonucleotides against miR-17-5p and miR-20a in lung cancers overexpressing miR-17-92. Oncogene 2007 Sep 6;26(41):6099-105.

[104] Garofalo M, Quintavalle C, Di Leva G, *et al.* MicroRNA signatures of TRAIL resistance in human non-small cell lung cancer. Oncogene 2008 Jun 19;27(27):3845-55.

[105] Krutzfeldt J, Rajewsky N, Braich R, *et al.* Silencing of microRNAs in vivo with 'antagomirs'. Nature 2005 Dec 1;438(7068):685-9.

[106] Parkin DM, Bray F, Ferlay J, Pisani P. Global cancer statistics, 2002. CA: a Cancer Journal for Clinicians 2005 Mar-Apr;55(2):74-108.

[107] Williams MD, Sandler AB. The epidemiology of lung cancer. Cancer Treatment & Research 2001;105:31-52.

[108] Belinsky SA. Gene-promoter hypermethylation as a biomarker in lung cancer. Nature Reviews 2004 Sep;Cancer. 4(9):707-17.

[109] Zochbauer-Muller S, Minna JD, Gazdar AF. Aberrant DNA methylation in lung cancer: biological and clinical implications. Oncologist 2002;7(5):451-7.
[110] Tsou JA, Hagen JA, Carpenter CL, Laird-Offringa IA. DNA methylation analysis: a powerful new tool for lung cancer diagnosis. Oncogene 2002 Aug 12;21(35):5450-61.
[111] Momparler RL. Epigenetic therapy of cancer with 5-aza-2'-deoxycytidine (decitabine). Semin Oncol 2005 Oct;32(5):443-51.
[112] Marquez VE, Kelley JA, Agbaria R, *et al.* Zebularine: a unique molecule for an epigenetically based strategy in cancer chemotherapy. Annals of the New York Academy of Sciences 2005 Nov;1058:246-54.
[113] Mufti G, List AF, Gore SD, Ho AY. Myelodysplastic syndrome. Hematology Am Soc Hematol Educ Program 2003:176-99.
[114] Momparler RL, Bouffard DY, Momparler LF, Dionne J, Belanger K, Ayoub J. Pilot phase I-II study on 5-aza-2'-deoxycytidine (Decitabine) in patients with metastatic lung cancer. Anti-Cancer Drugs 1997 Apr;8(4):358-68.
[115] Carmichael J, DeGraff WG, Gazdar AF, Minna JD, Mitchell JB. Evaluation of a tetrazolium-based semiautomated colorimetric assay: assessment of chemosensitivity testing. Cancer Res 1987 Feb 15;47(4):936-42.
[116] Wang J, Wang B, Chen X, Bi J. The prognostic value of RASSF1A promoter hypermethylation in non-small cell lung carcinoma: a systematic review and meta-analysis. Carcinogenesis 2011 Mar;32(3):411-6.
[117] Wang Y, Yu Z, Wang T, Zhang J, Hong L, Chen L. Identification of epigenetic aberrant promoter methylation of RASSF1A in serum DNA and its clinicopathological significance in lung cancer. Lung Cancer 2007 May;56(2):289-94.
[118] Zou Y, Ling YH, Van NT, Priebe W, Perez-Soler R. Antitumor activity of free and liposome-entrapped annamycin, a lipophilic anthracycline antibiotic with non-cross-resistance properties. Cancer Res 1994 Mar 15;54(6):1479-84.
[119] Zou Y, Yamagishi M, Horikoshi I, Ueno M, Gu X, Perez-Soler R. Enhanced therapeutic effect against liver W256 carcinosarcoma with temperature-sensitive liposomal adriamycin administered into the hepatic artery. Cancer Research 1993 Jul 1;53(13):3046-51.
[120] Jones PA, Taylor SM. Cellular differentiation, cytidine analogs and DNA methylation. Cell 1980 May;20(1):85-93.
[121] Juttermann R, Li E, Jaenisch R. Toxicity of 5-aza-2'-deoxycytidine to mammalian cells is mediated primarily by covalent trapping of DNA methyltransferase rather than DNA demethylation. Proc Natl Acad Sci U S A 1994 Dec 6;91(25):11797-801.
[122] Digel W, Lubbert M. DNA methylation disturbances as novel therapeutic target in lung cancer: preclinical and clinical results. Critical reviews in oncology/hematology 2005 Jul;55(1):1-11.